Orthopaedic Physical Therapy

Orthopaedic Physical Therapy

Edited by

ROBERT DONATELLI, M.A., P.T.

Instructor, Graduate Programs in Physical Therapy
Division of Allied Health Professions
Emory University
Orthopaedic Physical Therapist
Physical Therapy Associates of Metro Atlanta
Co-Founder, Clinical Education Associates of Atlanta
Atlanta, Georgia

MICHAEL J. WOODEN, M.S., P.T.

Instructor, Graduate Programs in Physical Therapy
Division of Allied Health Professions
Emory University
Orthopaedic Physical Therapist
Physical Therapy Associates of Metro Atlanta
Co-Founder, Clinical Education Associates of Atlanta
Atlanta, Georgia

Churchill Livingstone
New York, Edinburgh, London, Melbourne   1989

Library of Congress Cataloging-in-Publication Data

Orthopaedic physical therapy.

   Includes bibliographies and index.
   1. Orthopedic. 2. Physical therapy. I. Donatelli, Robert. II. Wooden, Michael J.
[DNLM: 1. Orthopedics. 2. Physical Therapy. WE 168 0769]
RD736.P47079   615.8′2   88-25675
ISBN 0-443-08554-4

© **Churchill Livingstone Inc. 1989**

Distributed in the United Kingdom by Churchill Livingstone, Robert Stevenson House, 1–3 Baxter's Place, Leith Walk, Edinburgh EH1 3AF, and by associated companies, branches, and representatives throughout the world.

Accurate indications, adverse reactions, and dosage schedules for drugs are provided in this book, but it is possible that they may change. The reader is urged to review the package information data of the manufacturers of the medications mentioned.

The Publishers have made every effort to trace the copyright holders for borrowed material. If they have inadvertently overlooked any, they will be pleased to make the necessary arrangements at the first opportunity.

Acquisitions Editor: *Kim Loretucci*
Assistant Editor: *Leslie Burgess*
Copy Editor: *Margot Otway*
Production Supervisor: *Sharon Tuder*

Production services provided by Bermedica Production

Printed in the United States of America

First published in 1989

To my family,
Joni Marie Whelchel-Donatelli and Rachel Marie Donatelli,
for their support and love
R.A.D.

To my wife, Mary Lee,
whose love and understanding sustain me;
to my children Gena, Trevor, and Alec,
who give me so much joy;
and to my parents,
Helen R. Wooden and the late Harold W. Wooden,
my most special teachers
M.J.W.

Contributors

Turner A. Blackburn, Jr., M.Ed., P.T., A.T.C.
Adjunct Assistant Professor, Columbus College; Chief, Sports Physical Therapy, Rehabilitation Services of Columbus, Inc., Columbus, Georgia

William G. Boissonnault, M.S., P.T.
Clinical Assistant Professor, Program in Physical Therapy, College of Allied Health Sciences, University of Tennessee, Memphis, Tennessee; Physical Therapist, Physical Therapy Orthopaedic Specialists, Inc., Minneapolis, Minnesota

Jean M. Bryan, M.A., M.P.T.
Assistant Professor, US Army-Baylor University Graduate Program in Physical Therapy, Baylor University; Major, US Army Medical Specialist Corps, Fort Sam Houston, Houston, Texas

Robert Donatelli, M.A., P.T.
Instructor, Graduate Programs in Physical Therapy, Division of Allied Health Professions, Emory University; Orthopaedic Physical Therapist, Physical Therapy Associates of Metro Atlanta; Co-Founder, Clinical Education Associates of Atlanta, Atlanta, Georgia

Peter I. Edgelow, M.A., P.T.
Core Faculty, Kaiser Orthopaedic Physical Therapy Residency Program; Owner, Hayward Physical Therapy, Hayward, California

Mary Engles, M.S., P.T.
Instructor, Physical Therapy Assistant Program, Mesa College; Independent Contractor, San Diego, California

John C. Garbalosa, M.M.Sc., P.T.
Physical Therapist, Physical Therapy Associates of Metro Atlanta, Atlanta, Georgia

Gary W. Gray, P.T., A.T.C.
Director and Owner, Gary Gray Therapy Clinic, Adrian, Michigan

Bruce Greenfield, M.M.Sc., P.T.
Instructor, Graduate Programs in Physical Therapy, Division of Allied Health Professions, Emory University; Physical Therapist, Physical Therapy Associates of Metro Atlanta, Atlanta, Georgia

Rick Hammesfahr, M.D.
Clinical Associate Professor, Department of Orthopaedics, Emory University School of Medicine; Director, Orthopaedic and Sports Medicine Associates, Atlanta, Georgia

Scot Irwin, M.A., P.T.
Associate Professor, Department of Physical Therapy, Georgia State University, Atlanta, Georgia; Director, Physical Therapy and Rehabilitation, Clayton General Hospital, Riverdale, Georgia

Steven C. Janos, M.S., P.T.
Assistant Professor, Northwestern University Medical School Programs in Physical Therapy; private practice, Physical Therapy Ltd., Chicago, Illinois

Stanley Kalish, D.P.M.
Associate Professor, Department of Surgery, New York College of Podiatric Medicine, New York, New York; Attending Podiatrist, and formerly Chairman of Residency Education, HCA/Doctor's Hospital, Tucker, Georgia; Staff Podiatrist, Henry General Hospital, Atlanta, Georgia; Diplomate, American Board of Podiatric Surgery

Steven L. Kraus, P.T.
Clinical Assistant Professor, Orthodontic Residency Program, and Part-Time Faculty, TMJ/Facial Pain Clinic, Emory University School of Dentistry; Adjunct Faculty and Clinical Educator, Orthopedic Physical Therapy Master's Program, Emory University; Co-Director, Physical Therapy Associates of Metro Atlanta, Atlanta, Georgia

Shirley Kushner, M.Sc., B.Sc.P.T., BPE, Level 3 S.P.D.
Physiotherapist, Canadian Ski Jumping and Nordic Combined Teams, and Alberta Ballet Company; Physiotherapist, Meadowlark Physiotherapy, Edmonton, Alberta, Canada

Christine A. Moran, M.S., P.T.
Assistant Clinical Professor, Graduate Studies in Physical Therapy, Virginia Commonwealth University Medical College of Virginia, Richmond, Virginia; Adjunct Assistant Clinical Professor, Program in Physical Therapy, Old Dominion University, Norfolk, Virginia; Director, The Richmond Upper Extremity Center, Richmond, Virginia

Robert M. Poole, M.Ed., P.T., L.A.T.
Adjunct Clinical Professor, Department of Sports Medicine, Columbus College; Physical Therapist, Rehabilitation Services of Columbus, Columbus, Georgia

David C. Reid, M.D., M.Ch. (orth), F.R.C.S. (C)
Professor of Orthopedic Surgery, Department of Surgery, and Director, Continuing Medical Education, University of Alberta Faculty of Medicine; Director, The Glen Sather University of Alberta Sports Medicine Clinic, Edmonton, Alberta, Canada

David Rouben, M.D.
Clinical Professor, Department of Physical Therapy, Georgia State University; Staff Orthopaedic Surgeon, Georgia Baptist Medical Center, Atlanta, Georgia

Robert B. Sprague, Ph.D., P.T., G.D.A.M.T.
Professor, Department of Physical Therapy, Ithaca College; Senior Partner, Sprague & McCune Physical Therapy, Ithaca, New York

Rick K. St. Pierre, M.D.
Director, Gwinnett/Dekalb Sports Medicine and Orthopaedic Surgery, Atlanta Center for Athletes, Atlanta, Georgia

Steven A. Stratton, Ph.D., P.T., A.T.C.
President, Alamo Physical Therapy Resources, Inc.; Clinical Associate Professor, Department of Physical Therapy, University of Texas Health Science Center at San Antonio; Athletic Trainer, San Antonio Racquets Professional Team Tennis, San Antonio, Texas

Robert W. Sydenham, B.Sc., Dip.P.T., M.C.P.A., M.A.P.T.A., R.P.T.
Member, Canadian Orthopaedic Manipulative Therapists; Director, URSA Foundation, Edmonds, Washington; Director, R.W. Sydenham and Associates Physical Therapy Services, Edmonton, Alberta, Canada; Owner, Academy Place Physical Therapy Ltd., Edmonton, Alberta, Canada

David Tiberio, M.S., P.T.
Assistant Professor, Physical Therapy Program, University of Connecticut, Storrs, Connecticut; Consultant, Physical Therapy and Sports Medicine Associates, West Hartford, Connecticut; Director, On Site Biomechanical Education and Training, Storrs, Connecticut

George Vito, D.P.M.
Resident, HCA/Doctors Hospital, Tucker, Georgia

Randy Walker, Jr., Ph.D., P.T.
Assistant Professor, Department of Physical Therapy, Georgia State University, Atlanta, Georgia

Joseph S. Wilkes, M.D.
Assistant Clinical Professor of Orthopaedic Surgery, Department of Orthopaedics, Emory University School of Medicine; Orthopaedic Surgeon, Orthopaedic Associates of Atlanta, P.C., Atlanta, Georgia

Allyn L. Woerman, M.M.Sc., P.T.
Lieutenant Colonel, Army Medical Specialist Corps; Assistant Chief, Physical Therapy, Reynolds Army Community Hospital, Fort Sill, Oklahoma

Michael J. Wooden, M.S., P.T.
Instructor, Graduate Programs in Physical Therapy, Division of Allied Health Professions, Emory University; Orthopaedic Physical Therapist, Physical Therapy Associates of Metro Atlanta; Co-Founder, Clinical Education Associates of Atlanta, Atlanta, Georgia

Preface

As a result of a growing body of knowledge, physical therapy has undergone over the past ten years a process of specialization like that in the medical profession. Orthopaedics has emerged as the largest specialty group. Specialization and advanced educational programs have led to new methods of evaluation, treatment, and prevention of musculoskeletal injuries, and thereby to better patient care.

This book is written for physical therapy practitioners and students specializing in orthopaedic physical therapy. It will also be a valuable reference text for physicians, osteopaths, podiatrists, and nonmedical practitioners specializing in the treatment of orthopaedic dysfunction.

The book is divided into three sections: Fundamental Principles, The Upper Quarter, and The Lower Quarter. The fundamental principles section discusses the response of tissues and body systems to trauma, immobilization, and movement, and gives guidelines for safe and effective treatment.

The division of the rest of the text into sections on the upper and lower quarters is intended to emphasize the fact that the clinician must treat the entire individual, not just the site of dysfunction. Because idiopathic dysfunction syndromes often develop as a result of abnormal postures or movement patterns, the entire region containing the dysfunctional area should be evaluated. For example, in the lower quarter, abnormal foot or ankle mechanics can result in such problems as shin splints and nonspecific knee pain.

Within each section, the interrelation and interdependence of anatomy, mechanics, and kinesiology are discussed. Gait analysis and upper quarter posture are reviewed, with emphasis on the interrelation of the parts during movement. Following these general discussions, the specific pathologies and common dysfunctions of each region are presented, including reviews of normal anatomy, local tissue response to pathology and overuse syndromes, and physical therapy evaluation and treatment. Surgical options for restoring normal movement are also discussed. Each section ends with an overview of mobilization techniques for the limb.

Our goal has been to present the current state of orthopaedic physical therapy practice as it has been influenced by specialization, advanced education, and research. We believe that the best care of the patient depends on a total regional approach, incorporating an understanding of the orthopaedic fundamentals, regional interdependences, and clinical physical therapy treatment and mobilization. We trust that, through the excellent contributions written by the authors, this book will lead to improved patient care.

We would like to thank the staffs of the Clinical Education Associates and the Physical Therapy Associates of Metro Atlanta for their continued dedication and help in maintaining the highest quality of education and patient care.

Robert Donatelli, M.A., P.T.
Michael J. Wooden, M.S., R.P.T

Contents

SECTION 3
THE LOWER QUARTER

FUNDAMENTAL PRINCIPLES

1

Tissue Response

MARY ENGLES

In studying the human body and its response to its environment, we quite naturally proceed from the normal to the abnormal. Normal body tissues are grouped into four categories according to similarities of function and structure. In orthopaedic physical therapy we are most concerned with three of these: connective tissue (including bone, tendon, ligament, and fascia); muscle; and nerve. The fourth category epithelium, is left to other specialists. Let us have a brief look at the normal structure and function of each of these tissues before moving on to examine the tissue-specific responses to mechanical stress, immobilization, and remobilization.

NORMAL TISSUE
Muscle

Muscle is that tissue type which most completely expresses cell contractility.[1] It is a composite structure consisting of muscle cells or fibers, and the connective tissue network that transmits the pull of the muscle cells.[1,2] The sarcomere, the basic contractile unit that makes up most of the muscle cell, is composed of actin and myosin.[1] These contractile proteins are arranged in a specific pattern, which gives muscle tissue its characteristic striated appearance. Sarcomeres are further arranged in parallel to form myofibrils (muscle fibers or cells), which in turn are arranged in bundles to form fascicles and finally a whole muscle (Fig. 1-1). Other qualities of the muscle structure, particularly the contents of the sarcoplasm, cause muscle fibers to be classified as red, white, or intermediate.[1] These characteristics affect not only the contractile properties of the mus-

cle fiber but also its response to exercise and immobilization. Chapter 2 of this book and other works describe the response of muscle to exercise.[3-5] The noncontractile element of the muscle, the connective tissue, is manifest at every level of muscle organization. Thin sheets of connective tissue surround each muscle fiber, becoming thicker as they surround each fascicle and finally enveloping the exterior of the muscle itself (Fig. 1-2). These delicate sheets of tissue provide a mechanical framework for contraction and a conduit for blood vessels and nerve fibers to reach the interior of the muscle. At each end of the muscle, collagen fibers extend beyond the muscle itself and blend with the connective tissue that forms the tendon, fascia, or aponeurosis, which anchors the muscle to its end point.

With the advent of electron microscopy in the early 1950s, the exact arrangement of the actin and myosin filaments within the sarcomere was discovered (Fig. 1-1C). By comparing micrographs of muscle in the relaxed and the contracted state, H. E. Huxley and co-workers in 1954 developed the "sliding filament" theory, which immediately gained widespread acceptance.[1] The manner in which this sliding occurs has been the subject of much study. When the muscle is relaxed, the lateral projections of the myosin filaments lie close to their parent filament, whereas in contraction they project to contact the adjacent actin strands. In contracted muscle the actin filaments slide, in relation to the myosin, toward the center of the sarcomere, bringing the attached Z bands closer together and thus shortening the whole contractile unit (Fig. 1-3). This and many other observations indicate that muscle contraction may be caused by the successive

3

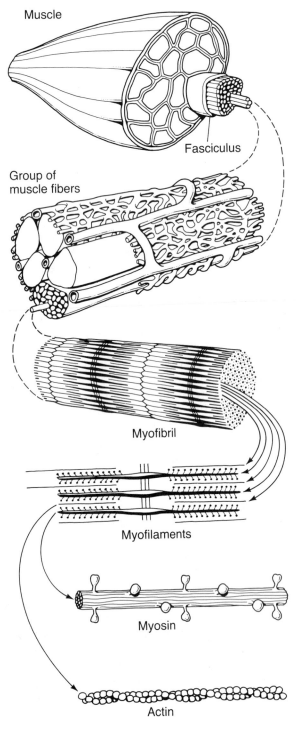

Fig. 1-1. Levels of organization within a skeletal muscle. (From Warwick and Williams,[2] with permission.)

making and breaking of cross-connections between thick myosin and thin actin filaments in a cyclical fashion, pulling the actin between the myosin toward the sarcomere center.[2] If contraction is continued, actin filaments may overlap each other in the middle of the A band, and the Z bands may meet the ends of the myosin filaments. As the length of the sarcomere changes, so does the amount of overlap between the actin and the myosin. Since the numbers of possible cross links between the two depend on the amount of overlap, it might be expected that a muscle would generate different tensions if it were made to contract at different lengths without being allowed to shorten.[2,5] Measurements confirm this expectation (Fig. 1-4).

The three types of muscle contraction—isotonic, isometric, and eccentric—can be correlated with the behavior of the fine structure of the contractile mechanism of actin and myosin. In isotonic contraction, in which a muscle shortens under a constant load to perform positive external work, actin and myosin cross-bridges are active in causing mutual sliding of the filaments. In isometric contraction, cross-bridges are made and broken repeatedly

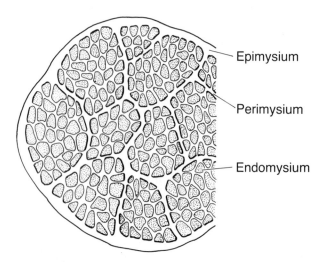

Fig. 1-2. Striated muscle in cross section, showing its connective tissue components and organization into bundles of muscle fibers. Epimysium encloses the entire muscle, perimysium surrounds each bundle of fibers, and endomysium lies in between individual muscle fibers. (From Ham and Cormack,[1] with permission.)

MUSCLE

A

SHORTENED
FIBERS

NORMAL FIBERS

LENGTHENED
FIBERS

B

SINGLE FIBER

C

A band
I band
H zone   Z line

D

Sarcomere

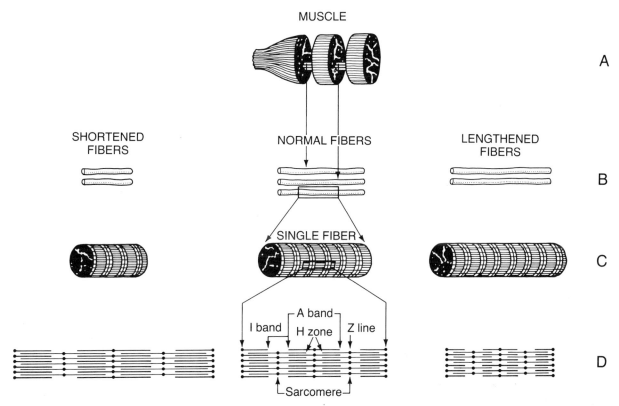

Fig. 1-3. The structure of normal muscle (center) and the changes that occur when a muscle is in a shortened (left) or a lengthened position (right). A, skeletal muscle; B, single muscle fibers; C, myofibrils; D, actin and myosin myofilaments. Note increased and decreased sarcomere length in the shortened and lengthened fibers, respectively. (From Gossman et al.,[6] MR: with permission of the American Physical Therapy Association.)

to maintain a constant muscle length under an external load. In eccentric contraction, a muscle generates tension while it is being actively lengthened by an external load. The precise behavior of the filaments has not been established in this type of contraction, but it is probable that cross-bridges are active in the usual manner while the actin and myosin are sliding apart.[2,6]

The last factor to be considered in the basic understanding of muscle structure and function is its innervation. Efferent, or motor, nerves supply each muscle via numerous axons. One axon may supply one or many muscle fibers by means of branching. The ratio of muscle fibers to axons in a muscle determines the fineness of the motion capabilities of

that muscle. A single motor neuron and its axons together with all the muscle fibers it innervates is called a motor unit.[2,7] When stimulated, the fibers belonging to a single motor unit contract either completely or not at all—the "all or none" law. The force of contraction can vary because of circumstances as well, such as the physiologic state of the fibers and the length-tension relationship. Within any one motor unit all the fibers can be either red or white but not both.[1]

Sensory nerves also supply muscles, signaling their degree of contraction to the central nervous system (CNS). Information from muscle spindles and other sensory receptors provides awareness of the position and rates of movement of our body

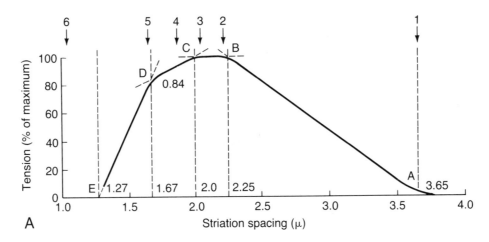

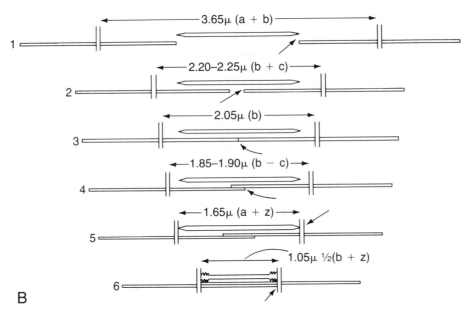

Fig. 1-4. Composite showing the relationship of sarcomere length to the length-tension curve. A = 1.60 m, b = 2.05 m, c = 0.015 to 2.0 μm, z = 0.05 m. (From Gordon AM: The variation in isometric tension with sarcomere length in vertebrate muscle fibers. J Physiol 184:185, 1966, with permission.)

parts. These sensory organs can be classified under the broad category of mechanoreceptors because they respond to mechanical deformation or stimulation.[8] Another category of receptors, called nociceptors, signals painful events, either mechanical or chemical, to the CNS. Nociceptors are found more abundantly in skin, connective tissue, and blood vessels than in the muscle belly itself.[7,8]

Connective Tissue

Connective tissue is found nearly everywhere in the body. It functions as a fibrous container for softer tissues, as a mechanical and chemical barrier, and as a highway for blood vessels and nerves (Fig. 1-5). Connective tissue is generally classified as loose or dense, regular or irregular, depending on the ar-

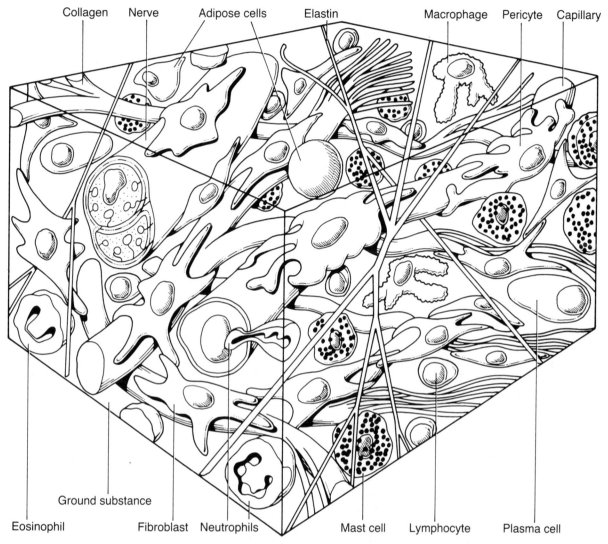

Collagen   Nerve   Adipose cells   Elastin   Macrophage   Pericyte   Capillary

Eosinophil   Ground substance   Fibroblast   Neutrophils   Mast cell   Lymphocyte   Plasma cell

Fig. 1-5. A diagrammatic reconstruction of loose connective tissue showing the characteristic cell types, fibers, and intercellular spaces. (From Warwick and Williams,[2] with permission.)

rangement and quantity of collagen fibers within it (Fig. 1-6). Tendons and ligaments are considered to be dense connective tissue. Structurally, dense connective tissue is 80 percent water, 20 percent collagen fibers, and 2 percent cells and glycosaminoglycans (GAG).[1] Collagen represents 80 percent of the dry weight of connective tissue and is the only tensile resistant protein in ligaments, tendon, and joint capsule.[9] The tensile strength of collagen has been estimated at 50 to 125 newtons/mm² depending on

the specimen tested.[10] Some studies of human collagen report loads at failure of 91 kilograms/force (kgf) for plantar fascia and 40 kgf for anterior cruciate ligament.[11,12] Clinically speaking, a dense, regular connective tissue structure such as a tendon is very strong. It usually ruptures from its bony attachment rather than tearing within its substance. The other major components of connective tissue are water and GAG. They impart very important biomechanical properties to the tissue. GAG is a large,

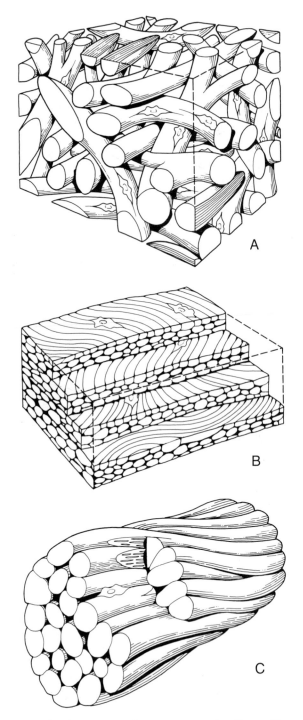

Fig. 1-6. Three types of arrangement of collagen fibers. **(A)** Dense irregular connective tissue; **(B)** a ligament; **(C)** a tendon. (From Warwick and Williams,[2] with permission.)

featherlike molecule with a great affinity for water. This affinity greatly increases its space-occupying capabilities.[9,13,14] Water and GAG create a gel-like material that acts as a lubricant and spacer between the collagen fibers and imparts important physical and mechanical properties to the composite. Having an adequate tissue matrix between the collagen fibers decreases friction and maintains the inter-fiber distance necessary for the normal sliding movement that occurs between fibers.[9,14,15]

Collagen and GAG are produced by fibroblasts, the cells of connective tissue (Fig. 1-7). A collagen precursor molecule is assembled within the fibroblast and then secreted as tropocollagen.[1,16] Tropocollagen is then assembled in series via intermolecular bonds, or cross links, to form collagen fibrils. The unique one-quarter overlap of this formation gives collagen its characteristic banded appearance.[1,17] The collagen continues to aggregate into bundles as needed, by means of strong chemical bonds, or intramolecular cross links, finally forming a whole structure such as a tendon or a ligament (Fig. 1-8). Individual bundles can be seen to have a wavy appearance, which permits small physiologic deformities to occur without placing the tissue under any stress.[17]

Physiologically, collagen is a rather sluggish substance.[13] In most forms it is quite inert and has a slow turnover rate.[17] As fibers mature, the cross links increase in strength. Attempts to modify its structure or alignment must therefore be prolonged and be made early after injury or immobilization.[18] As collagen ages, more intermolecular cross links form, and existing bonds become stronger.[9,17,18] The tissue thus becomes less extensible and more brittle. GAG has a more rapid turnover rate and more active metabolism than collagen and thus appears to be more easily influenced by changes in the mechanical or chemical environment.[14,15]

Connective tissue does have abundant afferent innervation.[8,19] Although incapable of active movement, connective tissue does lengthen passively in response to internally or externally applied forces. These changes in length and tension are reported to the CNS by the various sensory receptors found within the tendons, ligaments, and articular capsule surrounding a joint. Wyke classified these into four categories by size, structure, location, and function

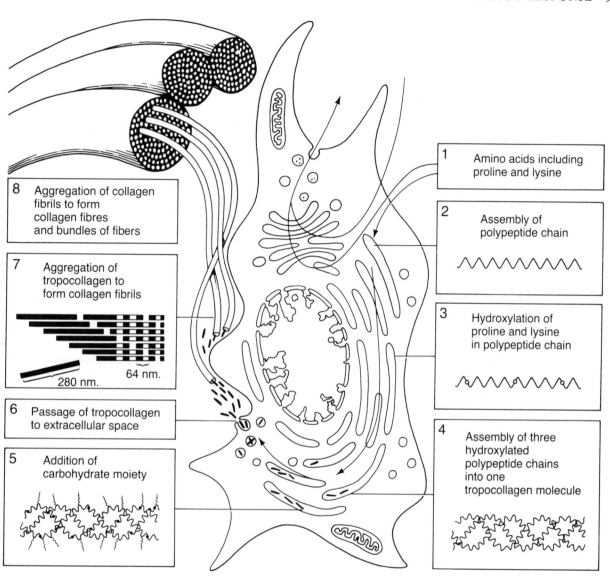

Fig. 1-7. The major steps in collagen synthesis by fibroblasts in connective tissue. (From Warwick and Williams,[2] with permission.)

(Table 1-1).[20] This rich supply of nerve endings, coupled with the muscle spindle endings, allows the CNS to constantly monitor the internal state of a particular joint. Type I, II, and III mechanoreceptors, via static and dynamic input, signal joint position, intra-articular pressure changes, and the direction, amplitude, and velocity of joint movements.[8] It is of note that type II receptors are structurally contained in a thick, multilayered connective tissue capsule, which would be subject to the same changes during immobilization that affect other connective tissue structures. Type III mechanoreceptors are the homologues of the Golgi tendon organ. Functionally, the articular mechanoreceptors have been shown to influence muscle tone, specifically the resistance of muscle to passive stretch.[21] Wyke stated that type I and II mechanoreceptors synapse with fusimotor (gamma) moto-

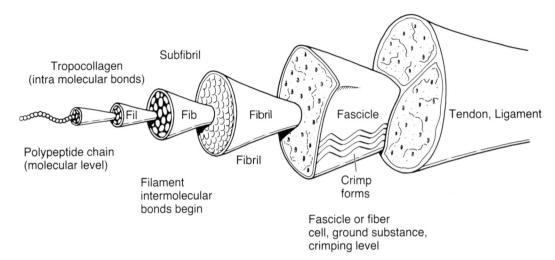

Fig. 1-8. Organization of a tendon from tropocollagen to filament, fibril, fascicle, and whole tendon. Note the presence of crimping or waveforms at the fascicle level. (Redrawn from Betsch and Bauer,[17] with permission.)

neurons via internuncial neurons. Type III receptors, being similar to Golgi tendon organs, can totally inhibit the excitability of the alpha motoneuron in nearby muscles when they are strongly stimulated. D'Andrade demonstrated this inhibitory effect on the quadriceps muscle with an experimentally induced joint effusion.[22] We see this clinically as the quadriceps "lag" after a knee injury or surgical procedure.

Freeman and Wyke investigated the electromyographic (EMG) and stretch reflex responses of the

tenotomized gastrocnemius muscle of the cat to passive ankle motion.[21] When the ligaments and capsule were intact, the EMG activity and myotatic response of the muscle increased during passive ankle dorsiflexion, indicating facilitation. In contrast, the responses of the antagonistic tibialis anterior decreased. Local anesthesia of the ankle joint abolished these responses. Direct stimulation of the posterior joint capsule by means of gradual compression showed a progressive increase in the EMG activity of the gastrocnemius. This gradually returned to baseline with sustained gentle compression. Freeman and Wyke concluded that mechanoreceptors provide valuable afferent pathways to indirectly influence muscle tone through mechanical stimulation of joint structures.

Peripheral Nerves

Peripheral nerves, like muscle, have both specialized cell components and a supporting connective tissue network (Fig. 1-9).[1,23] The fine structure of nerve fibers, or axons, follows the basic structure of the cell. The long processes of these nerve cells become the fibers that make up the peripheral nerve.[1,2] Although organized in a bundled manner similar to muscle and connective structures, nerve fibers, are unique in being surrounded by the fine cytoplasmic sheath called the neurolemma or

Table 1-1. Classification of Articular Receptor Systems

Type	Morphology	Behavior
I	Fibrous capsule of joint (mainly superficial layers)	Static and dynamic receptors, low threshold, slow adapting
II	Fibrous capsule of joint (mainly deeper layers) Articular fat pads	Dynamic mechanoreceptors, high-threshold, rapidly adapting
III	Joint ligaments	Dynamic mechanoreceptors, high-threshold, very slowly adapting
IV	Fibrous capsule Articular fat pads Ligaments Blood vessel walls	Pain receptors, high threshold, non-adapting

(Modified from Wyke B,[20] with permission.)

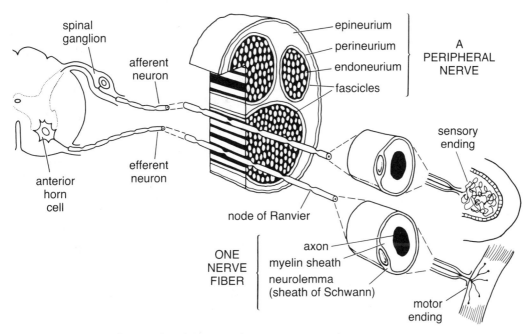

Fig. 1-9. Organization of a peripheral nerve and its various parts. (From Ham and Cormack,[1] with permission.)

sheath of Schwann (Fig. 1-10).[1] Some nerve fibers have a thick layer of the substance myelin between the nerve and the neurolemma (myelinated fibers), whereas others no not (nonmyelinated fibers).[23] The myelin sheath is probably formed by the Schwann cell wrapping itself successively around the axon, gradually squeezing its own cytoplasm toward its nucleus so that its cell membranes fuse with each other. Unmyelinated fibers are merely invaginated into the Schwann cell rather than being wrapped in layers.[1] Junctures between adjacent Schwann cells, down the length of an axon, form indentations called nodes of Ranvier.[1,2] These seem to facilitate conduction of impulses. Other functions attributed to the Schwann cell include collagen formation, materials transport in the cell, transport of metabolites, protection of the nodal region from deformation, and maintenance of the ionic milieu.[23]

The connective tissue component of peripheral nerves consists of tubular sheaths, which encase successively the nerve fibers (endoneurium), fascicles (perineurium), and the whole nerve (epineurium) (Fig. 1-9).[2] This is similar to the arrangement

of muscle fibers into whole muscles. The connective tissue surrounding nerves serves not only as a mechanical protector but as a chemical one as well. It acts as a diffusion barrier, maintains internal pressure for axoplasm flow, provides for uniform tensile strength, and maintains the conductile properties of the nerve.[23] Thickenings due to an increase in connective tissue are observed along the course of the axon where nerves cross bones or are near joints.

Within the nerve fascicles are different kinds of nerve fibers: sensory, motor, and sympathetic.

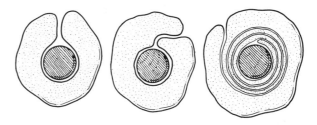

Fig. 1-10. Early stages of the formation of a myelin sheath by a Schwann cell of the peripheral nervous system. (From Ham and Cormack,[1] with permission.)

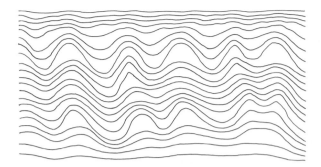

Fig. 1-11. Drawn from a high-power photomicrograph of a longitudinal section of a small peripheral nerve, showing the snake-like appearance typical of such sections. (From Ham and Cormack,[1] with permission.)

These vary in quantity and arrangement.[2,23] As the nerve proceeds to its final destination, these components repeatedly unite and divide, forming plexi. Nerves can also be seen to have the same wavy pattern seen in connective tissue, even after the removal of all the connective components of the nerve (Fig. 1-11).[23] As with connective tissue, this waviness disappears when gentle traction is applied.

Bone

Bone is essentially a highly vascular, constantly changing, mineralized connective tissue (Fig. 1-12). Bone can be thought of as a passive system made up of collagen, stiffened by an extremely dense filling of calcium phosphate interspersed with small amounts of water, amorphous proteins, and cells. Or it can be seen as consisting most importantly of cells imbedded in an amorphous and fibrous organic matrix permeated by inorganic bone salts.[1,14] The model we choose in considering the tissue we call bone depends upon which of its functions we choose as our focus: its function as the rigid support system for the body, or as the mineral reservoir.[1,14] Structurally, bone is similar to other forms of connective tissue in its major constituents but differs in both the quantity of the different components and the exact type of the component. Bone has mineralized ground substance whereas connective tissue contains water and GAG. Bone receives a greater nutritional supply via its own blood vessels than do other connective tissues, which are largely avascular. Bone also has more cells per unit area than the other connective tissues. Because of this greater vascularity and cellularity, bone is capable of more rapid change, including healing and remodeling, than the other connective tissues.

The fine structure of bone varies widely with the age, location, and natural history of the tissue. Its collagen fiber framework varies from an almost random network of bundles to a highly organized system of parallel-fibered sheets or helical bundles. The inorganic matrix may exist as irregular dense masses with scattered bone cells, or it may be arranged as a series of thin sheets (lamellae) in a variety of patterns. Both types often develop as minute cylindrical masses (osteons), each with a central vascular canal. For our purposes, we can classify bone by the organization of its collagen fibers or by its general microstructure (Table 1-2).

It is difficult to understand bone as a tissue without some knowledge of its formation. The collagen of bone is produced in the same manner as that of ligament and tendon, but by a different type of cell, the osteoblast. Collagen is laid down and then aggregates to form three distinct forms of bone: woven bone, lamellar bone, and parallel-fibered bone.[24] The collagen in woven bone is very fine and oriented almost randomly, like that of the skin. Woven bone contains many osteocytes and blood vessels. The spaces around the vessels are extensive, in contrast to lamellar bone.[1,24] The bone cells, called osteocytes, are contained inside mineralized cavities (lacunae) and connect via fine processes through channels (canaliculi) with each other and neighboring blood vessels.

Table 1-2. Classification of Bone

Organization of collagen fibers
  Woven-fibered bone (coarse-bundled bone) has an irregular collagen network, includes embryonic bone, occurs in isolated patches in adults, is also formed during fracture repair.
  Parallel-fibered bone includes all forms of lamellar bone and primary nonlamellar osteons.
General microstructure
  Nonlamellar bone includes early woven-fibered bone and primary osteons.
  Lamellar bone: almost all mature bone.

(Modified from Warwick and Williams,[2] with permission.)

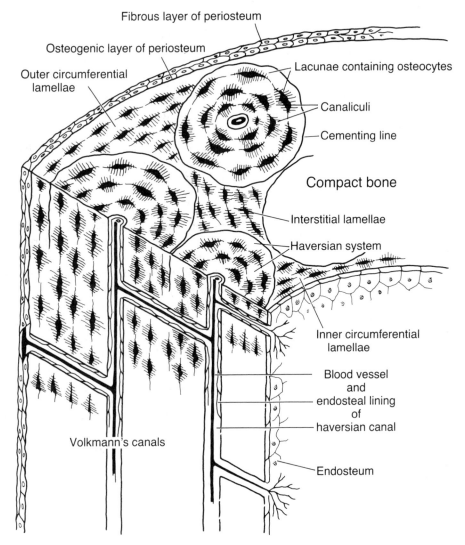

Fibrous layer of periosteum

Osteogenic layer of periosteum

Outer circumferential
lamellae

Lacunae containing osteocytes

Canaliculi

Cementing line

Compact bone

Interstitial lamellae

Haversian system

Inner circumferential
lamellae

Blood vessel
and
endosteal lining
of
haversian canal

Volkmann's canals

Endosteum

Fig. 1-12. Appearance in cross and longitudinal section of the components of the structure of the cortex of a long bone. In an actual bone there would be many more Haversian systems than shown here. (From Ham and Cormack,[1] with permission.)

Woven bone, or primary bone, is often replaced by lamellar bone during fetal growth and fracture repair. The collagen of lamellar bone is more precisely arranged than that of woven bone. The collagen and its ground substance are laid down in parallel sheets with much less ground substance between layers. The fibers are aligned within the plane of the lamella and are all oriented in the same direction. Within one lamella, however, there may be various domains of parallel-oriented fibers, similar to the arrangement of collagen in ligaments. Bundles of collagen may branch and are much thicker than in woven bone. Parallel-fibered bone is structurally intermediate between woven bone and lamellar bone. It is highly calcified, but the collagen fiber bundles are less randomly arranged than in woven bone. It is found in particular bones in particular situations.[24]

Lamellar bone also exists in a separate form called a Haversian system, or osteon.[2] Bone around a blood vessel is gradually eroded by the bone-destroying cells, the osteoclasts, leaving a central cavity. Bone is then deposited on the inner surface of this cavity in concentric lamellae (Fig. 1-13). The end result looks in cross-section like an onion, with discernible cylindrical layers. Bone modeling and remodeling within this system occur via bone deposition and resorption, mediated by osteoblasts and osteoclasts, respectively.

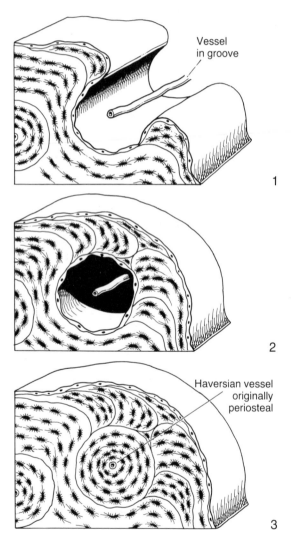

Fig. 1-13. A representation of how the longitudinal grooves on the exterior of a growing bone shaft form tunnels and finally Haversian systems. (From Ham and Cormack,[1] with permission.)

The next higher order of structure is the mechanically important distinction between compact and cancellous bone. Cancellous bone is a framework of united bone spicules or trabeculae. During fetal development, a layer of osteoblasts forms deep to the outer dense sheath of connective tissue, the periosteum, which surrounds a whole bone. These osteoblasts deposit layers of bone, again called lamellae, beneath the periosteum. Near the time of birth, some locations of primary cancellous bone become compact bone. The trabeculae thicken by the addition of concentric lamellae around osteocytes and by rearrangement of the trabeculae into Haversian systems (Fig. 1-13). With the formation of many of these Haversian systems the cancellous bone becomes compact bone. Osteoclasts remove bone centrally around the interior blood vessel of the Haversian system.[1] Changes in bone occur in the same way during immobilization and remobilization.

All bones have an outer shell of compact, or cortical, bone and an inner mass of cancellous, or trabecular, bone. In some instances, the trabecular bone may be replaced by the medullary cavity or an air space. Compact bone is further distinguished from cancellous bone by the amount of mineralized tissue per total bone tissue volume. Compact bone is 5 to 30 percent porous, or nonmineralized, whereas cancellous bone is 30 to 90 percent porous.[15,24,25] The mineralized portion of cancellous bone appears as a three-dimensional lattice work of trabeculae such as that seen in the head and neck of the femur (Fig. 1-14). Dense portions of cancellous bone also appear as plates such as those found in the pubis and lateral angle of the scapula. Other examples of dense portions of cancellous bone are the epiphyseal plates and the patellae.[26]

Mechanically, trabecular bone structure is designed to provide support along the shaft of a long bone, thus resisting tension and bending. Plate structure gives more support near articular surfaces, which are subjected to compression and shear stresses. The collagen fibrils, which are evident in the trabecular and plate portions of cancellous bone, are usually aligned to present optimum resistance to the loads placed on that particular area. In areas subject to tension, collagen fibers are arranged parallel to the tensile load.[15] This orientation can be readily seen where tendons and ligaments attach to a bone and in areas subjected to tension under a bending load, such as the head and neck of the femur.[15]

The strength of bone is directly correlated with its degree of mineralization and the number and organization of its osteons.[15] Demineralized bone has only 5 to 10 percent of the strength of mineralized bone.[27] The strength and strain of bone decrease as the number of osteons increase because of the relative weakness of the cement lines between them.[1] Indeed, areas of bonding between osteons provide for more elastic and viscoelastic deformation.[14,27] The three types of osteons have different tolerances for compression and elastic deformation depending on the organization of the collagen fibers in each.[14] Compressive strength is greatest in type 1 and least in type 3. Since collagen fibers resist tension along their axes, a longitudinal or steeply spiraling arrangement shows the greatest tensile strength, whereas a transverse arrangement (type 1) has greater compressive strength.[14] See Table 1-3 for a summary of the differences between compact and cancellous bone. Since most whole bones are a

Table 1-3. Mechanical Stresses in Cancellous and Cortical Bone

Cancellous	Cortical
Compression	
Trabeculae are aligned according to compressive stresses. Greatest strain is available in lateromedial direction.	Longitudinal sections are strongest, then transverse, tangential, and radial. Ultimate compressive strength is greater than ultimate tensile strength. Strain is greatest in transverse section. Ultimate compressive strain is greater than ultimate tensile strain.
Tension	
Ultimate tensile strain is less than ultimate compressive strain. Ultimate strength is less than in cortical bone.	Longitudinal sections are strongest by 8 times. Ultimate tensile strain is less than ultimate compressive strain.
Shear	
Trabeculae may be aligned according to direction of principal shear stress.	Longitudinal sections loaded perpendicularly are twice as strong as transverse sections loaded in parallel.

(Modified from Reigger,[14] with permission.)

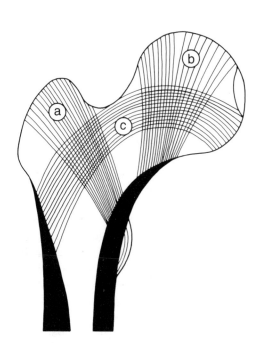

Fig. 1-14. The trabeculae of the head and neck of the femur. (From Rydell N: Biomechanics of the hip joint. Clin Orthop 92:6, 1973, with permission.)

combination of these two types of bony tissue, whole bone strength is greater than that of either tissue type alone.

Innervation of bone is supplied via finely distributed nerves within the periosteum, especially that of the articular extremities of the long bones, the vertebrae, and the larger flat bones.[2] Fine myelinated and unmyelinated nerve fibers also accompany blood vessels into the interior of bones. These are nociceptors, which signal pain from mechanical and chemical irritation.

RESPONSE TO MECHANICAL STRESS

Biologic tissue responds to mechanical stress by deforming according to specific mechanical and physical principles. The mechanical properties of biologic tissue containing large amounts of collagen are elasticity, viscoelasticity, and plasticity.[10,13,28,29] The physical properties are stress relaxation, creep, and hysteresis. These will be defined in this section.

Tissue with large amounts of collagen, such as bone and connective tissue, has also been found to respond to mechanical deformation by generating an electrical polarity.[14,26,30] This is called the piezo-electric effect and is a characteristic of some substances with regular repeating molecular patterns such as collagen. Mechanical stress further triggers firing of various mechanoreceptors found in muscle, tendon, ligament, and joint capsule.[20-22,28] Intense mechanical deformation can also trigger the nociceptors found in these tissues.[20,28]

Clinically, when a load is applied, bone, muscle, ligament, and nerve respond by gradually lengthening. Because of their differences in collagen content, fiber arrangement, and inorganic components, these different tissues respond in slightly different ways. Individual collagen fibers deform very little. Instead the unique arrangement of collagen into bundles of varying sizes and directional alignment within a tissue permits the various forms of tissue to have both strength and stiffness in varying amounts. The presence of a gel-like matrix allows the collagen bundles to move to align themselves along lines of stress application. Bone, muscle connective tissue, and nerve also respond differently depending on the speed, duration, and magnitude of the applied load. Maximum stiffness for a tissue is available along the lines of stress application if the load is applied slowly enough to permit time for collagen bundle realignment. As we shall see, the alignment of collagen fibers along lines of normal stress is lost during immobilization and is gradually regained through therapeutic stress application. The composition and amount of connective tissue matrix present are important factors in this time-dependent realignment phenomenon. As we shall see, changes take place within connective tissue during immobilization that retard the realignment process.

Tissue-Specific Responses to Mechanical Loading

Connective Tissue

The mechanical response of a material to a load (stress) can be measured and plotted on a load-deformation (stress-strain) curve (Fig. 1-15).[13] This curve has been well studied in connective tissue

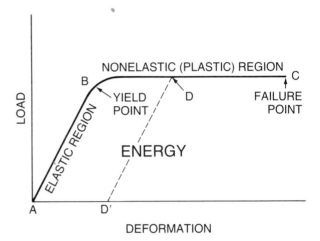

Fig. 1-15. Load-deformation curve of a somewhat pliable material. (From Frankel and Nordin,[15] with permission.)

structures. Specific regions have been identified that correspond to specific material and clinical behavior (Fig. 1-16). Connective tissue responds to mechanical stress in a time-dependent or viscoelastic manner.[10,13,17,26] Viscoelasticity is a mechanical property of materials that describes the tendency of tissue, in this instance, to deform at a certain rate regardless of the speed of the externally applied force. When the deforming force is removed, recovery of the original shape of the tissue occurs again at a tissue-specific rate.[8,25] In engineering, this slow, predictable rate of deformation is also known as "creep" (Fig. 1-17). If the rate of load application is increased, other mechanical responses change to maintain the rate of deformation constant. Thus a rapidly applied load will produce less deformation before failure than a slowly applied load. If the amount of deformation does not exceed the elastic range, the structure can return to its normal or original shape after the load is removed. If loading is continued into the plastic range, passing the yield point, the outermost fibers of the material will begin to tear (fail). Failure is thought to be a function of breaking of intermolecular cross links rather than rupture of the alpha chains of the collagen molecule.[31] If loading persists, ultimate failure for that structure is reached. An example of a load persisting until failure occurs, but where little deformation takes place, would be an injury in an individual who starts a sports activity without warming up. During

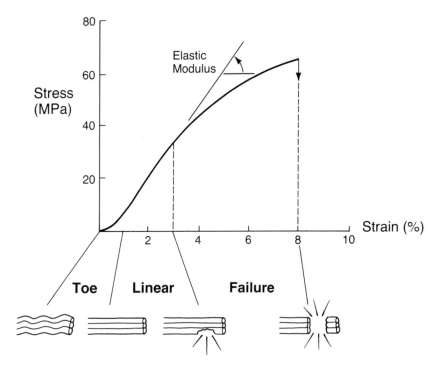

Fig. 1-16. Typical normalized stress-strain curve for collagen. The curve provides mechanical parameters that are independent of tissue dimensions. (From Noyes FR: Biomechanics of ligaments and tendons. Exc Sports Sci Rev 6:126, 1979, with permission.)

sports a large load is often rapidly applied to a connective tissue structure that has not been previously loaded in this way. Thus the stress perceived by the tissue is high, and the failure point is reached quickly before much tissue elongation has had time to take place. This is often seen clinically as a midsubstance ligamentous tear.[32] A load of equal magnitude applied more slowly results in failure at the bone-ligament junction, where the connective tissue structure is weaker as it blends into the bone.[32,33]

Repeated loading, or cyclic loading, shows a change in mechanical response beginning with the first cycle and stabilizing after the sixth cycle.[34] Changes reflect an increased compliance (softening) of the tissue, an increased early stiffness, and a decreased load to failure.[17,34] The softening of the tissue in the first cycle and subsequent cycles reflects a release of energy from the tissue, called hysteresis, which is perhaps due to internal friction. (Fig. 1-17C). Increased tissue temperature has been recorded during repeated loading; hence the term "warm-up" to describe repeated stretching before sports activities is particularly appropriate. Clinical experience also points to more connective tissue injuries occurring later in sports activities when ligaments and joint capsule are warmed, more compliant and less resistant to higher loads, and muscles are fatigued.[35] Connective structures thus take less time to reach their yield and failure points. This warming of the tissue can also be therapeutically induced by the external application of heat.[29,36]

If a tissue is held under a constant external load and at a constant length, force relaxation occurs (Fig. 1-17A).[10] Although the external load on the tissue and the length of the tissue remain the same, for example in a cylinder cast, the internal stress perceived by the tissue decreases. Thus, when the cylinder cast is removed the tissue remains at its new length instead of immediately returning to its former length. The actual ultrastructural changes occurring during force relaxation are as yet uninvestigated, but we can surmise that collagen fibers are realigning along the lines of stress and that ground substance is perhaps also being redistributed. These mechanical properties of collagen-bearing tissues are important parameters for the rehabilitation process and for mobilization procedures. No

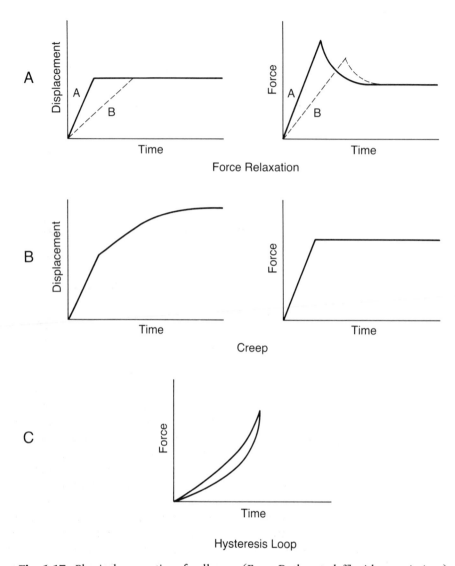

Fig. 1-17. Physical properties of collagen. (From Butler et al.,[27] with permission.)

specific or simple failure point can be stated for connective structures, as the specific mechanical behavior of a ligament or tendon depends on its individual cross section, length, and rate of loading in any situation. In general, connective tissue structures can tolerate 1.5 percent strain without any increase in stress; 1.5 to 3 percent is within physiologic limits, and 3 percent or greater begins to cause some mechanical failure.

Bone

As might be expected, bone is considerably stiffer (deformation resistant) than muscle, connective tissue, or nerve because of its inorganic matrix. Since the collagen component of bone is imbedded in this hard, mineralized matrix, it is not capable of rapid change in response to force application. As stated in Wolff's law, bone does respond to the forces placed upon it, but it requires more time, often weeks or months, to manifest this change. Bone strength also varies according to the direction of stress. It is nonuniform in construction, and it is strongest where it is most often exposed to loading, as are the more mobile forms of connective tissue. It is strongest in compression (the opposite of the nonossified connective tissues) and weakest in shear.[14] The weakness of bone in shear and its slow physiologic response to mechanical forces are important properties to remember when applying mobilization techniques on bones that may be weakened from immobilizational osteoporosis.

Muscle

Muscle responds to mechanical stress by lengthening passively and by a change in its ability to generate tension. This change has been well represented by the length-tension curve and its many variations.[5] The change in tension-generating ability is thought to be a result of both the elastic response of the connective tissue that surrounds the muscle and the change in position of the actin and myosin.[5] Electron microscopy has shown that the tension-generating capacity of actin and myosin filaments has a small tolerance for length variations (Fig. 1-4). Since different muscles have different fiber bundle arrangements, each muscle will have its own optimum length-tension position.[2,5] The combination of connective tissue response and active length-tension response partially explains why different muscles generate their maximum tensions at different joint angles.

Nerve

The mechanical responses of nerves to length changes appear to have been given little study. There is considerable clinical evidence that nerves have more tolerance for tension than compression before physiologic injury occurs. A study on the mechanical behavior of the sciatic nerve during the straight leg raising test was conducted by Fahrni in 1966.[38] He found that the straight leg could be elevated 30 to 40 degrees before all the slack was taken up in the peripheral portions of the sciatic nerve. Nothing was reported on the microscopic mechanical events. Sunderland reported that nerves can be

stretched to some extent without damage.[23] This may be because of the zigzag course of nerve fibers within a nerve. These waves are merely straightened out when a nerve is stretched to a certain point.

TRAUMA AND INFLAMMATION
Non-Tissue-Specific Response

Biologic tissue experiences mechanical trauma in the form of tension, compression. or shearing forces.[39] Muscle, nerve, connective tissue, and bone resist these mechanical stressors to differing degrees depending on the specific components of the tissue, the physiologic state of these tissues, and the magnitude, velocity, and direction of the force. Whatever the trauma, once mechanical damage has occurred, the initial biologic response is a generalized non-tissue-specific inflammatory process (Table 1-4).

The initial stages of this response are characterized by vascular changes.[16,39,40] The extent of these changes depends of course on the vascularity of the involved tissue; connective tissue has a lesser response than bone or muscle. Immediately following the injury there is a brief period of vasoconstriction lasting 5 to 10 minutes.[39] Vessel walls become lined with leukocytes, erythrocytes, and platelets.[16] Vasoconstriction is followed by active vasodilation of all local blood vessels and increased blood flow.

Table 1-4. Inflammatory Process

Reaction Phase
  1 to 3 days
  Vasodilation
  Edema
  Cell migration
  Debris removal

Repair Phase
  48 hours to 6 weeks
  Fibroplasia
  Wound closure
  Collagen content with random alignment
  Regeneration of small vessels

Remodeling Phase
  3 weeks to 12 months
  Reduction in wound size
  Increased wound strength
  Realignment of collagen
  Reduction of abnormal cross links

The small venules show an increase in permeability, allowing plasma to leak through into the site of injury. Edema or swelling then becomes apparent at the injury location. A highly cellular environment develops with active migration of leukocytes for "clean-up" of the damaged area.[41]

Once the debris has been removed by the leukocytes, the acute inflammatory process is completed and repair can begin.[40] Fibrocytes appear, possibly attracted by an electrical field within the wound area created by a local hypoxia.[42] Proliferation of collagen produced by the fibroblasts begins to close any gap or defect in the tissue. Collagen reaches a significant amount by the fourth or fifth day after injury and continues to increase for up to 6 weeks.[40] During this time, the injury site has very little tensile strength.[18] Immobilization is often needed to ensure an anatomically aligned repair.

In the absence of normal stress, collagen arrangement is random. Some resistance to tension can begin to develop about the second week.[18,40] Collagen synthesis has been briefly described in the section on normal tissue and illustrated in Figure 1-7. To review, the collagen molecule is a triple helical structure manufactured by the fibroblast. In its initial molecular form it is called tropocollagen.[1,16] The three chains making up the triple helix of tropocollagen are bonded by hydrogen bonds. Later, stronger chemical bonds form between the three chains. Outside the fibroblast, the tropocollagen units unite with each other in chains of longer length by overlapping their ends by one quarter. This is the "quarter-stagger array," which gives collagen its unique banded appearance.[1] Fibroblasts also produce the glycoproteins and GAG necessary for the ground substance of collagen.

Once a sufficient amount of collagen has been produced, the number of fibroblasts in the wound decreases. This marks the end of the proliferative or fibroplastic phase and the beginning of the maturation phase of wound healing. During the maturation phase, pronounced changes occur in the bulk, form, and strength of the scar tissue.[16] At the beginning of the phase, collagen is randomly oriented and the intermolecular bonds are weak. This appears to be the optimum time for applying gentle mobilization forces to reorient the collagen in a functional direction and to break any bonds that may have formed in

an abnormal pattern.[9,15] As tension across a wound site increases, reorientation of collagen fiber bundles and collagen phagocytosis also increase.[43] Remodeling may continue for years, although more slowly. Even after 40 weeks, normal organization and concentration of collagen are not yet present.[40,42]

It is important to remember that wound healing is a continuum. Inflammation, fibroplasia, and remodeling may overlap each other slightly in time. Judgment is required when mobilizing an injury that may still be undergoing fibroplasia, as overzealous movement may stimulate further collagen production and thicken the scar formation.[40,42]

Tissue-Specific Responses

Bone

Bone has a more specialized reaction to injury than do the soft connective tissues. Since there is soft tissue (periosteum) around the bone, which may be torn in an injury, the same non-tissue-specific response does occur in this area. Since bone contains large quantities of specialized osteocytes, rather than fibroblasts, there is repair of the bone with actual bone tissue rather than scar tissue.

Any trauma that fractures a bone results in the development of a callus: new tissue that forms around and between the ends of the fracture line or fragments.[1] Within the first few days after a fracture, osteogenic cells begin to proliferate in the deep periosteum close to the fracture site, much as in the proliferative phase of connective tissue healing. Eventually these cells form a collar around the fracture and begin to differentiate. The cells closest to a new blood supply become osteoblasts and form new bony trabeculae in this region.[1] Cells farther away from a blood supply, in the more superficial parts of the collar of callus, become chondrocytes. As a result, cartilage develops in this outer part of the collar of callus. The callus becomes a three-layered structure consisting of the outer proliferating portion, a middle cartilaginous layer, and an inner area of new bony trabeculae (Fig. 1-18). Growth of the collars of callus continues until the two sides of the fragment meet and fuse. The callus also undergoes a remodeling phase, as do the soft

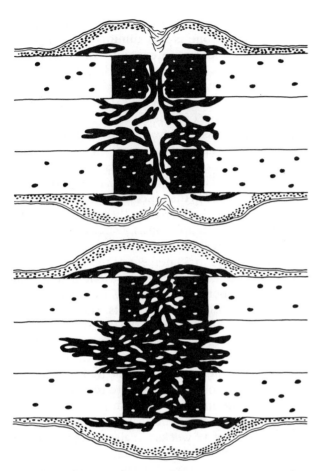

Fig. 1-18. Process by which periosteal collars form, approach one another, and fuse in the repair of a fracture. Living bone is depicted in light gray, dead portions in dark gray, and new bone in black. (From Ham and Cormack,[1] with permission.)

tissues. Cartilage is eventually replaced with bone as the intercellular substance deposited between the chondrocytes becomes calcified and the cells die. The trabeculae of bone that have formed close to the original fragments become firmly cemented to them and eventually to each other, thus bridging the fracture. The matrix of dead bone is gradually removed by osteoclasts. Osteoblasts move into the spaces opened by removal of dead bone and deposit new living bone. By replacing the cartilage of the callus with bone and converting cancellous bone into compact bone, the callus is gradually remod-

eled. Eventually the original line of the bone may be so well restored by this process that the fracture is almost undetectable by x-ray or palpation.

Nerve

Nerve also has a tissue-specific response to trauma because of its special tissue components and capabilities for repair. There is still the generalized inflammatory response and fibroplasia of the connective tissue component of the peripheral nerve. The degree of injury then dictates how much degeneration and time. This results in interference with function for a few days to several weeks. Sensory nerves are more easily affected than motor nerves, and peripheral fibers are affected before inner fibers. Second-degree injuries result from pressure over a longer period of time and lead to axon death, especially distal to the injury.[1,16] Complete severance of a nerve produces anatomic and metabolic changes both proximal and distal to the point of injury. The generalized traumatic response of the nerve includes degeneration of the myelin sheath with subsequent removal of debris by macrophages. New cytoplasm is synthesized, fibroblasts proliferate to bridge any defect created by the injury, and Schwann cells increase to restore the myelin sheath.[1,16] The Schwann cells grow in cords across the gap in the traumatized nerve. These cords provide guidance for any growing axons. The area of the damaged nerve may show enlargement due to fibroplasia for up to 3 weeks after injury. The severed axon degenerates both proximal and distal to the injury in the process called Wallerian degeneration. The axon then undergoes enlargement and budding. Excessive scar formation can deter the course of the growing axon buds to their target organs. Whether the axon reaches its proper destination at the distal end depends on the amount of scar tissue that has grown over the gap in the injured nerve.

Muscle

Muscles are often injured in compression, with a resulting contusion as evidenced by intramuscular bleeding and disruption of muscle fibers.[39] Muscle spasm, whether neurologic from the ensuing pain, or physiologic from the resulting fluid and cellular proliferation of the inflammatory response, may occur. This spasm limits the range of motion of the nearby joints. The amount of limitation may serve as an indication of the severity of the injury. A severe muscle contusion may result in myositis ossificans: the formation of bone tissue within the muscle. Caution must be used in mobilizing and exercising a severely contused muscle, as repeated trauma seems to stimulate the ossification process.[44]

Excessive tension may also injure a muscle; this is called a muscle strain. This strain may tear collagen fibers as well as muscle tissue itself if the failure point for that tissue is reached. The generalized inflammatory response of acute inflammation, repair, and remodeling occurs. Since muscle tissue has a limited potential for regeneration, any defect is usually filled with connective tissue scar. Some contractile function and thus strength may be lost, depending on the size of the defect.

IMMOBILIZATION

The effects of immobilization have been well studied in bone, connective tissue, and muscle and to a much lesser extent in nerve.[9,45-54] The general consequence of immobilization is loss first of tissue substrate and later of the most basic tissue components. In connective tissue, randomization of collagen fiber arrangement also occurs. The net result of these physiologic changes is always a loss of the basic function of the tissue in question. The amount of loss depends on the degree of the loss of tissue components. In bone, support and mineral reservoir capacities are diminished; in muscle, strength is compromised; in connective tissue, extensibility and tension resistance are reduced; and in nerve, sensitivity of some of the connective tissue-encapsulated receptors is reduced.

Bone

Bone accretion and absorption are maintained in equilibrium by weightbearing and muscular contraction.[45,55-59] Within 10 to 15 days of immobilization, the rate of bone turnover changes. Some sources report an initial increase in bone formation and absorption, with an eventual predominance of bone resorption by the 15th day.[45,55-58] The mineral content of the bone is also diminished and is reflected by an increase in excretion of urinary calcium. Increased excretion of hydroxyproline, an amino acid involved in collagen cross linking, indicates destruction of the organic as well as the inorganic components of bone.[45]

A localized loss of bone, such as that present in the distal fragment of a fractured long bone, is detectable on radiography when it constitutes a loss of 2 percent of total body calcium. This osteoporosis is most pronounced in the cancellous bone of the metaphysis and epiphysis, especially beneath the joint cartilage. True osteoporosis, a decrease in the total mass of the bony skeleton, is not detectable on radiography until 40 to 50 percent of the mineral content of the skeleton has been lost. The mechanical properties of bone also change with the loss of its organic and inorganic components. The hardness of bone steadily decreases with the duration of immobilization. By 12 weeks it is 55 to 60 percent of normal.[45] The elastic resistance also declines, and the bone becomes more brittle and thus more easily fractured. Most of these losses are recoverable in a comparable period of time if immobilization lasts 4 weeks or less. Components lost during an immobilization period of 12 weeks are also recoverable but require a longer recovery period.

Causes of osteoporosis have been associated with a change in blood flow during immobilization and a lack of normal mechanical stimulation.[45,55] Geiser and Trueta's study of immobilized rabbits showed a decrease in filling of osseous blood vessels after 4 to 5 days. For the next 4 to 6 weeks, bone became hypervascular and both bone formation and absorption increased. This was followed by a period of hypovascularity during which all activity declined. Cancellous bone showed only a network of thin, atrophic trabeculae. It was postulated that lack of muscle contraction reduced the suction effect on venous outflow and thus deprived distal areas of new blood.[55,56] The piezoelectric effect, thought to be important in maintaining normal bone activity, would also be lost in proportion to the loss of muscular activity.[57] Burr and Frederickson found that intracast muscle stimulation with implanted electrodes significantly altered the bone turnover rate in rabbit limbs immobilized for 17 days.[59] Oscillating beds, which provide full weightbearing and thus muscle contraction, when used for brief periods urinary calcium loss by 50 percent.[45] Supine exercises and quiet sitting did not have the same effect.[45] Demineralization was less responsive to weightbearing if the subject was paralyzed, although paraplegics who used crutches at least 1 hour per day seemed to be able to prevent the development of osteoporosis.[45]

Muscle

Changes with immobilization in muscle have been well investigated. Cooper's classic article investigated ultrastructural changes in muscle from the limbs of cats immobilized from 2 to 22 weeks in plaster casts.[46] Changes began appearing within 2 weeks, manifesting as a decrease in fiber size due to loss of myofibrils. Sarcomere elements lost their normal configuration and alignment. The mitochondria decreased in size and number. As degeneration progressed, debris from the breakdown of these cellular elements accumulated as myelin figures and lipid droplets. In some fibers all the myofilaments degenerated and the fibers became shrunken. Cell membrane and basement membranes enfolded deeply and later became fragmented or separated from each other. As degeneration progressed, rows of nuclei appeared, forewarning of impending nuclear degeneration. Total nuclear degeneration left only a mass of chromatin. Adjacent to degenerating cells, macrophages increased in number. A fibrofatty infiltrate and connective tissue accumulated in the degenerating muscle. Wet weight of the muscles decreased 25 percent, and total weight decreased 32 percent. As muscle weight decreased, the ability to generate tension also decreased in a greater proportion. Muscle contraction and relaxation times increased, perhaps because of the development of cross links between filaments that were not allowed to move normally.[46]

Neural elements such as muscle spindles, motor nerves, and motor end plates appeared unaffected. Tabary found that muscle immobilized in a shortened position for 4 weeks lost 40 percent of its original sarcomeres and required an equal length of time for recovery.[47] In this same study, muscles immobilized in a lengthened position gained 20 percent

more sarcomeres and sustained no changes in the normal length-tension curve. Individual sarcomeres were found to have a decreased length, although total fiber length increased. There was no change in the response to resistance to passive tension. Muscles immobilized in the shortened position showed the opposite reaction: Sarcomeres were reduced in number but showed either no change or an increase in length. Fiber length increased and there was an increase in resistance to passive tension. Muscles immobilized in the shortened position did lose weight more rapidly than those casted at resting length. Slow fibers appeared to be lost first.

Other researchers confirm the findings of Cooper and provide clinical relevance to his research.[47-49] Booth, in his review of the biochemical effects of immobilization on muscle, stated that there are lower levels of resting glycogen and ATP and more rapid depletion of ATP during exercise beginning as early as the sixth hour after immobilization.[48] He noted that there is also an increase in lactate during work and a decreased ability to oxidize fatty acids. The greatest loss of muscle mass occurs early in the immobilization period, evidently during the first 5 days. Lindboe stated that muscle fiber size is decreased by 14 to 17 percent after 72 hours of immobilization in humans.[49]

Connective Tissue

Akeson and his associates (San Diego, California) have been studying the effects of immobilization on connective tissue for many years.[9,50-52] In 1980 they presented the results of a study of the effects of immobilization on rabbit knee joints and formulated some theories on the pathomechanics of joint contracture.[9] They found changes both in the collagen fibers of the connective tissue around the immobilized joints and in the intercellular substance of GAG and water (Table 1-5). In the intercellular substance, water content was decreased by 3 to 4 percent, and the connective tissue appeared "woody" rather than smooth and glistening. An even greater decrease in concentration, 20 percent, was seen in the GAG portion of the intercellular substance. In contrast, total collagen remained unchanged. They theorized that this loss of water and

Table 1-5. Biochemical Observations on Fibrous Connective Tissue from Immobilized Joints

	Results of Immobilization
Collagen	Mass reduced by about 10% Increased turnover Increased degradation rate Increased synthesis rate Increased reducible collagen cross links
Glycosaminoglycans	Total GAG reduced 20% Hyaluronic acid reduced 40% Sulfated GAG reduced 20%
Water content	Reduced 3–4%

(Modified from Akeson et al.,[89] with permission.)

GAG, while total collagen remained the same, would decrease the space between collagen fibers in the connective tissue and thus alter free movement between the fibers. This lack of free movement would tend to make the tissue less elastic, less plastic, and more brittle. Further, in the absence of normal stress during the immobilization period, collagen fibers would be laid down in a random pattern, and cross links might form in undesirable locations, inhibiting normal gliding movement (Fig. 1-19). Since the loss of intercellular substance

would bring fibers closer together, cross links might form more easily.[9]

In support of the findings of Akeson et al. on the loss of connective tissue elasticity with immobilization, LaVigne and Watkins reported that joints immobilized at 90 degrees for 0 to 64 days required increasing amounts of force to be moved through the normal arc of motion.[53] Capsular structures also failed at lower loads than control joints. Changes in the force required for motion and in the load at failure were not evident until after 16 days of immobilization (Tables 1-6 and 1-7). Ligaments immobilized for 8 weeks showed a decrease in maximum load to failure, a decrease in energy absorbed at failure, and an increase in extensibility.[60]

The clinical implications for tissue that has been immobilized are many. Bone that has undergone local osteoporosis after fracture or immobilization is less able to bear weight or withstand normal forces of compression, tension, and shear. Caution must be exercised when applying manual techniques to a joint that has been immobilized or is near a fracture site, particularly the small joints of the fingers. The phalanges are small, and the therapist's hands can easily grasp both the dorsal and palmar surfaces of the phalanx. Often, patients with the common problem of adhesive capsulitis are older and may have a combined osteoporosis of age and immobilization. Again, care must be taken to

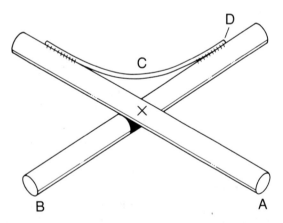

Fig. 1-19. An idealized model demonstrating the interaction of collagen cross links at the molecular level. A and B represent pre-existsing fibers, C represents the newly synthesized fibril, D represents the cross links created as the fibril becomes incorporated into the fiber, and X represents the nodal point at which adjacent fibers are normally freely movable past each other. (From Akeson,[9] with permission.)

Table 1-6. Gross and Microscopic Changes of Synovial Joints Observed After Prolonged Immobilization

Tissue	Results of Immobilization
Synovium	Proliferation of fibrofatty connective tissue into the joint space
Cartilage	Adherence of fibrofatty connective tissue to cartilage surfaces Loss of cartilage thickness Pressure necrosis at points of contact when compression has been applied
Ligament	Disorganization of the parallel arrays of fibrils and cells
Ligament insertion site	Destruction of ligament fibers attaching to bone
Bone	Generalized osteoporosis of cancellous and cortical bone

(Modified from Akeson et al.,[89] with permission.)

Table 1-7. Biomechanical Observations and Joint Structures from 12-Week-Immobilized Joints

Tissue	Results of Immobilization
Joint composite	Range of motion on an arthrograph indicates that the force required for the first flexion-extension cycle is increased more than 12-fold.
Ligament	Stress-strain diagrams of collateral ligaments show increased deformation with a standard load (i.e., greater compliance).
	Tensile failure tests of collateral and cruciate ligaments show failure at a lower load as well as lower energy-absorbing capacity of the immobilized bone-ligament complex (to about one-third of controls).

(Modified from Akeson et al.,[89] with permission.)

grade compression forces within the patient's pain tolerance and mechanical force absorption capabilities. As no studies are available as yet on the forces applied during specific mobilization maneuvers or manual therapy techniques, the grading of forces applied to joints or over osteoporotic bone is still a matter of therapeutic judgment.

Muscles that have been immobilized will be weak because of loss of the intercellular constituents that are necessary for muscle contraction and because of decreased storage of energy-producing substrates. Muscles may also be tight if immobilized in a shortened position because sarcomere numbers will be reduced and intramuscular connective tissue may have formed abnormal cross links. Since slow twitch fibers appear to be lost first, fatigue and low endurance will be most evident in postural activities and activities requiring sustained contraction. As muscle fatigues, its ability to absorb shock and protect neighboring joints is compromised. In short, muscle that has been immobilized or injured does not have the same contractile capacity as normal muscle, and therapeutic regimes must be altered and progressed accordingly.

Connective tissue likewise is compromised in strength, stiffness, and deformability after immobilization. This may be used to therapeutic advantage as in stretching abnormal connective tissue or scar tissue, or it may limit the amount of stress that can be placed on an injured joint capsule, ligament, or tendon. A thorough knowledge of the time frame of connective tissue healing, the stress-strain curve, viscoelastic tissue behavior, and the extent of soft tissue injury is absolutely essential to be able to exercise good therapeutic judgment in remobilization.

REMOBILIZATION

Mobilization of musculoskeletal injuries has changed greatly in some clinical practices in recent years.[61-66] The advent of the concept and technology of continuous passive movement in the late 1970s and early 1980s brought new dimensions to the prevention of deformity and limited movement after injury and to the promotion of healing of articular cartilage and connective tissue.[63-71] Modern surgery, antibiotics, and the use of cast bracing and intracast electrical stimulation have decreased the length of time of immobility needed for adequate healing.[48] Physicians, physical therapists, and patients are requesting early mobilization of injuries, within acceptable constraints of adequate healing and stability. It is hoped that prevention rather than treatment of the sequelae of musculoskeletal injury and prolonged immobilization will gradually become the norm. Until this comes to pass, however, therapists will have to be prepared to evaluate and treat muscles, joints, ligaments, and tendons that have undergone the changes inherent in the inflammatory and immobilizational processes.

Muscle, Bone, and Connective Tissue

Most studies available on the response of muscle to mobilization concentrate on the effects of exercise in normal subjects.[3,4] This topic is treated at length in Chapter 2 of this text. For purposes of comparison, it is of note that muscle regeneration begins within 3 to 5 days of the start of a reconditioning program after injury.[39,46] Within the first week, muscle weight increases. Some fibers may have completed regeneration of their contractile elements by 1 to 3 days.[46] One week after release from immobilization, muscle fibers of cats immobilized for various lengths of time showed intense regenerative activity, although no evidence of mitosis. Fibers began to return to normal via endomysial proliferation. The sarcoplasm started showing evidence of fibrils, which then formed myofibrils. Mitochondria increased in number, and contractile proteins were added. Sarcomeres began forming randomly within a cell, and fiber regeneration also proceeded randomly in terms of geographic distribution. Sarcomeres were initially longer than normal, and A bands were not aligned in register until later in the regenerative process. As regeneration proceeded, sarcomere size became normal, alignment became normal and thick, and then filaments became more definite. Normal contraction and relaxation times were regained within the first week after release from immobilization.[46] Muscle weight was not quite normal by 6 weeks, but several authors reported normal weight and ultrastructure by 3 months.[72,73] Cooper estimated that linear regeneration took place at the rate of 1 to 1.5 mm/day.

Recovery in muscle takes place at a faster rate and begins substantially sooner after immobilization or trauma than in bone or connective tissue, most likely because of the superior vascular supply of muscle tissue.[39] Muscle immobilized for 4 weeks required an equal amount of time for recovery, as did bone that was immobilized the same period of time.[45,47] Bone immobilized for longer periods of time, however, required proportionately longer periods for complete recovery. Connective tissue is the slowest of the tissues under consideration to return to normal after immobilization or injury. This may be because of its slow turnover rate, poor vascularity, or both. Ligaments that have been injured begin to regain tensile strength about the fifth week after injury, depending on the severity of the injury.[74] A healing ligament may have about 50 percent of its normal strength by 6 months after injury, 80 percent after 1 year, and 100 percent only after 1 to 3 years, depending on the type of stresses placed upon it and the prevention of a repeated injury.[75] Thus, stressing a connective tissue structure during remobilization is important for full recovery and yet must be properly graded to avoid reinjury. Patients with ligament injuries or reconstructions need to be cautioned about returning gradually to preinjury activities. Since few studies are available as to the exact stresses that functional and sports activities

place on connective tissue structures, this is again a matter of clinical judgment. Because healing ligaments have a poor nerve supply, pain cannot be the only guiding factor as to the appropriateness of any particular activity. Joint surfaces are also vulnerable to injury with a sudden increase in functional load.[76-80] Since the effects of periodic short immobilizations appear to be cumulative, it is important to avoid overstressing a recently mobilized limb to avoid reinjury and another period of immobilization.[79]

Studies are available on the response of articular cartilage injuries, total joint replacements, tendon lacerations, tendon transplants, and soft tissue injuries to intermittent and continuous movement.[63-67,69-71] All reported enhanced rate of healing, earlier recovery of normal range of motion, and improved strength over immobilized controls. Several researchers found that regular exercise and stress had the beneficial effect of increasing the mass of ligaments and tendons and rendering them more stiff and able to tolerate heavier loads at failure.[75,81-86] Biomechanical changes in reconditioned ligaments showed an increase in the stress at the yield point, a longer plastic region of deformation, and an increase in the maximum load capacity and energy at failure.[74,82] Early mobilization of healing tendon repairs decreased adhesion formation and thus increased mobility.[87] Strength was also enhanced when compared to the immobilized controls.[83] Microscopic examination showed an increase in the size of collagen fibrils.[81]

Collagen is known to align along lines of stress application, especially during healing or reconditioning after immobilization.[31,43,87] Again, early during the repair phase of the healing process or soon after immobilization is the optimum time to begin any reconditioning program for connective tissue structures, whether it be a program of continuous passive movement, graded active exercise, manually applied passive movement, or supervised functional activity. Therapeutic intervention can be more effective when collagen is immature and intermolecular bonds are weak. Specific procedures that concentrate directly on the tissue structures involved would certainly be preferred over general activities, especially at the beginning of a program.

When procedures are more specific, forces can be continually controlled and modified according to the response of the tissue and the patient. Without knowledge of the normal structure of the tissues we are dealing with; of the changes in these tissues with injury, immobilization, healing, and remobilization; and of the response of these tissues to the mechanical forces placed on them during physical therapy procedures, treatment is at best only minimally therapeutic.

REFERENCES

1. Ham AW, Cormack DH: Histology. 8th Ed. JB Lippincott, Philadelphia, 1979
2. Warwick R, Williams PL: Gray's Anatomy. 35th British Ed. WB Saunders, Philadelphia, 1973
3. Astrand P-O: Textbook of Work Physiology: Physiological Basis of Exercise. McGraw-Hill, New York, 1977
4. Golnick P, Armstrong RB, Saubert CW IV, et al: Enzyme activity and fiber composition for skeletal muscle of untrained and trained men. J Appl Physiol 33:312, 1972
5. Soderberg GL: Kinesiology: Application to Pathological Motion. Williams & Wilkins, Baltimore, 1986
6. Gossman MR, Sahrman SA, Rose S: Review of length associated changes in muscle. Phys Ther 62:1800, 1982
7. Brodahl A: Neurological Anatomy in Relation to Clinical Medicine. 3rd Ed. Oxford University Press, New York, 1981
8. Wyke B: The neurology of joints. Ann R Coll Surg 41:25, 1967
9. Akeson WH, Ameil D, Woo SL-Y: Immobility effects of synovial joints: the pathomechanics of joint contracture. Biorheology 17:95, 1980
10. Viidik A: On the rheology and morphology of soft collagenous tissue. J Anat 105:184, 1969
11. Van Brocklin JD, Ellis DG: A study of the mechanical behavior of toe extensor tendons under applied stress. Arch Phys Med 46:369, 1965
12. Kennedy JC, Hawkins RJ, Willis RB, et al: Tension studies of human knee ligaments. J Bone Joint Surg 58A:350, 1976
13. Donatelli R, Owens-Burkhardt H: Effects of immobilization on the extensibility of periarticular connective tissue. J Orthop Sports Phys Ther 3(2):67, 1981
14. Reigger CL: Mechanical properties of bone. p. 3. In Davies GJ, Gould JA (eds): Orthopedic and Sports Physical Therapy. CV Mosby, St. Louis, 1985
15. Frankel VH, Nordin M: Basic Biomechanics of the Skeletal System. Lea & Febiger, Philadelphia, 1980
16. Bryant WM: Wound Healing, Clinical Symposia. Vol. 29:3. CIBA Pharmaceutical, West Caldwell NJ, 1977
17. Betsch DF, Bauer E: Structure and mechanical properties of rat tail tendon. Biorheology 17:84, 1980
18. Arem AJ, Madden JW: Effects of stress on healing wounds. 1. Intermittent noncyclical tension. J Surg Res 20:93, 1976
19. Rowinski M: Afferent neurobiology of the joint. p. 50. In Davies, GJ, Gould JA (eds): Orthopedic and Sports Physical Therapy, CV Mosby, St. Louis, 1985
20. Wyke B: Articular neurology: a review. Physiotherapy 58:94, 1972
21. Freeman MAR, Wyke B: Articular reflexes at the ankle joint: an electromyographic study of normal and abnormal influences of ankle-joint mechanoreceptors upon reflex activity in the leg muscles. Br J Surg 54:12, 1967
22. de Andrade JR, Grant C, St J Dixon A: Joint distension and reflex muscle inhibition in the knee. J Bone Joint Surg 47A:313, 1965
23. Sunderland S: Nerves and Nerve Injuries. 2nd Ed. Churchill Livingstone, New York, 1978
24. Currey J: The Mechanical Adaptations of Bones. p. 24. Princeton University Press, Princeton NJ, 1984
25. Ackerman LV, Spjut HF, Abell MR: Bones and Joints by 24 Authors. International Academy of Pathology Monograph #17. Williams & Wilkins, Baltimore, 1976
26. Bassett CAL: Electrical effects in bone. Sci Am 18:213, 1965
27. Butler DL, Grood ES, Noyes FR, et al: Biomechanics of ligaments and tendons. Exerc Sport Sci Rev 6:126, 1979
28. Zachezewski JE: Flexibility for the runner: specific program considerations. Top Acute Care Trauma Rehab 10:9 1986
29. Sapega AA, Quadenfeld TC, Moyer RA, et al: Biophysical factors in range of motion exercise. Phys Sports Med 9:57, 1981
30. Fukuda E: Mechanical deformation and electrical polarization in biological substances. Biorheology 5:199, 1968
31. Hirsch G: Tensile properties during tendon healing. Acta Orthop Scand, suppl. 153, 1974
32. Crowninshield RD, Pope MH: Strength and failure characteristics of rat medial collateral ligament. J Trauma 16:99, 1969

33. Noyes FR, DeLucas JL, Torvik PJ: Biomechanics of anterior cruciate ligament failure: an analysis of strain-rate sensitivity and mechanics of failure in primates. J Bone Joint Surg 56A:236, 1974

34. Rigby BJ, Herai N, Spikes JD, et al: Mechanical properties of rat tail tendon. J. Gen Phys 43:265, 1959

35. Weismann MS, Pope MH, Johnson RJ: Cyclic loading in knee ligament injuries. Am J Sports Med 8:1, 1980

36. Lehmann JF, Masock ASJ, Warren CG, et al: Effect of therapeutic temperatures on tendon extensibility. Arch Phys Med Rehab 51:481, 1970

37. Welsh RP, MacNab I, Riley V, et al: Biomechanical studies of rabbit tendon. Clin Orthop 81:171, 1971

38. Fahrni WH: Observations on straight leg raising with special reference to nerve root adhesions. Can J Surg 9:44, 1986

39. Zarins B: Soft tissue injury and repair: biomechanical aspects. Int J Sports Med 3:9, 1982

40. Kellett J: Acute soft tissue injuries: a review of the literature. Med Sci Sports Excerc 18:5, 1986

41. Wilkerson GB: Inflammation in connective tissue, etiology and management. Athletic Training, Winter:298, 1985

42. van der Meulen JCH: Present state of knowledge on processes of healing in collagen structures. Int J Sports Med 3:4, 1982

43. McGaw WT: The effect of tension on collagen remodelling by fibroblasts: a stereological ultrastructural study. Connect Tissue Res 14:229, 1986

44. Turek SL: Orthopaedics: Principles and Their Application. 4th Ed. JP Lippincott, Philadelphia, 1984

45. Steinberg FU: The Immobilized Patient: Functional Pathology and Management. p. 33. Plenum Medical Books, New York, 1980

46. Cooper RR: Alterations during immobilization and regeneration of skeletal muscle in cats. J Bone Joint Surg 54A:919, 1972

47. Tabary JC, Tabary C, Tardieu C, et al: Physiological and structural changes in the cat's soleus muscle due to immobilization at different lengths by plaster casts. J Physiol 224:231, 1972

48. Booth FW: Physiologic and biochemical effects of immobilization on muscle. Clin Orthop 219:15, 1987

49. Lindbo CF, Platou CS: Effects of immobilization of short duration on the muscle fibre size. Clin Physiol 4:183, 1984

50. Akeson WH: An experimental study of joint stiffness. J Bone Joint Surg 43A:1022, 1961

51. Akeson WH, Ameil D, LaViolette D: The connective tissue response to immobility: a study of the chondroitin 4- and 6-sulfate and dermatin sulfate changes in periarticular connective tissue of control and immobilized knees of dogs. Clin Orthop 51:183, 1967

52. Akeson WH, Ameil D, LaViolette D: The connective tissue response to immobility: an accelerated aging response. Exp Gerontol 3:239, 1968

53. LaVigne AB, Watkins RP: Preliminary results on immobilization-induced stiffness of monkey knee joints and posterior capsule. In: Perspectives in Biomedical Engineering. Proceedings of a Symposium, Biological Engineering Society, University of Strathclyde, Glasgow, June 1972. University Park Press, Baltimore, 1973

54. Noyes FR, Torvik PJ, Hyde WB, et al: Biomechanics of ligament failure II: an analysis of immobilization, exercise and reconditioning effects in primates. J Bone Joint Surg 56A:1406, 1974

55. Geiser M, Trueta J: Muscle action, bone rarefication and bone formation. J Bone Joint Surg 40B:282, 1958

56. Little K, De Valderama JF: Some mechanisms involved in the osteoproptic process. Gerontologia 14:109, 1968

57. Hardt AB: Early metabolic responses of bone to immobilization. J Bone Joint Surg 54A:119, 1972

58. Hulth A, Olerud S: Disease of the extremities: II. A microangiographic study in the rabbit. Acta Chir Scand 120:338, 1961

59. Burr D, Frederickson R, Pavlinch C, et al: Intracast muscle stimulation prevents bone and cartilage deterioration in cast-immobilized rabbits. Clin Orthop 189:264, 1984

60. Dehne E, Torp RP: Treatment of joint injuries by immediate mobilization. Based on the spinal adaptation concept. Clin Orthop 77:218, 1971

61. Perry J: Contractures: a historical approach. Clin Orthop 219:8, 1987

62. Nicholas JA, Friedman MJ: Sprains and dislocations of joints and related structures. In Denton JR (ed): Orthopedics, Goldsmith Practice of Surgery 2:1. Harper & Row, Philadelphia, 1984

63. Salter RB, Simmonds DF, Malcolm BW, et al: The biological effect of continuous passive motion on the healing of full thickness defects in articular cartilage. J Bone Joint Surg 62A:1232, 1980

64. Salter RB, Hamilton HW: Clinical application of basic research on continuous passive motion for disorders and injuries of joints: a preliminary report of a feasibility study. J Orthop Res 1:325, 1984

65. Coutts RD, Kaita J, Barr R, et al: The role of continuous passive movement in the post operative rehabilitation of the total knee patient. Orthop Trans 6:277, 1982

66. Hamilton HW: Five years experience with continuous passive motion (CPM). J Bone Joint Surg 64B:259, 1982

67. O'Driscoll SW, Kumar A, Salter RM: The effect of continuous passive motion on the clearance of a hemarthrosis. Clin Orthop 176:305, 1983

68. Salter RB: Motion vs rest: why immobilize joints? Presidential address to the Canadian Orthopedic Association. J Bone Joint Surg 64B:251, 1982

69. Salter RB, Bell RS: The effect of continuous passive motion on the healing of partial thickness lacerations of the patellar tendon in the rabbit. Orthop Trans 5:209, 1981

70. Salter RB, Harris DJ, Bogoch E: Further studies on continuous passive motion (abstract). Orthop Trans 212:292, 1978

71. Salter RB, Minister RR: The effect of continuous passive motion on a semitendinosus tenodesis in the rabbit knee. Orthop Trans 6:292, 1982

72. Lash JW, Holtzer H, Swift H: Regeneration of mature skeletal muscle. Anat Rec 128:679, 1957

73. LeGros Clark WE: An experimental study of regeneration of mammalian striped muscle. J Anat 80:24, 1946

74. Frank G, Woo SL-Y, Amiel D, et al: Medial collateral ligament healing. A multidisciplinary assessment in rabbits. Am J Sports Med 11:379, 1983

75. Tipton CM, James SL, Mergner W, et al: Influence of exercise on strength of medial collateral knee ligaments of dogs. Am J Physiol 218:894, 1970

76. Tipton CM, Matthes RD, Maynard JA, et al: The influence of physical activity on ligaments and tendons. Med Sci Sports 7:165, 1975

77. Videman T: Connective tissue and immobilization: key factors in musculoskeletal degeneration? Clin Orthop 221:26, 1987

78. Videman T: Experimental osteoarthritis in the rabbit: comparison of different periods of repeated immobilization. Acta Orthop Scand 53:339, 1982

79. Videman T, Michelsson J-E: Inhibition of development of experimental osteoarthritis by distraction during immobilization. Int Res Commun Syst Sci 5:139, 1977

80. Shimizu T, Videman T, Shimazaki K, et al: Experimental study on the repair of full thickness articular cartilage defects. J Orthop Res 5:187, 1987

81. Woo SL-Y, Gomez MA, Young-Kyun W, et al: Mechanical properties of tendons and ligaments II: the relationship of immobilization and exercise on tissue remodeling. Biorheology 19:397, 1982

82. Clayton ML, Weir GJ: Experimental investigation of ligament healing. Am J Surg 98:373, 1959

83. Gleberman R, Woo SL-Y, Lothringer K, et al: Effects of early intermittent passive mobilization on healing canine flexor tendons. J Hand Surg 7:170, 1982

84. Downey JA, Darling RC: Physiologic Basis of Rehabilitation Medicine. WB Saunders, Philadelphia, 1971

85. Viidik A: Tensile strength properties of Achilles tendon systems in trained and untrained rabbits. Acta Scand Orthop 40:261, 1969

86. Evans P: The healing process at a cellular level: a review. Physiotherapy 66:256, 1974

87. Evans EB, Eggers GWN, Butler JK, et al: Experimental immobilization and remobilization of rat knee joints. J Bone Joint Surg 42A:737, July 1960

88. Cohen RE, Hooley CJ, McCrum NG: Viscoelastic creep of collagenous tissue. J Biomech 9:175, 1976

89. Akeson WH, Amiel D, Abel MF, et al: Effects of immobilization on joints. Clin Orthop 219:33, 1987

2

Exercise Treatment for the Rehabilitated Patient: Cardiopulmonary and Peripheral Responses

SCOT IRWIN

Rehabilitation after an injury often does not take into consideration the final state of fitness of the individual. There are several stages involved in completing this part of a rehabilitation program. Once the injured extremity has achieved an appropriate level of function, program goals should be adjusted to achieve a state of fitness equivalent to the preinjured state.

This chapter discusses the completion of rehabilitation through exercise training. Exercise training requires the therapist to adhere to some basic principles of exercise physiology, including: (1) designing a specific exercise program using an appropriate exercise mode to achieve the desired results, (2) recognizing the innate genetic limitations of each individual and thus the amount of improvement that can be expected, (3) developing cardiovascular conditioning by long-duration, continuous exercise of large muscle groups, and (4) increasing strength and power with high-intensity, short-duration bursts of activity.

These are principles, not laws. Each of these principles continues to be rigorously investigated, but for now they are considered solid standards of exercise that can be followed with reasonable confidence. These principles are affected by several external variables that can influence the conditioning program and thus the desired outcomes. These factors include, but are not limited to, age, initial state of fitness, sex, temperature, altitude, medications, and individual motivation.

The purpose of this chapter is to highlight the principles, evaluation methods, and desired effects of exercise training programs used to complete the rehabilitation process following an injury. To achieve this purpose, the chapter is divided into four sections covering the effects of bed rest and deconditioning, the evaluation of cardiovascular condition, the principles of exercise prescription, and the effects of training.

BED REST AND DECONDITIONING

Most extremity injuries, especially lower extremity injuries, are accompanied by a reduction in activity. Severe injuries, such as fractures and ligamentous tears, often result in short periods of complete bed rest and prolonged periods of inactivity.

The detrimental effects of inactivity in the form of bed rest have been heavily chronicled, especially in studies on the effects of weightlessness.[1] The effects of bed rest vary according to duration[2-4], prior state of conditioning,[5] and the activity conducted during bed rest[2] (e.g., isometric or isotonic exercises, bathroom privileges). The time course of some of these changes is presented in Table 2-1.[2-5]

Many of the effects of bed rest occur within 3 days or less (Table 2-1). These changes are primarily attributed to changes in plasma volume, fluids and electrolytes, and venous compliance. With prolonged bed rest, the detrimental effects become more numerous and severe. They include losses in body weight, calcium, muscle strength, and maximum oxygen consumption. Maximum oxygen consumption is perhaps the best single measure of fitness. Some additional detriments of bed rest include constipation, atelectasis, orthostatic hypotension, and osteoporosis.[6] On the other hand, some authors have demonstrated a significant increase in forced vital capacity and total lung capacity after bed rest of 11 to 12 days.[7] These data have been challenged by other researchers, who found no significant changes in static volumes following bed rest.[2]

There are numerous and sometimes conflicting reports on the effects of isometric and isotonic exercises on reducing the detrimental effects of prolonged inactivity.[2,8] A summary of the effects of bed rest of 7 to 14 days on young males can also be found in Table 2-1.

Knowledge of the detrimental effects of bed rest will have an influence on the treatment program chosen. The reader should not equate decreased activity with bed rest, for even modest activity like sitting in a chair or performing mild isotonic or isometric exercise can reduce the detrimental effects of bed rest.[2] A normalization from the effects of bed rest can be achieved in only 7 days with an exercise conditioning program,[8] but in effect most of the losses are reversible with normal activities.[8] The less time a person is subjected to bed rest or reduced activity, the less time it takes to return to a fit level.

Individuals in a higher state of fitness as measured by their maximum oxygen consumption, such as trained athletes, lose a greater percentage of their maximum oxygen consumption during periods of inactivity than the average sedentary individual, and have to retrain themselves to regain the same relative state of fitness.[5] The higher the state of conditioning required, the greater the need for an individualized exercise prescription. The rehabilitation process is not complete simply because normal joint motion and muscular strength have returned. An individual, especially an athlete, should retrain his muscles, joints, and cardiopulmonary system to their premorbid state before resuming athletic endeavors. Untrained individuals may cause themselves further injury and produce suboptimal performances.

Table 2-1. Effects of Bed Rest on Young Males

Effect	1 Hour/Day Isotonic	7–14 Days No Exercise	1 Hour/Day Isometric
Changes in body composition	Increases fat loss Decreases lean loss Total weight loss is determined by diet	Loss of lean and fat mass	Total body weight loss may actually be greater
Plasma volume loss	Attenuates loss to 7–8%	Plasma volume decreases by 300–500 ml (12–13%)	Attenuates loss to 11%
VO$_2$	Decreases loss by about one-third (8–5%)	10–12%[a]	Decreases loss to about 4–5%
Glucose tolerance	Reduces glucose intolerance	Glucose tolerance worsens	Reduces glucose intolerance
Plasma calcium[b]	Attenuates loss to 4%	11% loss continues steadily over 36 weeks	Attenuates loss to 7%

VO$_2$, maximum oxygen consumption.
[a] Depends on initial state of fitness. Men's rate of loss is less than women's.
[b] See references 2–5.

EVALUATION

Each individual should have a specifically designed exercise prescription based on a thorough evaluation of his maximum physical work capacity and postural and musculoskeletal limitations.

Physical work capacity can best be evaluated by performing an exercise test. This test can be as simple as a 12-minute walk or as sophisticated as a symptom-limited maximum thallium treadmill test. The choice of testing method should match the mode of exercise to be prescribed and be as sophisticated as the individual's age, cardiac risk factors, sex, and medical problems require. For example, if the mode of training is going to be biking, then the exercise test should be performed on a bike. If the patient plans on participating in activities that require maximum cardiovascular performance, then a symptom-limited maximum exercise test should be performed. Generally, if the patient is a man over 35, he should be thoroughly screened by his physician before beginning an exercise program.[9] If he is younger than 35 but has multiple risk factors for heart disease, he should also be cleared by his physician before initiating an exercise training program.[9]

A multitude of testing and evaluation modes are available. General guidelines for exercise testing can be found in the American College of Sports Medicine guidelines for testing and training.[9] Perhaps more important than the choice of testing methods is the interpretation of the test. It is not within the scope of this chapter to give a thorough discussion of exercise test interpretations. For an in-depth discussion of this topic see Astrand's *Textbook of Work Physiology*[10] and Ellestad's text *Stress Testing.*[11]

A typical symptom-limited maximum exercise test completed on a 40-year-old man is depicted in Figures 2-1 and 2-2. This test was performed on a treadmill using a Bruce protocol.[12] Although this protocol is not ideal for exercise prescription, it is commonly used in exercise testing laboratories throughout the United States, especially for ruling out coronary disease. It is strongly recommended that any patient who is going to begin a walking, walk-jog, or higher intensity exercise program have a symptom-limited maximum test. If the patient is

over 35, this test should be completed in a formal exercise testing lab with the appropriate personnel present. A study by Cahalin et al. has demonstrated the safety of this type of testing when completed independently by specially trained physical therapists.[13] There are several exercise test protocols (Fig. 2-3).

A symptom-limited maximum exercise test gives us the following vital information: (1) actual symptom-limited maximum heart rate, (2) presence or absence of normal cardiopulmonary responses to exercise, (3) presence or absence of EKG abnormalities, (4) limiting symptoms, and (5) predicted physical work capacity.[12]

Despite attempts to formulate exercise prescriptions directly from the treadmill exercise test,[14] I can state that, clinically, direct translation from a test to an exercise prescription is rarely possible. These tests should be considered as part of the patient's evaluation and as a screening process to rule out potentially dangerous pathologies. An exercise test can also be used to measure the extent of patient progress. Some protocols will enhance the therapist's ability to detect improvements because they have smaller incremental increases in each stage of the test (Fig. 2-3).

Alternative forms of testing include biking and arm ergometry. The format for these tests is quite different. Treadmill testing is a continuous test, whereas most arm or bike tests are intermittent. Participants are allowed to rest or pedal against a lower resistance between 2- to 4-minute bouts of progressively harder exercise. Bike testing generally does not produce as high a cardiopulmonary response as treadmill testing because leg muscle fatigue occurs before maximum cardiopulmonary levels are attained. If your clinic does not have access to an exercise testing laboratory, then simpler submaximal tests can be completed. A 12-minute walk test can be a useful evaluation, especially for people who have poor exercise tolerance. To complete this test, simply mark off a known distance and have the patient walk as far as he can in 12 minutes. Record the patient's resting and peak heart rates and blood pressures and any symptoms noted, and measure the distance the patient walked. This information can be used as a baseline for exercise prescription and repeated to assess improvement. This test can

TREADMILL TEST WORKSHEET
Clayton General Hospital

Name _____ Hosp. No _____ Date __1/12/87__ Age __40__

Sex __M__ Weight __212__ Height __6' 0"__ Diagnosis __0__ _____

Reason for test __Fitness Program__ Protocol _____

ECG Interpretation __Normal__ _____

Time __9:00 A.M.__ Medications __None__ _____

Time last dose __None__ Time last cigarette __None__ Time last meal __6:00 P.M.__

Physician: _____

_____

TEST RESULTS

Minutes Completed __7' 52"__ Limiting Factors __Leg fatigue, S.O. B.__ _____

Resting Heart rate __78__ Max. Heart rate __176__ Resting BP __108/78__

Max. BP __190/86__ BP Response __normadaptive__ _____

_____

Chest Pain __0__ _____

_____

Summary ST Segment Changes __negative test to HR 176__ _____

_____

_____

Heart Sounds __normal__ Arrhythmias __rare PVC's post exercise__ _____

_____

Physical Work Capacity __Fair-Good FAI 25% below predicted for a sedentary male__

_____

Remarks/Recommendations _____

_____

_____

_____

Fig. 2-1. Treadmill test interpretation.

STAGE	MPH	GRADE	MINUTE	HR	BP	ARRHYTHMIAS	SYMPTOMS
PRE-EX							
SUPINE			1	76	110/70	0	0
SUPINE			2	78	118/78	0	0
BREATH-HOLD			1	66	102/70	0	0
HYPERVENT.			1	78	120/76	0	0
SITTING			1	78	130/70	0	0
STANDING			1	84	140/80	0	0
MPH	%	SEC.					
1.7	10		1	100	144/80	0	0
			2	110	150/78	0	0
			3	110	150/78	0	0
2.5	12		1	126	156/84	0	0
			2	136	166/84	0	0
			3	144	170/80	0	0
3.4	14		1	160	186/86	0	S.O.B., leg pain
		52"	2	176	190/86	0	
			3				
			1				
			2				
			3				
			1				
			2				
			3				
IMMEDIATE POST-EX.							
SUPINE			1	175	174/76	Rare PVC	
			2	160	156/70		
			3	140	148/72	xx	
			4	114	144/72		
			5	96	136/70	x	
			6	88	130/88		
			7	88	136/78		
			8				
			9				
			10				

Fig. 2-2. Treadmill test worksheet.

FUNCTIONAL CLASS	CLINICAL STATUS	O₂ REQUIREMENTS ml O₂/kg/min	TREADMILL TESTS			BICYCLE ERGOMETER
			BRUCE* 3-min stages	KATTUS+ 3-min stages	BALKE# %grade at 3.4 mph	For 70 kg body weight kgm/min
NORMAL AND 1	PHYSICALLY ACTIVE SUBJECT	56.0			26	
		52.5		mph %gr	24	
		49.0	mph %gr	4 22	22	
		45.5	4.2 16		20	1500
		42.0		4 18	18	1350
		38.5			16	1200
	SEDENTARY HEALTHY	35.0		4 14	14	1050
		31.5	3.4 14		12	900
		28.0		4 10	10	750
	DISEASED, RECOVERED / SYMPTOMATIC PATIENTS	24.5	2.5 12	3 10	8	600
		21.0			6	
II		17.5	1.7 10	2 10	4	450
		14.0			2	300
III		10.5				150
		7.0				
IV		3.5				

Fig. 2-3. Classification and oxygen requirements for various workloads on treadmill and bicycle ergometers; gr, grade. (Modified from Fortuin and Weiss,[25] with permission.)

be modified by reducing the time; however, it is not advisable to reduce the time to less than 6 minutes.

Before developing an individualized exercise prescription, a thorough postural and musculoskeletal evaluation should be completed, including a posture analysis with special attention to the strength, flexibility, and symmetry of the individual to be trained. For example, a patient that is going to start a walking or walk-jogging program should have a careful evaluation of lower extremity strength, range of movement, and gait, especially foot and ankle biomechanics (see previous chapter). A posture analysis and an individualized muscle test are necessities. Elaboration of this part of the evaluation can be found in Kendall and Kendall-McCreary.[15]

Any joint, strength, or postural asymmetries should be corrected before initiating, or as a part of, the patient's conditioning program. From my clinical experience, this will reduce subsequent complaints of pain and encourage continued exercise compliance. Routine reassessment of the program intensity should also include a quick musculoskeletal screen to ensure that no detrimental changes have occurred as a result of training. Common clinical findings with walking and walk-jogging programs include shin splints, runner's hip, tightening of the hamstrings, achilles tendinitis, and calf pain. In some cases, a change in training mode is required. Biking and swimming are good alternatives, but reassessment and testing is required.

PRINCIPLES OF EXERCISE PRESCRIPTION

We live in a society that is becoming health conscious. Wellness is not a notion but a reality, but the forms of exercise that are sold on every street corner by all levels of educated and uneducated individuals may not be the answer. In fact, the incidence of exercise-related injury has increased dramatically in recent years. Generalized exercise prescription, based on the idea that what is good for the instructor is good for all, may well be the reason.

Individualized exercise prescription requires more than that. An individualized exercise prescription must be based on a thorough evaluation, and take into consideration the mode, intensity, frequency, and duration of the exercise.

Selecting the mode of exercise is easy but is often poorly done. The mode of exercise should be chosen by approximating the individual's actual athletic endeavors as closely as possible. It should include methods of training that incorporate strengthening, improved flexibility, and endurance training. Emphasis on one of these three areas should be encouraged if the evaluation findings have identified a specific area of weakness. The mode of exercise should be specific. The principle of the specificity of exercise cannot be overstated. If an individual is unable to train by performing the actual activity he wants to participate in, a mode of training that closely imitates that activity should be chosen. For example, a person suffering from a loss in physical work capacity because of prolonged bed rest or restricted activity needs a mode of exercise that most closely approaches his daily activities. This is usually best achieved by walking. On the other hand, a football star needs a program that incorporates modes of training to improve strength, flexibility, and endurance for repeated bouts of short-duration, high-intensity exercise.

Once the mode or modes of exercise have been chosen, the next part of the exercise prescription is to decide the intensity of the exercise. Often at this point in a chapter about exercise prescription the reader is exposed to a series of formulas and graphs. These formulas depict a reasonable but generally wide and unindividualized range of exercise target heart rates based on age. This information is avail-able in almost any textbook on exercise physiology, and so a brief summary will suffice here.

Heart rate is linearly related to oxygen consumption, especially between 40 and 90 percent of maximum effort. Cardiovascular fitness training is felt to best occur somewhere between 70 and 90 percent of an individual's maximum heart rate. This heart rate is predictable from a formula of 220 minus the person's age. The training heart rate can thus be computed by obtaining a maximum predicted heart rate ($220 - $ age) and multiplying it times a fixed percentage. This formula uses the individual's resting heart rate, training percentage, and maximum heart rate to obtain a training heart rate. For example, a 30-year-old man with a resting heart rate of 60 would need to achieve a training heart rate of 151 to be training at a 70 percent intensity $[(190 - 60).70 + 60]$[16] (190 is 220 minus age). All these formulas and numbers are entirely accurate and can even be used on a normal, relatively active, well motivated, healthy population of young people under 30. Exercise prescription for the rest of us is not that easy and should be carefully individualized to take into consideration each patient's current state of fitness, presence of disease (especially cardiopulmonary diseases), age, sex, altitude, temperature, and motivation.

In my clinical experience, these formulas are often not applicable. People recovering from injuries, bed rest, heart attacks, or surgery cannot and will not adhere to these generalized heart rate formulas. There are several reasons for this including, but not limited to, medication, age, prior exercise habits, side effects of surgery, and motivation. So how does one determine an appropriate, useful intensity for an individual's exercise prescription? One of the best methods is to evaluate the person's response to his exercise program. This can be achieved by having the person carry out the program with you. I have found that many people, even after bypass surgery or a heart attack, can exercise continuously for 30 minutes. This is an adequate duration for the beginning. The intensity is then increased according to the individual's response. For example, a patient returning to basketball after a foot injury needs endurance training. The patient is instructed to walk beginning at 2.5 mph for 30 minutes. The therapist continuously assesses the patient's responses to this intensity and adjusts the speed up or down accordingly. Maximum walking speed for most men is about 4.0 mph. Beyond this speed most patients are more comfortable jogging.

There are two other ways to increase intensity using a treadmill. One is to maintain the speed and steepen the grade. I have found this to be effective before moving a patient to a jogging program. The maximum grade I use is 5 percent. Steeper grades at high speeds tend to cause injuries, shin splints, calf pain, and knee pain. Another method for increasing intensity is to have the person jog. This can even be done at low speeds of 3.6 to 4.0 mph. Jogging will increase the intensity even though the speed may not have changed. I will have a person begin jogging with a low-speed walk-jog program. After the patient can comfortably walk at 3.6 to 4.0 mph on a 3 to 5 percent grade for 30 to 45 minutes, he will begin a walk-jog program consisting of a 1-minute job followed by a 5-minute walk at 3.6 to 4.0 mph on a level surface. The jogging duration is then gradually increased to a 5-minute job alternating with a 10-minute walk for a total of 30 to 45 minutes on a level surface. Continuation of this process will result in the patient eventually achieving an intensity that can be sustained without injury. I do not use a grade with jogging, as this seems to enhance the risk of injury, especially in people over 40.

By integrating continuous musculoskeletal evaluation with a progressive method of assessing intensity, each person can achieve an exercise prescription with an appropriate mode, duration, and intensity for his personal needs. Frequency is determined by the individual's response to training and the individual's goals. When training patients to improve cardiovascular fitness, I use a frequency of 4 to 5 times a week as a minimum. Often with low-level programs (2.0 to 3.0 mph), I will have a patient exercise twice a day 4 to 5 times a week. This requires that patient carry out the greater part of the program at home. The therapist must therefore teach the patient about walking surfaces, shoes, and climate. Each of these variables can affect compliance and the incidence of injuries. Once a person has achieved an acceptable level of training, the frequency can be reduced to 2 to 4 times per week, although compliance can easily fail at this juncture. People tend not to comply if too great a time lapses between exercise days. Lifelong training may be as frequent as daily, although, again, the incidence of illness and injury will often make this impossible.

So, how has our exercise prescription evolved? For improving aerobic capacity, the mode is specific, the intensity individualized and intimately related to the duration. Finally, the frequency is determined by the goals of exercise, maintenance, improved fitness, or lifelong training. With these concepts in mind, the clinician should be able to complete the rehabilitation of an injured person regardless of age, sex, state of fitness, or type of injury.

EXERCISE TRAINING EFFECTS

A chapter on exercise training would be incomplete without some discussion of the potential benefits of exercise. On the other hand, an in-depth analysis could encompass an entire text. Thus, this part of the chapter is dedicated to a condensed version of the specific effects of an exercise training program using the principles already described.

The effects of exercise training fit nicely into two broad categories: central (cardiovascular) and peripheral effects. Each of these categories contributes to the net effect, which is an improvement in maximum oxygen consumption and physical work capacity.

The central or cardiovascular effects of exercise conditioning are well documented. An untrained individual can expect to achieve a 10 to 30 percent increase in maximum oxygen consumption over a 3- to 6-month period of training.

The primary central training effects are an increase in stroke volume, an increase in maximum cardiac output, a decrease in resting heart rate, and a decrease in heart rate and blood pressure at a given workload. These effects may require a minimum of 6 months of training or longer to achieve. In other words, at a workload of 4.0 mph a person before training may exhibit a heart rate of 120, and blood pressure 170/80 mm Hg, whereas after training the heart rate and blood pressure at that same workload will be significantly lower. The amount of improvement depends upon several variables, including but not limited to the state of fitness of the individual before beginning exercise, the intensity and duration of training, the age of the individual, and the presence or absence of any systemic pathology. Those individuals who are most deconditioned before initiating an exercise program tend to have the greatest percentage improvement when compared to more fit individuals. Low-intensity programs, where heart rates do not exceed 60 percent of maximum, may not produce the expected improvements in maximum oxygen consumption that a higher level of exercise training would. The effects of training on elderly men and women appear to be very similar despite somewhat lower intensities in the elderly.[17-22] Cardiopulmonary patients with severe ventricular dysfunction or advanced obstructive or restrictive lung disease may not demonstrate the same central training effects and thus increases in their maximum oxygen carrying capacity, but functional improvements can be dramatic. For an in-depth review of the effects of training on cardiopulmonary patients, see the work by Irwin and Techlin.[23] Patients with coronary artery disease may never demonstrate improvement in stroke volume, although a small number of studies have demonstrated improvement after 12 months of training or more.[24]

The peripheral effects of training are more numerous and perhaps more rapidly attained. The initial effects of training are created peripherally. These effects include an increase in arterial oxygen extraction at the tissue level [the $(a - V)O_2$ difference], an ability to withstand higher levels of lactic acid accumulation, increased concentrations of oxidative enzymes, increased numbers of mitochondria, increased muscle capillary density, and increased lean body mass. In addition, there is a decrease in fat body mass.

These changes often account for the majority of the effects of exercise because they occur within the first 3 to 6 months of training.

SUMMARY

The general state of fitness of most adults in the United States is perhaps fair at best. Following an injury, bed rest, and prolonged inactivity, this condition may be significantly worsened. This chapter has reviewed (1) the causes of this loss of fitness (in particular, bed rest), (2) methods for evaluating the condition of the individual through musculoskeletal screening and exercise stress testing, (3) the characteristics of a unique method for producing an individualized exercise prescription, and (4) the effects that exercise training should have on an individual's general state of fitness. Clinically, physical therapists should try to incorporate some form of exercise training into their patient care programs. This is especially true for individuals who are returning to vigorous recreational or athletic activities and for therapists who wish to complete the rehabilitation process.

REFERENCES

1. Brannon EW, Rockwood CA, Potts P: The influence of specific exercises in the prevention of debilitating musculoskeletal disorders; implication in physiological conditioning for prolonged weightlessness. Aerospace Med 34:900, 1963
2. Greenleaf JE, Kozolowski S: Physiological consequences of reduced activity during bed rest. Exerc Sport Sci Rev 10:84, 1982
3. Goffney FA, Nixon JV, Karlscom ES, et al: Cardiovascular deconditioning produced by 20 hours of bed rest with head-down tilt (−5°) in middle aged healthy men. Am J Cardiol 56:634, 1985
4. Winslow EH: Cardiovascular consequences of bed rest. Rev Cardiol 14:236, 1985
5. Saltin B, Blomquist CG, Mitchell JH, et al: Response to exercise after bed rest and after training. Circulation, suppl. III: VII-1, 1968
6. Krolner B, Toft B: Vertebral bone loss: an unheeded side effect of therapeutic bed rest.
7. Beckett WS, Vroman DN, Thompson-Gorman, et al: Effect of prolonged bed rest on lung volume in normal individuals. J Appl Physiol 61(3):919, 1986
8. DeBusk RF, Convertino VA, Hung J, et al: Exercise conditioning in middle-aged men after 10 days of bed rest. Circulation 68(2):245, 1983
9. American College of Sports Medicine: Guidelines for Graded Exercise Testing and Exercise Prescription. 2nd Ed. Lea & Febiger, Philadelphia, 1975
10. Astrand R: Textbook of Work Physiology. 3rd Ed. McGraw-Hill, New York, 1986
11. Ellestad MH: Stress Testing: Principles and Practices. 2nd Ed. FA Davis, Philadelphia, 1980

12. Bruce RA: Maximal oxygen uptake and normographic assessment of functional aerobic impairment in cardiovascular disease. Am Heart J 85:346, 1973

13. Cahalin LP, Blessey RL, Kummer D, et al: The safety of exercise testing performed independently by physical therapists. J Cardiopulmonary Rehab 7:269, 1987

14. Foster C, Lembarger K, Thomson N, et al: Functional translation of exercise responses from graded exercise testing to exercise training. Am Heart J 112(6):1309, 1986

15. Kendall FP, Kendall-McCreary E: Muscle Testing and Function. 3rd Ed. Chapter 8: Muscle Function in Relation to Posture. Williams & Wilkins, Baltimore, 1983

16. Karvonen MJ, Kentola E, Mustola O: The effect of training on heart rate: a longitudinal study. Ann Med Exp Fenn 35:307, 1957

17. Thomas SG, Cummingham DA, Rechnitzer PA: Determinants of the training response in elderly men. Med Sci Sports Exerc 17(6):667, 1985

18. Despres JP, Bouchard C, Tremblay A: Effects of aerobic training on fat distribution in male subjects. Med Sci Sports Exerc 17(1):113, 1985

19. Savage MP, Petratis MM, Thompson WH: Exercise training effects on serum lipids of prepubescent boys and adult men. Med Sci Sports Exerc 18(2):197, 1986

20. Gossard P, Haskell WL, Taylor BC, et al: Effects of low- and high-intensity home based exercise training on functional capacity in healthy middle-aged men. Am J Cardiol 57:446, 1985

21. Posner JD, Gorman BS, Klein HS: Exercise capacity in the elderly. Am J Cardiol 57:52C, 1986

22. Krisha AM, Boyles C, Cauley JA: A randomized exercise trial in older women: increased activity over two years and the factors associated with compliance. Med Sci Sports Exerc 18(5):557, 1986

23. Blessey R: The beneficial effects of aerobic exercise for patients with coronary artery disease. In Irwin S, Techlin JS (eds): Cardiopulmonary Physical Therapy. CV Mosby, St. Louis, 1985

24. Hagberg JM, Ehsani AA, Holloazy JO: Effect of 12 months of exercise training on stroke volume in patients with coronary artery disease. Circulation 67:1194, 1983

25. Fortuin N, Weiss JL: Exercise stress testing. Circulation, 56:suppl. 5, 699, 1977

THE UPPER QUARTER

3

Upper Quarter Evaluation: Structural Relationships and Interdependence

BRUCE GREENFIELD

Lesions of the motor system often result in secondary joint and soft tissue changes. The major areas of dysfunction—the cervical spine, the shoulder complex, the thoracic outlet, and the craniomandibular complex—may be involved simultaneously, especially in chronic conditions. Muscle imbalances and postural abnormalities may predispose to or perpetuate a particular musculoskeletal lesion.

The myriad changes related to musculoskeletal lesions often confuse clinicians and hamper treatment. The discussion in this chapter of the interrelationships of structure and function in the upper quarter is designed to rectify this confusion. Elements of an upper quarter screening evaluation are reviewed as a systematic method of evaluating all structures that could contribute to or be the sole cause of the patient's chief complaint.

STRUCTURAL INTERRELATIONSHIPS IN THE UPPER QUARTER

The upper quarter includes the occiput, the cervical and upper thoracic spine, the shoulder girdle, the upper extremities, associated soft tissues, and related nerves and blood vessels. The relationships among these structures are such that changes in the position and function of one structure may influence the position and function of another. A cursory review of functional anatomy will help clarify these relationships.

Functional Anatomy

The shoulder girdle, which consists of the clavicle, humerus, and scapula, is largely suspended by muscles in order to allow mobility. The only direct connection of the shoulder girdle to the axial skeleton is through the clavicle. The clavicle articulates at its medial and more movable end with the sternum, and at its lateral end, through a slightly movable sliding joint, with the scapula.[1]

The clavicle is important as a brace that keeps the shoulder joint positioned far enough laterally to allow movements of the humerus. The movements of the scapula and humerus are dependent upon each other. Limited excursion of the free limb at the glenohumeral joint is under normal circumstances dependent on movements of the scapula. Forward, upward, and downward movements of the humerus are typically accompanied by a turning of the glenoid cavity in the corresponding direction. The mobility of the scapula in turn depends in part upon the mobility of its one bony brace, the clavicle.[1]

The occiput, mandible, cervical spine, and shoulder girdle are joined by numerous soft tissue and muscular attachments. The deep superficial fibers of the cervical fascia join the superior nuchal line of the occipital bone, the mastoid process, and

43

the base of the mandible above to the acromion, clavicle, and manubrium sterni below. Muscles partly responsible for scapular movement, namely, the upper fibers of the trapezius and the levator scapulae, connect the occiput and cervical spine to the superior lateral and superior medial borders of the scapula, respectively. Anteriorly, the sternocleidomastoid muscle attaches from the mastoid process of the cranium to the sternum and clavicle.[2]

The deep muscles in the cervical and thoracic spine can be divided anatomically and functionally into a longer and a shorter group.[3] The muscles of the longer group, which includes the iliocostalis, longissimus, and spinalis muscles, originate and insert across several segments. These muscles function as prime movers for spinal extension, as well as counteract, during upright posture, the forces of gravity in the spinal column.

The shorter group, which includes the multifidus, rotatores, interspinales, and intertransversarii, arise from and insert more closely to the intervertebral joints. These muscles function during spinal movement by stabilizing and steadying the bony segments.[3-4] According to Basmajian, during movement and standing, the shorter or intrinsic muscles in the back act as dynamic ligaments by adjusting small movements between individual vertebrae.[4] Movements of the vertebral column probably are performed by the larger muscles with better leverage and mechanical advantage.[4]

Deep suboccipital muscles connecting the axis, atlas, and occipital bones are the rectus capitis posterior minor and major, and the obliquus capitis superior and inferior.[3] These muscles have a high innervation ratio, with approximately three to five fibers innervated by one neuron. These muscles, therefore, rapidly alternate tension within milliseconds, allowing for subtle postural adjustments in the head and neck during standing.[3] Joint stiffness or degenerative joint disease that alters suboccipital joint mobility influences suboccipital muscle function. Muscle dysfunction commonly accompanies degenerative joint disease. Jowett and Fiddler demonstrated, in the presence of degenerative spinal disease, histochemical changes in the multifidus muscle resulting in an increase from the normal in slow twitch muscle fibers.[5] These authors concluded that the multifidus, in the presence of spinal

segmental instabilities and joint disease, functioned less as a dynamic spinal stabilizer than as a postural muscle.[5] One may speculate that degeneration in the craniovertebral joints may alter the phasic capabilities of the suboccipital muscles to a more postural mode. The result may be a loss in the quick muscle reaction necessary for normal upper quarter equilibrium and control.

An important area of soft tissue connections is that between the cranium, mandible, hyoid bone, cervical spine, and shoulder girdle. The cranium and the mandible are joined by the temporalis and masseter muscles. The mandible is joined to the hyoid bone by the suprahyoid muscles including the digastric, stylohyoid, mylohyoid, and geniohyoid. The infrahyoid muscles connect the hyoid bone to the shoulder girdle, and indirectly, through soft tissue connections, to the cervical spine.[2] These muscles include the sternohyoid, sternothyroid, thyrohyoid, and omohyoid. Specifically, the hyoid bone is joined to the scapula by the omohyoid muscle, and to the sternum and clavicle by the sternohyoid muscle.[2]

Brodie displayed, using a model substituting pieces of elastic for muscles, how tension in one group of muscles may result in tension in another group.[6] The mandible, during normal orthostatic standing posture, remains balanced to the cranium through tensile forces produced by normal function of the supra- and infrahyoid muscles.[7] The activity of these muscles is related to those of the neck and trunk, as well as to the direction of the gravitational forces acting on the system. Changes in head position in a relaxed subject will alter the rest position of the mandible. When the head is inclined backward, the mandible moves away from the maxilla into a retruded position.[8] The influence of the cervical spine on the position and function of the mandible is well documented.[9-12] Further discussion follows later in this chapter and in Chapter 4.

Specialized mechanoreceptors are numerous in the cervical facet joint capsules, as well as in the skin overlying these joints.[13] Essential afferent impulses for the static and dynamic regulation of body posture arise from the receptor systems in the connective tissue structures and muscles around these joints.[14] Muscle tone is regulated via these and other afferent impulses in upper quarter joint structures including capsules, synovial membrane, ligaments, and tendons. Activation of these specialized receptors and pain receptors during musculoskeletal dysfunction may alter motor activity in the neck and limb musculature. Subsequent change in muscle tone about the head, neck, and shoulder girdle may result in distortions in posture, movement patterns, and joint mobility.

Summary

The upper quarter is a complicated mechanical unit, interconnected by numerous soft tissue links. These links, or articulations, are functionally and reflexly interdependent on one another. The simple act of picking up a pencil involves movement at the head, neck, shoulder, elbow, hand, and fingers. Performance of a precision task requires adequate freedom of motion in the various joints (arthrokinematics), proper muscle control and length, and proper neurophysiologic responses. The relative alignment of body segments influences motor function. Alignment of body segments is a function of postural control. Normal posture is that state of muscular and skeletal balance which protects the supporting structures of the body against injury and deformity and occurs in the presence of normal joint and soft tissue mobility.[15] Maintaining good alignment in the upper quarter, therefore, is necessary for normal function. Good alignment allows for normal joint integrity and muscle balance and promotes normal arthrokinematic movements. Long-term changes in normal postural alignment resulting in muscle imbalances and compromising joint arthrokinematics may result in motor dysfunction and pathology.

NORMAL POSTURE

Posture is defined by Steindler in terms of the relationship of the parts of the body to the line and center of gravity.[16] The ideal normal erect posture is one in which the line of gravity drops in the midline between the following bilateral points: (1) the mastoid processes, (2) a point just in front of the shoulder joints, (3) the hip joints (or just behind), (4) a point just in front of the center of the knee joints, and (5) a point just in front of the ankle joints (Fig. 3-1).

The maintenance of normal posture is influenced by the forces of weightbearing (e.g., leg length difference, uneven terrain) and several physiologic processes including respiration, deglutition, sight, vestibular balance, and hearing.[17-19] Solow and Tallgren found, during cephalometric postural recording, that subjects looking straight into a mirror held their head and neck approximately 3 degrees higher than did subjects using their own feeling of natural head balance.[17] Vig et al. demonstrated that experimental nasal obstruction in humans resulted in progressive extension of the head, and that removal of the obstruction resulted in a return to the normal baseline head position.[18] Cleall et al. demonstrated that a consistent pattern of head extension and flexion during normal swallowing is altered in

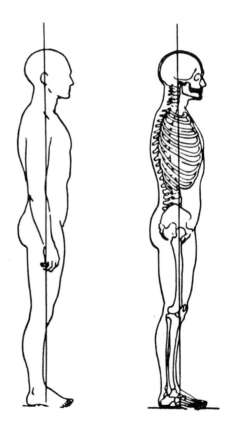

Fig. 3-1. Erect posture relative to the line of gravity. (From Basmajian,[4] with permission.)

subjects with a grade II malocclusion and tongue thrust.[19]

Normal posture, therefore, is dynamic, requiring constant neurophysiologic and accommodative adjustments. These normal adjustments maintain balance of equal weight in front of and behind the central gravity line. In more accurate mechanical terms, the moment of the forces anterior to the central gravity line must equal the moment of forces posterior to that line.[20] Therefore, if more weight of a body part is displaced forward of the central gravity line, there must be an equal shift of another body part backward. Thus, if the pelvis shifts anteriorly, the lumbar lordosis is increased and the thoracic kyphosis is also increased. The cervical spine shifts forward, resulting in a decreased midcervical lordosis. Backward bending occurs in the occipitoatlantal joint, so that one is in a position to look straight ahead.[20]

Body weight similarly must be equally divided between the two legs, and in the normal posture an equal weight is supported by each foot. Quite a considerable margin of lateral shift of the central gravity line is possible, however, because each leg can take the whole of the body weight at any time. A lateral shift, in the presence of uneven terrain or a leg length difference, of parts of the body away from the central gravity line results in compensatory shifts somewhere else. For example, if one side of the pelvis drops, a lateral curve is created in the lumbar spine to the opposite side and a compensating convexity to the same side higher up in the spine.[20] These accommodative shifts maintain the upper quarter within the central gravity line, allowing for normal balance and function.

Neurophysiology and Normal Posture

Vestibular sensation results in part from the orientation of the semicircular canals in the head. The head is held so that the horizontal semicircular canals are actually in a horizontal plant. Proprioceptive impulses from nerve endings in ligaments, joint capsules, tendons, and muscles also form a very large part of the input pattern and are most closely related to postural tone.[13-14] Muscle spindles of the proprioceptors are the specialized receptors involved in tendon reflexes. Postural or antigravity muscles are richly supplied with muscle spindles. When muscles are lengthened—for example, the posterior cervical muscles when the central gravity line in the cervical spine shifts forward—the parallel muscle spindles also are lengthened. This lengthening stimulates the muscle spindles to send afferent impulses to the homonymous alpha motor neurons, which carry excitatory impulses to the related muscles. Afferent impulses may also send, through interneurons, inhibitory impulses to alpha motor neurons of antagonistic muscles, causing a reflex inhibition of the anterior cervical or prevertebral muscles.[14,20]

Other afferent fibers from the muscle spindles carry impulse patterns about muscle length to the central nervous system, where these patterns are integrated in higher centers with patterns of changing tension and position that have originated in other proprioceptors.[14]

Summary

Normal posture during weightbearing consists of subtle accommodative movements to maintain the body segments along the central gravity line. Normal posture, therefore, depends on a variety of factors including normal joint arthrokinematics, muscle balance, and normal neurophysiologic responses. Muscular contractions, required to maintain normal balance, are controlled and coordinated by the nervous system. Changes in joint range of motion or muscle function may interfere with the normal accommodative responses necessary to maintain normal posture. Poor accommodative responses may result, in turn, in long-term postural deviations, pain, muscle imbalances, and pathologic conditions.

INTERDEPENDENCE OF FUNCTION AND STRUCTURE DURING NORMAL POSTURE

An excellent example of the interdependence of function and structure in the upper quarter is provided during shoulder elevation.

Shoulder elevation, or elevation of the humerus, is commonly described with reference to several different body planes: the coronal or frontal plane, the sagittal plane, and the plane of the scapula.[21] The plane of the scapula is approximately 30 to 45 degrees anterior to the frontal plane.[21] Movement of the humerus in this plane allows the muscles surrounding the glenohumeral joint to function in an optimal length-tension relationship.

Elevation of the humerus in the plane of the scapula depends on smooth, synchronous motion involving every component of the shoulder girdle complex. Normal scapulohumeral rhythm requires full range of motion at each joint and well-coordinated muscle balance. The ratio of humeral to scapular motion is a matter of controversy, but many authors agree that the humerus and scapula move in rhythm so that, for every 15 degrees of elevation of the arm, 10 degrees is provided by elevation at the glenohumeral joint and a corresponding 5 degrees by rotation of the scapula. Thus, full overhead elevation of the arm (180 degrees) requires 60 degrees of scapular rotation and 120 degrees of glenohumeral elevation.[22]

Movement of the scapula is accompanied by movement of the acromioclavicular (AC) and sternoclavicular (SC) joints. Movement of the SC joint is most evident from 0 to 90 degrees of elevation, and that of the AC joint primarily before 30 degrees and beyond 135 degrees. Half of the scapular rotation (30 degrees) is reached by clavicular elevation. The remaining 30 degrees occurs by rotation of the crank-shaped clavicle exerting pull on the coracoid process through the coracoclavicular ligaments.[22-23]

Elevation of the humerus results from a series of muscular force couples acting at the glenohumeral and scapulothoracic joints. A force couple is formed when two parallel forces of equal magnitude but opposite direction act on a structure, producing rotation.[24]

Rotation at the glenohumeral joint is produced by the upward pull of the deltoid and by the combined inward and downward pull of the rotator cuff muscles. Similarly, scapular rotation results from the upward pull of the upper fibers of the trapezius and the downward pull of the lower fibers of the trapezius. The serratus anterior also helps to rotate the scapula along the thoracic wall.[22]

Elevation of the upper extremities results in motion in the cervical and upper thoracic spine, as well

as in the atlantoaxial joint.[25-26] Unilateral elevation of an upper extremity in the plane of the scapula results in rotation of the midcervical spine to the ipsilateral side.[26] Pure rotation does not occur in the midcervical spine but is accompanied by side flexion to the ipsilateral side. Contralateral side flexion with ipsilateral rotation occurs at the occipitoatlantal joint and upper thoracic spine to enable the head to remain in the sagittal plane. This counterrotation only occurs in the axially extended or neutral position. In the presence of a forward head posture, these compensatory motions are lost and excessive forces are placed on the midcervical spine.[25]

Overhead work requiring bilateral elevation of the upper extremities results in extension of the head and thorax. This "habitual extension" induces flexion of the upper thoracic spine, extension of the midcervical spine, and extension of the craniovertebral region, thus restoring the weight of the skull in the line of gravity.[25] Specifically, during midcervical extension the superior articular facets slide posteriorly and inferiorly on the inferior facets, as well as tilt posteriorly, thus increasing the anterior interspace of the facet joint.[25] The posterior tilting of the related spinal segment is restrained by the intervertebral disc and its associated longitudinal ligaments and by the osseous impact of the posterior neural arches as well as the capsule of the facet joints.[25-26]

Additionally, the forces generated during limb, trunk, and neck movements are responsible for the repeated piston-like movement of the nerve complex in the intervertebral foramen of the cervical and upper thoracic spine. Overstretching of the nerve roots, according to Sunderland, is prevented by the nerves' elastic properties, as well as by their attachment by fibrous slips to gutters in the corresponding transverse processes.[27] Overstretching or friction on the nerve roots often occurs in the presence of postural deviations, such as the forward head posture.

POSTURAL DEVIATION AND DYSFUNCTION

A musculoskeletal lesion, according to Janda, produces a chain of reflexes that involve the whole motor system.[28] The reflex changes and functional impairment not only may result in clinical manifestations of pain arising from impaired function but also may influence the results of the whole process of motor re-education.

Changes in muscle function play an important role in the pathogenesis of many painful conditions of the motor system and are an integral part of postural defects. Certain muscles usually respond to dysfunction by tightness or shortening, whereas others react by inhibition, atrophy, and weakness. Muscles that have become tight tend to pull the body segments to which they attach, causing deviations in alignment. The antagonistic muscles may become weak and allow deviation of body parts due to their lack of support. These muscle responses follow typical patterns and have been described by Janda.[28]

The structures of connective tissue, bone, and muscle adapt to alterations in function. When stresses are applied to a bone, the trabeculae within that bone develop and align themselves to adapt to these lines of stress (Wolff's law).[29] Pressure within the physiologic limits of force exerted by the musculature stimulates or enhances osteogenesis.[30] Excessive pressure causes necrosis with delayed osteogenesis. Pressure exerted perpendicular to the axis of a long bone is more likely to cause resorption of bone, whereas pressure acting in the line of the bone axis is more likely to cause osteogenesis.[29] Therefore, postural deviations causing malalignment and asymmetrical stresses on bone and cartilage can result in reabsorption and degeneration.

Continued asymmetrical stresses on soft tissues can result in degeneration. Salter and Field found in animal models that continuous compression of opposing joint surfaces causes pressure necrosis of articular cartilage.[31] Tabary et al. experimentally shortened soleus muscles in guinea pigs and demonstrated resultant hypoextensibility and a decreased number of sarcomeres.[32] These authors suggested that reduction of total sarcomeres in a shortened muscle is an adaptation to faulty posture. The connective tissue response to immobility is well documented.[33-34] Changes in the joint capsule include loss of glycoaminoglycan and water, random deposition of newly synthesized collagen with abnormal cross-linking, and infiltration in joints of fibrofatty material. The results are increased joint stiffness and altered arthrokinematics. Similar changes may occur in joint capsules shortened as a result of long-term postural deviations.

Abnormal Posture and Shoulder Dysfunction

The forward head posture typifies a postural deviation reflective of muscle imbalance. The altered posture is characterized by protracted and laterally rotated scapulae, internal rotation of the glenohumeral joints, increased kyphosis of the upper thoracic spine, and increased anterior cervical inclination with flattening of the midcervical spine and craniocervical backward bending.[9]

The muscles and other soft tissues of the upper quarter change in response to the forward head posture. Excessive compression of the facet joints and posterior surfaces of the vertebral bodies occurs, as well as excessive lengthening with associated weakness of the anterior vertebral neck flexors and tightness of the neck extensors. Additional changes include shortening of the suboccipital and suprahyoid musculature and lengthening of the infrahyoid muscles with elevation of the hyoid bone. Increased tension in the suprahyoid muscles pulls the mandible posteriorly and inferiorly, increasing the distance between the maxilla and the mandible. The temporalis, masseter, and medial pterygoid muscles must contract against the shortened antagonistic muscles to close the jaw. Excessive tension in the muscles of mastication can result in myofascial strain and painful trigger points.[35] Chapter 4 further discusses stomatognathic problems.

Elevation of the hyoid increases tension on the omohyoid muscle and its attachment to the upper portion of the scapula. With the head moving anteriorly and the posterior aspect of the occiput moving posteriorly and inferiorly, there is shortening of the upper trapezius muscle and of the levator scapulae. Shortening of these muscles results in scapular elevation.[6]

The increased thoracic kyphosis tends to abduct or protract the scapulae and lengthen the rhomboid and lower trapezius muscles, while shortening the serratus anterior, latissimus dorsi, subscapularis, and teres major muscles. In addition, the increased scapular abduction shortens the pectoralis major and minor muscles, which, by their attachment to the coracoid process of the scapula, tend to pull the scapula over the head of the humerus. The humerus internally rotates, shortening the glenohumeral ligaments and the anterior shoulder capsule.[36]

Muscle tone changes in response to afferent impulses from the joint capsule, resulting in inhibition or facilitation of selected muscles. Numerous muscle imbalances result, because a tight muscle inhibits its antagonist.[28] Weakness of the lower trapezius muscle may result from shortening of the upper trapezius, levator scapulae, and serratus anterior muscles, whereas inhibition of the rhomboid muscles may occur in response to the shortening of the teres major muscle. Increased glenohumeral internal rotation will shorten the glenohumeral medial rotators, with lengthening and inhibition of the lateral rotators. These changes in normal muscle length may result in alteration in the normal scapulohumeral rhythm.

Weakness of the supraspinatus, infraspinatus, and teres minor alters the force couple at the glenohumeral joint during elevation of the humerus. The function of these muscles in maintaining the humeral head at the glenoid fossa and resisting the upward pull of the deltoid is lost. Repetitive upward pull of the deltoid during glenohumeral elevation results in abutment of the humeral head and associated soft tissues against an unyielding coracoacromial ligament. Impingement of the rotator cuff tendons may result in inflammation with subsequent pain and loss of function.[37]

Diminished scapular rotation during elevation of the humerus results from muscle imbalances at the scapulohumeral articulation. Increased strain is placed on the rotator cuff muscles to elevate the arm overhead. The result may be inflammation of the rotator cuff tendons. Overactivity of the rotator cuff muscles to compensate for reduced scapular rotation results in painful trigger points.[38]

Abnormal Posture and the Cervical Spine

Forward head posture produces compensatory motions in the cervical and upper thoracic spine, as well as in the atlantoaxial joint. Unilateral elevation of an upper extremity, as mentioned previously, results in rotation with ipsilateral sidebending in the midcervical spine.[25] Compensatory contralateral side flexion with ipsilateral rotation occurs in the upper thoracic spine and in the occipitoatlantal joint to maintain the head and neck in the central gravity line. However, these compensatory motions occur only in the axially extended or neutral position. The forward head posture results in increased flexion in the upper thoracic spine and extension in the upper cervical spine. Compensatory motions, therefore, are lost, and excessive forces are placed on the midcervical spine during unilateral elevation of the upper extremity. Traumatic changes in the intervertebral disk and neural arches may result in transverse intradiskal tears, most commonly seen at the C5–C6 and C6–C7 segments. Degeneration of the intervertebral disk leads to reabsorption and approximation of the related segments.[25,30] Osteophytic spurs may develop in the uncovertebral joints as well as the posterior facet joints. The result during repetitive extension and rotation of the degenerated midcervical spine is friction of the nerve roots by osseofibrous irregularities in the intervertebral foramen or traction on nerve roots fixed in the gutters of the related transverse processes.[25,27]

Pressure or traction on a nerve can result in mechanical irritation of that nerve, producing pain and dysfunction.[27] The initial response of a nerve to mechanical irritation, according to Sunderland, is an increase in the intrafunicular pressure in the nerve, obstructing venous drainage and slowing capillary drainage.[27] Capillary circulation slows and intrafunicular pressure rises. The incarcerated nerve fibers are compressed, and their nutrition is impaired by hypoxia to the point that they become hyperexcitable and begin to discharge spontaneously.[27] Spontaneous firing of selective large myelinated fibers occurs, resulting in hyperesthesia in the related dermatome. A steady increase in the amount of intrafunicular pressure can result in spontaneous firing of gamma efferents leading to hypertonicity of the segmentally related muscles.

Chronic anoxia damages the capillary endothelium with leakage of protein through the capillary walls, fibroplasia, and intraneural scarring.[27] In patients with a long history of recurrent sciatica, Lindahl and Rexed observed histologic changes at the L5 and S1 nerve roots including hyperplasia of the perineurium with infiltration of lymphocytes and degeneration of nerve fibers.[39] Resultant demyelination of selected nerve fibers may increase the sensitivity of segmentally related structures. According to Gunn, deep muscle tenderness may be secondary to denervation sensitivity of nociceptors at the neurovascular hilus.[40] Long-term denervation can result in decreased total collagen in the segmentally related soft tissues and muscles.[40] Muscle atrophy occurs, with progressive destruction of the fiber's contractile element resulting in decreased fiber diameter and decreased speed of muscle contraction. Changes in collagen content and degenerated muscle fibers can increase the susceptibility of the related tissues to micro- or macrotears, resulting in inflammation and dysfunction. Lee has suggested denervation of the C6 nerve root in the cervical spine as a possible extrinsic cause of lateral epicondylitis.[25] Examination of a musculoskeletal lesion should therefore include the local contractile and noncontractile tissues, as well as the integrity of the related spinal and/or peripheral nerve.

Abnormal Posture and Entrapment Neuropathies

Thoracic Outlet

Compression of the nerves of the brachial plexus and of the great vessels in the region of the thoracic outlet may occur in a variety of ways, some due in part to poor posture.

The clavicle holds the shoulder up, out, and back, thus producing a short, broad outlet canal. The angle between the anterior and middle scaleni muscles is broad enough to allow passage of the nerve roots of the brachial plexus. The loss of muscle tone and drooping shoulders seen in forward head posture can result in depression of the anterior chest wall. The depression of the sternum pulls the anterior thoracic cage downward. This, in turn, pulls the shoulder girdle down, forward, and closer to the chest wall. As a result, the angle between the scaleni muscles is decreased, and the outer end of the clavicle and the shoulder girdle are pulled closer to the lateral chest wall as well as down and forward. These changes decrease the width and increase the length of the outlet canal, which makes the nerve trunks of the brachial plexus and the subclavian artery more vulnerable to compression or kinking as they pass through the scaleni triangle (Fig. 3-2).[41] Chapter 5 further discusses thoracic outlet problems.

Dorsal Scapular Nerve

The dorsal scapular nerve arises from the upper trunk of the brachial plexus and pierces the body of the scalene medius muscle. The scaleni muscles are prime movers of the cervical spine. When the myoligamentous system, that is, the stabilization mechanism for the vertebral function, is inadequate, the prime movers go into compensatory hyperactivity.

Myoligamentous laxity may result from increased tension in the anterior cervical spine in a forward head posture. Hyperactivity and hypertrophy of the scalene muscle may result in entrapment of the dorsal scapular nerve. When the dorsal scapular nerve is compressed at the entrapment point in the scalene medius muscle, the slack necessary to compensate for head and arm motion is prevented.[36] A tense nerve moving against taut muscles can set up the initial mechanical irritation in the nerve.[27] The resultant nerve ischemia, as outlined previously, can result in scapular pain, as well as diffuse pain that radiates down the lateral surface of the arm and forearm.[27,33,39] Soft tissue changes in response to denervation neuropathy may result along the segmental distribution of the nerve.[40]

Suprascapular Nerve

The suprascapular nerve is derived from the upper trunk of the brachial plexus which is formed from the roots of C5 and C6. The nerve passes through the suprascapular notch at the upper border of the scapula. The notch is roofed over by the transverse scapular ligament. This nerve supplies the supraspinatus muscle, the glenohumeral and acromioclavicular joints, and the infraspinatus muscle.

The forward head posture, resulting in increased scapular abduction and lateral rotation, may cause traction in the brachial plexus at the origin of the suprascapular nerve (Fig. 3-3).[36,38] The abducted position increases the total distance from the origin of the nerve to the suprascapular notch, thus placing tension on the suprascapular nerve.

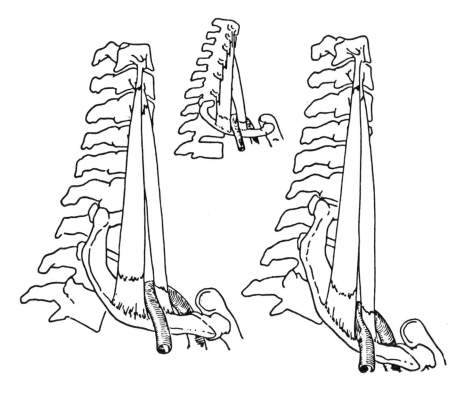

Fig. 3-2. The descent of the sternum with maturation and aging. **(A)** Position at birth; **(B)** position in an adult man; **(C)** position in an adult woman. (From Overton,[41] with permission.)

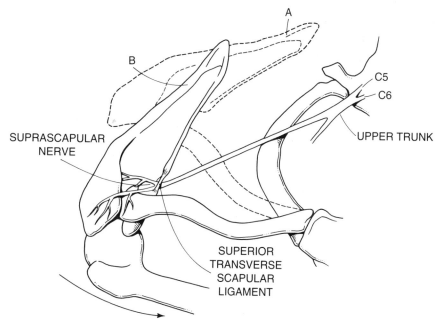

Fig. 3-3. The effect of shoulder abduction on the course of suprascapular nerve. **(A)** Position of scapula when arm is in the anatomic position; **(B)** position of scapula when scapula is abducted across the thoracic wall. (From Thompson and Kopell,[51] with permission.)

SUPRASCAPULAR NERVE

SUPERIOR TRANSVERSE SCAPULAR LIGAMENT

C5

C6

UPPER TRUNK

Changes in normal scapulohumeral rhythm in such conditions as frozen shoulder may result in suprascapular nerve neuropathy. Limitation of glenohumeral motion in frozen shoulder forces a greater range of scapular motion for a desired degree of shoulder motion. This abnormal excursion of the scapula may induce a neuropathy at the entrapment point of the suprascapular nerve. Pain may be felt in the lateral and posterior aspects of the shoulder with secondary radiation down the radial nerve axis to the region of the common extensor group.[36]

Summary

Dysfunction in the upper quarter may result in, and from, postural deviations. The interdependence of the motor system suggests that a functional disturbance produces a chain of reflexes that may involve the whole upper quarter. Therefore, although upper quarter dysfunctions appear locally, the subsequent success of treatment may necessitate evaluation of the motor system as a whole.

UPPER QUARTER EVALUATION

Elements of an upper quarter evaluation offer a systematic method of evaluating all structures that could contribute to or be the sole cause of the patient's chief complaint. A history should precede the evaluation. Proper interpretation of each test designed to differentiate tissues and structures is based on our knowledge of anatomy, mechanics, and typical etiologic and pathologic processes, as well as our clinical processes.

History

History taking procedures for individual joints and joint complexes have been described elsewhere.[42-44] Routine questions are asked to determine the onset of the problem, the area and nature of the pain, previous treatment, functional impairment, and associated health problems.

Common musculoskeletal disorders usually manifest with pain.[42] Because the various lesions that produce pain and dysfunction about the shoulder and upper extremities may have their origin in the cervical spine, the thoracic outlet, the craniomandibular area, or the arm itself, the clinician must have knowledge of the patterns of pain referral.

Embryology

Many structures are innervated by nerve fibers from more than one spinal segment. Limb buds in the developing embryo comprise a mass of undifferentiated mesenchymal cells. The anterior primary divisions of the spinal nerves invade the developing limb buds to innervate the early muscle masses. Because of the intertwining of segmental nerves throughout the regional plexus, and because the early muscle masses tend to divide or fuse with one another, a muscle typically receives innervation from more than one segment, and a segmental nerve tends to innervate more than one muscle.[2]

Overlapping of myotomes, dermatomes, and sclerotomes results from a change in orientation of the developing limb buds from a position in the frontal plane at approximately 90 degrees abduction, with the palms facing forward, to the fetal position.[2] The growth of the arm bud draws the lower cervical and uppermost thoracic segments out into itself. The scapula and surrounding muscles are derived from the middle and lower cervical segments, whereas the overlying skin and ribs are formed from the thoracic segments. Therefore, pain felt in the upper posterior part of the thorax into the shoulder and upper limb has a cervical or scapular origin, and pain felt in the upper posterior thorax radiating into the upper chest has an upper thoracic origin.[44]

Patterns of Pain Referral

Several authors have investigated the patterns of pain referral.[38,45-48] Robinson found that similar patterns of referred pain in the upper extremity area were reproduced by stimulating different structures in the cervical spine.[45] Robinson exposed the anterior portions of the cervical vertebrae and the adjacent muscles of patients under local anesthesia. The same referred pain was reproduced by plucking with a needle the anulus fibrosus of more than one intervertebral disk. Similarly, identical pain was reproduced by plucking the edge of the longus colli muscle. Feinstein et al. studied patterns of deep somatic pain referral after paravertebral injections of 6 percent saline solution from the occiput to the sacrum.[46] Pain distributions were found to approximate a segmental plan, although the pain patterns overlapped considerably and differed in location from the conventional dermatomes.

Studies by Kellgren identified specific reproducible patterns of pain activated when selective connective tissues and muscle structures were irritated (Figs. 3-4 and 3-5).[47] Inman and Saunders demonstrated that pain resulting from the stimulation of joints and other structures deep to the skin had no superficial component.[48] These authors used needles with or without hypertonic saline to produce

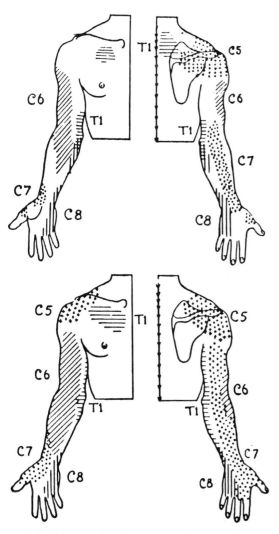

Fig. 3-4. Mappings of referred pain from local irritation of the rhomboids (crosses), the flexor carpiradialis (oblique hatching), the abductor pollicis longus (stippling), the third dorsal interosseus (vertical hatching), and the first intercostal space (horizontal hatching). (From Kellgren,[47] with permission.)

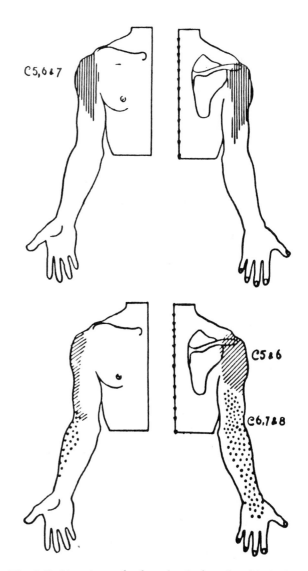

Fig. 3-5. Mappings of referred pain from local irritation of the serratus anterior (vertical hatching) and the latissimus dorsi (stippling). (From Kellgren,[47] with permission.)

pains that commonly arise from the deeper structures. Such a pain, Inman and Saunders concluded, unlike that of a cut in the skin, cannot be localized with any precision. The distance of radiation, they found, varied proportionately with the intensity of the stimulus. Activation of trigger points in muscles about the shoulder and neck were shown by Travell and Simons to consistently refer pain into the hand, wrist, and elbow, as well as produce pain at the site of the lesion.[38]

To summarize, pain arising from the muscles, deep ligaments, and joints of the cervical spine and shoulder girdle area will tend to be referred segmentally. Because of the similarity of the type and the distribution of pain referred to the upper extremities from various structures, the clinician should consider every case with careful attention to all potential pain-producing structures and tissues.

Upper Quarter Screening Examination

The following screening examination was developed by Personius at the Medical College of Virginia (Fig. 3-6). The goal is to scan quickly the entire upper quarter to rule out problems and note areas that need more specific testing. The entire examination should require no more than 5 minutes.

The first three steps are self-explanatory. The fourth step requires a brief explanation on how the arm is held and used. For example, a patient with a painful stiff shoulder will tend to hold the arm adducted and internally rotated across the body. Elevation at the glenohumeral joint may be compensated by increased elevation at the scapula.

Postural evaluation in step five requires observations for postural deviation such as a forward head posture. From behind, the therapist should observe the positions of the scapulae for protraction, retraction, elevation, or winging of the medial border, and the relative positions of the cervical spine on the thorax and the cranium on the cervical spine. Deviations from the midsagittal spine (scoliosis, rotation, or tilting of the head and neck) should be recorded.

Laterally, the alignment of the upper quarter segments should be compared to the hypothetical plumb mentioned previously. Increased cervical in-

clination and backward bending of the cranium on the cervical spine or abnormal axial extension with reversal of the normal cervical lordosis indicates postural deviations and potential dysfunction. Anteriorly, the position of the cervical spine and cranium should again be noted relative to the midsagittal plane. Positional changes at the shoulder (internal or external rotation, elevation, or depression) together or relative to each other are recorded.

In the next step, the function of the cervical spine is examined with respect to the mechanics (degree and quality of motion) and pain (location and severity). After each active motion, overpressure is applied while the pain is located and its severity assessed. Janda has suggested that rotation should be tested in ventro- and dorsiflexion, as well as in the vertical position.[49] If the cervical spine is maximally flexed, the segments from C2 and C3 are blocked, and therefore the movement restriction is a sign of dysfunction of the upper cervical segments. Conversely, during maximum dorsiflexion the upper segments are blocked. The limitation of rotation is then a symptom of dysfunction of the segments distal to C2 and C3.[49] In addition, axial compression (Fig. 3-7) and axial distraction (Fig. 3-8) are applied manually by the clinician to provoke or change the patient's symptoms. The cervical spine tests are performed to identify or exclude pathology originating in the cervical region.

The neurologic, sensory, and vascular examinations have been described elsewhere.[20-21] The vascular examination includes tests (Adson's, costoclavicular, hyperabduction) to rule out vascular or neural entrapment in the areas of the thoracic inlet.[50]

Each peripheral joint is tested for mechanics (M) and pain during overpressure (OP). The locking position (Fig. 3-9) and the quadrant position (Fig. 3-10) are performed on the shoulder to test for impingement and anterior capsule, respectively. Reproduction of the patient's symptoms is recorded.

Palpation should be added to the screening evaluation to differentiate and recognize changes in skin, subcutaneous tissue, ligaments, and muscles.[49] Patterns of pain referral should be recorded. Special attention should be paid to the muscles. Spasm, tenderness, hyperirritability, tightness, or hypotonia should be noted. A characteristic and specific chain

Patient _____

Date _____

Observation and Inspection
1. Body build: endo _____ , ecto _____ , meso _____ ; ht _____ ; wt _____
   Unusual features _____
2. Assistive devices _____
3. Skin _____
4. Upper Quarter Functions
   Position _____
   Use _____
5. Posture
   Lateral _____
   Posterior _____
   Anterior _____

Function Tests
1. Cx ROM   active   OP
   FB   ___ M ___ : ___ P _____ ___ P _____
   BB   ___ M ___ : ___ P _____ ___ P _____
   LRot   ___ M ___ : ___ P _____ ___ P _____
   RRot   ___ M ___ : ___ P _____ ___ P _____
   LSB   ___ M ___ : ___ P _____ ___ P _____
   RSB   ___ M ___ : ___ P _____ ___ P _____
   Comp   ___ M ___   ___ P _____
   Trac   ___ M ___   ___ P _____
2. Neuro
   Motor
         C1   ___
         C2,3   ___
         C3,4   ___
         C5   R ___   - L ___
         C6   ___   -   ___
         C7   ___   -   ___
         C8   ___   -   ___
         T1   ___   -   ___
   Sensory
         Dizziness: yes   no
         Tinnitus: yes   no
         Light Touch & Pinprick   R   LT   L   R   PP   L
         C4   ___ - ___   ___ - ___
         C5   ___ - ___   ___ - ___
         C6   ___ - ___   ___ - ___
         C7   ___ - ___   ___ - ___
         C8   ___ - ___   ___ - ___
         T1   ___ - ___   ___ - ___
   Reflex   R   -   L
         C5,6   ___   -   ___
         C7   ___   -   ___
3. Vascular
   Radial Pulse
   Thoracic Outlet
4. Peripheral Joints
   Shoulder
      UE Elevation   ___ M ___ : ___ P _____   (OP) _____
      Locking Position   ___ M ___ : ___ P _____
      Quadrant Position ___ M ___ : ___ P _____
   Elbow   (OP)
      Flex RL   ___ M ___ : ___ P _____ ___ P _____
      Ext   ___ M ___ : ___ P _____ ___ P _____
   Forearm
      Sup   ___ M ___ : ___ P _____ ___ P _____
      Pro   ___ M ___ : ___ P _____ ___ P _____
   Wrist
      Flex   ___ M ___ : ___ P _____ ___ P _____
      Ext   ___ M ___ : ___ P _____ ___ P _____
      RD   ___ M ___ : ___ P _____ ___ P _____
      UD   ___ M ___ : ___ P _____ ___ P _____

Fig. 3-6. Upper quarter screening examination. (Courtesy of Walter J. Personius, Department of Physical Therapy, Medical College of Virginia. From Donatelli,[43] with permission.)

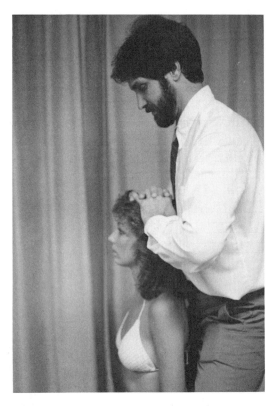

Fig. 3-7. Axial compression as part of the screening evaluation.

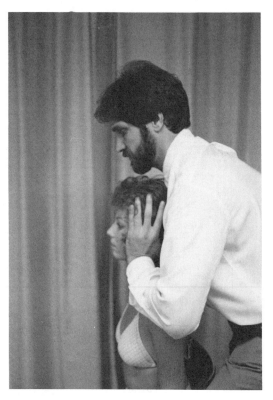

Fig. 3-8. Axial distraction as part of the screening evaluation.

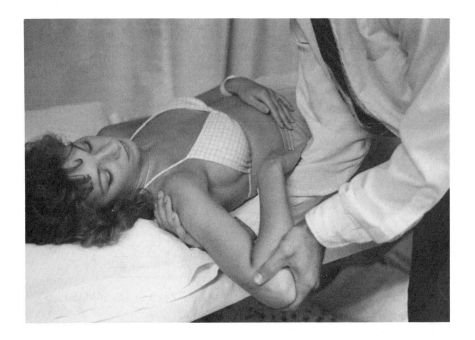

Fig. 3-9. Locking maneuver: internal rotation and abduction of the shoulder.

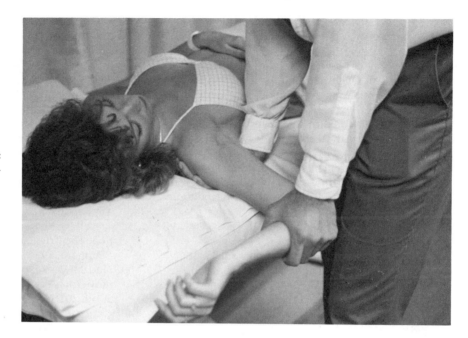

Fig. 3-10. Quadrant position: external rotation and abduction of the shoulder.

of muscle changes and imbalances should be assessed. A proposed sequence of palpation in the head and neck is as follows: trapezius and levator scapulae, followed by the scaleni, sternocleidomastoid and suprahyoid muscles, followed in turn by the lateral and medial pterygoid, masseter, and temporalis muscles.[49]

In conclusion, the screening examination affords the clinician a quick, precise scan of upper quarter structure and function. A specific test that provokes the patient's symptoms alerts the clinician to the potential site of the musculoskeletal lesion, to be followed by a thorough evaluation of that area.

REFERENCES

1. Hollinshead WH: The Back and Limbs. Anatomy for Surgeons. Vol. 3. Harper & Row, New York, 1969
2. Warwick R, Williams P (eds): Gray's Anatomy. 35th British Ed. WB Saunders, Philadelphia, 1973
3. Grieve GP: Common Vertebral Joint Problems. Churchill Livingstone, New York, 1981
4. Basmajian JU: Muscles Alive. 4th Ed. Williams & Wilkins, Baltimore, 1979
5. Jowett RL, Fiddler MW: Histochemical changes in the multifidus in mechanical derangements of the spine. Orthop Clin N Am 6:145, 1975
6. Brodie AG: Anatomy and physiology of head and neck musculature. Am J Orthod 36:831, 1950
7. Rocabado M: Biomechanical relationship of the cranial, cervical and hyoid regions. J Craniomandib Pract 11:3, 1983
8. Mohl NO: Head posture and its role in occlusion. NY State Dent J 42:17, 1976
9. Ayub E, Glasheen-Wray M, Kraus S: Head posture: a study of the effects on the rest position of the mandible. J Orthop Sports Phys Ther 5:179, 1984
10. Gresham H, Smithells PA: Cervical and mandibular posture. Dent Record 74:261, 1954
11. Darling PW, Kraus S, Glasheen-Wray MB: Relationship of head posture and the rest position of the mandible. J Prosthet Dent 16:848, 1966
12. Goldstein DF, Kraus SL, Williams WB, Glasheen-Wray MB: Influence of the cervical posture on mandibular movement. J Prosthet Dent 52:3, 1984
13. Wyke B: Neurology of the cervical spinal joints. Physiotherapy 85:3, 1979
14. Guyton AC: Organ Physiology: Structure and Function of the Nervous System. 2nd Ed. WB Saunders, Philadelphia, 1976
15. Kendall HO, Kendall FP, Boynton D: Posture and Pain. Robert E Krieger, Huntington NY, 1977
16. Steindler A: Kinesiology of the Human Body: Under Normal and Pathological Conditions. 5th Ed. Charles C Thomas, Springfield, IL, 1955

17. Solow B, Tallgren A: Natural head position in standing subjects. Acta Odontol Scand 29:591, 1971

18. Vig PS, Showfety KJ, Phillips C: Experimental manipulation of head posture. Am J Orthod 77:3, 1980

19. Cleall JR, Alexander WJ, McIntyre HM: Head posture and its relationship to deglutition. Angle Orthod 36:335, 1966

20. Bailey HW: Theoretical significance of postural imbalance, especially the "short leg." JAOA 77:452, 1978

21. Johnston TB: Movements of the shoulder joint—plea for use of "plane of the scapula" as plane of reference for movements occurring at the humeroscapula joint. Br J Surg 25:252, 1937

22. Calliet R: Shoulder Pain. 2nd Ed. FH Davis, Philadelphia, 1981

23. Poppen N, Walker P: Normal and abnormal motion of the shoulder. J Bone Joint Surg 58A:195, 1976

24. Frankel VH, Nordin M: Basic Biomechanics of the Skeletal System. Lea & Febiger, Philadelphia, 1980

25. Lee D: Tennis elbow. J Orthop Sports Phys Ther 8:3, 1986

26. Kapandji IA: The Physiology of Joints. 2nd Ed. Vol 3. Churchill Livingstone, London, 1974

27. Sunderland S: Traumatized nerves, roots and ganglia: Musculoskeletal factors and neuropathologic consequences. p. 137. In Korr IM (ed): The Neurobiologic Mechanisms in Manipulative Therapy. Plenum, New York, 1978

28. Janda V: Muscles, central nervous motor regulation and back problems. p. 29. In Korr IM (ed): The Neurobiologic Mechanisms in Manipulative Therapy. Plenum, New York, 1978

29. Turek SL: Orthopaedic Principles and Their Application. 3rd Ed. p. 48. JB Lippincott, Philadelphia, 1977

30. Eggers GWN, Shindler TO, Pomerat CM: Osteogenesis: Influence of the contact-compression factor on osteogenesis in surgical fractures. J Bone Joint Surg 31:693, 1949

31. Salter RB, Field P: The effects of continuous compression on living articular cartilage: an experimental investigation. J Bone Joint Surg 42A:31, 1960

32. Tabary JC, Tardieu C, Tardieu G, Tabary C: Experimental rapid sarcomere loss with concomitant hypoextensibility. Muscle Nerve 4:198, 1981

33. Akeson WH, Amiel D, Mechanis GL, Woo SLY, Harwood FL, Hamer ML: Collagen cross-linking alterations in joint contractures: changes in the reducible cross-links in periarticular connective tissue collagen after nine weeks of immobilization. Connect Tiss Res 5:15, 1977

34. Woo S, Matthews JU, Akeson WH, Amiel D, Convery R: Connective tissue response to immobility: correlative study of biomechanical and biochemical measurements of normal and immobilized rabbit knees. Arthritis Rheum 18:3, 1975

35. Manns A, Miralles R, Santander H: Influence of the vertical dimension in the treatment of myofascial pain dysfunction syndrome. J Prosthet Dent 50(5):700, 1983

36. Kopell HP, Thompson WAL: Peripheral Entrapment Neuropathies. 2nd Ed. Robert E Krieger, New York, 1976

37. Penny JN, Welsh MB: Shoulder impingement syndromes in athletes and their surgical management. Am J Sports Med 9:11, 1981

38. Travell JG, Simons DG: Myofascial Pain and Dysfunction. The Trigger Point Manual. Williams & Wilkins, Baltimore, 1984

39. Lindahl O, Rexed B: Histologic changes in spinal nerve roots of operated cases of sciatica. Acta Orthop Scand 20:215, 1951

40. Gunn CC: Prespondylosis and some pain syndromes following denervation supersensitivity. Spine 5:2, 1980

41. Overton LM: The causes of pain in the upper extremities: a differential diagnosis study. Clin Orthop Rel Res 51:27, 1967

42. Kessler RM, Hertling D: Management of Common Musculoskeletal Disorders. Harper & Row, Philadelphia, 1983

43. Moran CA, Saunders SA: Evaluation of the shoulder: a sequential approach. p. 17. In Donatelli R (ed): Physical Therapy of the Shoulder. Churchill Livingstone, New York, 1987

44. Cyriax J: Textbook of Orthopaedic Medicine. 7th Ed. Vol 1. Bailliere Tindall, London, 1979

45. Robinson RA: Brachalgia: a panel discussion. Proceedings of the International Congress on Orthopaedics and Trauma, Paris, France, 1966

46. Feinsten B, Langton JNK, Jameson RM, Shiller F: Experiments of pain referred from deep somatic tissues. J Bone Joint Surg 36A:5, 1954

47. Kellgren J: Observations of referred pain arising from muscle. Clin Sci 3:175, 1938

48. Inman VT, Saunders JB: Referred pain from skeletal structures. J Nerv Ment Dis 99:660, 1944

49. Janda V: Some aspects of extracranial causes of facial pain. J Prosthet Dent 56:4, October, 1986

50. Ridell DH: Thoracic outlet syndrome: thoracic and vascular aspects. Clin Orthop Rel Res 51:53, 1967

51. Thompson WAL, Kopell HP: N Engl J Med 260:1261, 1959

4

Influences of the Cervical Spine on the Stomatognathic System

STEVEN L. KRAUS

Physical therapists see patients presenting with a variety of upper quarter symptoms. Treatment for such symptoms may be helped by addressing the dysfunction of the cervical and thoracic spine, the shoulder girdle, and/or the upper extremity. During treatment of upper quarter dysfunction, the physical therapist should ask the patient if the treatments offered are affecting his symptoms. The patient's response will depend on the area and degree of dysfunction, the age and overall physical condition of the patient, and the skills of the therapist rendering the treatments.

During the initial evaluation or during treatment, the physical therapist may question the reliability of a patient who complains of certain symptoms that may not be thought of as associated with upper quarter dysfunction. The patient may even suggest that these symptoms are being affected either for better or for worse as the upper quarter dysfunction is treated. Such unrelated symptoms cannot always be explained on the basis of referred pains or pathologic involvement. For the therapist trying to determine whether such unrelated symptoms are clinically possible, an understanding of how the cervical spine influences the stomatognathic system may provide some answers.

The suggestion that a specific dysfunction (e.g., of the cervical spine) can cause or contribute to a dysfunction that results in specific symptoms in an adjacent region (stomatognathic) must be made cautiously. The actual experience of symptoms by an individual and their expression involve a very complicated and detailed series of events that is yet to be fully understood. These events involve a variety of excitatory and inhibitory reflexes occurring at the spinal cord, the brain stem, the thalamus, and the cortex of the central nervous system. With such a complex series of events occurring, the clinician seldom observes a specific dysfunction contributing to a specific symptom. A precise correlation between signs of dysfunction and symptoms is the exception rather than the rule. Dysfunction, in fact, can exist in the absence of any subjective complaints.

The treatment goals that physical therapists establish for patients vary depending on their clinical experience and expertise. A common treatment goal is to achieve normal function and position for the area being treated. But what are the normal values for the upper quarter region? For example: what is normal head-neck-shoulder girdle posture? What is normal muscle tone? What is normal active-passive mobility of the cervical spine? The word *normal* implies conformity with the established norm or standard for its kind. If one were to apply this definition to an asymptomatic population, one would probably find that what is "normal" or average is actually varying degrees of dysfunction. By definition, then, when we attempt to restore normal function we may actually be treating toward an ideal condition that does not commonly exist.

These elaborations on normalcy may seem to be a lot of rhetoric. The point, however, is that goals established for patients should be what is functional and not what is normal. It is not clinically possible to resolve all dysfunction. Achieving as much mobility as is consistent with stability, and educating the patient on appropriate exercise and means of prevention, would be reasonable goals for most patients. These goals will help the patient to help himself to maintain his individual physiologic adaptive range.

The treatment techniques used and their sequence depend largely on the experienced judgment and level of expertise of the physical therapist. Caution should be exercised before asserting that one treatment approach is better than another for a particular dysfunction or symptom. The effectiveness of physical therapy treatments in a clinical environment has seldom been evaluated through rigid experimentation. Clinically controlled studies also need to consider the measurement of pain, which remains elusive. Rather, the application of a particular technique or treatment approach is largely based on clinical opinions. Sicher warned us many years ago that "clinical success does not prove anything but the acceptability of the method employed; any attempt to prove an anatomical concept by clinical success is merely a rationalization and certainly is not to be regarded as truly scientific evidence."[1] The approach to treatment for functional involvement should be reversible, unless of course pain, dysfunction, and neurologic signs suggest otherwise. Treatment should not be given if the clinician is not willing to treat the complications that may result.

The objective of this chapter is to heighten the reader's awareness of the influence the upper quarter has on the stomatognathic system. The clinical symptoms associated with the dysfunction of the stomatognathic system are discussed. Cervical spine dysfunction indicates altered mobility and position of the cervical spine. Altered positioning of the cervical spine often is recognized by the acquired forward head posture (FHP). However, patients can have good position of their cervical spine but lack proper mobility. Conversely, patients can have what is suspected to be improper positioning of the head and neck due to congenital and/or genetic factors but have good mobility. The emphasis in treatment of the cervical spine should be on mobility and not just position.

I do not want to mislead the reader into believing that the following interrelationships have been documented. Documentation does confirm that a neurophysiologic and anatomic relationship exists between the cervical spine and portions of the stomatognathic system. References on the "normal" functional relationships are provided when possible. Any conclusions drawn about dysfunctional relationships and associated symptoms and any mention of treatments are entirely a matter of clinical opinion.

THE STOMATOGNATHIC SYSTEM

The word *stomatognathic* is one that is not often used and probably not understood by physical therapists. *Stoma* is the Greek word for "mouth", and *stomato* denotes relationship to the mouth.[2] *Gnathos*[2] likewise means "jaw," and *gnathology*[3] refers to the study of relationships of the temporomandibular joint, the occlusion (teeth), and the neuromusculature. The phrase *stomatognathic system* refers to the muscles of mastication (the mandibular and cervical musculature), the tongue, the temporomandibular joint (TMJ), the occlusion, and all of the associated vessels, ligaments, and soft tissues.

The stomatognathic system functions continuously during breathing and in the maintenance of an upright postural position of the mandible and tongue. The daily activity of this system is intermittently increased during such activities as chewing, talking, yawning, coughing, and licking the lips.

The following areas of the stomatognathic system are suggested to be directly influenced by cervical spine dysfunction:

The upright postural position of the mandible
The upright postural position of the tongue
Swallowing
Occlusion (In reference to the mandibular teeth and their initial contact with the maxillary teeth during jaw closure.)

The Upright Postural Position of the Mandible

The rest or upright postural position of the mandible (UPPM) is maintained nearly 23 hours a day. When the mandible is in this position, the teeth are held slightly apart. The vertical space (freeway space) between the tips of the mandibular anterior teeth and the maxillary anterior teeth is on the average about 3 mm. The anteroposterior relationship of the UPPM to the maxilla is with the mandibular teeth positioned below the point of occlusion (maximum intercuspation) of the maxillary teeth (Fig. 4-1).

The muscles and soft tissues attaching to the mandible are in a state of equilibrium in the UPPM.[4] The least amount of muscle and soft tissue effort is then needed to elevate the mandible from the UPPM to maximum intercuspation. Once movement of the mandible has occurred such as to make tooth-to-tooth contact, or following any other functional movements of the mandible, the mandible will return to the UPPM. Essentially all movement begins and ends in the UPPM.[5] Individuals who talk or eat excessively or have acquired certain habits such as chewing gum or biting their fingernails will spend less time with the mandible in the UPPM. Individuals who brux or clench their teeth will spend even less time with the mandible in this position. Less time spent in the UPPM means more muscle and soft tissue activity is occurring. Such an increase in muscle activity over a period of time is not therapeutic.

Cervical Spine Influences

Many short- and long-term factors have been suggested to influence the UPPM.[6] However, head posture appears to have the most significant and immediate effect upon the UPPM.[7] Several studies have demonstrated that changes in the UPPM occur in response to short term changes in the position of the head on the neck.[8,9] Cervical spine dysfunction (FHP) influences the UPPM.[10] Long term positioning or mobility changes as seen in cervical spine dysfunction has not yet been entirely documented.

The mandible can be visualized as being engulfed in the web of muscles and soft tissue attaching to it. The FHP plus the influence of gravity changes the mandibular position by altering the tone and tension of the muscle and soft tissue attaching to the mandible.[10] This altered muscle and soft tissue tone is suggested to develop a force of elevation and retrusion on the mandible.[10] This force can vary from person to person as well as within the same person. To what degree and for how long a change in the vertical and or anteroposterior positioning occurs with the UPPM will depend upon the degree of cervical spine involvement.[10]

Symptoms

A common symptom relating to a change in the UPPM is the patient's complaint that "I don't know where to rest my jaw." This complaint may result from a change in head positioning influencing the UPPM. Cervical spine dysfunction changing the UPPM may give the patient the perception of not knowing where to position his jaw.

This perception may be exaggerated in those individuals who have a very keen sense of their teeth. Studies have shown significant differences between

Fig. 4-1. The upright postural position of the tongue and mandible. (From Kraus,[54] with permission.)

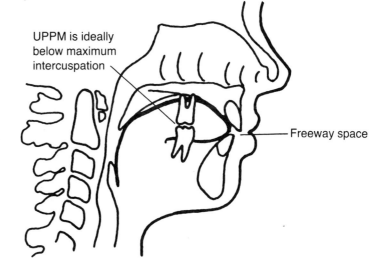

UPPM is ideally below maximum intercuspation

Freeway space

individuals with respect to the occlusal receptors' sensory threshold.[11] Occlusal receptors provide a great deal of proprioceptive feedback to the mandibular muscles, which in turn influence the UPPM.[11] As previously stated, the anteroposterior position of the UPPM should be below maximum intercuspation. Patients who have a keen sense of their occlusion will not allow for much variability in their UPPM. Cervical spine dysfunction changes both the vertical and horizontal positions of the UPPM. The end result is both the occlusion (whether "normal" occlusion or malocclusion) and cervical spine dysfunction influence the mandible to position itself in different ways. The altered proprioceptive feedback from muscles, soft tissue and occlusion may influence the ability of the patient to know where to position the mandible.

A consequence of not knowing where to rest the mandible may be that the patient tries to "brace" the mandible. The patient may brace the tip of the anterior mandibular teeth against the posterior part of the anterior maxillary teeth. Bracing the mandible gives the patient some point of reference for jaw positioning. Bracing does require an isometric contraction of the mandibular muscles, but should not be confused with bruxism, which is covered later. Some patients, however, place their teeth in maximum intercuspation as another way of having some point of reference with their mandible. The symptoms expressed by such a patient would be those associated with muscle hyperactivity (myalgia) of the mandibular muscles. In addition, the patient may complain of a decrease or tightness in jaw movement as observed clinically.

The Upright Postural Position of the Tongue

The tongue is composed of two muscle groups, the extrinsic and intrinsic muscles. The extrinsic muscles suspend the tongue from the skull (styloid process) to the anterior portion of the mandible. The mandible itself is also suspended from the skull. The intrinsic tongue muscles begin and end within the tongue and have no attachment to skeletal structures. The only intrinsic muscle of the tongue to be mentioned is the genioglossus, since it is the only muscle that protrudes the tongue,[12] and the majority

of electromyographic (EMG) documentation has been done on the genioglossus. Clinical observations to be covered will emphasize tongue protrusion.

The tongue is active during almost all oral and mandibular functions. When the stomatognathic system is in a state of equilibrium, the upright postural position of the tongue (UPPT) is up against the palate of the mouth.[13] In this position, the tip of the tongue will touch lightly, if at all, against the back side of the upper incisors (Fig. 4-1). The UPPT enhances the UPPM. As Fish has stated,[14] ". . . the rest position of the mandible is related to the posture of the tongue . . ."

Cervical Spine Influences

The FHP is proposed to influence the UPPT in several ways. The main supports of the extrinsic tongue muscles are the styloid process at one end and the front of the mandible at the other end (Fig. 4-2). The tongue can be visualized as being suspended like a sling between the styloid process and the mandible.[15] As the head moves forward (FHP), the cranium extends (rotates posteriorly) on the upper cervical spine.[16] The styloid process, being a part of the cranium, moves anteriorly as posterior rotation of the cranium occurs as a result of the FHP (Fig. 4-2).

Forces of elevation and retrusion are placed on the mandible during the acquired FHP. The FHP causes the two points of attachment of the extrinsic muscles to come closer together (Fig. 4-2). This positional change of both the styloid process and the mandible causes the tongue to "drop" from the top of the palate (the UPPT) to the floor of the mouth. A change in the resting length of the extrinsic muscles of the tongue will more than likely change the resting length of the intrinsic muscles.

In addition to a change in the length of the extrinsic muscles, a change in EMG activity of the genioglossus secondary to a change in head-neck positioning will occur. Studies have documented that a change in mandibular position will alter genioglossus (intrinsic muscle) activity mediated through the TMJ receptors.[17,18] Mandibular position is altered by a change in head position. It is conceivable, then, that a change in head posture that alters the UPPM

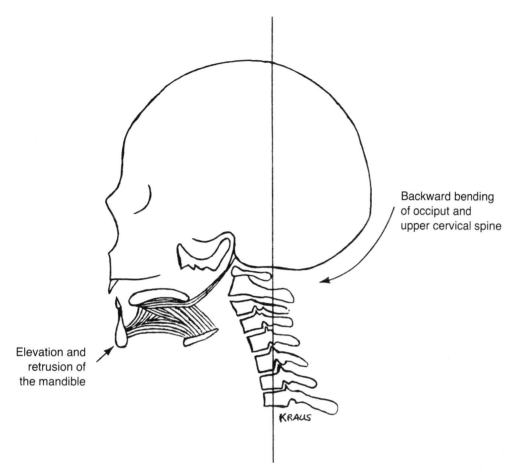

Backward bending
of occiput and
upper cervical spine

Elevation and
retrusion of
the mandible

KRAUS

Fig. 4-2. FHP with a cutaway section of the mandible for easier viewing of the tongue and its muscles. The primary insertions of the extrinsic tongue muscles are to the styloid process and the anterior portion of the mandible. The arrows represent the proposed anatomic positional changes that occur secondary to FHP. The result is that the two points of insertion for the extrinsic muscles come closer together, thereby influencing the UPPT.

will in turn alter the TMJ receptors influencing genioglossus activity.

A second way in which head and neck position may alter genioglossus activity is through the tonic neck reflex. Extension of the head on the neck has been shown to produce an increase in genioglossus activity.[19] Backward bending (extension) of the head on the upper cervical spine occurs in the FHP (Fig. 4-2). Therefore, the previous discussion suggests that the FHP can cause an increase in genioglossus activity, either indirectly through the TMJ receptors or directly through the tonic neck reflex.

Cervical spine dysfunction (FHP) will result in the tongue lying on the floor of the mouth, with the tip of the tongue pressing against the posterior side of the anterior mandibular teeth.

Symptoms

Patients often are not aware of where they position their tongues until they are asked. When cervical spine dysfunction is present, the patient often states that his tongue is lying in the floor of his mouth with the tip of the tongue pressing against the back side of his bottom teeth. Some patients, when asked to place the tongue up against the palate of the mouth (in the UPPT), may say that such a position feels awkward or difficult.

An altered tongue position contributes to symptoms of fullness or tightness in the floor of the mouth and/or the front of the neck. The pressing of the tongue against the teeth contributes to discomfort felt in the angle of the mandible. This discomfort is often mistaken for discomfort stemming from the TMJ. The reader can experience such discomfort by pressing the tip of the tongue against the front teeth for a period of time.

Maintaining the UPPT will keep the teeth out of the maximum intercuspated position. If the teeth were to come together, then the patient could not maintain the UPPT. Such a natural phenomenon of the tongue up and teeth apart is enhanced in the majority of patients by overbite, where the maxillary anterior central incisors overlap the mandibular anterior central incisors by approximately 1 to 1½ mm. If the patient maintains the correct UPPT, he must keep his teeth apart or he will either bite the tip of the tongue or move the tongue away from its upright postural position. Therefore an altered rest position of the tongue (usually in the floor of the mouth) secondary to cervical spine dysfunction allows the teeth to come together, resulting in hyperactivity of the elevator muscles of the mandible as observed clinically. Patients may then complain of myalgia of the mandibular muscles.

Finally, in the supine position, the tonic activity of the genioglossus is markedly increased.[20] This increased activity plays an important role in maintaining an open air passage in the oropharyngeal region in the supine position.[20] It is generally agreed that supine sleeping with proper support is best for the cervical spine. However, cervical spine dysfunction with or without proper cervical support influences the UPPT. To maintain an adequate airway, the patient may lie on his stomach in order to keep the tongue out of the oropharyngeal area. The prone-lying position, which places a great deal of stress on the cervical spine tissues, may produce or increase cervical symptoms. One way to discourage the prone-lying position is to maintain the tongue in its upright postural position, thereby maintaining an open airway. Training of the patient to maintain the UPPT will have to be done first during the conscious waking hours. Achieving good mobility and positioning of the cervical spine, educating the patient on the normal UPPT, and providing good cervical support at night will encourage supine and/or side-lying sleeping postures.

Swallowing

Although it is generally acknowledged that swallowing involves nearly all the muscles of the tongue, the muscles that seem to be of particular importance are the geniohyoid, the genioglossus, the mylohyoid, and the anterior digastric.[21] Of these four muscles, emphasis will be on the activity of the genioglossus. Swallowing or deglutition is the process by which a fluid or solid is passed from the mouth to the stomach. There are three stages of swallowing: oral, pharyngeal, and esophageal.[22] The oral stage is voluntary and involves the passage of the bolus to the fauces (the passage from the mouth to the pharynx). The other two stages of swallowing are involuntary. During a 24-hour period, we swallow subconsciously many times. The amount of subconscious swallowing added to the number of times we swallow during eating and drinking adds up to a significant amount of muscle activity even when done correctly.

The oral stage is the only stage of swallowing for which some documentation is available regarding the influence of positional changes of the head and neck. It is also the only stage over which we have conscious control in order to correct altered swallowing patterns. For these reasons, the oral stage will be the only stage covered.

During the normal oral stage of swallowing (Fig. 4-3), once the fluid or solid is in the mouth, the tip of the tongue moves forward and upward to contact the palatal mucosa behind the upper incisors.[23] Then, like a wave in the ocean, the tongue reaches the junction of the hard and soft palate.[24] At this point the oral stage of swallowing ends, with the tongue returning to its upright postural position.

Cervical Spine Influences

The UPPT has been described as the foundation of all swallowing movements.[24-26] Cervical spine influence on the UPPT has been discussed previously. Because the swallowing begins and ends in the

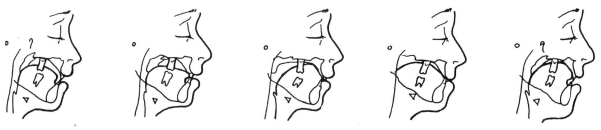

Fig. 4-3. Normal sequence of swallowing described in five stages. (From Kraus,[54] with permission.)

UPPT, the entire oral stage of swallowing will be altered in the presence of cervical spine dysfunction.

During an altered sequence of swallowing, the patient often will push the tip of the tongue off the back side of the upper or lower incisors. The tongue pressing anteriorly diminishes the effectiveness of the middle and posterior parts of the tongue in pressing up at the junction of the hard and soft palate. Continuation of an altered sequence of swallowing contributes to an increase in the duration of swallowing. The duration of normal swallowing ranges from 1.42 to 2.74 seconds.[27] It has been suggested that swallowing can occur with the teeth together or apart.[28] It is the author's belief that in the presence of good mobility and positioning of the cervical spine swallowing should occur without tooth contact. Cervical spine dysfunction, by causing the oral stage of swallowing to be altered, contributes to an increase in tooth-to-tooth contact time for each swallow. Tooth contact lasting for a longer duration contributes to muscle hyperactivity of the tongue and mandibular muscles.

In a recent study involving 12 normal subjects, significant measurements of the genioglossus were noted as subjects assumed the FHP.[29] The duration of conscious swallowing and maximal genioglossus EMG activity were significantly greater in the FHP.

To appreciate the influence of head posture on swallowing, simply look up and swallow. You will find it difficult to swallow. However, you may find it to be slightly easier to swallow if you press the tip of your tongue firmly against the back side of your upper or lower incisors. This tongue position of course encourages more dysfunction. Now bring your eyes level but exaggerate the FHP. Again you will find it to be more difficult to swallow correctly with the middle to posterior third of the tongue pressing against the palate of the mouth.

Symptoms

Symptoms associated with an altered sequence of swallowing secondary to cervical spine dysfunction will consist of difficulty in swallowing (food gets caught in the throat or there is a fullness in the throat) or tightness in the front of the neck. Discomfort in the angle of the mandible associated with an altered UPPT will be further increased. Secondary symptoms will be related to myalgia of the tongue and masticatory muscles. Some patients will feel as though their tongue is swollen. Patients may complain of biting their tongue because of the lack of coordination between tongue positioning, swallowing, and chewing.

Occlusion

Occlusion in dentistry refers to the way teeth meet, fit, come together, or touch. Much has been written about malocclusion of the natural teeth and the relationship between occlusion and myofascial pain and/or TMJ dysfunction.[11,30–32] The modification of occlusal relationships is regarded by some dentists as a specific and definitive treatment for muscle and TMJ involvement.[33,34] Some individuals consider occlusal modification to be specific treatment because it deals directly with the presumed etiologic factor, and definitive because it eliminates or corrects the occlusal problem. On the basis of this concept, some clinicians treat patients with muscle and TMJ involvement by altering the occlusion in various ways. Occlusal relationships may be altered by any one or a combination of techniques including equilibration (selective grinding to modify the occlusion), orthodontics, or full-mouth reconstructions, to name a few.

The rationale behind altering the occlusion is based on several biomechanical hypotheses. Some believe that malocclusion causes displacement of the mandible, and that proper occlusal treatment allows repositioning of the mandible to its optimal position.[35,36] The other, more popular theory holds that malocclusion initiates neuromuscular reflexes of accommodative activity in the masticatory muscles. Such muscle activity in response to the malocclusion is suggested to lead to muscular fatigue and spasm.[37,38]

However, many individuals with obvious malocclusion have no dental, muscle, or joint complaints.[39,40] In fact, malocclusion is the rule rather than the exception. Because of this common observation a theory of physiologic versus pathologic of the occlusion has been espoused.[40] By definition,[40] a "physiologically acceptable occlusion is one free of patient complaints and recognizable pathological conditions, by the dentist, at the time of examination."

When to treat or not to treat the occlusion in the absence or, for that matter, the presence of symptoms becomes largely a clinical judgment. It has been shown that the same types of occlusal disharmonies are distributed equally among populations of patients with muscle and/or TMJ symptoms and randomly selected normal individuals.[41] It has also been shown that four out of five patients with muscle and/or TMJ symptoms are women; however, no consistent differences with respect to occlusion have been shown to exist between the sexes.[42]

When muscle and/or TMJ symptoms do appear, it becomes important for the dentist to use reversible treatments, for example, by utilizing an interocclusal appliance.[43,44] Other forms of treatment such as equilibration and orthodontics are irreversible. Interocclusal appliances must be designed, applied, and modified for each individual patient; otherwise orthodontic movement of the teeth can occur, which of course should be avoided in the symptomatic patient. It should be recognized that the patient's response to either occlusal adjustment or splint therapy is a complex interaction between the psychology of the patient, the type of treatment offered, and how the treatment may be influenced by other adjacent areas. Simply to suggest that a response by a patient to treatment of the occlusion, or for that matter of any dysfunctional problem, is a cause-and-effect phenomenon is not justified.[1,45]

With such differences in opinion as to the role of occlusion in producing symptoms, the dentist and physical therapist should be alert to other adjacent areas that influence how the teeth meet in maximum intercuspation. An area often overlooked by the clinician that may decrease the patient's ability to accommodate to a malocclusion is the cervical spine.[10,44] Treating patients with symptoms related to the muscle and/or the TMJ will require that more than just the occlusion be dealt with. To help the patient achieve a painfree functional physiologic adaptive range, treat not only the occlusion by reversible procedures but also those areas that influence the occlusion. One such area believed to influence how the teeth come into maximum intercuspation, is the cervical spine. There are of course other forms of malocclusions which are not a part of this discussion.

Cervical Spine Influences

How cervical spine dysfunction influences the occlusion can be understood by appreciating the influence the cervical spine has on the adaptive (habitual) arc of closure. The adaptive arc of closure is an arc directed by a conditioned reflex[40]: "The entire proprioceptive neuromuscular mechanism sets up the conditioned reflex and guides this arc of closure."[40]

What is obviously acknowledged by the dentist is that at one end of this arc is the occlusion. Ideally, the teeth should meet in maximum intercuspation as the mandibular teeth approach the maxillary teeth during closure. If any portion of a tooth or teeth makes contact prior to maximum intercuspation, this is considered a form of malocclusion. Such an interference or premature contact stimulates the mechanoreceptors of the periodontium (the tissues investing and supporting the teeth).[11] This in return causes abnormal recruitment of the muscles of mastication to reposition the mandible into a more favorable position as maximum intercuspation is approached.[11,44] The neuromuscular system, by positioning the mandible so as to avoid the interference, changes the adaptive arc of closure. A change in the adaptive arc of closure occurs at the expense of additional muscle activity.[44] As previously suggested, when such interferences cannot be accommodated by the neuromuscular system, muscular symptoms develop. Muscle hyperactivity contributes to symptoms arising from the muscle and is also believed to be a cause of temporomandibular disorders.

However, what is often totally overlooked in this ordering of events is the other end of the adaptive arc of closure. The end of the arc from which jaw closure begins is the UPPM. Posselt has stated, "the conclusion that the rest position can generally be considered a position on the path of closing movement is almost self-suggestive."[46] Changes in cervical spine position (FHP) change the UPPM.[10] As Mohl stated regarding head and neck posture, ". . . we must logically conclude that, if rest position is altered by a change in head position, the habitual path of closure of the mandible must also be altered."[47] Cervical spine dysfunction may alter the arc of closure to maximum intercuspation.[10] Such a change in the path of closure will cause premature contacts of the teeth prior to maximum intercuspation. If premature contacts secondary to a malocclusion may eventually cause muscle and/or TMJ symptoms, premature contacts secondary to cervical spine dysfunction may also result in muscle and/or TMJ symptoms. The neuromuscular system will try to accommodate for such interferences. When such accommodative responses are exhausted and muscle and/or TMJ symptoms develop, the cervical spine needs to be evaluated and treated.

Symptoms

Symptoms will be those that have been attributed to a malocclusion (interferences prior to maximum intercuspation). A physiologic occlusion may be present, yet there is interference of the mandibular teeth approaching the maxillary teeth to maximum intercuspation. Such an interference may be secondary to cervical spine dysfunction and would actually be a pseudomalocclusion.[10] Clinically, a combination of malocclusion and a pseudomalocclusion is usually more common, thus complicating the clinical picture even more.

Bruxism is considered by some a symptom of malocclusion. Bruxism is the clenching or grinding of the teeth when the individual is not chewing or swallowing.[48] Bruxism has been implicated in producing a variety of symptoms such as headache, TMJ and myofascial pain, tooth mobility, and occlusal wear.[49] Bruxism has been associated with the presence of occlusal interferences.[11] Cervical spine influences may contribute to occlusal interferences as teeth come into contact and therefore bruxism. Other causes of bruxism (muscle hyperactivity) have been suggested to be related to daily stress and emotional tension.[50]

Patients may also complain of their "bite" (occlusion) being off. The dentist may not find any indication that this patient's complaint is related to the occlusion. In this case the patient's perception is of a pseudomalocclusion caused by cervical spine dysfunction. Some patients may feel they cannot get their supporting teeth together (usually in the molar region) on one or both sides even after an occlusal adjustment or during splint therapy. Again the cervical spine may be implicated.

If a patient is undergoing splint therapy with a dentist and is not responding, several factors may be involved:[10]

1. The splint is not indicated, but therapy to the cervical spine is.
2. The splint is indicated, but due to the degree of cervical spine dysfunction present, accommodation to the splint is not possible.
3. The splint may have helped, but the patient cannot be weaned off of the splint without his symptoms returning. The cervical spine again may be a factor in such a response.

TREATMENT

The physical therapist should always perform an evaluation of the cervical spine to determine if treatment is needed. The specifics of the evaluation are not within the scope of this chapter; the reader is referred to the bibliography.[51] The type of treatment of the cervical spine used to reduce its influence on the stomatognathic system is the same treatment offered for involvement of the cervical spine alone. Even if the patient does not complain of any of the symptoms of dysfunction of the stomatognathic system, instructing the patient on the normal function of the stomatognathic system will enhance treatment of the cervical spine.

Awareness Exercises for the Stomatognathic System

The patient needs to be told what is normal jaw and tongue positioning at rest. First instruct the patient on the normal rest position of the tongue. The tongue should be up against the mouth, with the tip lightly touching, if at all, the back side of the upper central incisors (Fig. 4-1). Patients tend to overcompensate, so inform the patient not to press the tongue hard against the roof of the mouth.

The UPPM (rest position) is with the teeth apart. As was discussed earlier, if the patient's tongue is up and an overbite exists, the teeth will be apart. The patient should not be concerned with how far apart the teeth are. Inform the patient not to work hard at keeping the teeth apart ("Just let the jaw float"). Reassure the patient that the position with the tongue up and the teeth apart will become easier as the cervical spine dysfunction is treated.

Patients who have developed an altered sequence in swallowing secondary to cervical spine dysfunction will need to be instructed on the normal sequence in swallowing. Swallowing will be practiced with water. Inform the patient to practice swallowing with their teeth slightly apart.

In stage 1 (Fig. 4-3), the tongue drops from its normal rest position to allow water to enter into the mouth.

In stage 2, the tip of the tongue is directed to its rest position. Emphasize to the patient that no pressure should be felt from the tip of the tongue pressing upward or forward against the teeth.

In stage 3, the main force of swallowing occurs with the middle third (middle to posterior) of the tongue. From stage 2 to stage 3 the patient should feel the tongue moving like a wave in the ocean.

Stage 4 is essentially the end of stage 3, as the water is pressed into the pharynx, where involuntary control takes over.

Stage 5 is the completion of the swallowing cycle. The tongue is in its rest position and the teeth are apart.[52]

A pseudomalocclusion is treated by treating the cervical spine. The therapist should not dwell on the patient's perception of his occlusion too often after the initial evaluation. Occasionally asking the patient about how his bite feels is acceptable. Otherwise, the repeated mention of the bite, especially if the patient has a keen sense about the occlusion, may result in too much of an awareness by the patient. This is important to realize, because even after occlusal therapy malocclusion may still persist.

The awareness exercises should be practiced numerous times during the day. Awareness exercises must be practiced with good head and neck posture. If good head and neck posture cannot be achieved as yet, then the patient should practice with the existing head and neck posture at that time. Above all do not have the patient force a good head and neck posture.

SUMMARY

This chapter expresses clinical opinion about the influence of the cervical spine on key portions of the stomatognathic system, which are often not recognized by the clinician. By having an understanding of how the cervical spine influences the stomatognathic system, certain symptoms may be better understood.

The influence of the cervical spine on the TMJ has been covered indirectly. The cervical spine influences mandibular positioning and mobility, and thus indirectly the TMJ. Apart from symptoms related to minimal inflammation of the TMJ, the majority of cases of symptomatic capsular and intercapsular (disk-condyle derangements) involvement will more than likely require the use of an intraoral appliance from a dentist.[53] Where the cervical spine plays a key role in the treatment of a symptomatic TMJ is in the presence of muscle hyperactivity secondary to cervical spine dysfunction. In such cases the sequence and design of the intraoral appliance may need to be changed.[10]

Muscles of the stomatognathic system have been discussed only as needed, not to de-emphasize the importance of the muscles, because muscles are in fact the key to interrelating the cervical spine with the stomatognathic system. The topic of cervical spine influence on muscle activity of the craniomandibular region has been covered in detail elsewhere.[10]

The symptoms discussed in this chapter are only those symptoms of the stomatognathic system secondary to cervical spine dysfunction; the reader should be alert to referred symptoms from the cervical spine to the stomatognathic system.[10]

Treatment of stomatognathic dysfunction is through patient education in the application of the awareness exercises. Of course, treatment of cervical spine dysfunction must also be offered. Involvement of the masticatory muscles and the TMJ beyond that responsive to physical therapy treatment requires consultation with a dentist.

REFERENCES

1. Sichers H: Positions and movements of the mandible. J Am Dent Assoc 48:620, 1954
2. Dorland's Medical Dictionary. 26th Ed. WB Saunders, Philadelphia, 1981
3. Nasedkin J: Occlusal dysfunction: screening procedures and initial treatment planning. Gen Dent, 26:52, 1978
4. Yemm R: The mandibular rest position: the roles of tissue elasticiy and muscle activity. Journal of the Dental Associations of South Africa, Vol. 30 p 203, January 1975
5. Kazis H, Kazis A: Complete Mouth Rehabilitation. Henry Kimpton, London, 1956
6. Atwood DA: A critique of the rest position of the mandible. J Prosthet Dent 16:848, 1966
7. Mohl N: Head posture and its role in occlusion. Int J Ortho 15:6, 1977
8. Mohamed SE, Christensen LV: Mandibular reference positions. J Oral Rehab 12:355, 1985
9. Funakoshi M, Fujita N, Takehana S: Relations between occlusal interference and jaw muscle activities in response to change in head position. J Dent Res 55:684, 1976
10. Kraus S: Cervical spine influences on the craniomandibular region. p 367. In Kraus S: TMJ Disorders: Management of the Craniomandibular Complex. Churchill Livingstone, New York, 1988
11. Ramfjord SP, Ash M Jr: Occlusion. 2nd Ed. WB Saunders, Philadelphia, 1971
12. Sauerland EK, Mitchell SP: Electromyographic activity of intrinsic and extrinsic muscles of the human tongue. Tex Rep Biol Med 33:258, 1975
13. Proffit W: Equilibrium theory revisited: factors influencing position of the teeth. Angle Orthod 48:172, 1978
14. Fish F: The functional anatomy of the rest position of the mandible. Dent Practitioner 11:178, 1961
15. Grant JCB: A Method of Anatomy. 6th Ed. Williams & Wilkins, Baltimore, 1958
16. Kendall H, Kendall F, Boynton D: Posture and Pain. Robert E Krieger, Malabar FL, 1967
17. Lowe A: Mandibular joint control of genioglossus muscle activity in the cat and monkey. Arch Oral Biol 23:787, 1978
18. Lowe A, Johnston W: Tongue and jaw muscle activity in response to mandibular rotations in a sample of normal and anterior open bite subjects. Am J Orthod 76:565, 1979
19. Bratzlavsky M, Vander Eecken H: Postural reflexes in cranial muscles in man. Acta Neurol Belg 77:5, 1977
20. Sauerland E, Harper R: The human tongue during sleep: electromyographic activity of the genioglossus muscle. Exp Neurol 51:160, 1976
21. Hrycyshyn A, Basmajian J: Electromyography of the oral stage of swallowing in man. Am J Anat 133:333, 1972
22. Guyton AC: Textbook of Medical Physiology. 3rd Ed. WB Saunders, Philadelphia, 1967
23. Cleall J, Alexander W, McIntyre H: Head posture and its relationship to deglutition. Angle Orthod 36:335, 1966
24. Cleall J: Deglutition: a study of form and function. Am J Orthod 51:566, 1965
25. Barrett H, Mason R: Oral myofunctional disorders. CV Mosby, St Louis, 1978
26. Logemann J: Evaluation and Treatment of Swallowing Disorders. College-Hill Press, San Diego, 1983
27. Cunningham D, Basmajian J: Electromyography of genioglossus and geniohyoid muscles during deglutition. Anat Rec 165:401, 1969
28. Bole C: Electromyographic kinesiology of the genioglossus muscles in man. Thesis, Ohio State University, 1969
29. Milidonis M, Kraus S, Segal R, et al: Genioglossus muscle activity in response to changes in anterior/posterior head posture. Am J Orthod in press, 1988
30. Shore NA: Occlusal Equilibration and Temporomandibular Joint Dysfunction. JB Lippincott, Philadelphia, 1959
31. Mann A, Pankey LD: Concepts of occlusion. The PM

philosophy of occlusal rehabilitation. Dent Clin North Am p 621, November 1963

32. Dawson PE: Evaluation, Diagnosis and Treatment of Occlusal Problems. CV Mosby, St Louis, 1974

33. Krogh-Poulsoen WG, Olsson A: Occlusal disharmonies and dysfunction of the stomatognathic system. Dent Clin North Am 10:627, 1966

34. Posselt UOA: Physiology of Occlusion and Rehabilitation. 2nd Ed. FA Davis, Philadelphia, 1968

35. Granger ER: Occlusion in temporomandibular joint pain. J Am Dent Assoc 56:659, 1958

36. Dyer EH: Importance of a stable maxillomandibular relation. J Prosthet Dent 30:241, 1973

37. Ramfjord SP: Bruxism: a clinical and electromyographic study. J Am Dent Assoc 62:21, 1961

38. Zarb GA, Thompson GW: Assessment of clinical treatment of patients with temporomandibular joint dysfunction. J Prosthet Dent 24:542, 1970

39. Barghi N: Clinical evaluation of occlusion. Tex Dent J p 12, March 1978

40. Huffman R, Regenos J, Taylor R: Principles of Occlusion: Laboratory and Clinical Teaching Manual. 3rd Ed. H&R Press, Columbus OH, 1969

41. Posselt U: The temporomandibular joint syndrome and occlusion. J Prosthet Dent 25:432, 1971

42. Carraro JJ, Caffesse RG, Albano EA: Temporomandibular joint syndrome. A clinical evaluation. Oral Surg 28:54, 1969

43. Greene C, Laskin D: Splint therapy for the myofascial pain-dysfunction syndrome: a comparative study. J Am Dent Assoc 81:624, 1972

44. Razook S: Nonsurgical management of TMJ and masticatory muscle problems. p. 113. In Kraus S: TMJ Disorders: Management of the Craniomandibular Complex. Churchill Livingstone, New York, 1988

45. Goodman P, Greene C, Laskin D: Response of patients with myofascial pain-dysfunction syndrome to mock equilibration. J Am Dent Assoc 92:755, 1976

46. Posselt U: Studies on the mobility of the human mandible. Acta Odont Scand 10:1, 1952

47. Mohl N: Head posture and its role in occlusion. NY State Dent J 42:17, 1976

48. Ramjford SP, Kerr DA, Ash MM: World Workshop in Periodontics. p. 233. The University of Michigan, Ann Arbor MI, 1966

49. Solberg W, Clark G, Rugh J: Nocturnal electromyographic evaluation of bruxism patients undergoing short term splint therapy. J Oral Rehab 2:215, 1975

50. Rugh JD, Solberg W: Psychological implications in temporomandibular pain and dysfunction. Oral Sci Rev 7:3, 1976

51. Kaput M, Mannheimer J: Physical therapy concepts in the evaluation and treatment of the upper quarter. In Kraus S: TMJ Disorders: Management of the Craniomandibular Complex. Churchill Livingstone, New York, 1988

52. Kraus S: Physical therapy management of TMJ dysfunction. p. 139. In Kraus S: TMJ Disorders: Management of the Craniomandibular Complex. Churchill Livingstone, New York, 1988

53. Kraus S: Temporomandibular joint. p 171. In Saunders HD: Evaluation, Treatment and Prevention of Musculoskeletal Disorders. Viking Press, Minneapolis, 1985

54. Kraus S: Tongue-Teeth-Breathing-Swallowing: Exercise Pad. Stretching Charts, Inc., Tacoma WA, 1987

5

Dysfunction, Evaluation, and Treatment of the Cervical Spine and Thoracic Inlet

STEVEN A. STRATTON
JEAN M. BRYAN

Many patients present to physical therapy with complaints of pain due to cervical dysfunction. The cervicothoracic region is complex and requires a thorough evaluation to correctly and appropriately treat the disorder. The clinician must understand the applied anatomy and biomechanics of this region in order to recognize pathology. This chapter covers the pertinent anatomy and kinesiology of the cervical and upper thoracic spine, the evaluation procedure, and the correlation of findings to initiate treatment.

FUNCTIONAL ANATOMY

Upper Cervical Spine

The joints of the upper cervical spine region, also known as the craniovertebral joints, include the occipitoatlantal (OA) joint, the atlantoaxial (AA) joint, and the articulations between the second and third cervical vertebrae (C2–C3) including the facet joints, the intervertebral disk, and the joints of von Luschka. Clinically, the upper cervical spine is considered a functional region because of the interdependency of these joints associated with movement.

The Atlas

The first and second cervical vertebrae have characteristics that make them different from the more typical cervical vertebrae C3 through C7. The atlas (C1) is best thought of as a "washer" between the occiput and the axis (C2).[1] The two distinguishing features of the atlas are its long transverse processes and its lack of a spinous process. The superior articulating surfaces, which articulate with paired, convex occipital condyles, are concave both anteroposteriorly and mediolaterally. The articulating surfaces are oval (Fig. 5-1).[2]

The Axis

In addition to being the largest cervical vertebra of the upper cervical region, the axis (C2) has several other distinguishing features (Fig. 5-1). Its most striking landmark is the odontoid process (the dens), which passes up through the middle of the atlas, articulates with the anterior arch, and acts as a pivot for the OA joint. In addition, the axis has a large vertebral body. The superior articular facets face superiorly and laterally, are convex anteropos-

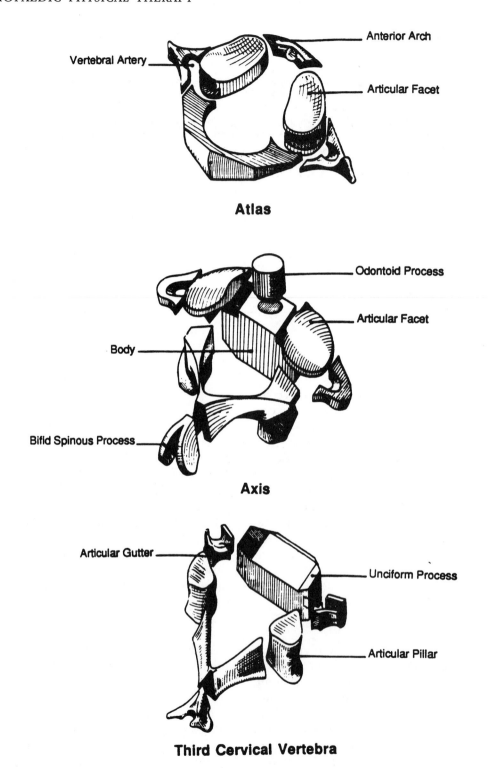

Fig. 5-1. The upper cervical vertebrae. (Modified from Kapandji,[2] p. 173, with permission.)

teriorly, and are flat transversely. The spinous process of the axis is bifid, like that of other cervical vertebrae, but is larger in mass. The inferior articular processes of C2 are attached below the pedicle, face inferiorly and anteriorly, and correspond to the superior articular processes of C3. Both the C1 and C2 transverse processes have a vertical foramen for the vertebral artery.[2]

The Occipitoatlantal and Atlantoaxial Ligaments

Alar Ligaments

The alar ligaments are irregular, quadrilateral, pyramid-like trunks that attach from the medial occipital condyle to the lateral surface of the dens (Fig. 5-2). The function of the alar ligament is to assist in controlling movements of extension and rotation.[1,3] During extension of the head, the alar ligament is stretched; during flexion it is relaxed. During rotation of the OA joint the ligament of the opposite side is stretched and drawn against the dens of the axis. For example, with rotation to the right, the left alar ligament is stretched and the right alar ligament is relaxed. During sidebending the alar ligament on the same side relaxes, and the opposite alar ligament causes a forced rotation of the axis to the side-bending side. The forced rotation is due to the attachment of the alar ligament to the dens[1,2] (Fig. 5-3).

Cruciform Ligament

The cruciform ligament consists of a horizontal transverse ligament of the atlas and the vertical attachments to the occiput and axis, respectively called the transverso-occipital and transversoaxial ligaments. The transverse ligament arises from the medial surfaces of the lateral mass of the atlas and functions to guarantee physiologic rotation of C1–C2 while protecting the spinal cord from the dens.[2] The other ligaments of the craniovertebral complex —tectorial membrane, the anterior longitudinal ligament, the OA ligament, the facet capsules, and the ligamentum nuchae—all help to provide support; however, only certain ligaments restrict flexion and extension[1] (Fig. 5-2, Table 5-1).

Occipitoatlantal Motion

The upper surface of the occipital condyles is concave; thus, arthrokinematically, movement of the occiput on the atlas requires opposite joint glide in relation to physiologic movement.[4] The articulations are divergent at approximately 30 degrees so

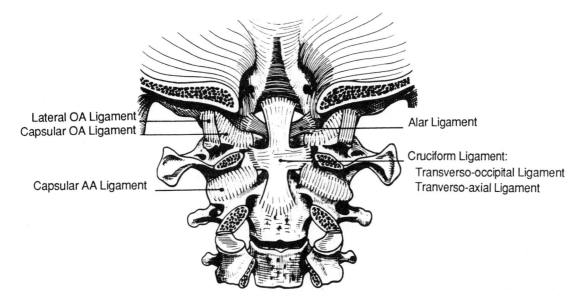

Fig. 5-2. Ligaments of the upper cervical spine complex. (Modified from Kapandji,[2] p. 189, with permission.)

Lateral OA Ligament
Capsular OA Ligament

Capsular AA Ligament

Alar Ligament

Cruciform Ligament:
Transverso-occipital Ligament
Tranverso-axial Ligament

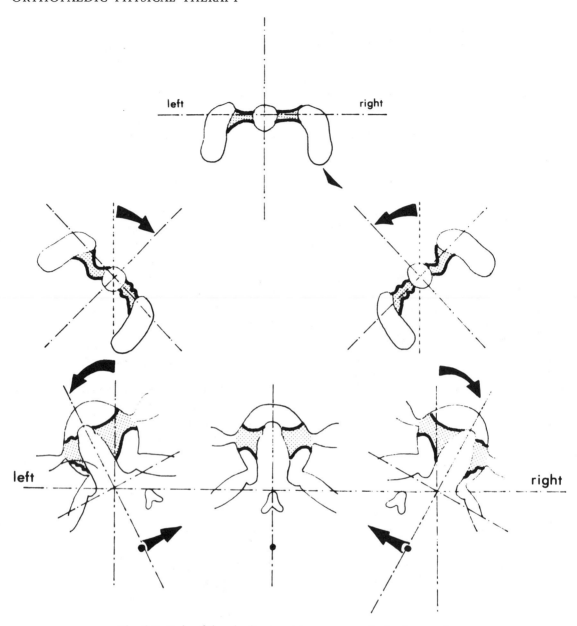

Fig. 5-3. Role of the alar ligament in upper cervical spine motion.

that the joint surfaces are not in a true sagittal plane. The sagittal axial angle of the joints is 50 to 60 degrees in the adult. The sagittal angle of the joint axes from the occipital condyles as described by Ingelmark[5] reveals a 28 degree divergence of the articular surfaces anteriorly (Fig. 5-4). Werne[3] described this joint as condyloid, with free flexion and extension

(nodding) and limited sidebending. Flexion and extension take place around a transverse axis and sidebending around a sagittal axis. Flexion and extension range from 16 to 20 degrees and are limited by bony structures. Sidebending measures approximately 4 to 5 degrees. Maximum sidebending is possible with the head in a slightly flexed position;

Table 5-1. Structures That Restrict OA and AA Joint Range of Motion About the Transverse Axis

Flexion	Extension
Bony limitation	Bony limitation
Posterior muscles of the neck	Anterior muscles of the neck
Longitudinal fibers of the cruciform ligament	Sternocleidomastoid and scalene muscles
Tectorial membrane	Tectorial membrane
Nuchal ligament	Alar ligaments
Posterior longitudinal ligament	Anterior longitudinal ligament

Table 5-2. Active Range of Motion of the Upper Cervical Spine

Vertebral Unit	Active Range of Motion (Degrees)			
	Flexion	Extension	Sidebending[a]	Axial Rotation[a]
C0–C1 (OA joint)	0–15	0–20	5–0–5	12–0–12
C1–C2 (AA joint)	0–10	0–10	3–0–3	50–0–50

[a] Range available on either side of neutral.

when the head is extended, sidebending is prohibited by the alar ligaments.[6]

Different findings have been reported in the literature regarding the possibility of rotation at the OA joint. Fielding,[6,7] White and Panjabi,[8,9] and Pen-

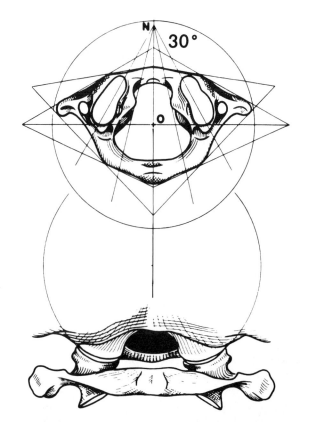

Fig. 5-4. OA joint sagittal axis from the occipital condyles. (Modified from Kapandji,[2] p. 181, with permission.)

ning[10] found no rotation, whereas Depreux and Mestdagh[11] contend that 5 degrees of rotation exists. Caviezel[12] clinically examined the passive terminal rotation of the atlas in testing resiliency. Attempts to explain this rotation often describe the atlas as a washer, interposed between the occiput and atlas like a meniscus, which would imply a gliding or linear movement[1] (Table 5-2).

Atlantoaxial Motion

The AA joint has four articulations for movement: the bursa atlantodentalis together with the middle and two lateral articulations. The bursa atlantodentalis is a space between the transverse ligament of the atlas and the dens of the axis. The middle AA articulation is located between the dens of the axis and the posterior surface of the anterior arch of the atlas. Most movement at the AA joint occurs at the lateral AA articulations, which are the superior articular surfaces between the atlas and axis.[2] The articular surfaces of the atlas are convex, and those of the axis are relatively flat.[1] The range of motion to each side is 40 to 50 degrees, which constitutes half of the total rotation of the cervical spine.[6] As in the OA joint, rotation is limited primarily by the alar ligaments. Only minimal (10 to 15 degrees) flexion-extension occur because of the bony geometry and the securing ligamentous structures. Sidebending between C1 and C2 is possible only with simultaneous rotation about the axis.[1] Lewit[13] and Jirout[14] described this movement as forced rotation that is mainly a result of the physiologic function of the alar ligaments. When forced rotation is produced there is a lateral displacement of the articular margin of the lateral joint of the atlas as compared with the lateral margin of the axis.[2]

Third Cervical Vertebra

The third cervical vertebra is typical of the remaining cervical vertebrae C3 to C7 (Fig. 5-1). The vertebral body is wider than it is high, and its superior surface is raised laterally to form the uncinate processes (uncovertebral joints or joints of von Luschka). The inferior vertebral surface resembles the superior surface of the inferior vertebra, and the anterior border shows a beak-like projection facing downward. These articular processes, which are part of the posterior arch, have both superior and inferior articulating facets. The superior facet is oriented superiorly and posteriorly and corresponds to the inferior facet of the overlying vertebra; the inferior facet faces inferiorly and anteriorly and corresponds to the superior facet of the underlying vertebra. These articular processes are attached to the vertebral body by the pedicles so that the spaces between the processes form the articular pillar. The transverse processes form a gutter and contain a transverse foramen for passage of the vertebral artery (Fig. 5-1). The two lamina, which are oblique inferiorly and laterally, meet in the midline to form the bifid spinous process.[2] In the upper cervical spine complex, the articular surfaces for the OA and AA joints are in a horizontal plane, but C2–C3 articular processes or facets have an abrupt frontal oblique slope.[15]

Motion of the C2–C3 Segment

Motion of the C2–C3 segment is representative of the typical cervical vertebral segment, with an intervertebral disk and eight plane articulations, including the four articular (apophyseal) facets and four uncovertebral joints (joints of von Luschka). The axis of motion is through the nucleus pulposus and allows freedom of movement in all three planes. Because of the orientation of the articular facets, sidebending and rotation occur concomitantly in the same direction.[2] Because of this concomitant motion, pure rotation or pure sidebending is impossible. The sliding of the joint surface depends on the rotation perpendicular to the axis. The relative amount of rotation or sidebending that occurs depends on the obliquity of the articular surfaces in the frontal plane. The more horizontal the joint surface, the more rotation will occur; the more vertical, the more sidebending will occur. At the second cervical vertebra, there are 2 degrees of coupled axial rotation for every 3 degrees of sidebending.[2] The most abrupt change in joint obliquity occurs at the C2–C3 facet. Grieve noted that all cervical facet joints are oriented so that the cervical facet joint surfaces converge in the region of the eyes.[15]

Motion of C3–C7

The midcervical spine allows the greatest ranges of motion in the neck (Table 5-3). The inclination of the facet surfaces of these vertebrae is 45 degrees to the horizontal plane. The lower segments are steeper than the upper segments. As in the C2–C3 segment, sidebending and rotation occur concomitantly in the same direction because of the oblique plane of the articular surfaces. However, at each motion segment there is opposite gliding of the articular surfaces. For example, with right rotation or right sidebending, the left superior articular facet glides superiorly and anteriorly while the right superior articular facet glides posteriorly and inferiorly on their adjoining inferior articular surfaces.[1] The total amount of sidebending in this region is 35 to 37 degrees, and total rotation is 45 degrees. With pure flexion and extension, both superior facets at each motion segment glide in the same direction. With flexion, both facets move superiorly, and with extension, both move inferiorly. Total range of flexion and extension in the lower cervical column is 100 to 110 degrees.[2]

Upper Thoracic Spine

The upper thoracic spine must be included in any discussion of the cervical spine, since the movement of the lower cervical spine occurs in conjunction with that of the upper thoracic spine. Gross cervical spine movements include upper thoracic spine motion as a result of the distal attachment of the cervical muscles to as low as T6 in the case of the splenius, longissimus, and semispinalis cervicis and semispinalis capitis muscles.[16] To accommodate

Table 5-3. Limits and Representative Values of Range of Rotation of the Middle and Lower Cervical Spine

Vertebral Unit	Flexion/Extension (X axis rotation)		Sidebending (Z axis rotation)		Axial Rotation (Y axis rotation)	
	Limits of Range (Degrees)	Representative Angle (Degrees)	Limits of Range (Degrees)	Representative Angle (Degrees)	Limits of Range (Degrees)	Representative Angle (Degrees)
C2–C3	5–23	8	11–20	10	6–28	9
C3–C4	7–38	13	9–15	11	10–28	11
C4–C5	8–39	12	0–16	11	10–26	12
C5–C6	4–34	17	0–16	8	8–34	10
C6–C7	1–29	16	0–17	7	6–15	9
C7–T1	4–17	9	0–17	4	5–13	8

(Data from White and Panjabi,[9] p. 71.)

the more frontal orientation of the thoracic articular facets, the seventh cervical vertebra makes a transition in its plane of facet motion. In addition to having all the characteristics of a typical vertebra, a thoracic vertebra has specific characteristics distinguishing it from a cervical vertebra. Thoracic vertebrae have no uncovertebral joints, bifid spinous processes, or intertransverse foramina. The attachments of the ribs to the thoracic vertebral bodies allow stability at the expense of mobility, with motion of the facet articulations occurring more in the frontal plane. The spinous processes incline inferiorly.[2]

Ribs

The first two ribs are atypical in that they have only one facet. The first rib is the most curved and is usually the shortest rib. This rib slopes obliquely downward and forward from the vertebra toward the sternum. Because of the costovertebral orientation primarily in the transverse plane, movements occur in a superior-inferior direction, with a resultant "pump handle" effect. The second rib is about twice the length of the first but has a similar curvature. The first rib is the site of insertion for the anterior and middle scalene muscles and the site of origin for the subclavius and the first digit of the serratus anterior. The second rib is the site of origin for the serratus anterior and the site of insertion for the posterior scalene and serratus posterior superior muscles.[16]

A typical rib has two articulations with the corresponding vertebra: The costovertebral joint articulates with demifacets on the vertebral bodies, and the costotransverse joint articulates between the rib tubercle and the transverse process of the underlying vertebra. The costovertebral joint is a synovial joint with condyloid movement, since the head of the rib is convex and moves on the concave costal facets of the vertebra. The costotransverse joint is a simple synovial joint, which allows a gliding movement. Both of these joints are reinforced by strong ligaments.[16,17]

During breathing, the axis of the costovertebral joints of the upper ribs lies close to the frontal plane, allowing an increase in the anteroposterior diameter of the thorax. Because of the fiber orientation of the scalene muscles superior to the first two ribs, these muscles can elevate these ribs and influence rib motion.[17]

Vertebral Artery

The vertebral artery enters the costotransverse foramen of C6 (sometimes that of C5) and traverses to the axis through the costovertebral foramina of the individual vertebrae. After entering the costotransverse foramen of the atlas, the artery exits and penetrates the atlanto-occipital membrane and dura mater in the region of the foramen magnum at the occiput.[16] Functionally, the vertebral artery is important because decreased blood supply in the basilar region of the brain stem diminishes one of the major blood supplies to the brain. Usually extreme rotation of the head will cause a decrease in the blood flow in the opposite vertebral artery at the OA junction. Typical neurologic symptoms of vertebrobasilar artery insufficiency include dizziness, tinnitus, visual disturbances, and nausea.[18,19] Occlusion of the vertebral artery may occur either at the suboccipital region or at the C6 level.[20]

Thoracic Inlet

Clinicians usually refer to the thoracic inlet as the thoracic outlet; however, from a strict anatomic point of view, the thoracic outlet is the opening at the inferior portion of the ribcage and the diaphragm.[16] The thoracic inlet is the superior opening of the ribcage, bounded posteriorly by the first thoracic vertebra, anteriorly by the superior border of the manubrium, and laterally by the first ribs. The structures that pass through the inlet include, centrally, the sternohyoid muscle, the sternothyroid muscles, the thymus, the trachea, the esophagus, and the thoracic ducts. Behind these ducts and just in front of the vertebral column are the longus colli muscles and the anterior longitudinal ligament. Laterally the inlet contains the upper lung and neurovascular structures, which join the lowest trunk of the brachial plexus. Within the thoracic inlet the vagus nerve deserves special attention since this nerve provides parasympathetic innervation to the pharynx and visceral organs.[16] The complex anatomy of the thoracic inlet and the intimate relationship of the bony, soft tissue, and neurovascular structures within the inlet provide multiple opportunities for compression. The term *thoracic inlet* (outlet) *syndrome* (TIS) refers to compression of arteries and/or the upper or lower trunk of the brachial plexus.[21]

MUSCULOSKELETAL DYSFUNCTION AND TRAUMA

Postural Abnormality

The most common postural deviation affecting the cervical spine is the forward head posture. This posture involves increased kyphosis of the thoracic spine, with resultant increased lordosis of the cervical spine and increased backward bending in the upper cervical complex.[22] Over time, persons with forward head posture adjust their head position and

decrease the midcervical lordosis.[23] The increased backward bend of the upper cervical complex results from the body's attempt to keep the eyes horizontal.[15] In doing so, the head is anterior to the vertical plumbline (the ideal postural alignment). This postural deviation puts abnormal stress on the soft tissues and changes the weightbearing surfaces of the vertebrae, especially in the suboccipital and cervicothoracic areas. Forward head posture causes muscle length adaptation, which results in altered biomechanics such that normal motions produce abnormal strain.[24] The muscles most often affected are the levator scapulae, upper trapezius, sternocleidomastoid, scalene, and suboccipital muscles.

Factors contributing to a forward head posture include poor postural habits and pain. We acquire these poor postural habits at a young age when we learn that slumping the upper back requires no energy expenditure. Adolescent girls who are taller and more developed than their peers also develop this posture. In older patients, this posture may be related to working at an incorrect height or in poor lighting. The second contributing factor to this posture is pain. Many patients with chronic cervical pain compensate by thrusting their head forward in an attempt to move away from their pain. Along with a forward head posture, patients present with associated postural changes in the head, neck, trunk, and shoulder region, and with a retruded mandible, rounded shoulders, and protracted scapulae with tight anterior muscles and stretched posterior muscles. Because of this direct relationship between pain and posture, postural correction is an appropriate treatment goal for most patients with chronic cervical pain[24] (Fig. 5-5).

Somatic Dysfunction

By far the most common cervical pathology seen by manual therapists is vertebral motion restriction or somatic dysfunction. The term *somatic dysfunction* is used by the osteopathic profession to refer to altered function of the component parts of the musculoskeletal system. Many terms such as "loss of joint play,"[25] "chiropractic vertebral subluxation,"[26] "joint dysfunction,"[25] "joint blockage,"[27] and "acute facet lock"[28] describe restrictions of vertebral motion. The osteopathic profession has adopted somatic dysfunction terminology to repre-

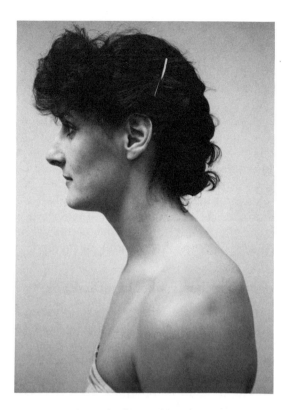

Fig. 5-5. The forward head posture.

sent a specific joint restriction in three dimensions. Specifically describing the loss of joint movement by its location in relationship to position or by its lack of movement allows treatment specific to the restriction to be administered.[29,30]

Many theories attempt to explain vertebral motion restriction. These theories range from entrapment of the synovial material[31] or a meniscoid,[32] to hypertonic contracted or contractured musculature,[33] to changes in nervous reflex activity such as sympathicotonia or gamma bias,[34] to abnormal stresses on an unguarded spine.[35] To date, no clear scientific evidence exists to explain what causes somatic dysfunction; however, one conceptual model, the biomechanical model, does help explain the clinically observable relationship between two vertebral segments or within a group of vertebral segments. This model conceptually defines the inability of the facet joints to open or close, either individually or bilaterally. This methodology allows consistency for a single examiner between patients

and between multiple examiners with the same patient. Probably the most important reason for using this model is that it is an excellent method for distinguishing structural and functional asymmetries.[29]

According to this manual medicine model, if some pathology interferes with the ability of both the right and the left facet of a given segment to open, that segment will have restriction of forward bending movement. Conversely, if some pathology prevents both facets from closing, there will be backward bending restriction of that segment. If only one facet is unable to open, forward bending movement will be restricted because the facet cannot open, but, in addition, sidebending movement to the contralateral side will be limited. In determining segmental vertebral motion, if both facets are functioning symmetrically, then the excursion of the paired transverse processes should be symmetrical through forward and backward bending.[36]

Cervical Spondylosis

Cervical spondylosis is the result of wear and tear on the weightbearing structures of the cervical spine. This degenerative process is generally considered to occur first in the articular cartilage but is not limited to the cartilage. This wear-and-tear phenomenon is attributed to repetitive microtraumas to cartilage from sustained impact loading on the bone.[17,30,37] Changes first occur in the deepest, calcified layer of cartilage, where subchondral bone hyperplasia begins as an irregular advance of ossification into the cartilage. This change becomes evident radiographically as increased bone density and sclerosis. At the vascular borders where cartilage, bone, synovium, and periosteum meet, a proliferation of bone formation begins, concentrated at the edges of the articular cartilage. These intra-articular osteophytes grow outward and tend to increase the lateral dimensions of the bone ends, increasing the joint cavity and stretching the capsule. These bony rims may trespass on pain-sensitive structures. These peripheral osteophytes are covered by a layer of fibrocartilage and are larger than they appear on radiographs because of this radiotranslucent covering. Typically degeneration occurs at the uncovertebral joints (joints of von Luschka), the facets, the intervertebral disks, the vertebral bodies, and the hyaline cartilage plates.[15]

Rib Dysfunction

Dysfunction of the upper costovertebral joints may cause pain in the cervical spine in the posterior triangle region. Greenman[17] stated that the first and second ribs, being atypical, can contribute to pain in the cervicothoracic region. Costovertebral motion allows both a "pump handle" and a "bucket handle" movement as described earlier. If the first and second ribs cannot complete a normal range of motion, several patterns of restriction are possible. The most common dysfunctions are inhalation and exhalation restrictions. If the first rib is not able to complete its anteroposterior range of motion, the motion of all the underlying ribs will be restricted. Most often a rib becomes dysfunctional as a result of the position assumed when a thoracic vertebra is asymmetrically restricted. The result is a slight rotation of a rib with rotation of the corresponding thoracic vertebra secondary to its inability to follow the rib in a straight plane. With rotation of the thoracic vertebra, the rib also rotates because of the attachment of the ligaments and intercostal muscles above and below the rib. If the vertebra remains rotated, soft tissue around the rib will compensate and adapt to this abnormal position so that the rib becomes immobile. If motion is restored to the vertebra, the rib may not return to its normal position because of this soft tissue adaptation. This situation is called a torsional rib dysfunction.[30]

The first rib can also subluxate superiorly since there are no structures above it to limit this superior excursion. This dysfunction can contribute to a myriad of symptoms including cervicothoracic pain, difficult deep breathing, restricted cervical rotation and sidebending, and possibly the numbness, tingling, and vascular complaints seen with thoracic inlet syndrome. Many times the fibromyositis described in the upper trapezius muscle is accompanied by dysfunction of the first and second ribs.

Thoracic Inlet Syndrome

As mentioned earlier, thoracic outlet syndrome should be termed thoracic inlet syndrome to be anatomically correct in describing the superior opening of the thoracic cavity. This syndrome represents a multitude of symptoms involving the neck and upper extremities, which are believed to be caused by proximal compression of the subclavian artery and vein and the brachial plexus. Probable etiologies for compression of the neurovascular structures include a cervical rib, a subluxated first thoracic rib, a shortened anterior scalene muscle, and anomalous fibromuscular bands. Other structures that can be involved in compression are any bony or soft tissue abnormality to include malunion of a fractured clavicle, Pancoast's tumor of the apex of the lung, altered posture, tight pectoralis minor muscles, and anomalous thoracic vertebral transverse processes. Secondary causes associated with thoracic inlet syndrome include trauma, occupational stress, obesity, and pendulous breasts.[21]

Vertebrobasilar Insufficiency

The vertebrobasilar arterial system supplies the spinal cord, the meninges, and the nerve roots, plexuses, muscles, and joints of the cervical spine. Intracranially, the basilar portion supplies the medulla, the cerebellum, and the vestibular nuclei.[16] This arterial system can be compromised at several points during its course as it passes through the transverse foramina of the upper six cervical vertebrae; as it winds around the articular pillar of the atlas; as it pierces the posterior OA membrane; or as it enters the foramen magnum to unite with the basilar artery. Blood flow can be diminished by a variety of mechanical disorders, which can be classified as either intrinsic or extrinsic. The most common intrinsic disorder is atherosclerosis. The basilar artery is the most commonly affected component, followed by the cervical portion of the vertebral artery. Usually seen as a complication of atherosclerosis, thrombosis of the vertebrobasilar arteries can result from an embolus, which usually lodges in the distal branches of the system, particularly the posterior cerebral artery.[15]

An extrinsic disorder compromises a blood vessel, restricting flow by compressing its external wall and thereby narrowing its lumen. This compression can result from:

1. An anomalous origin of the vertebral artery from the subclavian, causing the vertebral artery to be kinked and occluded during rotation of the neck

2. Constriction of the vertebral artery by bands of the deep cervical fascia during rotation of the neck

3. An anomalous divagation of the vertebral artery from its course through muscle and the transverse foramina of the vertebrae, or compression or angulation caused by projecting osteophytes. The most common site of compression is at the C5–C6 level, with a lower incidence at the C6–C7 level.

When this system is compromised, patients present with nystagmus, vertigo, blurred vision, giddiness, nausea, pallor, dysphagia, pupil dilation, and cervical pain.[15,19] Since compromise of the vertebral artery can occur both in the craniovertebral region and where the artery passes through the transverse foramen, all patients presenting with cervical pain should be screened for vertebrobasilar artery insufficiency. Manual therapists emphasize testing this system for patients with upper cervical complaints; however, serious compromise can also occur with damage to the middle and lower cervical regions.[15,20,38] A vertebral artery test for assessing vertebrobasilar insufficiency, described under the objective portion of the examination, must always be performed before any manual therapy is attempted on the cervical spine.

Cervical Disk

Cervical disk disease may cause symptoms similar to facet involvement and/or neurologic signs due to root or cord compression. The typical history involves insidious onset after performing a relatively minor physical activity or maintaining a prolonged position, for example after a long car trip, sleeping in an uncomfortable hotel bed, holding the phone with ones's shoulder, or working overhead. The pain is usually unilateral and may be felt anywhere in the cervical or scapular area.[39–41]

Cloward[42] described the typical referred pain pattern of cervical disk involvement. The pain usually starts in the cervical area and then diminishes and quickly extends to the scapula, the shoulder, the upper arm, and then possibly the forearm and hand.[41,42] The symptoms of a cervical disk lesion are provoked in a manner similar to a restricted facet joint, in that certain cervical movements will be painful while others are painfree; however, the pattern of painful and painfree movements does not follow the pattern for a restricted joint.[43]

Painful or restricted neck movements may be intermittent over a period of several months. Initially the patient may experience only a paresthesia, but when the nerve root becomes involved, the pain is more defined and can be reproduced with extreme neck movement. Sustained holding of these neck positions will exacerbate arm paresthesia and pain.[39] Clinical presentation of root involvement has been described as acute radiculopathy from a posterolateral bulging disk, an acute disk extrusion, or an exacerbation of pre-existing trespass in patients with radiographic evidence of a spondylosis. In addition to nerve root symptoms, the tendon reflex may be depressed or absent, or muscle weakness within the myotome may exist. If the disk material is extruded and occupying enough of the spinal canal to put pressure on the cord, the patient may demonstrate myelopathic signs such as spasticity, positive plantar response, clonus, and spastic quadriparesis or paraparesis.[40]

Trauma

All patients presenting with a history of trauma to the cervical region should have roentgenograms performed to rule out any fractures. Aside from fractures, discussion of which is beyond the scope of this chapter, a common clinical presentation of patients with cervical trauma is the whiplash syndrome. This term was introduced to describe the total involvement of the patient with whiplash injury and its effects.[44,45] The typical mechanism of injury involves flexion-extension injuries of the cervical spine, which result from sudden acceleration and deceleration collision forces on a vehicle in which the patient is riding. The magnitude of this collision force is determined by the mass of the vehicle and its rate of change of velocity. The shorter the impact time, the greater is the rate of change of velocity, or acceleration. As the acceleration becomes greater, the force of impact likewise increases. The faster a vehicle is moving at the time of impact, the greater will be the impact forces.[46]

A head-on collision causes deceleration injuries,

with the head and neck moving first into hyperflexion, terminating when the chin touches the chest. Following Newton's third law, after hyperflexion the head and cervical spine rebound into extension. These reciprocal flexion/extension movements continue until the forces are finally dissipated.

Side-on collisions cause lateral flexion of the cervical spine, with movement ceasing as the ear hits the shoulder. In rear-end collisions the car accelerates forward, causing the front seat to be pushed into the trunk of the occupant. This force causes the trunk to be thrust forward. The unrestrained head stays at rest, moving into relative backward bending as the trunk moves forward. This backward bending of the head and cervical spine continues until the occiput strikes the headrest or the thoracic spine. Many patients will describe the impact as being so great that their car seat was broken, or their glasses or dentures were thrown into the back seat, or the movement into hyperextension was so great that they came to rest facing the rear of the vehicle. Rebound into flexion occurs after the car stops accelerating and is complemented by contraction of the flexor muscles.[46]

The amount of actual damage to anatomic structures depends on the position of the head in space at the time of impact, the forces generated, and the histologic makeup of the tissues. In experimental studies simulating rear-end automobile accidents the following lesions occurred:

1. Tearing of the sternocleidomastoid and longissimus colli muscles
2. Pharyngeal edema and retropharyngeal hematoma
3. Hemorrhage of the muscular layers of the esophagus
4. Damage to the cervical sympathetic plexus
5. Tearing of the anterior longitudinal ligament
6. Separation of the cartilaginous endplate of the intervertebral disk
7. Tears of the facet joint capsules
8. Hemorrhage about the cervical nerve roots and spinal cord with possible cerebral injury.

The extent of damage seen in hyperflexion (head-on collision) injuries is similar. Damage can include tears of the posterior cervical musculature, sprains of the ligamentum nuchae and posterior longitudinal ligament, facet joint disruption, and posterior intervertebral disk injury with nerve root hemorrhage.[15,46]

Depending on the magnitude and direction of forces at the time of impact, patients may present with any combination of these hyperflexion and hyperextension injuries, as well as damage to the thoracic, lumbar, and temporomandibular joint (TMJ) regions. Onset of whiplash symptomatology is usually within 24 hours after the accident. The patient may describe headache, posterior neck pain, and referred scapular pain. Pain may radiate down the arm, mimicking thoracic inlet syndrome. Other complaints include upper thoracic and pectoral pain, weakness, dysphagia, dyspnea, TMJ dysfunction, and cerebral complaints such as insomnia, fatigue, nervousness, tenseness, decreased concentration span and memory, and hyperirritability. Many patients will describe dizziness, which may be associated with a high-frequency hearing loss. They may also have tinnitus and visual disturbances.[15]

Because of the complexity of this syndrome, if these patients are not evaluated thoroughly and treated appropriately, they may develop postural adaptations, psychogenic overlay, and chronic manifestation of any of the above symptoms.

Myofascial Pain Syndrome

Because of the use of a variety of terms to describe similar clinical findings, myofascial pain disorders have not been well understood. The different terms used may have the same, similar, or totally different meanings. Myofascial pain syndrome, also referred to as myofascial syndrome and myofascitis, involves pain and/or autonomic responses referred from active myofascial trigger points with associated dysfunction. Other terms such as myositis, fibrositis, myalgia, and fibromyositis have multiple meanings.[47] Some authors use these terms to identify myofascial trigger points; others have used them to label clinical manifestations.[48] To avoid further confusion, the definition of myofascial pain syndrome used here refers to the trigger point, as described by Travell.[47] A myofascial trigger point is "a hyperirritable spot, usually within a taut band of skeletal muscle or in the muscle's fascia, that is painful on compression and that can give rise to characteristic referred pain, tenderness, and autonomic phenomena."[47] Normal muscle does not have these trigger points.[47]

A clinical manifestation of myofascial trigger points is a typical referred pain pattern from the trigger point. On examination, findings include a local spot tenderness (the trigger point) and a palpably tense band of muscle fibers within a shortened and weak muscle. The trigger point may also respond to rapid changes of pressure; this has been described as the pathognomonic local twitch response. Direct pressure over a trigger point will reproduce the referred pain patterns. Travell[47] contends that a myofascial trigger point begins with muscular strain and later becomes a site of sensitized nerves, increased local metabolism, and reduced circulation. A myofascial trigger point is to be distinguished from a trigger point in other tissues such as skin, ligament, and periosteum. Myofascial trigger points are classified as either active or latent. An active trigger point causes pain, whereas a latent trigger point causes restriction of movement and weakness of the affected muscle and may persist for years after apparent recovery from an injury; however, a latent trigger point is predisposed to acute attacks of pain, since minor overstretching, overuse, or chilling of the muscle may cause a latent trigger point to become active. This symptomatology is not found in normal muscle.[47]

Referred Pain

Pain that is perceived in a location other than its origin is termed *referred pain*.[49] Nearly all pain is referred pain, referred either segmentally as in a dermatomal distribution, or specific to the tissue involved as in left upper extremity pain with myocardial infarction. Recognition of the embryologic derivation of tissues from the same somite is important in identifying many of the segmentally referred pain patterns. For example, as the upper limb bud grows, it draws the lower cervical and upper thoracic segments out into itself. Thus, the scapula and its muscles are derived from the middle and lower cervical segments, whereas the skin overlying the scapula and ribs is formed from the thoracic segments; therefore, pain perceived in the upper poste-

rior thoracic region may have a cervical origin. In addition, tissues other than visceral organs may have a specific reference pattern of pain that cannot be ascribed to segmental distribution.[43] Most practitioners are familiar with patients who complain of suboccipital headache and describe a reference pattern to the frontal region of the cranium.

Although clinical expectation is based on the assumption that a somatic nerve goes to a specific anatomic region, pain in that peripheral distribution can only be due to abnormalities of the spinal segment associated with that nerve. This assumption may be true; however, other pain patterns have been identified. Miller[50] suggested that pain does not really occur in the hands, feet, or head, but rather in the patient's conscious image of his hands, feet, or head. This theory suggests that pain and referred pain are central phenomena. A classic example is the phantom pain experienced by some amputees. Supporting this idea of referred pain as a central phenomenon, Harman[51] found that anginal pain referred to the left arm was not abolished by a complete brachial plexus block with local anesthesia. Referred pain has been experimentally evoked in areas previously anesthetized by regional nerve block.[52] Bourdillon[53] suggests that the central mechanism involves both the spinal cord and higher centers.

According to Cyriax,[43] if pain is segmentally referred, a lesion at a cervical level will produce pain in all or part of that cervical dermatome. For example, a C5 nerve root compression may produce pain in the neck, the midneck, the shoulder, and/or the lateral upper arm. All of these areas are supplied by the C5 dermatome. Although this relationship appears clear-cut, some research and clinical experience shows that the pain reference appears to be segmental in nature yet does not always correspond to dermatome or myotome distributions.[15,54-56] Because some referred pain patterns are not easily ascribed to particular segments, the clinician must perform a detailed, specific examination to determine the source of the pain. Experienced therapists are familiar with specific reference patterns that have several separate possible sources. An example is the clinical presentation of unilateral pain along the trapezial ridge (yoke area), which may be produced by dysfunction of the OA joint, the C4–C5

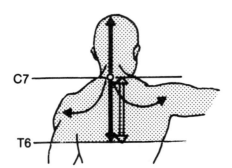

Fig. 5-6. Extrasegmental reference of the dura mater.

segment, or the joints of the first rib. Treatment of these dysfunctions may relieve the symptoms; however, any two or all three sites may have to be treated before the signs and symptoms are eliminated.[53]

Some general characteristics of segmentally referred pain are that the pain is usually referred distally from the cervical spine; the pain never crosses the midline; and the extent of the pain is controlled by the size of the dermatome and the location of the tissue involved. Again considering the C5 dermatome, a lesion at the nerve root level can result in a larger dermatomal reference pattern than a lesion of a C5-derived tissue at the shoulder level.[43]

A tissue that does not follow segmental reference is the dura mater. A lesion at the cervical level may cause pain anywhere from the head to the midthorax, and the pain often pervades several dermatomal levels. Symptoms are usually central or unilateral[43,49] (Fig. 5-6).

Other Pathologies

This discussion of cervical pathologies is by no means all-inclusive; other pathologies of nonmusculoskeletal origin can also elicit cervical pain. Some of these disorders, if not recognized, can have serious consequences. The clinical picture seen in these disorders differs significantly from symptoms of musculoskeletal origin. These differences include the presence of night pain as seen with metastatic disease; cord signs such as Lhermitte's sign, positive plantar response, and ankle clonus as seen in myelopathies; nuchal rigidity as seen in spinal meningitis or subarachnoid hemorrhage; and brachial plexus tension signs seen in brachial plexus neuritis or stretch injuries. Complaints of unrelenting, pulsating pain may be seen in a patient with an aortic aneurysm. Patients with advanced rheumatoid arthritis may present with the neck in the characteristic "cocked robin" position because of unilateral subluxation of the AA joint. Systemic infections may enlarge the lymph nodes and cause neck pain as seen in sinusitis, pharyngitis, otitis media, mediastinitis, and dental abscess. Other symptoms not usually seen with pain of musculoskeletal origin include unrelenting pain, severe symptoms after a trivial insult, and neurologic symptoms including blurred vision, visual field deficit, and loss of motor control.[57]

THE HISTORY AND PHYSICAL EXAMINATION

Patient History

The importance of careful and precise history taking cannot be overemphasized. The clinician will ultimately base a treatment plan on the patient's presenting signs and symptoms. The history should always precede the evaluation, since areas of emphasis during the examination will be determined by the history. Hoppenfeld[58] stated that this selective examination, based on a good history, produces the highest yield of information about clinical disease in the shortest time.

Asking concise, clinically relevant questions is a far more complex skill than the actual techniques of physical examination. Learning how to ask those questions by reading in textbooks or listening to lectures is difficult. Good history taking is both an art and a science. A closed-end question asks for a yes or no answer. Many practitioners, in an attempt to hurry the interview, will guide the patient in his answers by how they ask the questions. A yes or no response may reflect only a portion of what the patient may really want to say. The questioning process should use open-ended rather than closed-ended questions to allow the patient to answer in his own words. Instead of asking, "Do you have pain?" the question could be phrased, "Where do you have discomfort?" The second question requires the patient to formulate his own answer and will probably yield more useful information than the first question. This approach helps keep the examiner from jumping to conclusions and attends to the patient as a person and not as a disease entity.

While taking the history and performing the evaluation, the clinician should record the findings in a form that is easy to interpret and familiar to other health professionals. The SOAP (subjective, objective, assessment, and plan) note format meets these criteria. It can be used for initial evaluations, progress notes, and discharge summaries. Although notes are important for communicating with other professionals, this record is also invaluable to the clinician as a quick reference on each patient.

The patient's chief complaint or complaints should be documented carefully. Initially the patient should be allowed to tell his own story for several minutes without interruption; otherwise, important details may be pushed aside in his mind. The clinician may then need to guide the patient's comments with a question such as, "How did your neck problem begin?" in order to get a chronologic picture of the symptoms. The clinician needs to ask open-ended questions to find out important details about the symptoms such as the time of day they occur, the location of the pain, and the relation of symptoms to other events. For evaluating the cervical and upper thoracic spine, the clinician should follow the general rule of evaluating the joints above and below the joint being examined and should ask questions concerning the cranium, the TMJ, and the shoulder. The actual analysis of the patient's symptoms follows a logical sequence for any musculoskeletal evaluation.

Locating the Complaint

Locating the patient's cervical pain is a logical introduction to establishing rapport between the therapist and the patient. The total area in which the pain is felt needs to be documented; the area and depth of symptoms should be mapped out on a body chart for future reference. The patient should also be questioned about the type of pain. Typically, superficial electric shock-like pain is from a dermatomal reference; deep aching pain may be from either a myotomal or a sclerotomal reference.[43] Upper extremity numbness or tingling may help implicate a specific nerve root involvement.

Present History

Current history needs to be established before past history. The examiner should consider the precipitating factors related to the onset of current symptoms. Again, the patient should have the opportunity to say what he thinks may have caused the problem before the clinician begins systematic questioning. If a specific injury occurred, the clinician should try to determine the exact mechanism of injury. The clinician should also ask about the onset (whether immediate or delayed) and the degree of pain. This information will assist in implicating specific tissues. For example, injured muscle or vascular tissue will cause immediate pain, whereas injury to noncontractile structures may cause delayed onset of symptoms.[59] This information will allow the clinician to focus on what special tests should be performed during the examination.

Behavior of Symptoms

Asking the patient to describe his symptoms over a 24-hour period is valuable in establishing what activities aggravate or relieve the symptoms and how long the symptoms last, and also provides a baseline for future comparison. The clinician needs to know about the frequency and duration of the patient's symptoms, that is, whether they are constant or intermittent. If dysfunction is present, specific movements should exacerbate or relieve the symptoms, and rest should decrease them. The answers to the clinician's questions will reveal what positions, movements, and activities exacerbate the pain and provide additional information about the nature of the problem, the tissue source of irritation, and the severity of the condition. If rest does not relieve the symptoms, and the patient describes them as constant and unrelenting, the cause of the problem may well be other than musculoskeletal.

Past History

If the patient has experienced similar symptoms in the past, that information is vital to the examiner. Clear information about the frequency and onset of symptoms, the recovery period, and the treatment of previous episodes will help establish the correct diagnosis and treatment plan. Other past medical history such as cardiac problems and current medication may also be pertinent and affect treatment plans.

Systemic History

The patient's current symptoms can be easily influenced by visceral or neurologic involvement; therefore, the clinician needs to ask questions concerning gastrointestinal function, including recent weight loss, abdominal pain, change in bowel habits, or blood in the stool. Questions dealing with the genitourinary system include asking about polyuria, dysuria, blood in the urine, or problems with sexual function or menses. Questions pertaining to the cardiopulmonary systems include asking about ease of breathing, coughing, palpitations, hemoptysis, and chest pain. To rule out central nervous system disorders, the clinician should ask about lack of coordination, seizures, dizziness, tremors, and headaches.

All of the above information will give the practitioner a general idea about the patient's problems. However, the specific questions asked of patients presenting with cervical complaints will not only give information about the problem but also help rule out more serious pathologies.

1. Is the patient experiencing any headaches? Numerous disorders can cause headache; headaches from cervical spine problems, however, usually present with specific referral patterns. Problems at the first cervical level usually cause headaches in a characteristic pattern to the base and top of the head. The second cervical level tends to refer ipsilateral pain retro-orbitally in the temporal region. Lower cervical problems will frequently refer to the base of the occiput.[59]
2. Is the patient experiencing dizziness, especially upon rotation or extension of the spine? These symptoms may be due to vertebral artery occlusion or inner ear disorders.[60] Disorders of the cervical spine can also cause vertigo.[61]
3. Is the patient experiencing bilateral numbness or tingling of the hands or feet? Bilateral symptoms should lead the therapist to suspect either a large space-occupying lesion pressing on the spinal cord or a systemic disorder causing neuropathies, such as diabetes or alcohol abuse.[57]

4. Does the patient experience difficulty in swallowing? Anterior space-occupying lesions can cause retropharyngeal compromise. With a history of trauma, swelling may be the space-occupying lesion.[57]
5. Does the patient experience any electric shock-like pain? If the head is flexed and the patient experiences such pain down the spine, the therapist should consider the possibility of inflammation or irritation of the meninges (Lhermitte's sign).[41,57]
6. What kind of pillow does the patient sleep on? Cervical symptoms are often increased when a foam or very firm pillow is used, as a result of loss of cervical lordosis or abnormal pressure placed against the neck due to lack of support.[16]

Objective Testing

In addition to the upper quarter screening examination, the clinician needs specific objective information about the cervical spine. This information allows the practitioner to confirm the subjective findings and inculpate the area causing the patient's symptoms. Further, more specialized objective testing will help isolate the structure or structures at fault. As mentioned in the section on patient history, according to the upper quarter screen format, the TMJ, shoulder, and thoracic spine joints should be cleared during the cervical spine examination. The neurologic examination should include muscle stretch reflexes; sensation testing incorporating light touch, pinprick, and two-point discrimination; and specific muscle testing if weakness was found in the screening examination. The following special tests need to be performed only if warranted by patient history or findings during the upper quarter screen (Table 5-4).

Functional Active Testing

Several combined active movements can alert the practitioner to regions of the cervical spine that may be restricted. For example, in assessing the movement of the upper cervical spine, the OA joint can be grossly tested by fully rotating the cervical spine and asking the patient to nod his head while the clinician looks for asymmetrical movement between

Table 5-4. Schematic for Objective Examination of the Cervical and Upper Thoracic Spine

ROM Tests	Special Tests	Thoracic Inlet Syndrome Tests
Active ROM of cervical and upper thoracic spine	Cervical distraction	Adson's
Functional OA ROM	Cervical compression	Costoclavicular
Functional AA ROM	Vertebral artery	Hyperabduction
Foraminal closure Upper cervical Mid- and lower cervical	Layer palpation Transverse process Spatial orientation, upper thoracic spine	3-Minute elevated arm exercise
Passive mobility Translation OA, AA, midcervical Transverse process positioning through flexion/extension in upper thoracic spine Spring testing of ribs	Trigger points Neurologic examination Motor testing Sensation testing Muscle stretch reflexes	
Active respiratory motion	Radiographs	

ROM, range of motion.

sides (Fig. 5-7). A gross test of the AA joint is to ask the patient to sidebend as far as possible and, while sidebent, rotate the head in the opposite direction; the clinician looks for restricted movement (Richard Erhard, personal communication) (Fig. 5-8). To test motion in the midcervical spine, ask the patient to sidebend the head and, while maintaining that range, introduce flexion and extension. These tests only tell the practitioner whether further mobility testing is required.

In addition to these tests of combined functional movements, the clinician should test the normal active movements in the cardinal planes. If active movements are full and painfree, introduce over-pressure to further stress the structures in order to clear that specific range of motion. Observation of active cervical movements will give the clinician a general impression of movement dysfunctions. For example, active sidebending that is restricted in the first few degrees from neutral suggests a restriction in the upper cervical complex. In contrast, restriction at the end of sidebending suggests a restriction in the mid- to lower cervical region.[62]

Foraminal Closure Tests

Combined cervical rotation and sidebending to the same side together with extension narrows the intervertebral foramen and puts the mid- and lower cervical facet joints in the closed-packed position.[4,35,62] If this maneuver reproduces the patient's

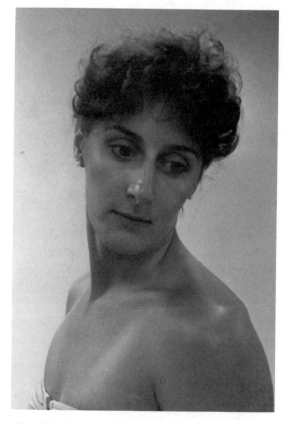

Fig. 5-7. Functional active testing of the OA joint.

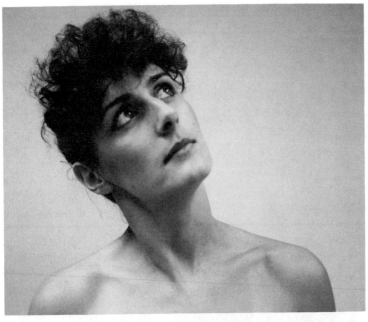

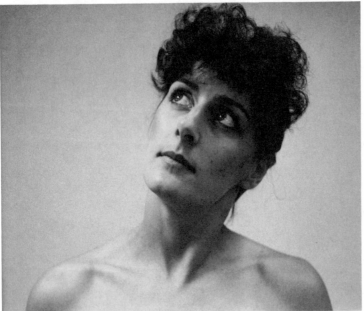

Fig. 5-8. Functional active testing of AA joint.

symptoms (i.e., neck, interscapular or upper arm pain), the cervical spine is implicated (Fig. 5-9). With respect to referred pain, the more distally the pain is referred from the cervical spine, the more impressive the test. To test the upper cervical spine, the neck is held in normal lordosis while actively backward bending the upper cervical complex and maintaining that position[62] (Fig. 5-10). If the patient's symptoms are reproduced, the test is positive.

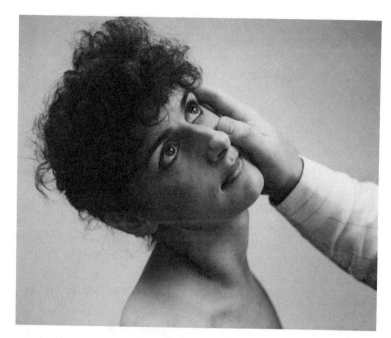

Fig. 5-9. Mid- and lower cervical foraminal closure test.

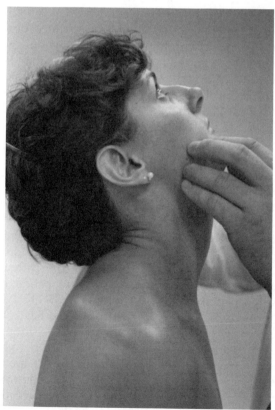

Fig. 5-10. Upper cervical foraminal closure test.

Cervical Compression/ Distraction Tests

The cervical compression test is performed by placing the head in slight flexion and sidebending and exerting a downward compressive force through the head[58] (Fig. 5-11). To further test the integrity of bony and soft tissue relationships, place the neck into a combined movement pattern of sidebending, extension, and rotation in the same direction and exert a compression force. This variation is done if the first procedure has not produced any symptoms. If no symptoms are produced by placing the neck into a closed-packed position and then exerting a compression force, the clinician can be satisfied that no major pathology exists. By approximating the articular surfaces, the compression test assesses foraminal patency and joint relationships. If a motion segment loses its normal anatomic spatial relationships, pain-sensitive tissue may be compromised. Therefore, the compression test is positive if this maneuver elicits articular or neural signs. Conversely, a distraction force, which separates the joint surfaces and stretches the adjacent soft tissues, should decrease symptoms from a tissue that was being compromised by compression. A cervical dis-

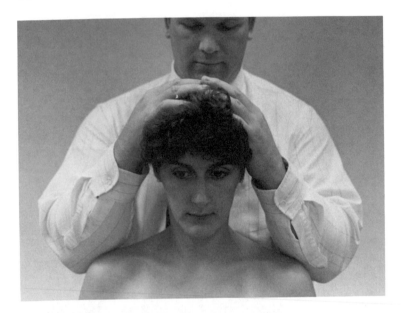

Fig. 5-11. Cervical compression test.

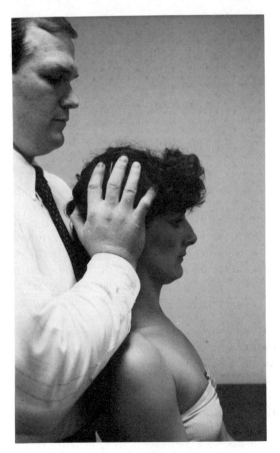

Fig. 5-12. Cervical distraction test.

traction test is performed by having the seated patient lean against the clinician, who stands behind the patient. The clinician lightly grasps the patient's head over the mastoid processes and, while maintaining the head and neck in a neutral position, lifts the patient's head so that the patient's body weight provides the distraction. This distraction test is positive when the patient's symptoms are decreased[59] (Fig. 5-12).

Vertebral Artery Test

Provocative testing of vertebrobasilar sufficiency is necessary if the head is going to be moved through extremes of motion. The vertebral artery should be tested in both a weightbearing and a nonweightbearing position.[20] The weightbearing position is done with the patient seated; place the patient's head in a neutral position and have the patient actively rotate the head to both sides (Fig. 5-13). If no symptoms are produced, then place the head and neck in extension and have the patient go through active rotation. If active movement does not produce symptoms, then the examiner slowly moves the head passively, asking the patient to report any symptoms experienced during the test. The nonweightbearing test is performed with the patient supine, the head supported by the examiner off the

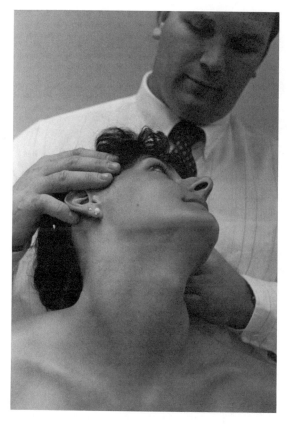

Fig. 5-13. Weightbearing vertebral artery test.

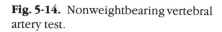

Fig. 5-14. Nonweightbearing vertebral artery test.

edge of the table. From this position, the head is passively extended and rotated to each side (Fig. 5-14). This position of extension and rotation is maintained for 10 to 15 seconds while the examiner observes the patient's eye movements (nystagmus) and looks for asymmetric pupil changes, and the patient reports any unusual sensations such as dizziness, giddiness, lightheadedness, or visual changes.[1,20] A variation of this test is to have the patient count backward out loud. If the patient has diminished blood flow, he will usually stop talking before other symptoms are manifested.

Upper Limb Tension Test

Elvy[63] demonstrated on cadavers during autopsy that movement of and tension on cervical nerve roots, their investing sheaths, and the dura occur with movement of the arm in certain planes. The maximum tension on the brachial plexus, C5, C6, and C7 nerve root complexes occurs with glenohumeral joint horizontal abduction and external rotation, elbow extension and wrist extension, forearm supination, shoulder girdle depression, and side-bending of the cervical spine to the opposite side. The upper limb tension test, also known as the brachial plexus tension sign, reproduces this stretch by positioning the patient supine with the arm placed into horizontal abduction and external rota-

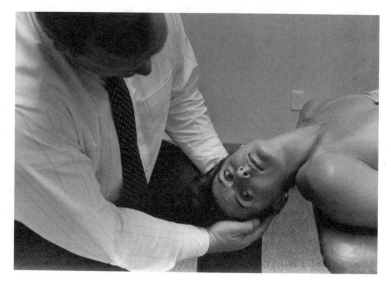

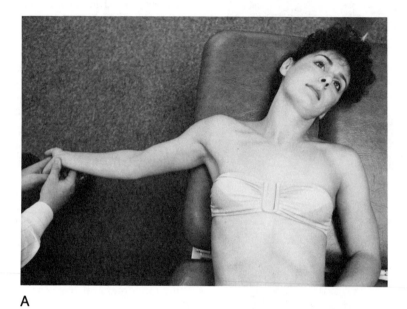

A

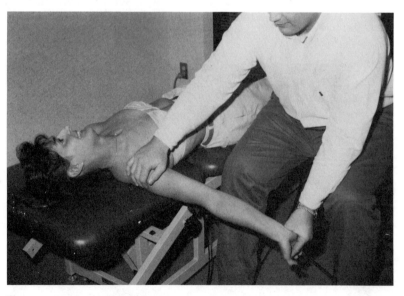

B

Fig. 5-15. Upper limb tension test. **(A)** Top view; **(B)** side view. The scapula should be depressed more than it is in these photographs.

tion at the glenohumeral joint while maintaining the shoulder girdle in a depressed position. The elbow joint is then passively extended with the wrist in extension and the forearm supinated. The cervical spine may be positioned in opposite sidebending to verify the results of the test by increasing tension on the nerve roots when a condition is relatively less sensitive to nerve root compression (Fig. 5-15). Magary[64] reported that in performing this test, when sidebending of the neck was toward the side of the arm being tested, the patient's symptoms decreased 70 percent of the time. This test assists the clinician in identifying the source of vague or recalcitrant shoulder or upper arm pain. If this maneuver reproduces the patient's arm pain, the test can be broken down into its parts to see which component actually insults the brachial plexus.[64,65]

Passive Mobility Testing

In addition to the physical examination of the cervical spine, the clinician needs to be able to assess passive motion from a manual medicine viewpoint. To understand the passive movement of the cervical spine, a review of spinal mechanics is appropriate.

Vertebral motion is described by facet function; however, the intervertebral disk and soft tissues also participate in motion. The motion available was described by Fryette[66] in terms of three basic laws of motion: The first law states that when the anteroposterior curve is in a neutral position (where facets are not engaged), sidebending to one side is accompanied by rotation to the opposite side. This law is in effect in typical thoracic and lumbar spines. The second law states that when the anteroposterior curve is flexed or extended, sidebending and rotation occur in the same direction. This law is seen exclusively in the typical cervical spinal segment and is in effect in the typical thoracic and lumbar spine. When motion is introduced in one direction, motion in all other directions is restricted. This is Fryette's third law. This law is evident when rotation in a forward head posture is compared with rotation with the head aligned over the trunk. Even though rotation occurs in the horizontal plane, rotation will be restricted with a forward head posture because of the accentuation of flexion of the lower cervical and extension of the upper cervical spine.[29,30]

Motion can be described in terms of the superior vertebra moving on the inferior vertebra of a motion segment. In the cervical spine, passive movement can be evaluated by using translation in the frontal plane. By sidegliding a cervical vertebra, the clinician imparts a sidebending force. For example, with left sideglide of C4 on C5, a right sidebending movement occurs. Since sidebending and rotation occur concomitantly, the clinician is also assessing rotation to the right. This translation maneuver allows the operator to assess quantity of movement as well as end-feel resistance. Since rotation and sidebending occur in the same direction in the midcervical spine, the ability to sidebend and rotate must be determined both in flexion and in extension. By comparing translation to the right and to the left, the clinician can assess the total movement available at that segment.[67]

Restricted motion can be described either by the location of the superior segment in space or by the motion that is restricted. The location or position of the superior segment is described using the past participle, for example extended, flexed, rotated, and sidebent. The suffixes used for physiologic motion restriction are flexion, extension, rotation, and sidebending. For example, when describing C4 vertebral motion on C5 for right sidebending, the right inferior articular process of C4 biomechanically would glide inferiorly and posteriorly on the superior articular process of C5. At the same time, the left inferior articular process of C4 would glide anteriorly and superiorly on the superior articular process of C5 (Fig. 5-16). If right sidebending is restricted, the superior segment (C4) would be left sidebent or in a relative position of left sidebending. The positional diagnosis would be described in terms of the restriction in three planes. If right sidebending was restricted, then right rotation at that segment would also be restricted, since rotation and sidebending are concomitant movements in the midcervical spine. The motion in the sagittal plane that would cause the superior segment to glide down and back is extension.

At this point, the clinician assessing a patient with a right sidebending restriction at C4–C5 would not be able to ascertain whether the restriction is at the right or the left facet. However, by testing active movements, the clinician may be able to determine

NECK EXTENDED TO LEVEL

Restricted.
Ⓛ facet not able to glide down and back.

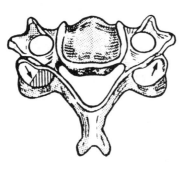

Not restricted since both facets able to move.

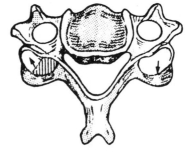

➡️ Translate right   ⬅️ Translate left

NECK FLEXED

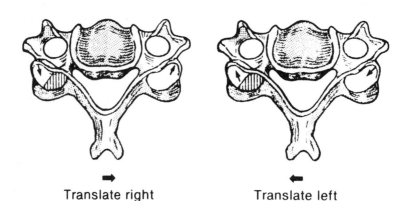

➡️ Translate right   ⬅️ Translate left

THE FACETS IN OPEN POSITION ARE ABLE TO GLIDE BOTH DIRECTIONS FREELY.

DX: FRS(R) with minor motion restriction.

↓ Arrows show direction of superior facet moving on inferior facet.

Ⓦ Shows area of joint restriction (loss of range).

Fig. 5-16. Translation of C4 on C5 illustrating motion barrier.

which facet is restricted. For example, a patient who has restricted and painful right sidebending will probably also have restricted and painful right rotation. Evaluating extension and flexion will help determine right or left involvement. If the right facet is unable to go through its full active range of motion, then extension movement will also be restricted; however, if the left facet is unable to glide up and forward, then flexion will be restricted and painful. In theory, this presentation is plausible; however, patients do not always present in this classic mode since accommodation for loss of active movement can be accomplished at adjacent segments.[36]

When discerning the loss of passive mobility, feeling the end-feel resistance will assist the examiner in determining what tissue or structure may be limiting the range of motion. Describing the end-feel as a barrier that is restricting motion may be helpful. This restriction may be due to one or more factors: skin, fascia, muscle, ligament, joint capsule, joint surface, or loose bodies. The examiner must be able to differentiate normal from abnormal barriers. A normal barrier at the limit of active motion will have a resiliency to passive movement that is caused by stretch of muscle and fascia. If the examiner imparts a passive stretch to the anatomic limits of the tissue, a harder end-feel will be noted. Passive stretch beyond the anatomic limits will result in violation of the tissue—a ligamentous tear, a fracture, or a dislocation. By learning to recognize normal restriction to passive movement, the examiner can identify resistance within the normal limits of cervical range of motion. With practice, the examiner can objectively assess and quantify this resistance.[68] (For more information on end-feels, see Chapter 6.)

For the purpose of passive motion testing, the cervical spine can be divided into atypical cervical joints (i.e., the OA and AA joints) and the typical cervical joints from the inferior surface of C2 to C7. In testing the OA joint, the examiner holds the patient's head between his or her palms and thenar muscles while using the index fingers to palpate for movement of the atlas. This position will assure the operator that movement is localized between the occiput and the atlas. By introducing translatory movement, sidebending can now be assessed. If the OA joint is localized in flexion by acutely tipping

the head forward, translation can be performed both to the right and to the left. Flexion of the neck and right translatory movement of the head tests for restriction of flexion, left sidebending, and right rotation. The motion restriction is felt when resistance is encountered during the translatory movement. To test for backward bending restriction, the OA joint is localized by acutely tipping the head upward, making sure that extension has not occurred below the level of the atlas. From this position, translatory movement is introduced to each side (Fig. 5-17). The examiner is testing the ability of the OA joint to produce extension together with sidebending-rotation movement to opposite sides. Backward bending and translation to the left tests for extension, right sidebending, and left rotation movement of the occiput at the atlas. These four maneuvers, translating the head to the right and left in both the flexed and extended positions, test for all of the motion restrictions found within the OA joint.[67]

Since rotation is the primary motion available at the AA joint, passive mobility evaluation of this joint will be confined to testing rotation.[6] To test rotation at C1–C2, the head is flexed in an attempt to block as much rotational movement as possible in the typical cervical spine, and rotation is then introduced to the right and to the left until resistance is encountered. If resistance is encountered before the expected end range, a presumptive diagnosis of limited rotation of the atlas on the axis can be made.[67]

To test for movement of the typical cervical segments (C2–C7), translation is performed in the flexed and extended positions. For testing purposes, the examiner palpates the articular pillars of the segment to be tested. Then the cervical spine is either flexed or extended to the level being tested followed by translation to the right or the left. With the examiner's palpating fingers on the articular pillars of C2, the head is carried into extension, and right translation is introduced until C3 begins to move under the examiner's finger. This tests the ability of the left C2–C3 facet joint to close (extension, left sidebending, and left rotation). The segment is also evaluated in flexion with right and left translation (Fig. 5-18). These translatory movements can be repeated at all remaining cervical segments.[67]

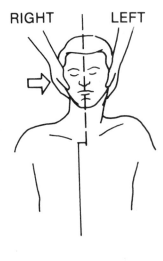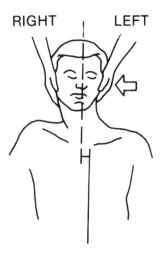

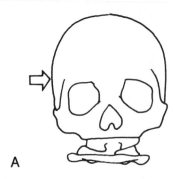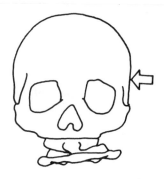

A

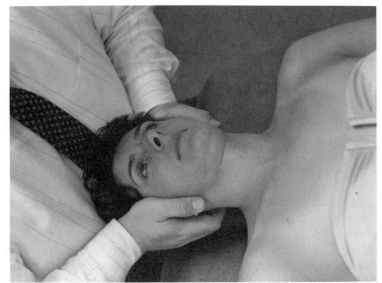

B

Fig. 5-17. **(A)** OA joint translation; **(B)** Translation of the OA joint in extension.

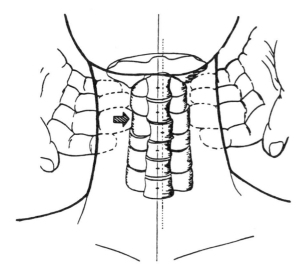

Fig. 5-18. Hand positioning for translation of the midcervical spine (C3 on C4).

The upper thoracic spine can be assessed for motion restriction by locating the transverse processes of a vertebral segment and determining their position in space through full flexion and extension. Using the second thoracic vertebra, the examiner's thumbs are placed on each transverse process, and, during forward and backward bending, the excursion of the paired transverse processes is assessed. If, during forward bending, the examiner notes that the right transverse becomes more prominent, and

with backward bending the two transverse processes become more equal, then the right facet is closed and cannot open. When the right facet is restricted in the closed position and is unable to open, that segment has restriction of forward bending, left sidebending, and left rotation.[30]

The upper ribs can also be assessed for their ability to move symmetrically. If the thoracic spine has been assessed and determined to be moving normally, then any asymmetrical motion of the ribs would be considered rib dysfunction. Two methods to assess restricted rib motion are springing of the ribcage and evaluating rib motion during full inspiration and expiration. Springing the thoracic cage is a gross measure of mobility; a resistance to spring alerts the examiner to dysfunction within that area of the ribcage. The second method is determining the key rib limiting the ability of the ribcage to produce an anteroposterior (pump handle) and a mediolateral (bucket handle) excursion. This test is performed by the examiner placing both open hands over the anterior chest wall, with the index fingers touching the clavicles. The patient is instructed to take a deep breath, and the examiner assesses the ability of the ribcage to move symmetrically throughout the pump handle motion (Fig. 5-19). If one side of the ribcage stops moving before the other, that restricted side is the dysfunctional side. To assess the bucket handle motion, the examiner places both cupped hands inferior to the clavi-

Fig. 5-19. Assessing upper ribcage pump handle motion.

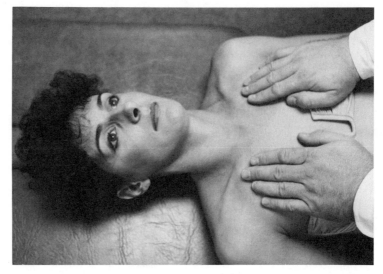

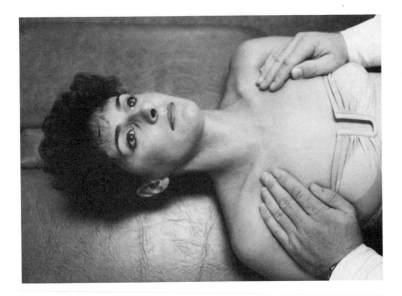

Fig. 5-20. Assessing upper ribcage bucket handle motion.

cle but superior to the nipple line. Again, asymmetrical motion is assessed during inspiration, and the side that stops first is considered the restricted side (Fig. 5-20). Although pump handle movement is the major motion in the upper ribcage, restrictions of bucket handle movement will be greater and easier to detect than the pump handle movement.[30] Then the examiner's fingers are placed on the first rib to determine if that is the segment that is restricting inhalation. Each segment is assessed until the level of asymmetry is found. That level is considered the key rib limiting motion (Fig. 5-21). Exhalation is assessed in the same manner; the side that stops moving first is considered restricted, and the key rib is then identified starting inferiorly and moving superiorly.[30]

Thoracic Inlet Tests

Many tests have been described to assess compromise of the thoracic inlet. The following provoca-

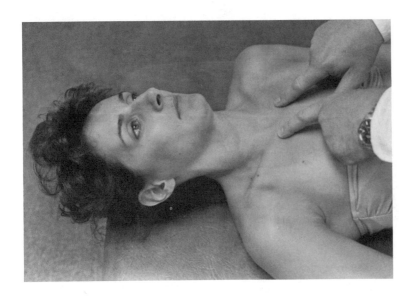

Fig. 5-21. Determining the key rib restrictor in pump handle movement.

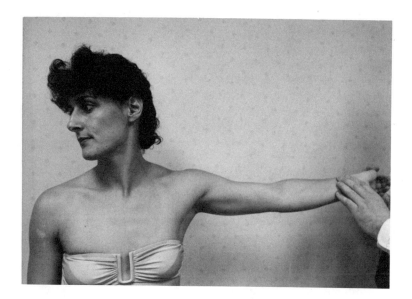

Fig. 5-22. Adson's test for thoracic inlet syndrome.

tive tests—the Adson's, costoclavicular, hyperabduction, and 3-minute elevated arm exercise tests—have been identified as the most sensitive in locating the site of the compromise. The Adson's test evaluates the anterior scalene muscle's role in compression of the subclavian artery. This test is performed by holding the arm parallel to the floor, turning the head first away and then toward the arm while holding a deep breath. Meanwhile the examiner monitors the radial pulse; a positive test is indicated by an obliteration or decrease in the pulse rate as well as reproduction of the patient's symptoms[69] (Fig. 5-22).

The costoclavicular test or exaggerated military position has been described as compressing the subclavian vessels and/or the brachial plexus in the narrow space between the first rib and the clavicle. To perform this test, the subject is seated with the arms held comfortably at the sides; the shoulder girdle is then retracted and depressed. Simultaneously the examiner monitors for a change in the radial pulse. A positive test is indicated by an obliteration of or decrease in pulse rate and/or onset of symptoms[70] (Fig. 5-23).

The hyperabduction maneuver involves passive circumduction of the upper extremity overhead while the examiner monitors the radial pulse. As with the Adson's test, this test is considered positive if the pulse rate changes and/or symptoms are elicited[71] (Fig. 5-24). The 3-minute elevated arm exercise test is performed with the patient seated, arms abducted and elbows flexed 90 degrees, and the shoulder girdle slightly retracted. The patient is then asked to open and close his fists slowly and steadily for a full 3 minutes. The examiner watches for dropping of the elevated arms or decreased exercise rate before onset of the patient's symptoms. Roos stated that this test evaluates involvement of all the neurovascular structures, and a positive test is indicated by the patient's inability to complete the full 3 minutes as well as the onset of symptoms[72] (Fig. 5-25).

Palpation

Cyriax[43] has advocated doing palpation as the last part of an examination to preclude premature conclusions and incomplete examinations. However, in testing passive cervical mobility, the examiner is also getting information on tissue tensions and specific structures. A thorough knowledge of cervical anatomy is necessary in order to perform a complete palpation examination. The examiner must view the anatomy in three dimensions before palpating any anatomic structure. Structures should be palpated from their origin to their insertion. Many structures cannot be differentiated when tissues are healthy; however, pathologically altered tissue can usually

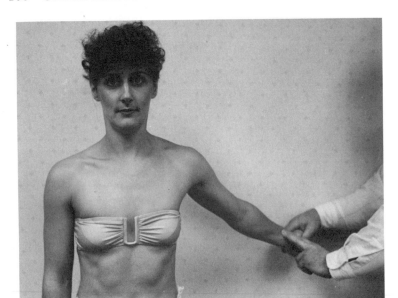

Fig. 5-23. Costoclavicular test for thoracic inlet syndrome.

be distinguished. The ability to palpate anatomic structures, especially in the cervical spine, takes hours of practice and concentration. The examiner should always palpate by layers, identifying every structure in one layer before attempting to palpate deeper structures. If the examiner has a good mental picture of all the muscles, ligaments, and soft tissues in the cervical area, he or she can identify individual structures.[1]

Palpation gives the examiner information about the size, consistency, temperature, and location of a structure, and about swelling, bony changes, or soft tissue changes such as nodules or scar tissue. Crepitus of bony surfaces can be easily detected, and tem-

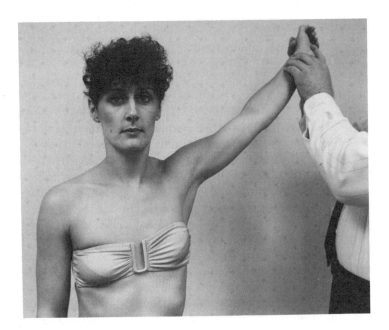

Fig. 5-24. Hyperabduction maneuver for thoracic inlet syndrome.

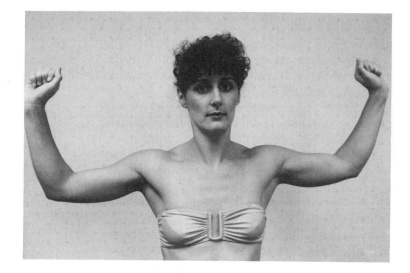

Fig. 5-25. Three-minute elevated arm exercise test for thoracic inlet syndrome.

perature changes can be appreciated. All of these clinical findings are important objective information. Palpation and point tenderness are viewed in terms of the patient's sensation, but more importantly the objective sensation of the examiner (what the examiner "feels") should be guided by sound anatomic knowledge and adequate application of pressure with regard to area, force, and direction. The clinician must remember, however, that point tenderness of a structure may also provide misinformation. Palpation should be done only after the tissue at fault has been identified by testing function. Treating point tenderness without identifying and treating the cause of the symptom is not an acceptable treatment approach.[43]

Correlation of Findings

After completing the objective examination, the clinician should be able to make assumptions about possible pathology or movement dysfunction that are corroborated by both the subjective and objective findings. The evaluation process depends on the clinician making inferences based on his or her knowledge and experience as well as the information obtained in the history and examination. The clinician's inferences are the basis for appropriate clinical decision making. With the information received from the patient and the objective examination, the clinician is now able to establish meaningful short- and long-term goals and to plan treatment to meet those goals.

TREATMENT

A complete, detailed description of treatment procedures for all cervical spine problems is beyond the scope of this chapter; rather, the intent is to alert the clinician to the various treatment procedures that are available.

Modalities

The decision to employ physical agents must be based on appropriate treatment goals; however, the use of physical agents alone will rarely alleviate the cause of the patient's complaints. Mennell[25] stated that the only problems that are "cured" by physical therapy are rickets treated with ultraviolet therapy and joint dysfunction treated with joint mobilization.[58] As with the rest of the spine, heat is still used as the treatment of choice for acute cervical problems, when in fact cryotherapy is more effective in acute situations to decrease pain, swelling, and muscle spasm.[73] Aside from these acute situations, any modality including both superficial and deep heat, electricity, and cold laser can be used as an adjunct therapy to decrease pain, promote relaxation, or to prepare the tissues prior to other therapeutic procedures.

Traction

Mechanical or manual traction of the cervical spine separates the cervical spine, affecting both articular and periarticular structures. Mechanical traction allows the clinician to give a specific poundage of traction over a given time, whereas manual traction allows the therapist to better localize the traction to the vertebral segments affected and requires less time for treatment. In setting up cervical traction, the therapist must be aware of several factors: the weight of the head, the angle of pull, the position of the patient, and the poundage of the traction pull. An accurate knowledge of these components is necessary to control in a particular direction the stress that is being applied to the cervical spine and soft tissues.[74,75] As a precaution, traction is usually initiated at a relatively low poundage and directed to the vertebral segments involved; therefore, a standard position for placing the cervical spine is not appropriate. Since most movement is achieved when a joint is positioned in its midrange, actual distraction will vary depending on the segment being treated. The OA and AA joints should be treated in a neutral or a slightly extended head and neck position.[76] By introducing more flexion, lower cervical spine segments can be isolated.[74]

Research reveals that traction forces above 20 pounds separate the vertebrae by 1 to 1.5 cm per space, with the greatest separation occurring posteriorly as flexion is increased. The normal cervical lordosis is eradicated with traction forces of 20 to 25 pounds. At a constant angle, a traction force of 50 pounds produces greater separation than 30 pounds, but the amount of separation is not significantly different at 7, 30, or 60 seconds.[75] Intermittent traction produces twice as much separation as sustained traction. If separation of vertebral bodies is desired, high traction forces for short periods of time will achieve that goal. When traction forces are removed, restoration of normal dimensions is four to five times quicker in the posterior structures; restoration anteriorly is much slower. As would be expected, less separation occurs in 50-year-olds than in normal 20-year-olds.[77-79]

The behavior of patient symptoms during traction is important, especially if the symptoms decrease. If traction reduces the patient's symptoms, there is no guarantee that the symptoms will remain relieved following treatment; however, relief of symptoms during treatment is a good prognostic sign that traction will be of benefit for that patient.

Soft Tissue Mobilization

Regardless of the cervical spine pathology, the clinician must always consider the soft tissue component of the problem. If body parts have maintained an abnormal relationship for some time, following Wolff's law,[80] soft tissue will adapt accordingly (see Chapter 1). All soft tissues must be recognized: skin, fascia, capsule, and muscle. Several soft tissue mobilization procedures are available and include stretching, myofascial release, fluoromethane spray and stretch, rolfing, deep massage, strain-counterstrain,[81] and craniosacral therapy.[82]

Joint Mobilization

Indications for joint mobilization include loss of active and passive range of motion, joint asymmetry, and tissue texture abnormality. Passive mobility testing during the evaluation will identify the joints to be treated. Chapter 6 discusses specific direct techniques such as oscillations, articulations, and muscle energy techniques. Indirect techniques such as strain-counterstrain, functional technique, and craniosacral therapy are also available.

Therapeutic Exercise

Active rehabilitation is of vital importance for restoration of function; however, patients cannot typically "work out" neck pain. An appropriate treatment plan progression should include restoration of normal, painless joint range of motion followed by correction of muscle weakness or imbalance, resumption of normal activities, and then prevention of recurrent problems. Too often treatment ends after normal, painfree motion is restored. Exercise restores adequate control of movement, and increased muscle strength provides increased dynamic support to the spine.

The choice of specific exercises is just as important as the decision to initiate postural exercise. The spinal musculature, which is comprised mainly of slow-twitch oxidative muscle fibers, has a role in maintaining body relationships. Following restoration of normal muscle length, appropriate strengthening exercise should include isometric and endurance activities.

Supports

Cervical collars and supports do have their place in treatment program planning; however, they are appropriate only in acute conditions and in segmental instability. The amount of external support needed should be dictated by the objective examination.

SUMMARY

A complete evaluation of the cervical spine must begin with a thorough understanding of its functional anatomy and biomechanics. With this background, the examiner will have a clear mental picture of the structures and the interdependency of the structures being examined. However, this mental image is sharpened and honed only with study, practice, and experience. The clinician must address all potential sources of the patient's complaints, which may go beyond just the physical sources. Psychological and psychosocial factors can play an important role in the patient's symptoms. A detailed discussion of all cervical and upper thoracic spine pathology is beyond the scope of this chapter; however, the clinician must always remember that not all cervical symptoms are musculoskeletal in origin. Those patients whose pain is not musculoskeletal in origin should be referred to the appropriate physician for further evaluation.

The cervical and upper thoracic spine is indeed complex, and no two patients are alike. Each patient presenting with cervical and upper thoracic pain must be evaluated according to his own signs and symptoms.

CASE STUDY

Rarely does the clinical presentation of cervical pain have a single underlying cause. The following case study describing an actual patient is a typical example of this point.

Subjective Examination

A 32-year-old Latin American woman presented to physical therapy with complaints of cervical-thoracic pain referring into the left upper extremity. She had been working as a computer word processing secretary; her symptoms started 6 months ago. She reported no specific incident that might have brought on her symptoms, except for sitting at a computer terminal 5 hours a day.

The patient's chief complaints were stiffness and pain in the posterior neck, traveling along the trapezial ridge into the left superior and lateral shoulder. She described a numbness along the lateral upper arm, forearm, and ulnar side of the left hand. The symptoms in her left upper extremity were aggravated when she attempted to lift a heavy object or use her arms over head. Her upper back pain was irritated when she sneezed. She related difficulty sleeping at night, with inability to find a comfortable position; she was using a down feather pillow.

Over a 24-hour period, the patient noticed stiffness on awakening in the morning, and as the day progressed, she would only experience discomfort if she was very active or sat too long (35 minutes or more) at the computer terminal without getting up.

Past history revealed a similar episode of pain in 1978, which lasted over 1½ years after she began working at a word processing machine. When she was promoted and no longer worked at a word processor, her symptoms disappeared. She had experienced no neck symptoms since that initial episode until this episode. She related a history of trauma to the cervicothoracic region 11 years ago when she fell off a motorcycle, landing directly on her buttocks. Ten months ago she fell down one flight of stairs with minimal musculoskeletal complaints. She denied any history of bowel or bladder dysfunction, headaches, dizziness, difficulty swallowing, weight loss, or being pregnant.

The patient was not currently being treated for any other medical condition, although she did have an epigastric hernia repair 6 years ago. She reported that stress plays an important role in how she feels; she noticed a direct relationship between increased stress and exacerbation of her symptoms. In her current job, she noticed less cervical pain after her boss bought her a Pos Chair (Congleton Workplace Systems, Inc., College Station, TX), which improved her head and neck alignment.

Objective Examination

The patient presented in no acute distress, but with guarded upper quarter movement. She had a forward head posture with rounding of the shoulder girdle complex. Active range of motion of both upper extremities was within normal limits; however, extreme elevation of the arms increased discomfort in the cervicothoracic region. Active range of motion of the cervical spine was restricted in left rotation (30 percent) and left sidebending (25 percent). Right rotation was full but produced pain along the left upper trapezius ridge. Backward bending was within normal limits but produced discomfort in the posterior neck region. Forward bending was restricted, with two fingerbreadths' distance between the chin and the anterior chest wall at maximum flexion. Right sidebending was full and painfree.

Neurologic testing revealed 2+ muscle stretch reflexes in both upper extremities. Sensation to light touch, pinprick, and two-point discrimination was intact in the upper quarter. Gross muscle testing revealed weakness in the following muscles: left biceps brachii, good minus (4-/5), and left triceps brachii, good (4/5). The triceps muscle contraction appeared to give way secondary to the pain felt by the patient in her cervicothoracic region.

Several special tests revealed positive findings. The foraminal closure test (quadrant) was positive for the lower cervical spine on the left and produced pain along the upper trapezius, and on the left the pain was reproduced in the right neck region. Left upper limb tension test was slightly positive with reproduction of neck and shawl pain. A cervical compression test was negative. A cervical distraction test decreased the patient's neck and shoulder pain. A vertebral artery test was negative. Clearing tests for the temporomandibular joint, shoulder, elbow, wrist, and hand were unequivocal.

Radiographs taken at the time of the examination revealed a flattening of the midcervical spine lordosis and posterior spurring of the vertebral body at the C4–C5 level, with foraminal encroachment at C4–C5 greater on the right than on the left (Fig. 5-26).

Passive mobility testing demonstrated restrictions at the left OA joint with translation to the left in flexion (extended, rotated right, sidebent left). The right AA joint was restricted with passive rotation to the right with the neck bent fully forward (rotated left). Translation of the cervical spine from C2 to C7 revealed restriction at the C2–C3, C4–C5, C5–C6, and C6–C7 levels. Translation of the C2–C3 level to the left in extension (flexed, rotated left, sidebent left) was diminished. The C4–C5, C5–C6, C6–C7 levels were restricted in translation to the right in extension (flexed, rotated right, sidebent right). Asymmetry of the upper thoracic region was revealed by palpation of the transverse processes at the T1–T2 and T2–T3 levels. The transverse process at T1 was more posterior on the left in flexion of the head and upper trunk (extended, rotated left, sidebent left) than when the neck and trunk were placed in extension. The T2 transverse process was more prominent on the right in flexion (extended, rotated right, sidebent right). Inhalation/exhalation testing of the anterior ribcage showed less movement on inhalation on the left, with the left first and second ribs revealing the most restriction.

Palpation revealed tightness in the posterior cervical musculature, the suboccipital muscles, the scalene muscles, and the trapezius, and levator scapulae muscles. Flexibility testing revealed tightness of the levator scapulae, the pectoralis major, and the scalene muscles. A trigger point was identified in the midsubstance of the upper trapezius muscle.

Assessment

The findings were consistent with cervical spondylosis with left C5 radiculopathy, upper cervical dysfunction, forward head posture, and upper rib and thoracic dysfunction.

Treatment Plan

Treatment goals included decreasing the patient's symptoms, improving posture, and increasing range of motion in the cervical and thoracic spine and

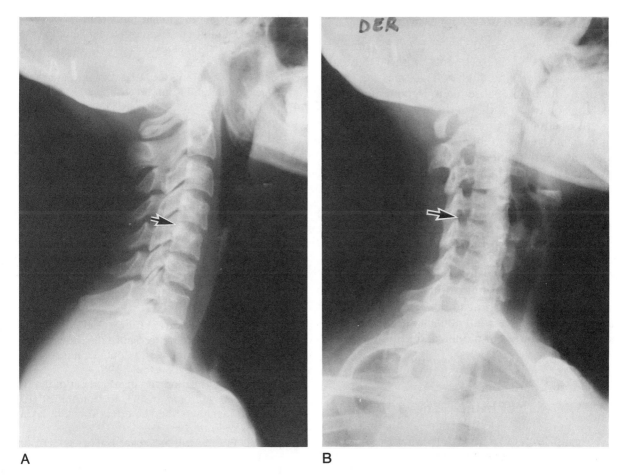

Fig. 5-26. Cervical radiographs. **(A)** Lateral view. Arrow shows C4–C5 spurring. **(B)** Oblique view. Arrow shows bony encroachment at the C4–C5 intervertebral foramen.

upper ribs. Other important treatment goals were patient education about work simplification, awareness of a need for lifetime postural correction, and avoiding potentially harmful activities.

To accomplish these goals the following treatment plan was administered:

1. Intermittent supine cervical traction using a Saunders[24] harness at 16 pounds, 30-second pull, followed by 12 pounds, 10-second pull, for a total treatment time of 20 minutes (static traction with intermittent increases)
2. High-voltage electrical stimulation massage of

the upper trapezius, upper thoracic, and posterior cervical regions for 10 minutes
3. Postural instruction in correct head and neck alignment in all activities
4. Basic instruction in proper sleeping postures; encouragement of continued use of down feather pillow
5. Soft tissue mobilization of the paracervical, suboccipital, levator scapulae, scalene, and upper trapezius muscles
6. Joint mobilization of the upper thoracic spine with the patient supine and the head supported; muscle energy technique to decrease upper cervical spine joint restrictions.

Treatment Progression

The patient was seen every other day, three times a week, for a total of six treatments. Initial treatment included traction and high-voltage massage and posture education. Subsequent treatments managed the soft tissue and joint dysfunctions. Following this treatment regimen, the patient was asymptomatic and resumed her normal activity level. Since this was the patient's first episode of radicular referred symptoms, home cervical traction would not be recommended unless the symptoms recurred.

ACKNOWLEDGMENTS

We wish to thank: my wife Nancy for her patience and love, and Brik, Benjamin, Brittany, Breanna, and Brock, who bring meaning to life (S.A.S.); my husband Rob for his love and understanding (J.M.B.); Patricia Wentworth, our model; and Laura Cox, our photographer.

REFERENCES

1. Dvorak J, Dvorak V: Manual Medicine Diagnostics. Thieme-Stratton, New York, 1984
2. Kapandji I: Physiology of the Joints. 2nd Ed. Vol III. The Trunk and Vertebral Column. Churchill Livingstone, Edinburgh, 1974
3. Werne S: Studies in spontaneous atlas dislocation. Acta Orthop Scand, suppl., 23:1, 1957
4. Kaltenborn FM: Mobilization of the Extremity Joints. Examination and Basic Treatment Techniques. 3rd Ed. Olaf Norlis Bokhandel, Oslo, 1980
5. Ingelmark BE: Ueber den craniocervicalen Uebergang bei Menschen. Acta Anat, suppl., 23:1, 1957
6. Fielding JW: Cineroentgenography of the normal cervical spine. J Bone Joint Surg 39A(6):1280, 1957
7. Fielding JW, Hawkins RJ, Hensinger RN, Francis WR: Deformities. Orthop Clin North Am 9:955, 1978
8. White A, Panjabi MM: The basic kinematics of the human spine. Spine 3:13, 1978
9. White A, Panjabi MM: Clinical Biomechanics of the Spine. JB Lippincott, Philadelphia, 1978
10. Penning L: Functional Pathology of the Cervical Spine. Excerpta Medica Foundation, Amsterdam, 1968
11. Depreux R, Mestdagh H: Anatomie functionelle de l'articulation sousoccipitale. Lille Med 19:122, 1974
12. Caviezel H: Klinische Diagnostike der Funktionsstörung an den Kopfgelenken. Schweiz Rundsch Med Prax 65:1037, 1976
13. Lewit K: Blockierung von Atlas-Axis und Atlas-Occiput im Robild und Klinik. Z Orthop 108:43, 1970
14. Jirout J: Changes in the atlas-axis relations on lateral flexion of the head and neck. Neuroradiology 6:215, 1973
15. Grieve GP: Common Vertebral Joint Problems. Churchill Livingstone, Edinburgh, 1979
16. Warwick R, Williams PL (eds): Gray's Anatomy. 35th British Ed. WB Saunders, Philadelphia, 1973
17. Greenman PE: Manipulative therapy for the thoracic cage. Osteop Ann 140:63, 1977
18. Tatlow TWF, Bammer HG: Vertebral artery compression syndrome. Neurology 7:331, 1957
19. Coman WB: Dizziness related to ENT conditions. p. 303. In Grieve GP (ed): Modern Manual Therapy of the Vertebral Column. Churchill Livingstone, Edinburgh, 1986
20. Grant ER: Clinical testing before cervical manipulation—can we recognize the patient at risk? Paper presented at the World Confederation of Physical Therapy, Sydney, Australia, 1987
21. Howell JW: Evaluation and management of the thoracic outlet syndrome. p. 133. In Donatelli R (ed): Physical Therapy of the Shoulder. Churchill Livingstone, New York, 1987
22. Kendall FP, Kendall-McCreary E: Muscles: Testing and Function. 3rd Ed. Williams & Wilkins, Baltimore, 1983
23. Rocabado M: Diagnosis and Treatment of Abnormal Craniocervical and Craniomandibular Mechanics. Rocabado Institute, Knoxville TN, 1981
24. Saunders, HD: Evaluation, Treatment and Prevention of Musculoskeletal Disorders. 2nd Ed. Viking Press, Minneapolis, 1985
25. Mennell JM: Joint Pain. Little, Brown, Boston, 1964
26. Schafer RC: Chiropractic Management of Sports and Recreational Injuries. Williams & Wilkins, Baltimore, 1982
27. Lewit K: Manipulative Therapy in Rehabilitation of the Motor System. Butterworths, Boston, 1985
28. Seimon LP: Low Back Pain: Clinical Diagnosis and Management. Appleton-Century-Crofts, East Norwalk CT, 1983
29. Greenman PE: Osteopathic Update Series 6, Vertebral motion. Mich Osteop J, p. 31, February 1983
30. Mitchell FL, Moran PS, Pruzzo NA: An Evaluation and Treatment Manual of Osteopathic Muscle Energy Procedures. Institute for Continuing Education in Osteopathic Principles, Valley Park MD, 1979

31. Bogduk N, Engel R: The menisci of the lumbar zyga-pophyseal joints: a review of their anatomy and clinical significance. Spine 9(5):454, 1984

32. Kos J, Wolf J: Die "Menisci" der Zwischenwirbelgelenke und ihre mögliche Rolle bei Wirbelblockierung. Manuelle Med 10:105, 1972

33. Janda V: Muscles, central nervous regulation and back problems. p. 27. In Korr IM (ed): Neurobiologic Mechanisms in Manipulative Therapy. Plenum Press, New York, 1978

34. Korr IM: Proprioceptors and somatic dysfunction. J Am Osteopath Assoc 74:638, 1975

35. Calliet R: Neck and Arm Pain. FA Davis, Philadelphia, 1981

36. Greenman PE: Osteopathic Update Series 7: Restricted vertebral motion. Mich Osteopath J, p. 31, March 1983

37. Hirsh LF: Cervical degenerative arthritis. Possible cause of neck and arm pain. Postgrad Med 74(1):123, 1983

38. Grieve GP: Manipulation therapy for neck pain. Physiotherapy 65(5):136, 1979

39. Bateman JE: The Shoulder and Neck. 2nd Ed. WB Saunders, Philadelphia, 1978

40. Brain WR, Nothfield D, Wilkinson M: The neurological manifestations of cervical spondylosis. Brain 75:187, 1952

41. Cloward RB: Cervical discography: a contribution to the etiology and mechanism of neck, shoulder and arm pain. Ann Surg 150:1052, 1959

42. Cloward RB: The clinical significance of the sinovertebral nerve. J Neurol Neurosurg Psychiatr 23:321, 1960

43. Cyriax JH: Textbook of Orthopaedic Medicine. 8th Ed. Vol I. Diagnosis of Soft Tissue Lesions. Bailliere Tindall, London, 1983

44. McNab I: The whiplash syndrome. Orthop Clin N Am 2(2):389, 1971

45. Hohl M: Soft-tissue injuries of the neck in automobile accidents. J Bone Joint Surg 56A(8):1675, 1974

46. Bower KD: The patho-physiology and symptomatology of the whiplash syndrome. p. 342. In Grieve GP (ed): Modern Manual Therapy of the Vertebral Column. Churchill Livingstone, Edinburgh, 1986

47. Travell JG, Simons DG: Myofascial Pain and Dysfunction: Trigger Point Manual. Williams & Wilkins, Baltimore, 1983

48. Yunus M, Masi AT, Calabro JJ, et al: Primary fibromyalgia (fibrositis): clinical study of 50 patients with matched normal controls. Sem Arthritis Rheum 11(1):151, 1981

49. Cyriax JH, Cyriax PJ: Illustrated Manual of Orthopaedic Medicine. Butterworths, Boston, 1983

50. Miller J: How do you feel? Listener 100:665, 1978

51. Harman JB: Angina in the analgesic limb. Br Med J 2:521, 1951

52. Feinstein B, Langton JNK, Jameson RM, et al: Experiments on pain referred from deep somatic tissues. J Bone Joint Surg 36A:981, 1954

53. Bourdillon JF: Spinal Manipulation. 3rd Ed. Heinemann, London, 1982

54. Inman VT, Saunders JB: Referred pain from skeletal structures. J Nerv Ment Dis 90:660, 1944

55. Campbell DG, Parsons CM: Referred head pain and its concomitants. J Nerv Ment Dis 99:544, 1944

56. Wall PD: The mechanisms of pain associated with cervical vertebral disease. p. 201. In Hirsch C, Zotterman Y (eds): Cervical Pain. Pergamon Press, Oxford, 1971

57. Collins RD: Dynamic Differential Diagnosis. JB Lippincott, Philadelphia, 1981

58. Hoppenfeld S: Physical Examination of the Spine and Extremities. Appleton-Century-Crofts, New York, 1976

59. Gould JA, Davies GJ (eds): Orthopaedic and Sports Physical Therapy. CV Mosby, St. Louis, 1985

60. Bogduk N: Cervical causes of headache. p. 289. In Grieve GP (ed): Modern Manual Therapy of the Vertebral Column. Churchill Livingstone, Edinburgh, 1986

61. Ryan GM, Cope S: Cervical vertigo. Lancet 2:1355, 1955

62. Maitland GD: Vertebral Manipulation. 4th Ed. Butterworths, London, 1977

63. Elvey RL: The investigation of arm pain. p. 530. In Grieve GP (ed): Modern Manual Therapy of the Vertebral Column. Churchill Livingstone, Edinburgh, 1986

64. Magarey ME: Examination of the cervical spine. p. 503. In Grieve GP (ed): Modern Manual Therapy of the Vertebral Column. Churchill Livingstone, Edinburgh, 1986

65. Kenneally M: The upper limb tension test: an investigation of responses amongst normal asymptomatic subjects. Unpublished thesis, School of Physiotherapy, South Australia Institute of Technology, 1983

66. Fryette HH: Principles of Osteopathic Technique. Academy of Applied Osteopathy, Carmel CA, 1954

67. Greenman PE: Osteopathic Update Series 8: Motion testing the cervical spine. Mich Osteopath J, p. 32, April 1983

68. Greenman PE: Osteopathic Update 3: Barrier concepts and structural diagnosis. Mich Osteopath J, p. 28, November 1982

69. Hirsch LF, Thanki A: The thoracic outlet syndrome.

Meeting the diagnostic challenge. Postgrad Med 77(1):197, 1985

70. Falconer MA, Weddell G: Costoclavicular compression of the subclavian artery and veins. Lancet 2:539, 1943

71. Wright IS: The neurovascular syndrome produced by hyperabduction of the arms. Am Heart J 29:1, 1945

72. Roos DB: Congenital anomalies associated with thoracic outlet syndrome. Am J Surg 132:171, 1976

73. Knight KL: Cryotherapy: Theory, Technique, and Physiology. Chattanooga Corp., Chattanooga TN, 1985

74. Colachis SC, Strohm BR: A study of tractive forces and angle of pull on vertebral interspaces in the cervical spine. Arch Phys Med Rehab 46:820, 1965

75. Colachis SC, Strohm BR: Cervical traction: relationship of traction time to varied tractive force with constant angle of pull. Arch Phys Med Rehab 46:815, 1965

76. Daugherty RJ, Erhard RE: Segmentalized cervical traction. p. 189. In Kent BE (ed): International Feder-ation of Orthopaedic Manipulative Therapists Proceedings, Vail CO, 1977

77. Valtonen EJ, et al: Comparative radiographic study of the effect of intermittent and continuous traction on elongation of the cervical spine. Ann Med Int Fenn 57:143, 1968

78. Colachis SC, Strohm BR: Effect of duration of intermittent cervical traction on vertebral separation. Arch Phys Med Rehab 47:353, 1966

79. Valtonen EJ, Kiurn E: Cervical traction as a therapeutic tool: a clinical analysis based on 212 patients. Scand J Rehab Med 2:29, 1970

80. Glimcher MJ: On the form and function of bone: from molecules to organs. Wolff's law revisited. p. 617. In Veis A (ed): The Chemistry and Biology of Mineralized Connective Tissues. Elsevier/North Holland, New York, 1981

81. Jones LH: Strain and Counterstrain. American Academy of Osteopathy, Colorado Springs CO, 1981

82. Upledger JE, Vredevoogd JD: Craniosacral Therapy. Eastland Press, Seattle, 1983

6

Mobilization of the Cervical and Upper Thoracic Spine

ROBERT B. SPRAGUE

Mobilization of the cervical or thoracic spine, with the intent of relieving pain or increasing range of motion, or both, may be done actively or passively using a variety of procedures and techniques, respectively. There is little evidence that passive techniques alone provide lasting relief of pain and a permanent increase in range of motion. Studies[1-3] of the effectiveness of spinal manipulation demonstrate the limitations of this form of treatment. Therefore, it seems logical, from both a clinical and an economic point of view, to provide the patient with a treatment protocol that will have a lasting effect. Physical therapists, in cooperation with their medical colleagues, have made significant progress toward providing such treatment.

This chapter presents an integrated approach to the assessment and treatment of the upper spine. The emphasis is on clinical assessment by the therapist and on treatment that fosters patient participation, self-treatment, and the prevention of recurrent bouts. The greater part of the chapter relies heavily on the approaches presented by Robin McKenzie,[4] Geoffrey Maitland,[5] and James Cyriax.[6] However, other methods of treatment borrowed from a variety of sources are introduced.

McKenzie proposed that therapists first use active movements performed by the patient, supplementing these with passive movements when required.[4] On the other hand, therapists may elect to first use passive movements supplemented by active movements as required.[5] It is quite possible that joints that are very stiff or very painful will require passive movement as a bridge to active movements. When active movements produce a desirable treatment effect, the patient is on his way toward improved function and independence.

The use of mobilization dates back to the days of Hippocrates.[7] The birth of orthopaedic medicine, according to Cyriax,[6] was in 1929. Orthopaedic manual therapy, as described by Cookston and Kent,[8] first became popular in Europe and Australia in the middle of the 20th century, largely as a result of the work of Freddy Kaltenborn, John Mennell, and Geoffrey Maitland. Robin McKenzie[9] first published his theories in 1972. Stanley Paris is thought by many physical therapists to be largely responsible for introducing mobilization concepts in the United States during the 1960s.

As one reflects on the evolution of specialization within physical therapy, which includes orthopaedic physical therapy as it is now called in the United States, one is impressed by the gradual assumption of leadership roles by physical therapists. Since orthopaedic physical therapy has been generally accepted within the physical therapy profession, there has evolved a tendency in some quarters to accept a single method of assessment and treatment. For example, one can easily become known as a Cyriax therapist or whatever label one assigns. It is quite possible that divisions within the profession could be generated, with loss of skills and treatment effectiveness being the worst outcome. To avoid such a tragic loss, it is suggested that we retain our focus on all approaches that allow each individual therapist to employ those skills that are most suitable to his or her personality and talents.

It is recognized that not all lesions of the upper spine are related only to the articulations. Thus, an effective program of treatment will often include other techniques for the soft tissue. It is also acknowledged that not all lesions of the upper spine are mechanical in nature. Thus, an effective program of treatment will frequently include physical agents or rest and analgesics for the treatment of chemical or inflammatory pain. It is beyond the scope of this chapter to discuss physical agents, connective tissue massage, cranial sacral therapy, or other approaches.

Generally speaking, a physical therapist may elect one of two approaches to assess a patient. One approach is to conduct a subjective assessment and a series of objective tests with the intent of reaching a definitive diagnosis, which in many cases leads to the identification of a specific structure at fault. The treatment is then aimed at this specific structure, and the therapist feels very comfortable and secure in addressing the problem in such a definite manner. In this approach, usually called the diagnostic approach, the techniques used in treatment confirm or deny the diagnosis and further define functional faults for treatment.

A second approach is to respect the medical diagnosis rendered by the referring physician, with appropriate precautions, and then to conduct a subjective assessment and a series of objective tests with the intent of recording the changes in the patient's signs and symptoms. No specific structure is designated as being at fault, and the treatment rendered is adjusted according to the patient's individual response. It is quite permissible to hypothesize what is at fault, but the nature and progression of the treatment depend on the clinical behavior of the patient's problem. This approach is usually called the signs-and-symptoms approach or the nonpathologic approach.

It is suggested that, from a historical perspective, diagnosis is subject to whims of the times. During the 1950s, for example, fibrositis was very popular; now there is some doubt whether that condition even exists. Then there is the chronic debate among practicing therapists concerning the relative guilt of the apophyseal joint and the intervertebral junction. It may well be that, in the next decade, the neuro-central joints of Von Luschka are the focus of our attention on the cervical spine. The current pathology appears to be subject to an eternal succession of changes.

From an academic and clinical point of view, physical therapists must understand diagnoses and pathologies. The stages of repair, referenced more thoroughly later in this chapter, are clearly related to treatment modes. It is proposed that individual therapists may employ either or both methods — the diagnostic approach or the signs-and-symptoms approach — depending on their preferences. In this chapter, the emphasis will be on the latter, with some reference to the diagnostic approach when appropriate.

THE McKENZIE AND MAITLAND APPROACHES

Some areas of agreement and difference between the approaches of McKenzie and Maitland are apparent. Both approaches are rooted in James Cyriax's principles. For example, in 1950 Cyriax[10] advocated the use of heavy lumbar traction coupled with the religious maintenance of the lumbar lordosis. In both approaches, there appears to be a bias in the direction of spinal extension. McKenzie's extension principle,[4,9,11] as compared to his flexion principle, is in some respects comparable to Maitland's central vertebral pressures or posteroanterior central vertebral movements.

It is acknowledged beyond any doubt, however, that the two approaches are different. Spinal traction is advocated more by Maitland than by McKenzie. The Maitland approach relies heavily on the use of passive movement performed by the therapist, whereas the McKenzie approach relies heavily on the use of active movement done by the patient himself. It is possible that the two approaches are not compatible.

Both approaches are largely nonpathologic in nature, with a heavy reliance on the treatment of the clinical signs and symptoms, as compared to treatment by diagnosis or using the theories of biomechanics. Consequently, in each approach there is a pervasive need for the therapist to be highly skilled in both types of assessment, objective and subjective. For example, subjective assessment of the changes in the patient's symptoms during treatment, based on information supplied by the patient, is essential in assessing the effects of the movements used during treatment. One clear exception to the nonpathologic nature of McKenzie's approach is the theory that the derangement syndrome is caused by deformation of the intervertebral disk. The theory that the disk is responsible for the derangement is in agreement with Cyriax's teachings. In fact, Cyriax[6] stated that the intervertebral disk is responsible for 90 percent of all low back pain.

It appears that neither McKenzie nor Maitland is willing to designate a specific structure as responsible for stiffness, hypomobility, or dysfunction in the spine. Both approaches see no need to join the endless debate regarding which specific structure is responsible for the patient's pain or stiffness. If the movement used in treatment is the correct movement, the symptoms and/or the signs will be influenced positively. For example, when treating the pain of derangement, if repeated passive or active sidebending to the painful side of the cervical spine reduces, centralizes, and eliminates the patient's pain, then the movement is a proper one and should be used as a major part of treatment until it is no longer effective. When treating stiffness, if the repeated sidebending away from the painful side, done either passively or actively, produces the patient's pain and subsequently increases his range, without an increase in symptoms (beyond treatment soreness), then the movement is a proper one and should be used as a major part of treatment until it is no longer effective.

DEFINITIONS

Most physical therapists, especially in communications with physicians, use standard medical terminology. However, the advent of specialization within the profession has generated a body of knowledge and, concurrently, a particular language peculiar to each specialization. For example, for many orthopedic physical therapists the term *dysfunction* has more specific meaning than simply the loss of function. To oversimplify, dysfunction in the

McKenzie approach means a lack of movement due to adaptive shortening of tissues. Provided that this definition is accurate as a clinical assessment, then the treatment rendered follows a particular pattern with certain expectations. Thus, it is imperative that therapists speak the same language to communicate their thoughts, theories, and treatment rationales.

In the sections that follow on assessment and treatment, certain terminology will be consistently used. Therefore, in the interests of clarity, the terminology will be defined and illustrated.

Mechanical and Chemical Pain

Pain is not a primary sensation, as are vision, hearing, and smell, but rather an abnormal affective state accurately described as an unpleasant emotional state. This emotional state is aroused by unusual patterns of activity within the nociceptive receptor system and is subject to various degrees of facilitation and inhibition.[12] The nociceptive receptor system is sensitive to mechanical and chemical tissue activity. Thus, if this largely inactive receptor system is stimulated by the application of sufficient mechanical forces to stress, deform, or damage it, mechanical pain is produced. On the other hand, if the system is irritated by sufficient concentrations of chemical substances such as lactic acid or potassium ions, chemical pain is produced. Thus, it is quite possible in a clinical situation to have either chemical or mechanical pain present, or both occurring concurrently.

Generally, mechanical pain is constant and variable or more intermittent and often is affected by movement or position. Movements, either passive or active, that reduce the mechanical deformation also reduce the patient's symptoms. Patients whose problem is mechanical in nature usually will report that there is some time during the day or night when they are symptom-free, or when their symptoms are significantly reduced or increased. Careful questioning by the therapist will frequently reveal that pain reported to be constant by the patient is, in fact, intermittent.

Chemical or inflammatory pain is more constant and is less affected by movement or position. Seldom is chemical pain reduced by either passive or active movements, because the movements have little positive effect on the chemical irritants. Chemical pain is often increased by movement and reduced by rest. Chemical pain is also obviously more responsive to medications that reduce the inflammatory process. For example, if a patient has active cervical arthritis, and his major complaint is a constant burning ache together with reduced range, even gentle attempts at increasing this range by movement may increase the ache, and either have no effect on the range or reduce it.

On the other hand, a second patient may present with the same medical diagnosis, correctly rendered, but whose major complaint is an intermittent pain coupled with reduced range. Attempts at increasing this patient's range of movement in the proper direction will decrease the pain and often concurrently increase the range. The latter patient often complains of increased symptoms, including occipital headache upon arising in the morning. His symptoms often are limited to the first hour in the morning. Further, he will report that his symptoms are either decreased or eliminated with movement, and frequently he only experiences his pain after periods of inactivity.

Many patients present with both a chemical and a mechanical component to their pain. These patients complain of both pain and stiffness. It is suggested that the two components of their pain, the chemical and the inflammatory, are closely related and interdependent; that is, one component, the chemical, may be the cause of the second component, the mechanical. With the presence of both mechanical and chemical components, the therapist is obligated to make a therapeutic decision to treat either one component or both. It is quite possible that reduction of one component will have a positive effect on the second. For example, gentle low-grade movements applied to an apophyseal joint that is mechanically deformed may reduce the deformation and consequently the mechanical pain. The movements have no obvious effects on the chemical irritation, but at least the chemical irritation is not increased. Since the mechanical component of pain has been reduced, the range is increased and the patient regains function without an exacerbation of his pain.

In this example, the therapist has chosen to treat the stiffness caused by the mechanical deformation and, concurrently, to respect (by not increasing) the patient's inflammatory pain. Provided that the patient retains some of his increased function, it is reasonable to assume that the same treatment should be repeated until the patient's progress plateaus. It is suggested that, in certain circumstances where the components of mechanical and chemical pain are favorably mixed, treatment of one component may have a positive effect on the second. Further, it is suggested that to treat only one component may result in an incomplete recovery. For example, treating only the chemical component of the patient's pain with physical agents may have no effect, or an incomplete effect, on his mechanical component. Thus, the stage is set for recurrent bouts of the same problem because of a likely regression of the patient's condition.

In summary, active, acute inflammatory pain in the cervical spine, as elsewhere, often requires rest, immobilization, and physical agents. As the healing process progresses and scar tissue forms, the area requires appropriate active or passive movement in proper doses. When the inflammatory stage abates and the patient presents with mechanical pain, the area requires more vigorous movement. Excellent and detailed discussions of the relationships among the healing processes and treatment modes may be found in writings by Cummings[13] and Evans.[14] A summary of the relationships among the stages of healing, joint reactivity to movement, and treatment modes is presented in Table 6-1.

Table 6-1. Treatment Modes Related to Reactivity and Stages of Scar Tissue Formation

Stages	Reactivity	Treatment
Inflammation	Pain, then resistance	Rest Immobilization Grade I and II movements
Granulation Fibroplastic (healing)	Pain and resistance simultaneous	Active range-of-motion exercises Grade I and II movements
Maturation	Resistance, then pain	Passive range-of-motion exercises Grade III, IV, and V movements

Elimination of the mechanical pain by proper treatment logically leads to the need to restore full function. Adequate muscle strength and flexibility to provide quality movement and reconditioning of the entire body for life's activities are essential. The use of appropriate treatment methods at the proper time for eliminating the chemical and mechanical pain, with progression through the reconditioning program, requires the skills of a talented therapist. In the author's opinion, this complete process done well is *real* physical therapy.

Three Syndromes: Pain and Stiffness and the Centralization Phenomenon

In the nonpathologic approaches, where changes in clinical signs and symptoms, with due respect for the medical diagnosis and contraindications, are used to select techniques and determine the progression of treatment, there are obvious principles and theories underlying the clinical assessments and treatments. The terms *posture, dysfunction, derangement,* and the *centralization phenomenon,* as described by McKenzie,[4] deserve explanation. Maitland[5] uses the terms *pain* and *stiffness,* which are, in some general way, related to derangement and dysfunction, respectively. The relationships among these terms provide some limited but clinically useful guidelines for assessment and treatment.

The terms *posture, dysfunction,* and *derangement* have very specific meanings in the McKenzie approach. Although not all patients fit neatly into a particular category, the use of the three terms provides a framework from which are generated essential clinical principles. For example, in treating dysfunction, defined in oversimplified terms as adaptive shortening of structures that hinders function, the purpose of the treatment is to lengthen the adaptively shortened structures to restore function. The patient's symptoms should be produced and the limitations of function established. In the treatment of derangement, defined simply as a disturbance of the normal anatomic relationship within the intervertebral disk, the purpose of the treatment is to reduce, centralize, and eliminate the patient's pain. Maintenance of the reduction, restoration of

function, and prevention of recurrences follow logically.

In the treatment of the posture syndrome, defined briefly as end-range strain on normal tissues, the purpose of the treatment is to remove the end-range strain by correction of the patient's poor posture. The patient must become keenly aware and convinced of the cause of his symptoms.

In the Maitland approach the therapist is obligated to decide, among other possibilities, whether he or she is treating the patient's pain or treating the patient's stiffness while respecting the pain. This decision is based on many subjective and objective assessment variables including joint irritability, the patient's perception of the nature of his problem, the relationship between range and pain, and the effects of passive movement or traction during treatment. If pain is the dominant factor of concern to the patient, and pain, not resistance or stiffness, prevents full range, then the therapist elects to treat the patient's pain. Thus, the success or failure of the treatment is based on the ability of the treatment to reduce, centralize (where applicable), and eliminate the patient's pain. This is not meant to imply that the treatment of pain in the cervical spine is limited to cases where the pain is produced by deformation of the intervertebral disk. There are other structures, in addition to the disk, commonly capable of producing sufficient pain to warrant the treatment of only the pain. The analogy between the two approaches in the treatment of derangement (McKenzie) and in the treatment of pain (Maitland) is definitely limited.

A very limited analogy between the two approaches in the treatment of dysfunction (McKenzie) and in the treatment of stiffness (Maitland) can also be postulated. In a case where lack of movement, for example, is theoretically caused by a decreased gliding of an apophyseal joint, and the patient complains mainly of stiffness or perhaps mild discomfort, treatment may be directed at the dysfunction or stiffness while respecting the discomfort. In this case, lack of movement concerns the patient the most. Thus, the therapist has the latitude to reproduce the patient's discomfort during treatment with the intent of increasing the patient's range and reducing stiffness. A positive treatment effect is possible using either approach, provided that the end-range pain or discomfort produced during treatment, by either active or passive exercises, does not linger unreasonably. A certain amount of post-treatment soreness is acceptable and expected. If there is no increase in range as a result of the stretching of adaptively shortened tissues after a reasonable number of treatments, then the treatment has been unsuccessful.

It is acknowledged that most patients present with both pain and stiffness, and the decision as to which is the dominant complaint is often complicated. If in doubt, treat the pain; only time is lost if the decision was incorrect. Subsequent assessments will reveal no gain from the treatment, and in most cases the role of the pain was probably exaggerated either by the patient or by the therapist, or both. With the new knowledge that the treatment of the pain was ineffective, therapist and patient may well decide to change the treatment and begin to treat the stiffness while respecting the pain. If this decision is made, it is most advisable that the patient be in agreement with the therapist. Patient compliance and understanding are both increased, not to mention happiness. An unhappy patient rapidly becomes a no-show or, worse, delivers an unfavorable message to the referring physician.

The three syndromes, as described by McKenzie,[4] are also described in handouts by the faculty of the McKenzie Institute at appropriate courses. Therapists are encouraged to refer to them. However, reading material is no substitute for course participation or supervised clinical practice.

McKenzie[4] described the centralization phenomenon as a movement of pain from the periphery toward the midline of the spine. This mechanical pain, originating from the spine and referred distally, centralizes as a result of certain repeated movements or the assumption of certain positions. The movements that cause this phenomenon then may be used to eliminate radiating and referred symptoms. Centralization occurs only in the derangement syndrome during the reduction of the mechanical deformation. This centralization of pain in patients whose symptoms are of recent origin may occur within a few minutes. When centralization takes place, there is often a significant increase of central spinal pain. For example, decreased arm pain is traded for a temporary increase in neck pain.

In a study of approximately 100 patients with low back pain, Donaldson[15] reported that occurrence of the centralization phenomenon had been documented. Centralization was found to be reliable in evaluating the nature of the disorder, selecting the appropriate mechanical treatment, and predicting eventual outcomes. Those patients whose pain centralized at the initial examination had an excellent prognosis for recovery, and those patients whose pain did not centralize or, worse yet, peripheralized, usually had a poor prognosis for recovery.

Although both authors reported the centralization phenomenon in regard to the lumbar spine, this author and others have repeatedly observed the same behavior in the cervical spine. Repeated movements, either active or passive, performed in one direction will often produce an increase in peripheral pain. Other movements, usually done in the opposite direction, will reduce the peripheral pain and centralize the symptoms. Cervical traction may be effective in some cases in producing the centralization phenomenon; however, the lasting effects of traction without other procedures in retaining centralization are open to question. On the other hand, patient procedures (active exercises), when successful in producing centralization, are preferred to cervical traction because of the ease with which self-treatment can be accomplished outside the therapist's office. There are circumstances when centralization is not possible with either active or passive exercises, and under these circumstances cervical traction may serve as a bridge to exercises. In other words, traction may be the treatment of choice until the exercises can produce a desirable effect. However, patients do not usually get better by traction alone.[16]

Active Procedures and Therapist's Techniques

Active procedures are those movements performed by the patient himself. They are similar to active exercises, but not identical, because some active procedures may be largely passive in nature. In the cervical spine, retraction and extension performed in the supine position, coupled with small rotations at the limit, are all assisted by gravity and may require little or no active muscle action in the cervical spine. If the patient applies overpressure, an active component is introduced into the procedure by the upper extremity muscle force. In the lumbar spine, the press-up movement is mainly a passive procedure without active involvement of the erector spinae or gluteal muscles. With active muscle contractions, full available range may not be obtained and the assessment becomes distorted. Sidebending or lateral flexion of the head performed in the sitting position is also obviously assisted by gravity, and relaxation of the muscles within the cervical spine often enhances a positive treatment effect.

The therapist is obligated to carefully instruct the patient in the proper method of performing the active procedures. It is often necessary to demonstrate the exact movement desired. Instruct the patient to report any changes in symptom behavior that take place during and immediately after the performance of the procedure. The precise status of the symptoms before performing the procedure is required for proper assessment. The consistency of test-retest (assessment) is affected by the patient's pretest posture.

Extension of the cervical spine should be performed starting in a retracted position. If consistency of the starting position (i.e., proper retraction) is not maintained, then the assessment may be inaccurate. A potentially successful procedure thought to be ineffective because of inaccurate instruction by the therapist is wrongly abandoned, or, worse yet, the approach is faulted.

Therapists' techniques are those movements performed on the patient by the therapist. They are passive in nature and, in most respects, are mobilizations using either passive physiologic techniques or passive accessory techniques. In the McKenzie approach, therapists' techniques are used as an adjunct to active procedures only when needed to produce a desired treatment effect. Philosophically, the application of therapists' techniques is believed to be one factor in promoting patient dependence on the therapist, and therefore their use may reduce the effectiveness of self-treatment. Therapists' techniques, in contrast to active procedures, provide an extrinsic force, whereas active procedures provide an intrinsic force generated by the patient himself. Since the patient may, in part, be responsible for his own problem, either by chronic poor posture or other self-inflicted abuse, it is the patient's responsibility to treat his own problem using active procedures. It is also believed that a well-educated patient who understands his problem, including an understanding of the mechanical model, will most likely be in a favorable position to effectively prevent or abort future deformations of his spine. Thus, he stands a reasonable chance of ending or reducing the classical, and boring, recurrent cycle of repeated bouts of spinal pain.

Therapist techniques are usually performed as repeated movements in the desired direction. Occasionally, movements are sustained when a sustained position produces the optimal effect of reducing symptoms or increasing range of motion. Sustained movements are also employed as provocative tests in an attempt to reproduce the patient's chief complaint or comparable sign, according to Maitland. Repeated movements, either physiologic or accessory, may be loosely compared to the Maitland oscillating techniques, except that the repeated movements in the McKenzie approach are not always graded. Both clinicians use the terms "pressure on" and "pressure off" to describe the rhythm of a technique. It appears at this writing that the degree of skill required to apply most of the techniques described by McKenzie is usually not as high as that required to apply the techniques described by Maitland. This is in no way meant to imply that one approach is superior, but is merely an observed difference between the two approaches. In the author's opinion, there is an appropriate place within the healing arts for both approaches. History will be the judge of any differences in effectiveness and efficiency. There is no room within our profession for exclusion based on the myth of elitism.

Direction of a Procedure or Technique

There are few, if any, absolutes or correct techniques or procedures based on theories. There are general guidelines and contraindications to provide the clinician with reasonably logical methods of selecting techniques or procedures. General guidelines and contraindications may be employed in determining the desirable direction of the forces. These guidelines are based on the correct mechanical diagnosis (rendered by the physical therapist) in the McKenzie approach. In general, the guidelines are based on current knowledge of pathology, the known mechanical disorders of the vertebral column, the medical diagnosis, and the changes in symptoms and signs. For the cervical and thoracic spine, Maitland[5] provides guidelines for the sequence of selection of techniques and primary uses for mobilizing techniques. He recommends the use of cervical traction for an acute cervical condition where there is severe arm pain with markedly limited neck movements to the painful side. Once the pain is under control with the use of traction, the therapist then may elect to change techniques to address the residual stiffness respecting the pain. This is not meant to imply that techniques are used only to treat stiffness, because the low-grade techniques (grades I and II) are used frequently and effectively to treat pain. The treatment of pain using passive movement is thoroughly described by Maitland.[5]

Some clinicians believe one of the advantages of the Maitland approach is its efficacy in treating pain. For example, passive accessory movements are frequently used in the part of the range that is totally free of any pain or discomfort. As the patient's pain decreases and movement signs improve, the technique can be taken further through the range and the amplitude of the technique increased. Some clinicians are surprised when gentle rotation movements of the cervical spine, often done away from the painful side in the painless part of the range, produce a significant improvement in the pain behavior and ranges on the painful side. The patient will often report only a mild strained feeling on the painful side during application of the technique. As this strain reduces, the active movement toward the painful side increases when assessed after treatment or between bouts of a technique. The stretching of the painful side in a carefully controlled manner by rotation away from the painful side is also described elsewhere.[17,18]

Guidelines for determining the direction of a technique are provided within the McKenzie[4] approach. These guidelines are reasonable, practical, and clinically effective, provided that the mechanical diagnosis is accurate. The term *mechanical diagnosis* is, in the author's opinion, synonymous with the phrase *clinical assessment*. The physical therapist classifies the patient as having a postural, dysfunction, or derangement syndrome. This classification is based in part on the physician's diagnosis appropriately weighed together with the information provided from the therapist's subjective and objective assessments. Both assessments are discussed later in this chapter.

In addition to providing guidelines for the direction of a technique, the teachings of McKenzie also provide a reasonable and logical rationale for the progression of a technique. The direction of a gentle therapeutic movement has been determined to be proper in advance of more vigorous techniques. For example, in treating a derangement, if movement in the direction of flexion of the lower cervical spine increases the patient's peripheral symptoms, then this is the wrong direction. Theoretically, and from a practical clinical standpoint, the flexion movement has made the patient worse by increasing the mechanical deformation. On the other hand, if movement in the direction of extension of the lower cervical spine decreases and centralizes the patient's symptoms, then this is the right direction to reduce the mechanical deformation. Theoretically, the extension movement has made the patient better by reducing the mechanical deformation of the anatomic structure causing the patient's pain. This illustration assumes, for the sake of clarity, that the lateral compartment's contribution to the pain is irrelevant; that is, it is unnecessary to effect movement in the frontal plane to gain centralization. This obviously is not always the case in the clinic. Provocation and reduction of symptoms generate useful information. If movement is provided in the correct direction, the patient will get better regardless of the underlying theories.

How then does the therapist determine the direction, vigor, and frequency of a procedure or technique? Part of the answer lies in the correctness of the mechanical diagnosis or clinical assessment. The three syndromes—posture, dysfunction and derangement—are all treated differently, and the intent of the procedure or technique is peculiar to each syndrome.

The posture syndrome has no pathology. In other words, the pain is produced by abnormal stress on normal tissue. Normal tissue, when stretched to the limit, produces pain. When the deformation or stretch is removed, the pain goes away. Any normal joint may be used to illustrate this fact, unless the end-range is limited by soft tissue as in knee and elbow flexion. The bent finger syndrome is commonly used to illustrate pain of postural origin, provided the metacarpophalangeal (MCP) joint is normal. Hyperextend the MCP joint of any finger and sustain this movement; the pain is produced by an abnormal stress acting on normal tissue. Remove the stress and the pain stops; the postural strain has been removed.

Since there is no structural anomaly and no loss of joint motion, there is no need to worry about the direction or progression of a technique. Such therapy is contraindicated, since there is nothing to stretch (no dysfunction) and nothing to reduce (no derangement). There is something to balance by removing the deforming stress off end-range strain. For example, assume the average head weighs 9 pounds and the average neck cephalad to C7 weighs 3 pounds. The total potential deforming force at C6–C7 is then equal to the total weight of 12 pounds times the lever arm distance from the center of gravity of the combined masses. Thus, if the head and neck mass is 2 inches forward of the fulcrum at C6–C7, then the moment of the force at C6–C7 is 2 foot-pounds.

If this deforming force is present 16 hours a day (during waking hours only), the stage is set for mechanical deformation, either elastic or plastic, depending on the time elapsed. Removal of this sustained end-range stretch of normal tissues will eliminate the patient's pain. Thus, correction of the patient's poor posture is all that is required to treat the posture syndrome effectively. No phonophoresis, manual techniques, or electrical currents are needed. The patient simply must learn how to remove the deforming force. Compliance, which is enhanced by a clear demonstration explaining the cause of the pain, is the key. The intent of the posture instruction is to remove the deforming force by teaching the patient how to sit, stand, and lie correctly in a balanced posture. Correct posture should be devoid of end-range strain.

In the derangement syndrome the intent of the technique or procedure is to reduce, centralize, and eliminate the patient's pain. The direction, mode (sustained or oscillating), and amplitude of techniques, procedures, and postures are dictated by selecting movements and positions that reduce the derangement. Reliance on the centralization phenomenon is essential. A temporary increase in central spinal pain, accompanied by a simultaneous decrease in peripheral pain, is acceptable.

In the dysfunction syndrome the intent of the technique or procedure is to reproduce the pain of dysfunction and to increase the range of motion as a result of appropriate repeated stretching. The direction of the procedure or technique is dictated by selecting movements that reproduce the pain of dysfunction. The adaptively shortened structures are stretched over a period of time, and function slowly improves. Treatment or exercise soreness is normal, but this soreness should not linger or interfere with subsequent exercise or treatment sessions. The pain of dysfunction or stiffness is slow to resolve, as is the pain of a "frozen shoulder."

SUGGESTED MECHANISMS FOR RELIEF OF PAIN AND INCREASE IN RANGE OF MOVEMENT

Nyberg[19] presented three possible mechanisms by which spinal manipulation may work: the mechanical effects, the neurophysiologic effects, and the psychological effects. The term *manipulation* has a multitude of meanings, and there is little agreement in the literature that could lead to universal acceptance. In this chapter, manipulation is defined in its broadest sense, which includes the use of refined motion performed either by the therapist (technique) or by the patient himself (procedure). Within the boundaries of this definition, we will explore the mechanical effects and the neurophysiologic effects. The psychological effects, although important, are beyond the scope of this chapter.

Mechanical Effects

It is established that new scar tissue can be influenced by movement applied at the appropriate time in the proper direction. Both Evans[14] and Cummings[13] have described the beneficial effect of remodeling new collagen. It is also quite possible that hypomobile joints that have been underexercised for an extended time can be influenced positively by movement. One possible mechanism is by the stretching or rupture of abnormal cross links that were formed between fibers.

Another mechanical effect, proposed by McKenzie,[4] is the influencing of annular or nuclear material by removing the forces causing the mechanical deformation and applying an appropriate reductive force. The mechanical deformation is reduced or eliminated by the use of repeated movements, usually performed in the direction opposite to the one that caused the mechanical deformation. For example, if the deforming force was flexion, then the reductive force would be extension, or vice versa. It is further hypothesized that, when the intervertebral disk is at fault, the pain is centralized, reduced, and eliminated in response to the appropriate repeated movements. Studies by Donaldson[15] addressing this centralization phenomena lend credibility to this theory. One advantage of the McKenzie approach is that, in most cases, the patient is able to perform these repeated movements himself, independent of the therapist.

One clinical problem frequently encountered in practice, which is largely mechanical in nature, is the common kyphus deformity in the lower cervical and upper thoracic spine. Older patients present with a markedly forward head and significant loss of movement. Younger patients present with the same deformity but only moderate loss of movement. One theory that may explain some of the differences between the two age groups involves the concept of plastic and elastic mechanical deformation.

Deformation in a material is defined as displacement of atoms from their equilibrium position as a result of a load.[20] The deformation is elastic in nature if the displaced atoms return to their equilibrium position when the load is removed, and plastic if they do not.[21] Thus, elastic deformation is nonpermanent and totally recovered upon release of the applied load, whereas plastic deformation is permanent and nonrecoverable after release of the applied load.[22]

It is suggested that, in the older patient with flexed lower cervical spine and extended upper cervical spine, recovery of full function is impossible, in part because of plastic deformation. The opposite results can be expected in most younger patients. It is also essential, in treating both age groups, to attain and retain proper posture with a desirable cervical lordosis. The proper posture will either correct the elastic deformation or reduce the progression of the plastic deformation. The elimination of chronic postural loads that most likely produce deformation of tissues is an essential part of a comprehensive treatment program.

Neurophysiologic Effects

Another theory dating back to the work of Korr[23] suggests that appropriate movements may have a positive effect on the neurophysiologic activity of the tissues. For example, in the cervical spine, according to Wyke,[24] there are three types of mechanoreceptors: type I receptors, in the superficial layers of the fibrous capsule of the joints, are stimulated by end-range movements of the joints; type II receptors, in the deeper layers of the fibrous capsule of the joints, are stimulated by midrange movements of the joints; and type IV, the nociceptive afferents, are responsible for producing the unpleasant emotional experience commonly called pain.

The stimulation of either type I or type II mechanoreceptors, through an involved network of neural connections, is believed to be capable of modulating the experience of pain. Repeated movements, either active or passive, when performed either at the end of range or in the midrange, are capable of reducing the pain and allowing for increased movement.

SUBJECTIVE ASSESSMENT

Skillful assessment separates the successful clinician from the technician. Without assessment, treatment is the mechanical application of techniques without guidelines; success is often a matter of luck, rather than the result of logical thought. Planning and progression are haphazard, without direction, and the therapist and the patient are often confused regarding the purpose or the expected outcome of the treatment. The individual practitioner, the patient, and the profession suffer needlessly. Some of our medical colleagues who rely only on the use of medications to treat mechanical problems of the spine are in need of a lesson on assessment.

Subjective assessment is more than a classical history. Although the information collected is gleaned from talking with the patient, as opposed to measuring objective changes, the quality of information needed far exceeds the recording of simple facts. For example, the accurate completion of a pain drawing or a body chart on a patient with an assortment of neck, head, upper extremity, and upper thoracic symptoms may consume 10 minutes of skilled questioning and clarification. The relationships, if any, among the different symptoms must also be sorted out. The present and past history of the disorder have yet to be addressed.

In general, the three major components of the subjective assessment (often abbreviated C/O, C, or S) are the area, behavior, and nature (including the type of disorder) of the patient's symptoms. Accurate definition of the area of symptoms includes the precise location on the body chart of all the patient's abnormal sensations, including their depth, their surface location, and the extent of the spread peripherally. It is often helpful, when the therapist has completed the body chart, to clarify where the symptoms stop, for example, "You mean that, below your elbow, your right forearm feels the same as your left forearm — there are no abnormal sensations in either forearm?" Clarification of the distal extent of the symptoms will then allow the therapist to refer to the elbow symptoms as the barometer for determining centralization in a derangement syndrome.

Symptom behavior, both diurnal and nocturnal, provides the therapist with an understanding of the nature of the problem. Are the symptoms constant or intermittent? If constant, do they vary in intensity? If symptoms caused by mechanical deformation are completely abolished during certain periods of the day, then the mechanical deformation has been removed. Once the symptoms appear to be mechanical in nature, then the effects of movement and posture on the symptoms can be established. For example, are the symptoms better or worse when the patient is sitting, moving, lying, or standing? Ask the patient to compare his symptoms in the morning with his symptoms in the evening. Is sleep disturbed? If so, to what extent? For example, "Are you unable to fall asleep or is your sleep disturbed?" If so, "How frequently are you awoken?" Pain at night may reflect inflammatory problems, other medical problems, or poor sleeping posture in need of correction. Coughing and sneezing increase intrathoracic pressure, and the behavior of symptoms during those maneuvers is essential information. If the patient's responses to questions about the behavior of his symptoms are not clear, possibly because of the chronic nature of his complaints or the minor nature of his problem, then the relative worsening of symptoms may be ascertained. It may be necessary to rephrase or repeat questions to get a clear picture.

The past or previous history, as compared with the recent history of current neck pain, is established. For recurrent problems it is important to clarify the severity and frequency of past bouts to determine if the problem is progressive in nature. Repeated progressive bouts with exacerbations in the absence of trauma strongly suggest a derangement syndrome. It is also helpful for the therapist to know the condition of the cervical spine before the most recent bout. If there have been repeated insults, from either intrinsic or extrinsic trauma, then it is quite possible that the neck may never move normally in response to the current treatment because of chronic hypershortened tissue or some other irreversible residual deformity.

Prior treatment for the same or previous conditions, and the efficacy of the prior treatment, may provide a clue as to what will be successful this time. It is also helpful to know what, if anything, has been done for the present problem and, of course, the effects, if any. Patients will frequently report that they get limited benefit from a particular exercise, and upon further investigation it is found that a fine tuning of the exercise produces a more positive treatment effect. For example, the direction of the self-treatment, discovered by the patient, may have been correct, but the depth of movement or frequency of exercises was insufficient. All that was needed was to go further into range more often.

Questions regarding special diagnostic tests such as radiography, CT, and magnetic resonance (MRI) should be unbiased; simply ask, for example, "Have you had recent x-rays?" The therapist would like to know the results and where the x-rays may be located in order to know if problems for which certain treatments are unsuitable have been ruled out. Cyriax[25] feels that radiographic findings can be misleading, as they often show an irrelevant abnormality not related to the present problem, or fail to show any soft tissue deformation. The patient is led to believe there is absolutely nothing wrong. There is no positive correlation between the findings on radiography and the clinical state of the patient.[26]

The patient's general health is explored with the intent of discovering serious pathology that may have been undetected by the referring physician, and to determine the relevance of known health problems. Does the patient look unwell, and has there been a recent unplanned weight loss? Is there a history of rheumatoid arthritis, which may suggest laxity of the transverse ligament? Are there any systemic diseases, including recent surgery and cardiorespiratory diseases, which will restrict the patient's ability to do active exercises? Are there symptoms of vertebral artery disease?

Questions regarding medications, including steroids, are asked to determine the effects of the medications on the patient's pain and to estimate any systemic effects of the drugs. The occasional use of mild analgesics that eliminate the pain suggests a moderately painful condition, whereas regular use of strong analgesics that only reduce the pain suggests a more painful condition. Long-term use of steroids may weaken the connective tissue. Patients who report suspected osteoporosis deserve gentle treatment, especially in the thoracic spine.

Upon completion of the subjective examination, the therapist has gleaned extensive and relevant information in an efficient manner to the extent that he or she is able to establish, in many cases, a tentative conclusion. When the questions and answers flow in a fluid and logical manner, a particular structure is often implicated. The assessment has been successful to this point. A summary of the subjective assessment is found in Table 6-2.

The objective assessment will confirm, deny, or modify the therapist's tentative conclusions. For example, headaches are well known to be associated with lower cervical spondylosis and upper cervical

Table 6-2. Summary of Subjective Assessment[a]

Type of disorder (pain, stiffness, weakness, etc.)

Location of the patient's symptoms, including the extent of peripheralization (recorded on the body or pain chart)

Nature of the symptoms, including frequency, original location, and degree of disability

Cause of the problem, if known (trauma, systemic disease, insidious)

Behavior of the symptoms over a 24-hour period, including the effects of different postures

Effects of changes in intrathoracic pressures

Present or recent history

Past history including treatment, if any

Patient's general health, results of any medical tests, and medications and their effect

Other relevant information peculiar to the patient

[a] It is assumed that the patient has already completed a brief medical history and that this information has been reviewed by the therapist.

joint arthrosis. Empirical evidence favors the upper joints as being at fault.[27] Clinically, many patients will complain of a stiff neck and a morning headache at the base of the occiput or late-in-the-day headaches behind the ipsilateral eye or on top of the head. Granted, there are many variations to these headache patterns, but let us assume that the occipital headache comes from the lower cervical spine, the headache behind the ipsilateral eye comes from C2, and the headache on top of the head comes from C1. The patient has indicated during the subjective examination the areas of her neck where she feels pain and the areas of her headaches. There are no upper extremity or interscapular symptoms. These areas are made clear (marked by a check) on the body chart. A reasonable clinical diagnosis is either lower cervical spondylosis or upper cervical arthrosis. Subsequent movement tests and palpations are aimed at reproducing the pain of the stiff neck and headache symptoms. It is most likely that the stiff neck and the headache are related, but it is possible that there are two separate entities. If the relationship was not clarified during the subjective examination, it will most likely be clarified during the objective examination.

In a review of cervical radiculopathy, Dillin[28] reported that cervical disk herniation is most common at the C5–C6 level, followed by C6–C7, C4–C5,

C3–C4, and C7–T1. Earlier, Cyriax[7] reported that protrusions were rare at C2–C3, uncommon at C4, C5, and C7, and very common at C6. Thus, it is likely that either the C6 or the C7 nerve root is involved.

There are many hypotheses regarding the proximate cause of these lower cervical lesions. Ligamentous lengthening with periosteal lifting, chronic lower cervical spine flexion deformation with weakening of the posterior annular wall, osteophyte formation, and alteration of the length and tone of the cervical musculature are explanations most frequently suggested.

It has been the author's experience that, regardless of the treatment approach favored by the therapist, most treatment is ineffective unless the patient assumes a balanced posture 24 hours a day. Thus, sitting, standing, and lying posture awareness is essential. Few patients, except in the acute state of a disorder, are unable to benefit from reduction of the chronic forward head posture. It is indeed a frustrating experience for both the patient and the therapist to see no consistent significant reduction of symptoms when the treatment is appropriate but the chronic stress of poor posture remains a dominant factor. In fact, many patients will get significant relief from their symptoms by posture correction alone.

OBJECTIVE ASSESSMENT
Definition

The objective assessment or physical examination is often abbreviated O (in the SOAP notation), O/A (objective assessment), or O/E (on examination). This part of the total assessment follows the subjective assessment in which the therapist has gathered a complete description of the patient's presenting symptoms. In general, the objective assessment is a series of appropriate active and passive movement tests aimed at collecting additional data that will confirm or deny the therapist's tentative conclusions reached during the subjective examination. A typical objective assessment consists of active physiologic movements, passive physiologic movements, passive accessory movements, and special tests, as needed.

Purpose

The general purpose of the examination is to assess movement, that is, limitations, deviations, aberrations, and the effects, if any, of the movements on the patient's symptoms. Any deviation from normal movement and any symptom changes are noted. Future changes in the patient's condition can then be measured against the benchmarks of objective signs and subjective symptoms. Movement loss may be graded as major, moderate, minor, or none. The loss may also be expressed as a percentage of normal or expressed in degrees.

In addition to assessing movement, a second purpose of the objective assessment, when treating dysfunction or stiffness, is to reproduce the patient's comparable sign. For example, if the patient's chief complaint is a moderate midcervical pain, this intermittent pain is reproduced by overpressure into the quadrant position. The same quadrant position may be used later to assess the effects of the treatment.

A third purpose of the objective assessment is to determine the proper direction of treatment movements. Repeated movements that reduce, centralize, and eliminate the patient's symptoms are the proper movements to use in treating derangements. Repeated movements that temporarily produce, but do not worsen, the patient's symptoms are the proper movements to use in treating dysfunction. If no movements, either passive or active, can be found that produce the desirable effect on the patient's symptoms, then the patient may not be a good candidate for this treatment.

Instructions to Patients

The relative vigor and extent of the examination depend upon the irritability of the patient's symptoms. If the cervical or thoracic spine is judged to be irritable, then the examination must be gentle and limited to a few appropriate movements. The patient with an acute nerve root irritation, with symptoms extending below the elbow, deserves a gentle examination. On the other hand, a nonirritable and moderately painful condition will require a more vigorous and extensive examination. Few patients require all the test movements to satisfy the purpose of the examination.

The therapist must know the status of the patient's symptoms immediately before starting the examination and at the conclusion of each test movement. Thus, the patient is asked to describe his pretest symptoms, and to report any change in his symptoms during and immediately following each test movement. It is also important for the patient to understand that, in most circumstances, some test movements may make the symptoms worse, and some may make them better. The more accurately the patient is able to convey any changes to the therapist, the more informative will be the examination, and, quite likely, the more effective will be the treatment.

Special Tests Before the Objective Assessment

If the symptoms extend below the elbow, a neurologic examination must be completed prior to conducting the objective assessment. When the neurologic examination is given prior to the objective assessment, the effects, if any, of the examination itself may be assessed at the conclusion of the objective assessment. Without a pretest there is no benchmark from which to measure.

If the patient complains of dizziness associated with movements of the head and neck, as compared to changes in body position (i.e., from sitting to standing), then an essential part of the examination consists of tests that estimate the integrity of the vertebrobasilar system. Other symptoms of possible vertebrobasilar artery involvement, besides dizziness, include severe head and neck pain at the limit of movements of the cervical spine, and fainting with unconsciousness.

Corrigan and Maitland[29] described two clinical tests of the vertebral arteries. The first is to sustain the three positions of rotation to each side and extension. Symptoms may occur while in the sustained positions or upon release. The second test is to have the patient rotate his trunk beneath the motionless head. For example, the therapist stabilizes the patient's head while the patient twists his trunk in the standing position fully from side to side, without moving his feet, or the movement is done with the patient sitting on a swivel chair. The second

test eliminates the effect of inner ear movement. Other tests for vertebral artery insufficiency, published by the German Association of Manual Medicine,[30] are the extension tests, Hautant's test, De Klejn's test, and Underberger's tests.

Dizziness and reflex disorders of posture and movement can also be caused by degenerative, inflammatory, or traumatic disorders of the joints and muscles of the cervical spine. These structures are richly supplied with proprioceptive nerve endings.[27,31,32] Thus, dizziness is not always vertebrobasilar in origin.

Proper radiographic evaluation of suspected atlantoaxial instability is imperative before any vigorous objective assessment is attempted. Afflictions of this joint do occur, especially in Down's syndrome, rheumatoid arthritis, ankylosing spondylitis, psoriatic arthritis, and post-traumatic conditions. Vigorous examinations or treatment, where instability exists, have had disastrous complications dating back to early reports by Blaine.[33]

According to Dvorak et al.,[34] it is not difficult to diagnose instability of the upper cervical spine caused by lesions of the transverse ligament. Functional radiographic studies, including CT scanning in maximal flexion of the cervical spine, provide indirect information about the integrity of the transverse ligament. In a cadaver study using 12 specimens, the same investigators reported that, after a one-sided lesion of the alar ligament, there was a 30 percent increase in original rotation to the opposite side. The increased movement was divided equally between C0–C1 and C1–C2. It was concluded that irreversible overstretching or rupture of the alar ligaments can result in rotatory hypermobility of the upper cervical spine. The alar and transverse ligaments could be differentiated on CT images in axial, sagittal, and coronal views.

Observation of the Cervical Spine

The patient is usually sitting on the narrow end of the treatment table to enable the therapist to observe from each side and from the front. Note the general sitting posture, static deformity, asymmetry, and skin condition. Also note the patient's willingness to move and any tenderness or swelling.

Test Movements

Before any test movements are assessed, the present symptoms in the sitting position must be recorded. For each test movement, estimate movement loss and the relationship between the patient's symptoms and his range. Pain within the range before the limit is more indicative of derangement, and end-range pain is more indicative of dysfunction. Pain at the limit of range that is only produced by prolonged, sustained positions is more indicative of the posture syndrome.

It is helpful, for the sake of consistency in recording data, for the therapist to establish a routine sequence. A routine in the order of testing movements also helps avoid omissions.

The normal method of testing active physiologic movements, in the McKenzie approach, is to test a movement once and then to repeat the same test movement 10 times. The joints must be moved sufficiently far into the range to produce a valid response to the test. The usual sequence of testing is as follows: protraction, flexion, retraction, retraction and extension, sidebend bilaterally, and rotation bilaterally.

Active movements may be sustained or oscillated to produce the desired effect. For the sake of patient education, it is often necessary to ask the patient to repeat a movement that makes him worse and then to repeat a movement that makes him better. The practical lesson learned by the patient creates a lasting impression, which will foster compliance.

For derangements, the test movement or combination of movements that centralizes, reduces, and eliminates the patient's symptoms is then selected as the treatment procedure. For dysfunctions, the test movement or combination of movements that reproduces the patient's symptoms is selected as the treatment procedure. The patient is then instructed how to do the exercise, given an exercise dosage and precautions, and asked to report details at the next visit. Proper performance of the exercise if verified.

The normal method of testing active physiologic movements, in the Maitland approach, is to have the patient move to his pain (when treating pain) or to move to his limit (when treating stiffness). The therapist must always relate and record the association between range and pain. The usual sequence of testing is as follows: flexion, extension, lateral flexion bilaterally in flexion and extension, if required, and rotation bilaterally in flexion and extension, if required.

Movements may be sustained and overpressured, when applicable. The quadrants (a combination of extension with sidebending and rotation to the same side) for the upper and lower cervical spine may be tested if previous tests have been negative. Compression and distraction are used when necessary. Passive physiologic movements may also be tested in supine lying. Tests of the pain-sensitive structures in the intervertebral canal and static tests for muscle pain are performed as applicable.

The patient is then placed in a prone-lying position for palpation tests including temperature and sweating, soft tissue palpation, position of vertebrae, and passive accessory intervertebral movement tests. The passive accessory intervertebral movements are described later in the section on Treatment Procedures and Techniques. The therapist marks important findings on the chart with an asterisk. The effects of the examination are then assessed both subjectively and objectively by retesting one or two movements. The patient's chart is also reviewed for reports of relevant medical tests.

For treating pain, the technique that reduces (and in many cases centralizes and eliminates) the pain is used as the treatment technique. For treating stiffness, the technique that produced the comparable sign, but did not make it worse, is used as the treatment technique. A concurrent increase in range is also an obvious desirable treatment outcome when treating stiffness. Following treatment the patient is reassessed.

The patient is then warned of possible exacerbations, requested to report details of the behavior of his symptoms between now and his next visit, and given instructions in neck care.

For both approaches, the complete objective assessment involves testing other joints, including the glenohumeral joints, which may be responsible for the production of the patient's symptoms. These tests involve active quick tests and passive accessory tests as needed.

Table 6-3.
Summary of the Objective Assessment[a]

Neurologic and vertebral artery tests

Active physiologic movements

Passive accessory movements

Passive physiologic movements

Special tests (i.e., quadrants and tension tests)

[a] Not all of these tests are performed on every patient. The therapist determines the extent of the examination on the basis of the information gleaned during the subjective assessment.

Not all of the active physiologic test movements are illustrated in this chapter. However, many of the procedures and techniques illustrated later in the chapter are used as part of the objective assessment.

The Thoracic Spine

Active physiologic and passive accessory movements are tested using the same principles of assessment as presented for the cervical spine. Techniques and procedures for the thoracic spine are presented later in this chapter.

A summary of the objective assessment is presented in Table 6-3.

TREATMENT PROCEDURES AND TECHNIQUES

Principles

In most cases the proper treatment procedures or techniques are selected by the therapist during the objective assessment. Confirmation or denial of the original selection takes place at the second visit. It may be necessary to fine tune the procedure by, for example, correcting faults in the patient's performance of the procedure. If the patient has made significant progress, both objectively and subjectively, at the second visit there is no need to modify the procedure. On the other hand, if the patient is the same or worse at the second visit, the therapist is obligated to re-evaluate the tentative conclusion reached at the initial visit, and revise the treatment as needed. The patient with derangement should be seen daily until the patient has his pain under control with active procedures.

The following general principles will help guide the therapist in the selection of techniques or procedures, in the progression of treatment, and in the estimation of expected progress:

1. Use procedures to reduce the symptoms of derangement or to produce the symptoms of dysfunction with the knowledge that the patient understands the purpose of the procedures. The symptoms of derangement are expected to reduce quickly and the symptoms of dysfunction to reduce slowly. In derangement, once the symptoms are reduced, the next three phases of treatment are the maintenance of the reduction, the restoration of function, and the prevention of recurrences.

2. In most cases, if not all, the learning of a new posture is essential to the success of a treatment program. For the patient to continue his poor posture habits, which perpetuate chronic mechanical deformation, will only delay recovery or produce treatment failures.

3. The use of therapist's technique, in general, promotes dependence on the therapist. Techniques are needed when the application of patient procedures has been exhausted or when the patient's progress has plateaued. Therapist's technique is useful in the treatment of derangement when the application of extrinsic forces is needed to gain or maintain a reduction. For dysfunction, the use of one therapist's technique per visit is acceptable when indicated. Accurate assessment of one technique is more reliable than attempts at assessing two or more techniques.

4. Regardless of the approach selected, active exercises done by the patient on a regular and continuing basis are one of the keys to preventing recurrent spinal pain and/or aborting future attacks of spinal pain. It is reasonable to expect that most patients are able, and willing, to do about four different exercises on a regular basis if they are convinced that the exercises are effective in maintaining function and preventing a recurrence.

5. One of the most difficult tasks faced by the practicing therapist is to create an effective and efficient home exercise program that will be religiously followed by a happy patient. This task is particularly challenging to both the therapist and the patient when it involves the conversion of a therapist's technique into an effective active exercise.

However, it is suggested that few patients will remain symptom-free only as a result of the application of therapist's technique.

6. In very general terms, it is reasonable to expect that most patients will retain, from one treatment session to another, about 50 percent of the gain that was achieved at a treatment session. Optimally, this gain will be both a subjective and an objective improvement. The actual rate of improvement achieved by individual patients will vary, but the average gain for each patient is useful in determining the prognosis. Patients are more secure and satisfied with their treatment program when they are aware of the expected outcome.

7. Not all patients are suitable candidates for physical therapy. All approaches have their limitations, and it is the therapist's responsibility to identify unsuitable candidates and to offer a reasonable explanation and suggested alternatives, if available. To do otherwise is irresponsible behavior.

8. The true success of an approach is not measured by the date of return to work or by symptom-free behavior. Spinal pain is self-limiting in a majority of the population. The true success of an approach is measured, in part, by the effectiveness of the approach in preventing or reducing the severity of recurrent bouts of spinal pain.

9. Physical therapists have in the past been guilty of seeing patients too often, but not long enough. Once the patient has control of his symptoms, the frequency of visits may be significantly reduced. However, to be confident that an effective program of prevention is actually working, it is necessary to see the patient for rechecks over a reasonable period of time. In other words, the simple relief of pain is not sufficient evidence for discharging a patient.

10. Lastly, and probably most controversially, physical therapists should remain within the framework of organized medicine. Although independent practice without referral is an attractive concept, it does not appear to be the ultimate answer for the profession or for the patient. Physical therapy has much to gain in terms of quality of care and professional respectability by retaining a cooperative relationship with physicians. I believe that we are on the brink of a new era in terms of effective treatment. Our professional research and clinical skills are reaching new heights. To separate from organized medicine, with all its faults, would in some respects put us into the role of "lay manipulators" as described by Cyriax.[6]

Techniques and Procedures

There are thousands of procedures and techniques. Maitland and McKenzie have described most of the ones that follow. They have contributed enormously toward the delivery of effective and efficient assessment and treatment.

The following techniques and procedures for the cervical and upper thoracic spine are those most frequently used by the author. This presentation is not intended to be comprehensive or exclusive. Although the proper application of procedures or techniques contributes to the success of the treatment, the relative importance of proper assessment far exceeds the importance of proper technique. There are no limits to the nature and variations of procedures and techniques, and what may work for one therapist may be ineffective for another.

Books and journal articles are poor methods for learning procedures or techniques because the communication between teacher and learner is one-way. Techniques and procedures are learned most effectively either in well-supervised workshops or in supervised clinical practice, where instant feedback is provided. Of the two methods of instruction, supervised clinical practice is preferred. Practicing techniques on an experienced therapist, who understands the intent of the technique, is an excellent teaching and learning situation. Treating patients, under supervision, is also invaluable.

Procedures for the Cervical Spine

The procedures illustrated in Figures 6-1 to 6-4 and 6-7 to 6-14 are described by McKenzie.[4,35]

Typical Slumped Posture

In the typical slumped posture (Fig. 6-1), the patient sits in an unbalanced posture with a loss of lumbar lordosis, increased thoracic kyphosis, and a protracted head. Such posture is believed to cause deformation of the spine. Correction of this poor posture, including the restoration of normal lumbar

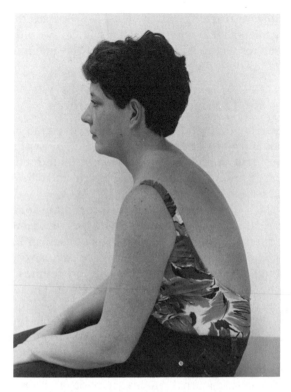

Fig. 6-1. Typical slumped posture with extended upper cervical and flexed lower cervical spine. Note also the absence of the lumbar lordosis, the marked forward head, and the protracted shoulders.

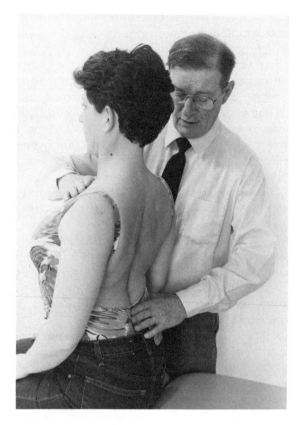

Fig. 6-2. Teaching the patient the proper lumbar lordosis, which for most people is about 10 percent off the end-range of extension.

lordosis, normal cervical lordosis, and normal thoracic kyphosis, is an essential part of the treatment program for all but a very few patients.

Teaching Proper Sitting Posture (Lumbar Lordosis)

The therapist assists the patient, either from in front or from the side, in attaining a normal lumbar lordosis (Figs. 6-2 and 6-3). This balanced lumbar posture provides a foundation on which to establish proper cervical and thoracic postures. Use of the slump overcorrection exercise, as described by McKenzie,[4] helps the patient become aware of his posture deficit. Removing the forces that cause mechanical deformation is key to successful treatment of mechanical spine pain. Restore the hollow and sit with a normal lordosis.

Cervical Retraction

Cervical retraction or posterior glide (Fig. 6-4) is done to help reduce the forward head posture. If the lower cervical spine is protracted, the retraction movement provides a desirable effect. It is normal for the patient to have some difficulty learning this procedure; therefore, the therapist must often demonstrate the proper method of doing the procedure and reinforce the proper execution of the exercise at subsequent visits. The patient may add overpressure to the movement by pushing on the maxilla or the mandible in a posterior direction. Cervical retraction is often combined with extension of the lower cervical spine and flexion of the upper cervical spine as a procedure for treating stiffness or reducing pain. Cyriax[36] described retraction as anteroposterior glide.

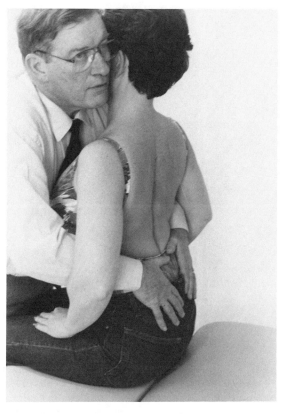

Fig. 6-3. Teaching the patient the proper lumbar lordosis by enhancing an anterior pelvic tilt. An awareness of this tilt is important in learning proper posture.

Flexion of the Upper Cervical Spine

Flexion of the upper cervical spine (Fig. 6-5) is usually done with the head in the retracted position. The purpose of this procedure is to stretch the upper cervical spine. The patient is able to provide overpressure by pushing on the maxilla or mandible in the direction of flexion. This procedure is often used to treat flexion dysfunction of the upper cervical spine. This procedure, like many other procedures, may also be done lying prone, with or without support (cervical roll) of the lower cervical spine.

Flexion of the Lower Cervical Spine

Flexion of the lower cervical spine (Fig. 6-6), in combination with flexion of the upper cervical spine, is done by having the patient move the chin

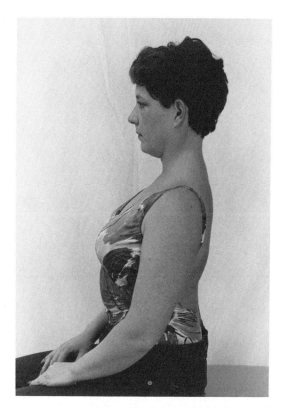

Fig. 6-4. Cervical retraction added to the proper sitting posture of normal lumbar lordosis.

toward the sternum. This procedure is used to treat flexion dysfunction of the lower cervical and upper thoracic spine. It is also used to reduce the pain in an anterior derangement and to restore flexion movement after the reduction of a posterior derangement. When treating the lack of flexion movement when a posterior derangement is stable, flexion of the lower cervical spine must be followed by retraction and extension movements to prevent a recurrence of the posterior derangement. When instituting flexion procedures, the expected strain-pain of dysfunction must not escalate or remain worse as a result of the procedure.

Sidebending or Lateral Flexion in Sitting

The patient performs generalized sidebending (Fig. 6-7), usually in the retracted position, as a physiologic movement. The movement may be used as a treatment procedure for sidebending dys-

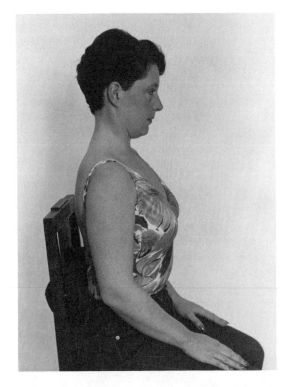

Fig. 6-5. Flexion of the upper cervical spine added to the retraction movement. The patient nods her head to produce a stretching of the upper cervical spine.

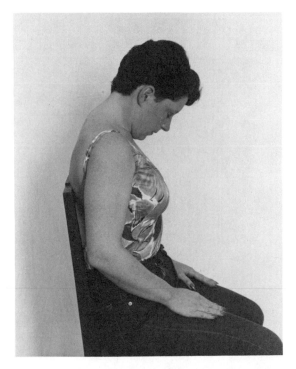

Fig. 6-6. Flexion of the lower cervical and upper thoracic spine done in sitting. The patient brings her chin toward her sternum, with her mouth closed, whereas in flexion of the upper cervical spine the chin is moved in the direction of the neck (nodding).

function, or to reduce and centralize the pain of derangement. Often, but not always, the symptoms of lower cervical spine derangement can be reduced by sidebending to the painful side. Likewise, the symptoms of dysfunction can be produced by sidebending away from the painful side. However, the direction of a procedure is always dictated by the desired changes in the signs and symptoms. Side-bending may also be done while lying supine.

Rotation with Overpressure

The patient applies overpressure in the direction of rotation, usually with the head retracted (Fig. 6-8).[35] This general physiologic movement is often restricted in the upper cervical spine by arthrosis and in the lower cervical spine by spondylosis. Generally, rotation is most effective in producing movement in the upper cervical spine, and sidebending is most effective in producing movement in the lower

cervical spine. Therefore, this procedure is often used to treat upper cervical spine dysfunction and derangement.

Lower Cervical Spine Extension Done in Retraction

The patient first retracts the head and then moves into extension (Fig. 6-9). One or both of these movements are frequently blocked in derangement. Retraction done in different positions of flexion, as needed, may be a required variation before extension is possible. This procedure is used to reduce posterior derangement. For extension dysfunction it is used to help restore lost movement into extension. Testing of the vertebral arteries is often required before using this procedure. The procedure may also be done supine. The patient should be encouraged to reach the full limit of the

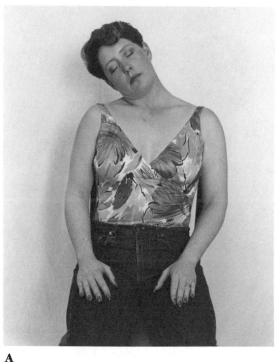
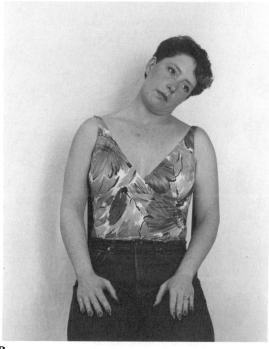

A   **B**

Fig. 6-7. Sidebending or lateral flexion of the cervical spine. The patient is instructed to bend sideways and bring her ear toward her shoulder, as opposed to rotation movements where she turns her nose toward her shoulder.[35] The curve of the neck, on the side away from the movement, is of superior quality in left **(B)** as compared to right **(A)** sidebending. Assessment of sidebending and rotation often yields similar results; therefore, it is not always necessary to assess both movements.

range and to perform small rotations at the limit of extension.[35]

Lower Cervical Spine Extension Done in Lying

In the lying position the effects of gravity are reduced compared to the sitting position (Fig. 6-10). The method of performing the procedure and the uses for the procedures are similar to those for extension done in retraction in the sitting position (Fig. 6-9).

Retraction in Lying

Retraction in lying (Fig. 6-11) is used mainly for the treatment of neck pain. This procedure as well as others may be done with a sustained position and/or oscillations with appropriate precautions. In treating derangement, always respect the centralization principle.

Sidebending or Lateral Flexion in Lying

Sidebending in lying must be a pure sidebend, but may be done at different angles of flexion for reduction and centralization of unilateral symptoms in derangement (Fig. 6-12). The patient usually has better control of this movement when lying rather than sitting. When treating dysfunction, movement is usually away from the painful side. There are times when this procedure will result in an increase of active flexion or extension movement.

Extension in Lying with Cervical Retraction

Cervical retraction and extension will usually produce movement down to T4, and repeated extension in lying will usually produce movement up to T4 (Fig. 6-13). Combining these procedures into one exercise is most useful in treating extension dysfunction of the spine.

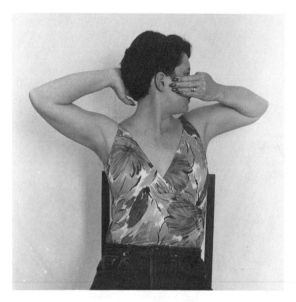

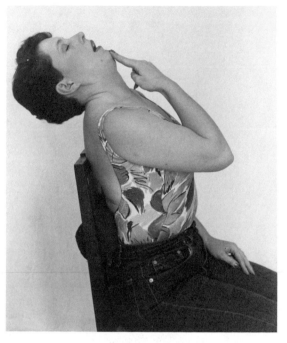

Fig. 6-8. Rotation overpressure to the left. The patient applies the end-range movement using both hands. The patient's left hand is placed on the maxilla in an attempt to reduce the stress on the temporomandibular joint. It is also important for the patient to keep her elbows in the position shown to facilitate feedback regarding the vigor of the overpressure. Movement of the upper cervical spine can often be enhanced by having the patient place her hands on the upper portion of the trapezius muscle to stabilize the middle and lower cervical spine (not illustrated).

Fig. 6-9. Lower cervical spine extension done in the retracted position. The patient is holding a finger on her chin as a reminder to retain the retraction while moving into extension. A high-backed chair, which stabilizes the middle thoracic spine, helps the patient to do this procedure correctly.

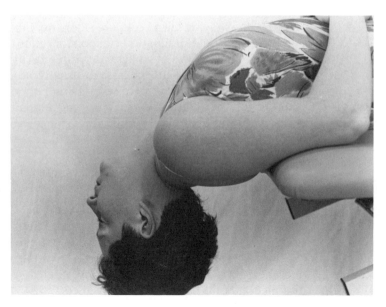

Fig. 6-10. Lower cervical spine extension done in lying. This procedure usually follows retraction in lying, and usually includes rotations done at the limit of extension.[35] It is important for the edge of the table to be at the level of T4 to allow for movement in the upper thoracic spine. When returning from the position of extension to neutral, the patient should lift her head with her hand and not perform the return movement actively. She should also rest in the neutral position on the table for about 30 seconds before sitting up. In sitting up, the patient should turn onto one side and sit up sideways to avoid neck flexion, instead of sitting straight forward.

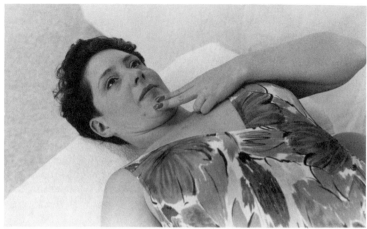

Fig. 6-11. Retraction in lying. The patient is lying flat on the table. Upper cervical spine flexion may also be performed in this position. Some patients who are unable to gain any positive treatment effects from doing this procedure in sitting will get benefit from doing this procedure in lying.

Retraction in sitting and in lying, extension in sitting and in lying, sidebending and rotation in sitting, and flexion in sitting are all well described in lay terms by McKenzie[35] in *Treat Your Own Neck*. This book is a most useful tool for patient education.

Patient Procedures for the Thoracic Spine

Thoracic Rotations in Sitting

To perform thoracic rotations in sitting (Fig. 6-14), the patient sits straddling the end of the table, facing the table. The intent of the procedure is to produce rotation in the thoracic spine and not to rotate the cervical spine. This procedure is used for unilateral pain and stiffness. Usually, the patient rotates toward the painful side when treating pain, and away from the painful side when treating stiffness. Centralization will occur in derangement syndromes only. Thoracic spine disorder as a cause of angina-like pain has been described by Lindahl.[37]

Thoracic Extension in Lying or Standing

The intent of thoracic extension in lying or standing (Fig. 6-15) is to enhance extension of the thoracic spine using the weight of the body against a bolster. The technique is useful for treating derangement when symptoms are centralized or for treating stiffness (extension dysfunction).

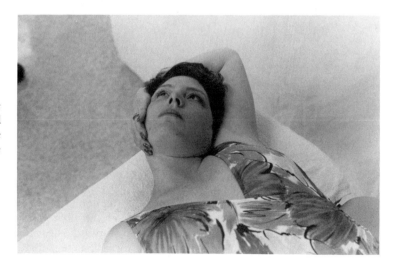

Fig. 6-12. Left sidebending in lying. The head is usually moved toward the desired side without allowing any rotation. The left arm is used, as illustrated, to provide overpressure when needed.

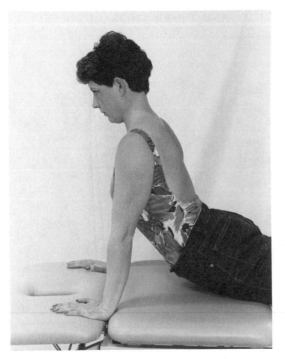

Fig. 6-13. Extension in lying with cervical retraction. This combined procedure is best taught in parts: The patient first perfects the lumbar procedure, then adds the cervical and thoracic procedures. Many patients extend their upper cervical spine when doing this exercise, sometimes with reckless abandon. Substitution of cervical retraction for upper cervical extension is helpful in preventing treatment soreness.

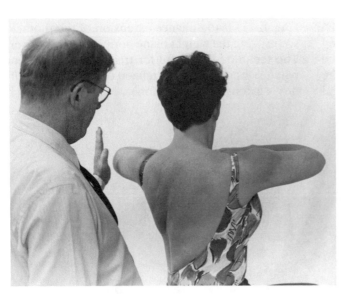

A

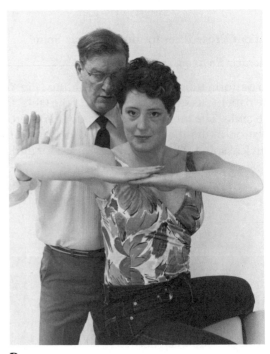

B

Fig. 6-14. Thoracic rotations in sitting. **(A)** Rotation to the left; **(B)** Rotation to the right. The patient in **B** straddles the end of the treatment table, facing the table. To reduce cervical rotations, the patient's head moves with the thoracic spine instead of facing forward. The patient must keep her chin in line with her hands as shown in **B**. End-range is accomplished by asking the patient to hit the therapist's hand with her elbow.

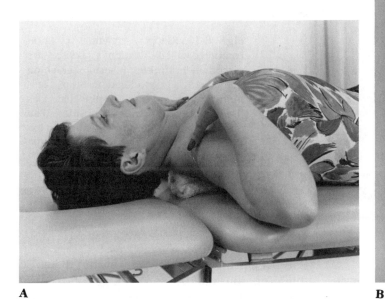
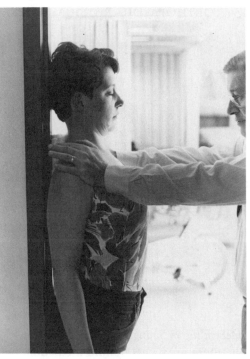

A
B

Fig. 6-15. Thoracic extension done in lying **(A)** and in standing **(B)**. In **A** the patient is lying supine on a firm surface with a bolster under the affected area. A bench press table (not illustrated) is most efficient because it is narrow and allows the patient to move into the posture correction position of shoulder horizontal extension. The patient should inhale when moving into horizontal extension. The same exercise may be done in standing **(B)** at the edge of a doorway. A bolster between the scapulae helps to localize the force. Overpressure may be added by the therapist or by a spouse by pushing on the shoulders bilaterally.

Klapp's Crawling Position (Prayer Position)

The crawling or prayer position (Fig. 6-16), when done properly, is a passive extension of the thoracic spine done in the prone position. The force is provided by the weight of the body. This procedure is used as an alternative or supplement to those previously described (Fig. 6-15).

Therapist's Techniques for the Cervical Spine

Palpation in Supine

The upper cervical spine is palpated with the patient lying supine (Fig. 6-17). In the neutral posture, with the patient supine, the therapist can often feel abnormalities of tissue tension and joint restriction. The cervical spine is also palpated effectively in the prone-lying position.

Manual Cervical Traction

Cervical traction, or longitudinal movement cephalad, may be applied manually or mechanically (Fig. 6-18). Manual traction is frequently used when very gentle movement is required, and/or as an assessment method to help determine the force, position, and mode (sustained or intermittent) for mechanical traction. There is evidence that traction can be both beneficial and harmful.[38]

Retraction and Extension in Lying

Retraction and extension in lying (McKenzie) is used in treating posterior derangements (Fig. 6-19). It is important to start the extension movement from the retracted position and to often precede the retraction movement with straight static traction. End-range extension is required, and overpressure is applied in small rotary movements.

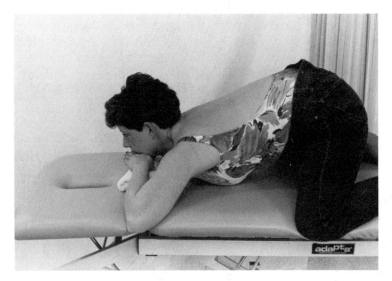

Fig. 6-16. Klapp's crawling position (modified). The patient's hands are placed under the chin instead of reaching out forward. The modified position places more force on the cervical spine than does the unmodified, or prayer, position. The thighs should be kept vertical, and an extension strain should be felt in the middle thoracic spine.

Sidebending in Sitting

The therapist stands behind the patient, who is sitting erect on a firm chair. The intent of the technique is to localize the sidebending at a particular level of the cervical spine. Figure 6-20 illustrates sidebending left of C7 on T1. A variation of the technique, to improve stabilization, is for the patient to sit on a treatment table with the therapist standing behind the patient. The therapist then places his or her foot on the treatment table adjacent to the patient's hip on the side of the intended movement.

The patient then rests the arm on the therapist's thigh (not illustrated).

This technique is useful when full-range sidebending is needed in the treatment of dysfunction. Since the spinous process of C7 moves left in normal right rotation, the technique is also useful in treating rotation dysfunction of the lower cervical spine. For example, to help restore right rotation, the spinous process of C7 is at first stabilized on the right, and the neck is sidebent to the right while the spinous process of C7 is moved left.

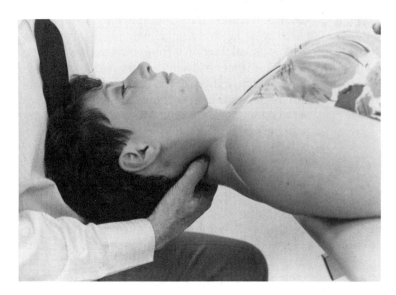

Fig. 6-17. Palpation in supine. The patient's head is comfortably supported by the therapist over the edge of the treatment table. Palpation for abnormal joint and muscle signs may be done in either the supine or the prone position (Figs. 6-23 to 6-28). Passive physiologic intervertebral movements may also be done in this position.

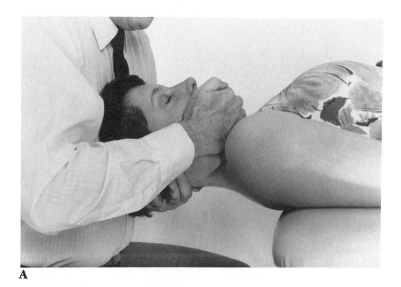

A

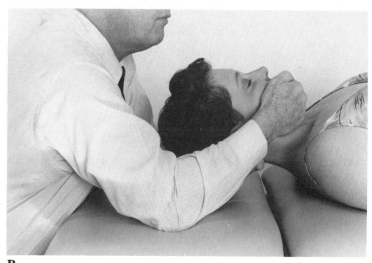

Fig. 6-18. Manual cervical traction done in the horizontal position using three different methods: **(A)** with the patient's head over the edge of the table; **(B)** with the patient lying on the table; **(C)** using pivotal traction. In **A**, the therapist provides the force by leaning backward. In **B**, the force comes from flexion of the therapist's elbows. In **C**, force comes from the patient's head pushing against the therapist's fingers.

B

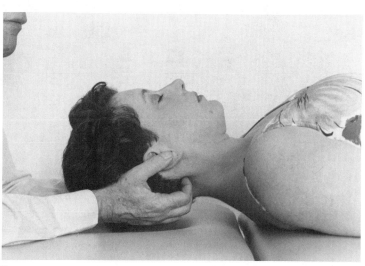

C

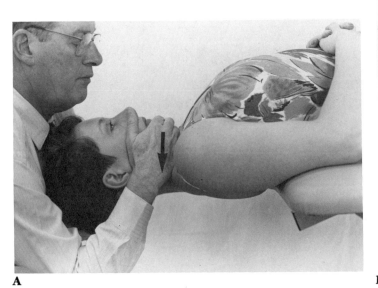 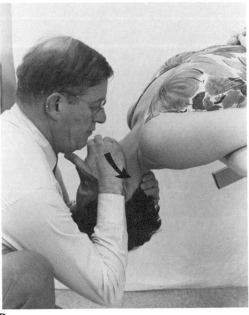

A   B

Fig. 6-19. Retraction and extension in lying. The patient is unsupported to about T4. **(A)** A traction force is applied and held, and then the neck is retracted; **(B)** while in the retracted position, the neck is slowly extended. Small rotary movements are frequently applied in overpressure. Continuous assessment of the changes in symptoms is essential.

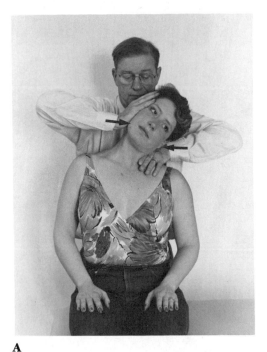 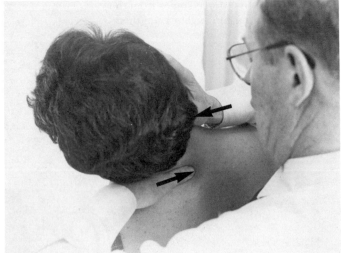

A   B

Fig. 6-20. Sidebending in sitting. The patient's neck is near, or at, the end of retraction. In left sidebending, the patient's head is sidebent to the limit of available range, and the force is applied by the therapist's right hand **(A)**. The spinous process of T1 is stabilized by the therapist's left thumb **(B)**. It is important for the therapist to hold his or her shoulders abducted with elbows out to the side **(A)**, to obtain optimum tactile feedback from the patient.

Sidebending in Lying on a Pillow

The patient is lying supine with the head on a pillow (Fig. 6-21). The therapist stands at the head of the table and supports the patient's neck from both sides. Positioning the head on a pillow allows the therapist to perform very gentle movements into sidebending while allowing the pillow to slide on the table. This technique is useful in treating pain when other positions are not tolerated.

Grade II and IV Rotations

The patient's head is properly cradled, and the therapist stands at the head of the treatment table (Fig. 6-22). Maitland[5] stated that rotation is one of the most useful techniques for the cervical spine. It is most useful in treating unilateral stiffness, with the movement usually in the direction away from the painful side. I believe that the restrictions causing the stiffness are being stretched when the painful

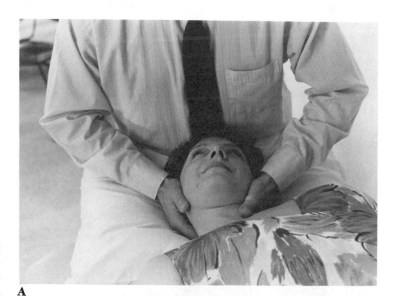

A

Fig. 6-21. Sidebending in lying on a pillow. **(A)** Left sidebending; **(B)** further left sidebending. The patient is lying supine on a pillow, and the therapist stands at the head of the treatment table. The patient's neck is supported from both sides. The therapist's left hand may act as a fulcrum for the sidebending. The force for the movement comes from the therapist's right hand. The left side is closed down and the right side is opened or stretched.

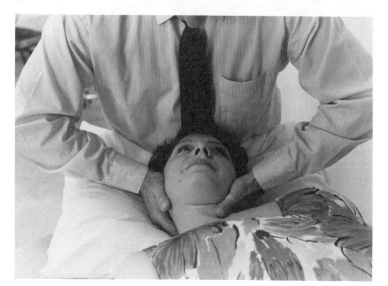

B

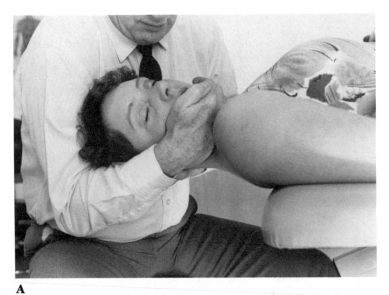

A

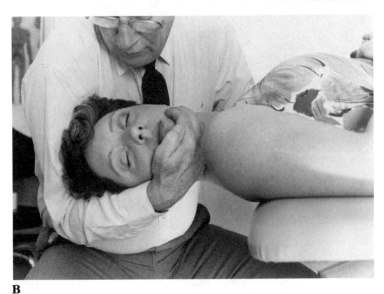

B

Fig. 6-22. Rotations of grades II **(A)** and IV **(B)**. The therapist cradles the patient's head at the occiput and at the chin. Grade II is a midrange rotation and grade IV an end-range rotation. The therapist should be able to do this technique with one hand at a time if the position is correct. Note that the patient's head is in contact with the therapist's chest and the anterior surface of his shoulder. Gentle oscillations are given at the proper position of range. The angle of flexion or extension may also be varied to produce an optimum treatment effect.

side is being opened by rotation away from the pain. Grade II movements are useful in the reduction of treatment soreness, and grade IV movements are useful in the treatment of stiffness, respecting the patient's pain. Grade I and grade III movements are also useful methods of treatment. (That grades I and III are not illustrated is not meant to imply lack of use of the techniques.)

Selected passive accessory intervertebral movements, as described by Maitland,[5] are presented in

Figures 6-23 to 6-29. Further information about these and other techniques is also presented by Maitland in his numerous writings.[39-51] Selected techniques are presented which provide a brief introduction to the approach. Examples are offered of how the techniques are used in concert with patient procedures. The skillful transfer between the use of therapist's techniques and the use of patient procedures is always challenging.

In all of the techniques presented in Figures 6-23

Fig. 6-23. Posteroanterior unilateral vertebral pressure to C0–C1 (↑⌐). Force is applied in the direction of the patient's ipsilateral eye. Therefore, the therapist must lean over the patient's head. The therapist's thumbs are placed on, above, or below the joint. Medial and lateral inclinations are also variations.

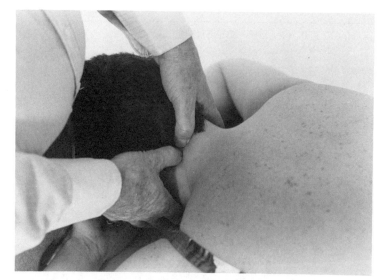

Fig. 6-24. Posteroanterior unilateral vertebral pressure to C2–C3. (↑⌐). Force is applied on the left articular pillar of C2 to move C2–C3. The patient's head is in neutral rotation. The therapist's arms are directed about 30 degrees medially to prevent the thumbs from slipping off the articular pillar.

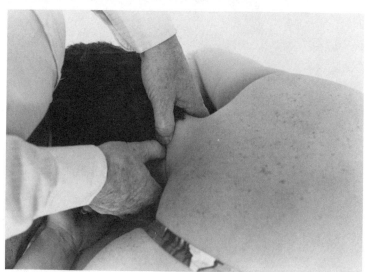

Fig. 6-25. Posteroanterior unilateral vertebral pressure to C1–C2 (↑⌐ in 30 degrees rotation left). Force is applied as in Figure 6-24 except that the patient's head is turned 30 degrees to the left. Rotation at C1–C2 is enhanced in this rotated position.

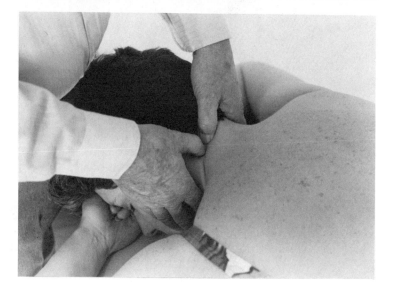

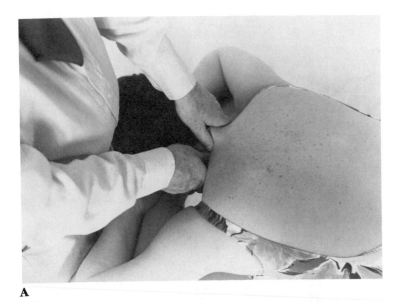

A

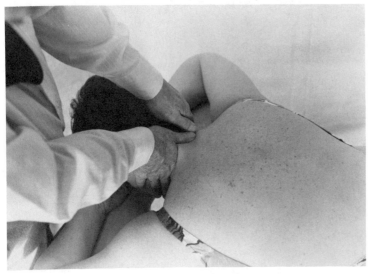

B

Fig. 6-26. Posteroanterior unilateral vertebral pressure to C5–C6 **(A).** These techniques may also be directed medially, laterally, **(B)** cephalad, or caudad as variations.

to 6-29, the patient is lying prone with the forehead resting on the overlapped and supinated hands. The therapist uses either the tips or the pads of the thumbs to provide an oscillating movement in the direction desired. The movement force is generated by movement of the therapist's shoulders and/or trunk, and this force is transmitted through the arms to the thumbs, which act as eccentric springs. No concentric muscle action should take place in the

therapist's thumbs, because accurate feedback from the patient is diminished by such action.

The Nelson Technique

The Nelson technique for traction and improved extension of the cervical-thoracic junction and upper thoracic spine (Fig. 6-30) is taught in the McKenzie approach. The Nelson technique is used

Fig. 6-27. Transverse vertebral pressures to C7 (←•—). Force is applied on the lateral surface of the spinous process of C7. Here the force is applied through the therapist's right thumb to the nonactive left thumbnail. The pad, not the tip, of the nonactive thumb is used for the patient's comfort. The therapist's right forearm should be held near parallel to the surface of the treatment table to provide movement in the desired direction. Often in treatment of stiffness, the patient rotates the neck to the limit of the available range. The technique is then performed at the pathologic limit (not illustrated).

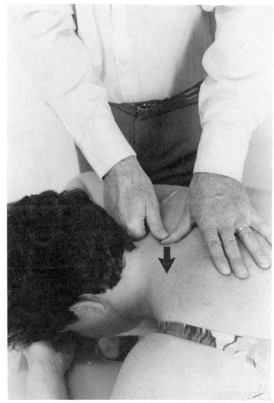

Fig. 6-28. Posteroanterior central vertebral pressures directed on C7 (↕). The therapist's two thumbs, often in contact with each other, cradle the spinous process, or, for gentle techniques, the tips of the thumbs may be used to localize the movement. To apply the technique in the painfree range, the neck may have to be placed in slight flexion. Prominent spinous processes are often the source of the patient's complaint.

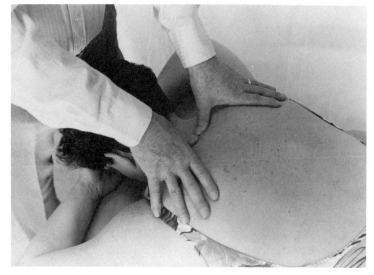

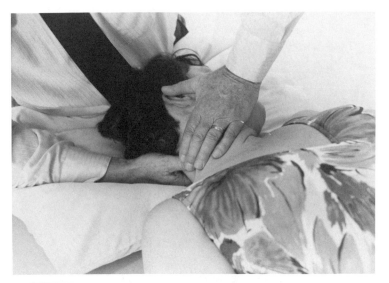

Fig. 6-29. A combined technique using left rotation and unilateral posteroanterior pressures on the right side of C2. Shown is an example of a physiologic and an accessory movement done simultaneously. It is frequently necessary to combine movements to reproduce the comparable sign. The same movements are then used as a treatment technique to reduce pain and/or increase range. In general, the technique done at the lowest grade that produces the desired treatment effect is preferred. The lowest grade provides for smooth and controlled, as opposed to rough and random, movement.

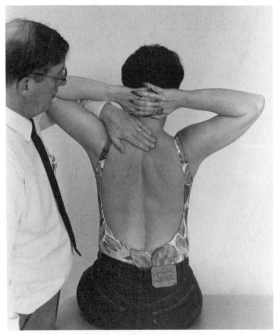

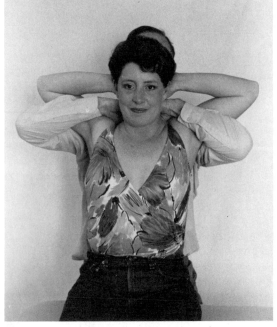

A **B**

Fig. 6-30. The Nelson technique for traction and improved extension of the cervical-thoracic junction and upper thoracic spine. The index and middle fingers of the therapist's left hand are placed over the spinous process of C7 **(A)**. The same two fingers of the therapist's right hand are then placed on top of these fingers. A posteroanterior force is directed cephalad by the therapist's arms and hands through the index and middle fingers of both hands. This force is generated by pushing on C7 and pulling the patient's shoulders into horizontal extension. The traction force is applied by attempting to lift the patient off the table. At the peak of the traction force, the therapist applies the extension force. Note that the shoulders of the therapist and the shoulders of the patient are at the same level **(B)**.

only after confirmed premanipulative testing, for providing extrinsic reductive or stretching forces in the lower cervical and upper thoracic spine. Other procedures or techniques, if required, are used prior to this technique to obtain and/or retain centralization of symptoms. This procedure cannot be done on patients with significant shoulder pathology because of the discomfort produced in moving the shoulders into end-range horizontal extension and external rotation. Well-muscled persons are very difficult to position properly. This technique is described by Laslett.[52]

Extension Mobilizations (NAGS)

The intent of the extension mobilization technique, also taught in the McKenzie approach, is to provide central posteroanterior movement of the segment

involved and gentle distraction. It is used on C2 through T4 to effect an extension movement. Asymmetrical variations are often used to treat unilateral or asymmetrical pain or stiffness. This technique is also described by Laslett.[52]

Thoracic Spine Techniques*

Transverse Vertebral Pressures on T4

The technique for applying transverse vertebral pressure to T4 ($\leftarrow\bullet-$) is similar to the technique shown for transverse vertebral pressures on C7 (Fig. 6-27). The technique is usually directed toward the

---

* Arrows indicate direction of technique; arrow pointing down is posterior/anterior.

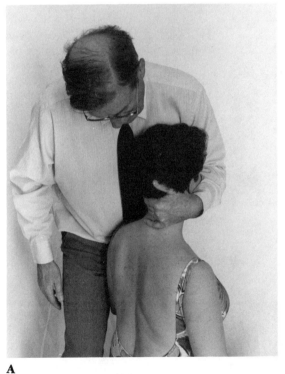

A

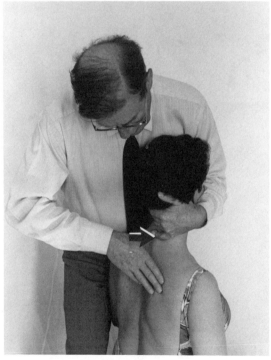

B

Fig. 6-31. Extension mobilization (NAGS). The patient should be sitting in a high-backed chair (not illustrated). The patient's head is cradled by the therapist's left hand and forearm against the therapist's chest. The therapist's little finger is placed on the spinous process of the appropriate vertebra **(A)**. The therapist's right thumb, or right pisiform-hamate groove, is then placed securely on his or her left little finger **(B)**. The movement desired is gentle traction, provided by the therapist's left arm, combined with posteroanterior central vertebral pressures, provided by the thumb or hand. The patient's head should remain stable.

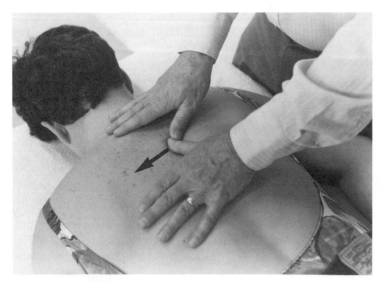

Fig. 6-32. Transverse vertebral pressures to T4 (←●—). Force is applied on the lateral surface of the spinous process of T4. In Figure 6-32, the force is applied through the therapist's right thumb to the nonactive left thumbnail. The pad, not the tip, of the nonactive thumb is used for the patient's comfort. Note that the patient's arms are at her sides to enhance relaxation of the thoracic spine.

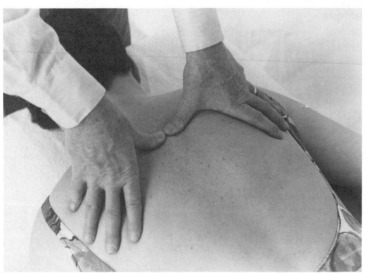

Fig. 6-33. Posteroanterior central vertebral pressures (●) to T4. The therapist's two thumbs, often in contact with each other, cradle the spinous process. For gentle techniques, the tips of the thumbs may be used to localize the movement.

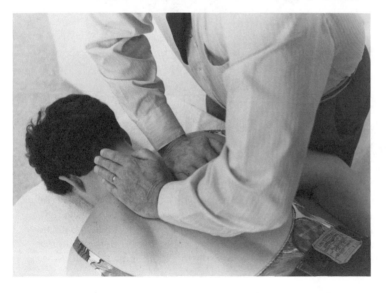

Fig. 6-34. Intervertebral rotatory posteroanterior movements of T1–T4. Force is applied bilaterally through the therapist's hypothenar eminences to the spaces between the spinous processes and the medial borders of the scapulae. A combination of clockwise and counterclockwise movements are applied in a posteroanterior direction. The force may also be directed cephalad, caudad, and laterally.

side of pain.[5] In cases of suspected derangements, the patient's symptoms often centralize when using this technique. When dysfunction is being treated, the patient's comparable sign is reproduced, and the range of physiologic movements is often increased. Although the accessory movement is in a frontal plane, physiologic movements in the sagittal plane (i.e., flexion or extension) are often improved.

Posteroanterior Central Vertebral Pressures to T4

The technique for applying posteroanterior central vertebral pressure to T4 (♦) is similar to that shown for posteroanterior central vertebral pressures on C7, except that in this case the force is not directed laterally at all (Fig. 6-33). This technique is used commonly for central or symmetrical symptoms,

and may be used for vague or generalized unilateral symptoms.[5] It is one of the most useful techniques for the thoracic spine and is often followed by a more vigorous technique, illustrated later.

Intervertebral Rotatory Posteroanterior Movements of T1–T4

The technique of intervertebral rotatory posteroanterior movements of T1–T4 provides a method for producing desirable movement without direct contact on the spinous processes (Fig. 6-34). It is suggested that localized movement can be produced in the costotransverse joints, the costovertebral joints, the intervertebral (apophyseal) joints, and the intervertebral junction. It is common for even gentle

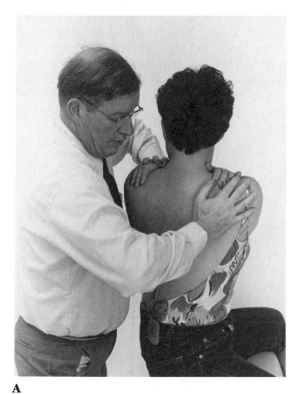

A

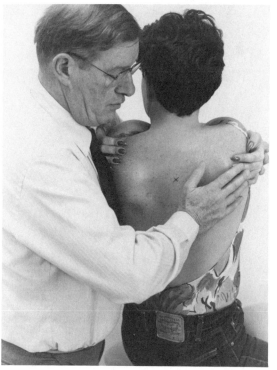

B

Fig. 6-35. Thoracic rotation to the left. **(A)** Generalized thoracic rotation. The patient sits straddling the end of the treatment table with arms folded in front of her chest. **(B)** More localized overpressure in the middle thoracic spine.

techniques to produce local sounds of release, and for the patient to gain rapid relief from symptoms using this technique.

Thoracic Rotations

Thoracic rotations may be tested with the patient standing (mostly lower movement), sitting (Fig. 6-35), and lying. For stretching stiff structures, rotation is often performed in the direction away from the symptomatic side. For reducing and centralizing the pain of derangement, rotation is often performed in the direction toward the painful side. However, as always, the clinical assessment of the individual patient and the response to movement tests dictate the proper direction.

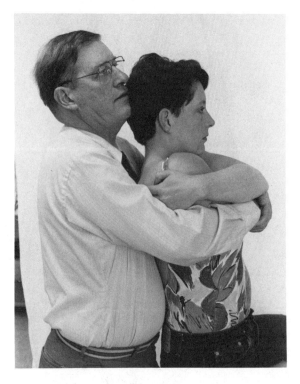

Fig. 6-36. Longitudinal movement and extension in sitting. The patient sits straddling the end of the treatment table. The longitudinal movement is provided by partially lifting the patient off the table. The extension movement is provided by the therapist leaning backward and applying overpressure (when desired) through his or her chest.

Longitudinal Movement and Extension in Sitting

The generalized technique of longitudinal movement and extension may be done with the patient sitting (Fig. 6-36) or standing. Because of the nonspecific nature of the technique, it is most useful in treating generalized stiffness of the middle thoracic spine. Greater specificity may be achieved with the technique described next.

Posteroanterior Manipulation of T4

The technique of posteroanterior manipulation of T4 ( ), which must be learned and practiced under the supervision of an experienced therapist, is one of the most useful techniques for the upper and middle thoracic spine (Fig. 6-37). When successful, the patient experiences dramatic relief. It is suggested not only that are stiff joints loosened, but that thoracic spine derangements may be reduced by selected use of this technique. Reduction, if achieved, must be retained by the religious use of patient procedures.

Thoracic spine disorders as a cause of angina-like pain have been described by Lindahl.[53] This technique has been useful in treating this type of disorder. This technique is described by both Maitland[5] and McGuckin.[54]

SUMMARY

An integrated approach for the assessment and treatment of the cervical and upper thoracic spine that relies heavily on the teachings of McKenzie,[4] Maitland,[5] and Cyriax[6] has been presented. Mechanical and chemical pain were described. The three syndromes of posture, dysfunction, and derangement as described by McKenzie[4] are loosely related to the treatment of pain and stiffness as described by Maitland.[5]

The individual therapist may elect to use active procedures followed by passive procedures, or passive procedures followed by active procedures, to relieve pain and restore function. Suggested mechanisms for the relief of pain and to increase range were described.

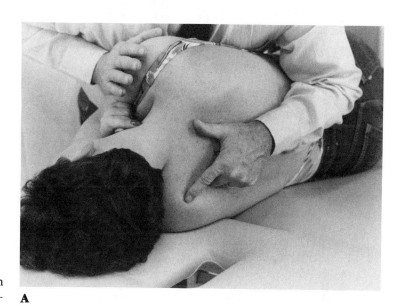

A

Fig. 6-37. Posteroanterior manipulation ( ) of T4. **(A)** Therapist's hand placement for the central technique; **(B)** therapist's hand placement for the unilateral technique. *(Figure continues.)*

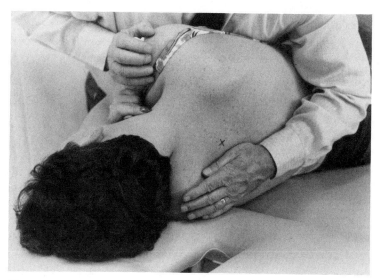

B

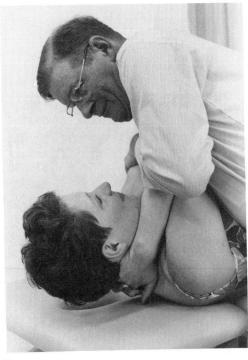

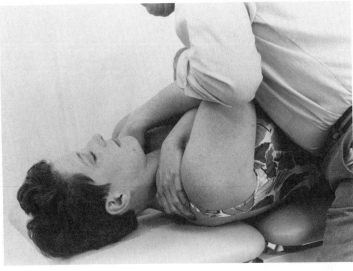

C

D

Fig. 6-37 *(continued)*. **(C)** Positioning of the patient in neutral flexion and extension for the level to be treated; **(D)** application of force through the patient's elbows. At this point the patient exhales. The hand of the therapist under the patient provides for the localization of the technique. In **C** and **D**, the therapist's right hand is under the patient.

Subjective assessment, objective assessment, and methods of treatment were described and illustrated. Guidelines and principles for the direction of a technique or procedure were presented. Further information regarding the details of these approaches may be found in the writings of McKenzie,[4,9,11,36,55] Maitland,[5,39–51] and Cyriax.[6,10,35,56]

REFERENCES

1. Laslett M: Use of manipulative therapy for mechanical pain of spinal origin. Orthop Rev 16:8, 65, 1987
2. Haldeman S: Spinal manipulative therapy: a status report. Clin Orthop Rel Res 179:62, 1983
3. Ottenbacher K, DiFabio R: Efficacy of spinal manipulation/mobilization therapy. Spine, 10: suppl. 9, 833, 1985
4. McKenzie R: The Lumbar Spine. Spinal Publications, Waikanae, New Zealand, 1981
5. Maitland G: Vertebral Manipulation. 5th Ed. Butterworths, London, 1986
6. Cyriax J: Textbook of Orthopedic Medicine. 6th Ed. Williams & Wilkins, Baltimore, 1975
7. Basmajian J (ed): Manipulation, Traction and Massage. 3rd Ed. Williams & Wilkins, Baltimore, 1985
8. Cookson JC: Orthopedic manual therapy—an overview. II. The spine. Phys Ther 59(3):259, 1979
9. McKenzie R: Manual correction of sciatic scoliosis. NZ Med J 76:484, 1972
10. Cyriax J: Treatment of lumbar disk lesions. Br Med J 2:1434, 1950
11. McKenzie R: Prophylaxis in recurrent low back pain. NZ Med J 89:22, 1979
12. Wyke B: The neurology of low back pain. p. 266. In Jayson M (ed): The Lumbar Spine and Back Pain. 2nd Ed. Pitman Medical, Kent, 1980
13. Cummings G, Crutchfield C, Barnes M: Orthopedic

Physical Therapy Series—Soft Tissue Changes in Contractures. Vol. 1. Stokesville Publishing, Atlanta, 1983

14. Evans P: The healing process at the cellular level: a review. Physiotherapy 66:256, 1980
15. Donaldson R: Centralization phenomenon: its usefulness in evaluating and treating sciatica. Presented at International Society for the Study of the Lumbar Spine, Dallas, 1986
16. Saunders H: Evaluation, Treatment and Prevention of Musculoskeletal Disorders. Anderberg-Lund, Minneapolis, 1986
17. Sprague R: The acute cervical joint lock. Phys Ther, 63: suppl. 9, 1439, 1983
18. McNair J: Acute locking of the cervical spine. p. 357. In Grieve G (ed): Modern Manual Therapy of the Vertebral Column. Churchill Livingstone, Edinburgh, 1986
19. Nyberg R: Role of physical therapists in spinal manipulation. p. 36. In Basmajian J (ed): Manipulation, Traction and Massage. 3rd Ed. Williams & Wilkins, Baltimore, 1985
20. Thornton P, Calangelo V: Fundamentals of Engineering Materials. Prentice-Hall, Englewood Cliffs NJ, 1985
21. Callister W: Materials Science and Engineering. John Wiley & Sons, New York, 1985
22. Smith C: The Science of Engineering Materials. 3rd Ed. Prentice-Hall, Englewood Cliffs NJ, 1986
23. Peterson B (ed): The Collection of Papers of Irvin M. Korr. American Academy of Osteopathy, Colorado Springs CO, 1979
24. Wyke B: Neurology of the cervical spine. Physiotherapy, 65: suppl. 10, 72, 1979
25. Cyriax J: Illustrated Manual of Orthopedic Medicine. Butterworths, London, 1983
26. Gore D, Sepic S, Gardner G, Murray M: Neck pain: a long term follow-up of 205 patients. Spine, 12: suppl. 1, 1, 1987
27. Bogduk N: Cervical causes of headache and dizziness. p. 289. In Grieve G (ed): Modern Manual Therapy of the Vertebral Column. Churchill Livingstone, Edinburgh, 1986
28. Dillin W, Booth R, Cuckler J, et al: Cervical radiculopathy: a review. Spine, 11: suppl. 10, 988, 1986
29. Corrigan B, Maitland G: Practical Orthopaedic Medicine. Butterworths, London, 1983
30. German Association of Manual Medicine: Memorandum on the prevention of accidents arising from manipulative therapy of the cervical spine. April 1979
31. Grieve G: Common Vertebral Joint Problems. Churchill Livingstone, Edinburgh, 1981
32. Wyke B: Articular neurology: a review. Physiotherapy 58:94, 1972
33. Blaine E: Manipulative (chiropractic) dislocation of the axis. J Am Med Assoc 1356, 1925
34. Dvorak J, Panjabi M, Gerber M, Wichmann W: CT-functional diagnostics of the rotary instability of the upper cervical spine. Spine, 12: suppl. 3, 197, 1987
35. McKenzie R: Treat Your Own Neck. Spinal Publications, Lower Hut, New Zealand, 1983
36. Cyriax J: Textbook of Orthopaedic Medicine. Vol. 2. Williams & Wilkins, Baltimore, 1971
37. Lindahl O, Hamberg J: Thoracic spine disorders as a cause of angina-like pain. Pract Cardiol. 10: suppl. 2, 62, 1984
38. DeLacerda F: Cervical traction. p. 683. In Grieve G (ed): Modern Manual Therapy of the Vertebral Column. Churchill Livingstone, Edinburgh, 1986
39. Maitland G: Application of manipulation. Physiotherapy 56:1, 1970
40. Hickling J, Maitland G: Abnormalities in passive movement: diagrammatic representation. Physiotherapy 3:105, 1983
41. Maitland G: The hypothesis of adding compression when examining and treating synovial joints. J Orthop Sports Phys Ther 2:7, 1980
42. Maitland G: Negative disc exploration. Aust J Physiother, 25: suppl. 3, 129, 1979
43. Maitland G: Manipulation: individual responsibility. Physiotherapy 1:2, 1972
44. Maitland G: The treatment of joints by passive movement. Aust J Physiother, 19: suppl. 2, 65, 1973
45. Maitland G: Relating passive movement treatment to some diagnoses. Aust J Physiother, 20: suppl. 3, 129, 1974
46. Maitland G: Palpation examination of the posterior cervical spine: the ideal, average and normal. Aust J Physiother, 28: suppl. 3, 3, 1982
47. Maitland G: Examination of the cervical spine. Aust J Physiother, 25: suppl. 2, 49, 1979
48. Maitland G: Manipulation-mobilization. Physiotherapy 52:382, 1966
49. Maitland G: Acute locking of the cervical spine. Aust J Physiother 24:103, 1978
50. Maitland G: Musculoskeletal Recording Guide. Virgo Press, Adelaide, South Australia, 1978
51. Maitland G: Peripheral Manipulation. 2nd Ed. Butterworths, London, 1970
52. Laslett M: The rationale for manipulative therapy in the treatment of spinal pain of mechanical origin. Unpublished workshop manual. Mark Laslett, 211-213 White Swan Rd., Mt. Rosekill, Auckland 3, New Zealand, 1986

53. Lindahl O, Hamberg J: Thoracic spine disorders as a cause of angina-like pain. Pract Cardiol 10: suppl. 2, 62, 1984

54. McGuckin N: The T4 syndrome. p. 370. In Grieve G (ed): Modern Manual Therapy of the Vertebral Column. Churchill Livingstone, Edinburgh, 1986

55. Stevens B, McKenzie R: Mechanical diagnosis and self treatment of the cervical spine. p. 271. In Grant R (ed): Physical Therapy of the Cervical and Thoracic Spine. Churchill Livingstone, New York, 1988

56. Cyriax J: Illustrated Manual of Orthopaedic Medicine. Butterworths, Boston, 1983

7
Dysfunction, Evaluation, and Treatment of the Shoulder

WILLIAM G. BOISSONNAULT
STEVEN C. JANOS

It is well recognized that pain in the shoulder and shoulder girdle is very common in the general population, with a reported prevalence of 15 to 25 percent in patients 40 to 50 years of age.[1,2] In industry, the prevalence of symptoms and disorders from the shoulder region is about 30 to 40 percent and has increased six times during the last decade.[3] With the contemporary explosion of physical fitness activities, these numbers will very likely increase.

This chapter presents a brief overview of the functional anatomy of the shoulder region, an examination scheme for the area, and an in-depth look at three common shoulder pathologies: frozen shoulder, rotator cuff injuries, and anterior glenohumeral joint instability. The description of the pathologies will include pathohistologic changes, common clinical signs and symptoms, and treatment considerations. Other chapters in this text present further information related to assessing and treating shoulder dysfunction.

FUNCTIONAL ANATOMY

The anatomic and biomechanical complexity of the shoulder region can make assessment and treatment of shoulder dysfunction difficult. Inman et al.[4] demonstrated the interdependency of glenohumeral joint and shoulder girdle motions for elevation of the upper extremity to 180 degrees. Using straps to prevent scapulothoracic motion and clavicular elevation, they showed that shoulder abduction was restricted to 90 and 120 degrees, active and

passive, respectively. Inman also manually prevented clavicular rotation, which limited active shoulder flexion and abduction to approximately 110 degrees. The fact that the glenohumeral, sternoclavicular, acromioclavicular, and scapulothoracic joints all contribute to shoulder movement makes a detailed clinical assessment of each of these joints and associated soft tissue structures a necessity. A working knowledge of the anatomy and mechanics of each of these regions is the basis for many of the examination techniques and for the understanding of many of the shoulder disorders seen clinically.

Stability

The price for the tremendous mobility of the shoulder complex has been poor stability. This is particularly true at the glenohumeral joint. In contrast to the hip joint, little support is supplied by the osseous elements, the humeral head and glenoid fossa. In fact, Sarrafian[5] stated that because the concave glenoid fossa is relatively flat and only one-quarter the size of the convex humeral head, there is no element of stability provided by the bony articulation. The orientation of the glenoid fossa in relation to the remainder of the scapula may be a factor in glenohumeral joint stability, however. Saha[6] related the retrotilted position of the glenoid fossa to a reduced inherent risk of anterior dislocation of the humeral head. The orientation of the scapula on the thorax may also influence glenohumeral joint stability regarding inferior dislocation of the humeral

151

head. With the upper extremity in a dependent position, the glenoid fossa faces laterally, anteriorly, and superiorly. Because of this superior inclination, for the humeral head to subluxate inferiorly it must also displace laterally.[7] Therefore, by preventing lateral displacement, structures oriented in the horizontal plane, such as the superior joint capsule and the coracohumeral ligament, could prevent inferior subluxation of the humeral head. Because of the horizontal orientation of the supraspinatus and the posterior deltoid, these muscles may also contribute to this mechanism.

The glenohumeral joint capsule is relatively thin, allowing approximately one-half inch of joint distraction in a dissected specimen.[8] The joint capsule is reinforced superiorly and anteriorly by the coracohumeral and glenohumeral ligaments, respectively. The middle and inferior portions of the glenohumeral ligament help prevent anterior dislocation of the humeral head with the glenohumeral joint positioned in abduction and external rotation.[9] The rotator cuff muscles also reinforce the joint capsule.[5,10] The subscapularis adds support anteriorly, especially when the arm is positioned near the body.[9] The teres minor and the infraspinatus help stabilize the posterior aspect of the glenohumeral joint[5]; the supraspinatus stabilizes the superior aspect. The inferior aspect of the joint is not reinforced by muscles or capsular ligaments, making it the weakest area.

Limiting superior displacement of the humeral head is the coracoacromial arch. This arch forms the superior border of the subacromial joint, a physiologic joint described by Kessel and Watson.[11] The rotator cuff tendons and the greater tuberosity of the humerus form the inferior border of this joint, and the subacromial bursa acts as the joint cavity. Soft tissue structures, such as the supraspinatus and infraspinatus tendons, lying between the two unyielding joint borders are at risk for impingement or compressive injuries in the presence of abnormal glenohumeral joint mechanics or trauma.

The anatomic joints of the shoulder girdle include the acromioclavicular and sternoclavicular joints; the latter is the sole bony connection between the upper extremity and the trunk. The fibrocartilaginous disk and the costoclavicular ligament are the principal stabilizers of the sternoclavicular joint.[12,13] Besides adding stability, the costoclavicular ligament is described as the fulcrum around which all sternoclavicular joint motion occurs.[13] The principal stabilizer at the acromioclavicular joint is the coracoclavicular ligament.[5,13] This ligament also plays a key role in shoulder girdle mechanics during shoulder elevation.

Shoulder Motion: Elevation

The most often studied shoulder movement has been elevation in the frontal plane or in the plane of the scapula. The plane of the scapula is described as being approximately 30 to 45 degrees anterior to the frontal plane.[14] Shoulder abduction is generally considered as consisting of 90 to 120 degrees of glenohumeral joint motion and approximately 60 degrees of upward scapular rotation.[4,15,16] There is agreement that the initial 25 to 30 degrees of abduction primarily occurs at the glenohumeral joint, while the scapula seeks a stable position.[4,16] Afterward both the shoulder girdle and the glenohumeral joint contribute to the movement in what has been described as scapulohumeral rhythm.

Poppen and Walker[14] studied the humeral head position in relation to the glenoid fossa during elevation of the arm in the plane of the scapula. The humeral head translated in a superior direction an average of 3 mm during the initial 30 to 60 degrees of the motion. Afterward the humeral head position on the glenoid was relatively constant, translating 1 to 2 mm in either a superior or an inferior direction. This finding was thought to be due to the medially and inferiorly directed pull of the teres minor, infraspinatus, and subscapularis muscles. These muscles form a functional group, which depresses the head of the humerus to counteract the superior and lateral pull of the deltoid.[4,10] The teres minor, the infraspinatus, and the subscapularis are active throughout the abduction range, as is the deltoid.[4] The deltoid and the supraspinatus are considered the prime movers for glenohumeral joint abduction. Each muscle is capable of elevating the arm independently, but with a resultant loss of power.[17] Glenohumeral joint external rotation is necessary for normal shoulder abduction. The rotation allows for the greater tuberosity and accompanying rotator cuff tendons to clear the acromion, the coracoacromial ligament,[10,16] and/or the superior ridge of the glenoid fossa.[18] Components of the rotator cuff—the teres minor and the infraspinatus—are thought to account for the external rotation as their activity increases throughout the abduction range, whereas the subscapularis activities tends to peak at around 90 degrees of the motion.[12] Extensibility of the inferior and anterior periarticular structures of the glenohumeral joint are necessary for the angular displacement of the humerus away from the inferior aspect of the glenoid with the corresponding inferior glide of the humeral head, and for the external rotation that must occur.

Shoulder girdle contributions to shoulder elevation are important for many reasons. Besides adding to the abduction range, the 60 degrees of upward scapular rotation on the thorax helps maintain an optimal length-tension relationship for muscles acting across the glenohumeral joint,[4,10,15] and allows the glenoid fossa to remain in a stable position in relation to the humeral head.[15,16] The amount of upward scapular rotation is equal to the amount of movement occurring at the clavicular joints.[4] Last described the initial 20 degrees of scapular rotation as occurring at the acromioclavicular joint as the scapula moves on the clavicle.[13] This produces tension within the coracoclavicular ligaments, resulting in clavicular rotation at the sternoclavicular joint. This clavicular rotation, which allows for another 40 degrees of upward scapular rotation, is therefore passive in nature, relying on normal acromioclavicular joint mechanics.[13]

Clavicular elevation occurring at the sternoclavicular joint during the initial 90 degrees of abduction is also important for the general position of the scapula on the thorax.[4] For clavicular elevation to occur, inferior displacement of the sternal end of the clavicle is necessary. This movement primarily occurs between the clavicle and the fibrocartilaginous disk.[13] The trapezius, the rhomboids, the serratus anterior, and the levator scapulae muscles form the axioscapular muscle group responsible for scapular stability and motion.[4] The serratus anterior, the lower and middle trapezius, and the rhomboids stabilize the medial border of the scapula, preventing winging from occurring during abduction.[4,10] In addition, the serratus anterior works in concert with portions of the trapezius to rotate the scapula upward on the thorax.[4,10]

The other shoulder motions have not been studied as extensively as abduction; therefore, only a brief comparison between flexion and abduction will be presented. Although flexion is somewhat like abduction in that similar contributions at the glenohumeral joint and shoulder girdle are necessary for full range, differences between the two movements exist. Inman[4] stated that approximately 60 degrees of flexion occurs before significant scapular motion begins, as opposed to 30 degrees of abduction. Inman demonstrated that there was less middle trapezius activity with flexion than with abduction, which would allow the scapula to migrate further laterally on the thorax during flexion.[4] Blakely and Palmer[19] found internal rotation of the humerus to be an important concurrent motion for full flexion to occur, whereas external rotation is important for full abduction to occur. Basmajian[12] stated that the anterior deltoid and the clavicular portion of the pectoralis major are the prime movers for flexion. Both these muscles are also internal rotators. Finally, Saha[18] described an anterior and superior movement of the humeral head on the glenoid during flexion, which again differs from the humeral head displacement noted during abduction.

Description of the other shoulder motions is beyond the scope of this chapter. These other motions, however, will be specifically related to shoulder dysfunction later in this chapter.

EXAMINATION AND EVALUATION OF THE SHOULDER

Evaluation of the shoulder follows the same principles used in examination of any joint in the body. It is assumed that a subjective examination and an upper quarter screening examination have been completed, and the findings have led to the decision to look at the shoulder in more detail. The cervical spine is an important region to be screened since local cervical dysfunction may cause referred pain to the shoulder. Kellgren[20] demonstrated the referral of pain to the glenohumeral joint area from the midline cervical and thoracic spine ligaments.

Table 7-1. Examination of the Shoulder Girdle

Observation/Inspection
  Standing
  Sitting
Palpation
  Standing
  Sitting
  Supine
  Prone
Active and passive range (Physiologic)
  Shoulder girdle
    Elevation
    Depression
    Protraction
    Retraction
  Glenohumeral joint
    Forward flexion
    Abduction
    Internal rotation
    External rotation
    Extension
    Horizontal flexion
    Horizontal extension
    Hand behind back
    Hand behind head
Accessory movements
  Glenohumeral joint
    Distraction
    Compression
    Anterior glide
    Posterior glide
    Inferior glide
  Subacromial joint
    Distraction
    Compression
  Acromioclavicular joint
    Anterior glide/distraction
    Posterior glide/compression
    Cephalic glide
    Caudal glide
  Sternoclavicular joint
    Distraction
    Compression
    Anterior glide
    Posterior glide
    Cephalic glide
    Caudal glide
  Scapulothoracic joint
    Distraction
    Cephalocaudal glide
    Mediolateral glide
    Mediolateral rotation
Resisted tests (isometric)
  Cardinal planes (shoulder/elbow)
  Specific manual muscle testing
Special tests
  Locking position
  Quadrant test
  Biceps tendon testing
  Apprehension test
  Drop arm test

Glenohumeral joint pain was primarily noted with irritation of the interspinous ligament associated with the C4–C5 motion segments but also with irritation of ligaments of the C7–T1 and T1–T2 segments. In a similar study, Campbell and Parsons[21] demonstrated pain referral to the shoulder area with irritation of ligaments and joints of the upper and midcervical regions. See Chapter 3 for a description of an upper quarter screening examination that indicates tests for the cervical spine. Table 7-1 gives a proposed examination scheme for the shoulder region.

Observation and Inspection

The initial observation and inspection of the shoulder are often referred to as the postural portion of the examination. It is important to remember not to diagnose a problem solely on the basis of a person's posture in a given area. The real importance of posture lies in its relationship to function, which is studied later in the examination. For the shoulder, it is important to look at trunk and neck position in both sitting and standing positions. The position of the scapula relative to the trunk should be inspected. Excessive protraction is probably most commonly seen, followed by excessive elevation. Next, the position of the humerus relative to both the scapula and the trunk should be noted. Often the humerus sits anterior relative to the scapula. Hypertrophy and atrophy of the musculature of the shoulder region should be noted, as should other soft tissue changes. In more chronic shoulder dysfunction, one will often note atrophy of the deltoid along with hypertrophy of the upper trapezius trying to compensate for this weakness. In observing soft tissue and bony landmarks, it is important that the patient be relaxed, and that the arms be free to hang at the side if possible. If the arm stays supported, one could miss a possible elevated clavicle indicative of an acromioclavicular separation.

Palpation

Palpation should start superficially and proceed to deeper structures. One should look for changes in soft tissue and bony contour, skin temperature and moisture, and swelling and thickening of soft tissue. Pain and tenderness are important findings but can be misleading. A systematic approach should be taken when palpating major bony and muscle landmarks around the shoulder. Alterations in muscle tone should be noted, as well as any hypertrophy of bony landmarks such as the greater tuberosity, the acromium, and the bicipital groove region when involved in a chronic impingement syndrome. The joint lines of the acromioclavicular, sternoclavicular, and glenohumeral joints should be found and palpated for abnormalities. The examiner should also assess soft tissue mobility of the muscles and tendons around the shoulder. This is analogous to accessory motion testing of joints. Normal mobility may be lost secondary to spasm, swelling, or fibrosis.

Active Range of Motion

Always start with the big picture. Look at what happens to the patient's entire body upon active range of motion of the shoulder girdle. As with active motion at any joint complex, one should look for provocation of symptoms and quantity and quality of movement. Poor quality may show itself as any of the following: a hitch during range; an arc of pain with impingement of the rotator cuff and subacromial bursa between 70 and 120 degrees of abduction; trunk over- or undercompensation; or improper rhythm of movement between the scapula

and the humerus. As an example, excessive protraction and upward rotation of the scapula upon elevation are common. The examiner must then determine if the problem is one of scapular muscle weakness, or if the scapula is merely compensating for a glenohumeral problem, or both. While the patient performs these movements, one should also palpate each of the joints of the shoulder girdle for quality of movement, crepitation, popping, clicking, or snapping.

Passive Range of Motion

Again one will look at quantity and quality of movement, as well as the end-feel imparted to the examiner's hands by the structures limiting the movement. Normal end-feels at the glenohumeral joint are classified as capsular.

For both passive physiologic and accessory movements, the examiner must be aware of the starting position for testing, as well as stabilization upon producing movement. As an example, in producing passive physiological abduction, the therapist needs to align the humerus in the plane of the scapula before abducting the humerus (Figs. 7-1, 7-2). If the arm is brought straight up in the body's frontal plane, in most cases the movement produced will be one of abduction as well as horizontal extension.

Proper stabilization is also of importance. When

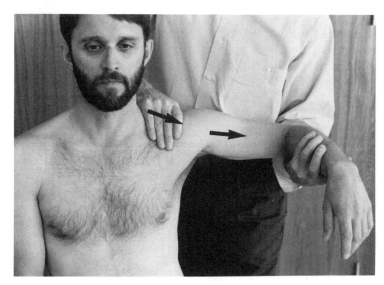

Fig. 7-1. Passive abduction. The humerus is elevated in the body's frontal plane, so that the movement is really abduction and horizontal extension at the glenohumeral joint.

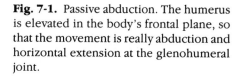

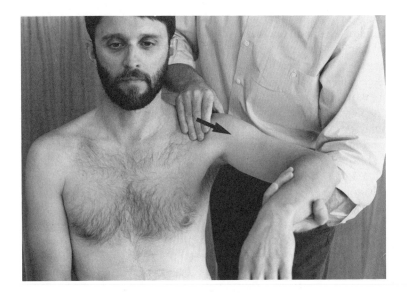

Fig. 7-2. Passive abduction. The humerus is in the same plane as the scapula (approximately 30 degrees flexion). This is closer to pure abduction.

looking at glenohumeral motion, the scapula must be well stabilized (Figs. 7-3 to 7-8). If it is not, the range of movement will be greater, the end-feel not as specific, and provocation of symptoms not as reliable. Ideally the examiner should move the shoulder through its range both with scapular stabilization for the glenohumeral joint, and without stabilization for the acromioclavicular, sternoclavicular, and scapulothoracic joints. For both active and passive range of motion, it should be noted if, with

restricted motion, a pattern exists. At the shoulder, the capsular pattern of restriction in order of limitation is external rotation, abduction, and internal rotation.

Resisted Testing

The two goals of resisted testing are the provocation of symptoms and the assessment of strength of the muscle-tendon unit. To be sure that reproduction of

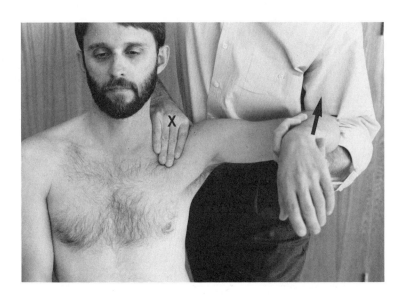

Fig. 7-3. Abduction overpressure at the glenohumeral joint.

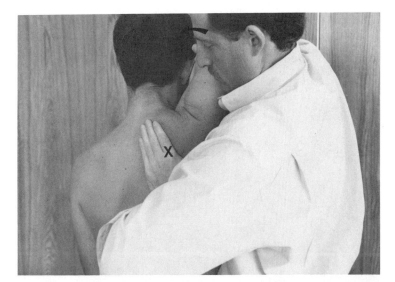

Fig. 7-4. Flexion overpressure at the glenohumeral joint.

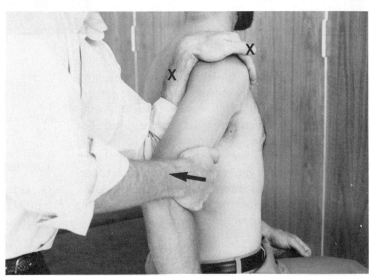

Fig. 7-5. Extension overpressure at the glenohumeral joint.

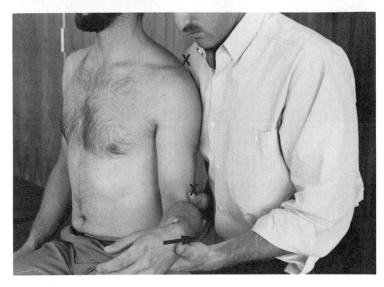

Fig. 7-6. External rotation overpressure at the glenohumeral joint.

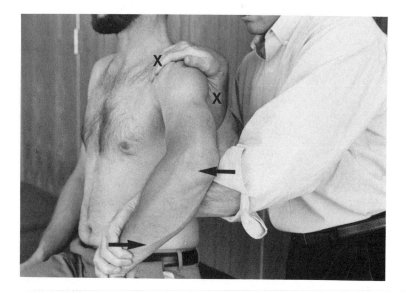

Fig. 7-7. Internal rotation overpressure at the glenohumeral joint. The arm is slightly abducted so that the hand will clear the patient's body.

pain is from the contractile unit involved, the examiner does not want any movement of the joint produced during testing. This can be especially difficult at the shoulder because of its great mobility. For resisted testing here, the humerus is placed at the patient's side in a neutral position. Resistance should be given slowly, while observing and palpating for possible movement. If pain is not an issue, standard manual muscle testing can be utilized to better assess specific muscle strength.

Special Tests

An assortment of special tests are used in the examination of the shoulder.

Locking and Quadrant Tests

Locking and quadrant tests are described by Maitland.[22] In the locking position (Fig. 7-9), the greater tuberosity and its rotator cuff attachments are caught

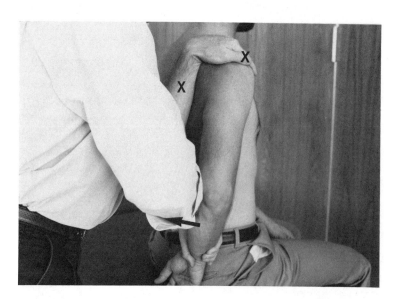

Fig. 7-8. Overpressure for the functional movement of placing the hand behind the back (extension, adduction, internal rotation).

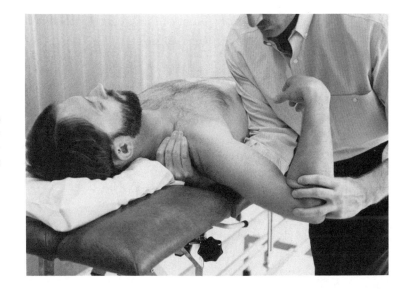

Fig. 7-9. Locking position. The scapula is stabilized, and the humerus is slightly internally rotated and placed in slight extension, then abducted until a firm stop is reached.

within the subacromial space so that any further movement into lateral rotation, abduction, or flexion is impossible. The quadrant position (Fig. 7-10) is a continuation from the locking position, this time allowing some flexion and external rotation as the arm is abducted. A small hill or arc of movement can be felt at approximately 30 degrees from the fully abducted position.

Biceps Tendon Testing

Tendinitis of the long head of the biceps tendon should be picked up with standard testing at the shoulder, but occasionally the information is confusing. Additional testing may include resisted testing of shoulder flexion with the elbow flexed and supinated. Weakness and pain in the anterior aspect

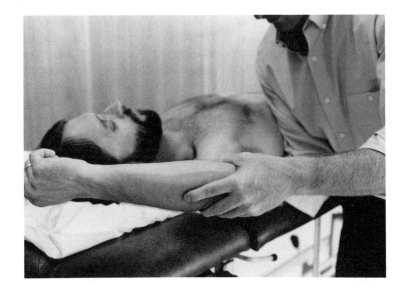

Fig. 7-10. Quadrant position. From the locking position, the humerus is allowed to slightly externally rotate and flex while the arm is slowly abducted. A small hill or arc of movement will be felt at approximately 30 degrees from the fully abducted position. Both the locking and quadrant positions place stress on the subacromial structures (rotator cuff, bursa, coracoacromial arch), as well as on the glenoid labium. Both tests are used to provoke symptoms and to determine the feel of the joint at the point of resistance.

of the shoulder suggest involvement of the biceps tendon. Another test is to have the patient resist elbow flexion and supination while externally rotating the shoulder. If the biceps tendon is unstable in the bicipital groove, it may subluxate, and the patient will experience pain.

Apprehension Test

To test for chronic anterior glenohumeral dislocation, slowly abduct and externally rotate the patient's arm to a position where it may easily dislocate. If the shoulder is ready to dislocate, the patient will begin to hesitate and guard against the movement. He should also be asked if this reproduces the sensation when the shoulder pops out.

Drop Arm Test

The drop arm test is used to diagnose complete tears of the supraspinatus tendon. It is positive if the patient is unable to slowly lower the arm from a position of 90 degrees of abduction.

It is not just the performing of all of these tests that makes for a good shoulder examination, but performing them well. There is a wealth of information to be gained from each part of the examination if one is sensitive with both eyes and hands.

FROZEN SHOULDER

The diagnosis of frozen shoulder provides the therapist with little information except that the patient usually has a stiff and painful shoulder. The condition, whose onset is often insidious and idiopathic,[23] is usually progressive in nature. There is general agreement that the glenohumeral joint capsule is the site of the lesion, although some authors hypothesize that bicipital tenosynovitis[24,25] and rotator cuff injuries[24,26,27] precede the capsular involvement.

Pathologic changes in the glenohumeral joint capsule are often cited to result in the shoulder stiffness.[24,28-30] Neviaser[28] described a condition, adhesive capsulitis, which included a thickened, fibrotic glenohumeral joint capsule adhered to the humeral head and an obliteration of the capsular axillary pouch. DePalma[29] also described a loss of

the axillary pouch in the early stages of frozen shoulder. Arthrography supports the contention there is a loss of glenohumeral joint capsule extensibility in these patients. Normal shoulder joint volume capacity is 20 to 30 ml, whereas a capacity of 5 to 10 ml was present in patients with frozen shoulder.[23,31] Arthrography has also demonstrated a loss of the axillary pouch, the subscapular bursa, and the long head of the biceps sheath.[31] Histologic events that could result in the loss of capsular extensibility may include abnormal cross-bridging between newly synthesized collagen fibers and pre-existing fibers, and loss of critical fiber distance due to a significant decrease in hyaluronic acid and water content.[32] In addition, authors have described a postimmobilization fatty fibrous connective tissue scar creating intra-articular adhesions within synovial joints, which could also result in decreased mobility.[32-34]

A capsular pattern of restricted passive motion and abnormal glenohumeral joint accessory movements are among the physical examination signs that suggest glenohumeral joint capsule involvement. Cyriax defined joint capsule dysfunction as arthritis, which at the shoulder is represented by external rotation as the most limited motion followed by abduction and internal rotation.[30] The arthrographic evidence of loss or reduction of the axillary pouch and anterior joint capsule extensibility[31] corresponds to external rotation and abduction being the most restricted movements, since normal extensibility of these portions of the joint capsule is necessary for the two motions to occur.[35] The arthrographic findings also correspond to the commonly restricted glenohumeral joint accessory movements, namely, inferior and anterior glides. This does not preclude other accessory movements from being restricted, including lateral distraction, which stresses the entire capsule.

The therapist must consider other factors besides the glenohumeral joint capsule when assessing shoulder stiffness. Acromioclavicular, sternoclavicular, and scapulothoracic joint dysfunction may contribute to the decreased or painful shoulder motion. Fibrotic changes and adhesions affecting the rotator cuff, the long head of the biceps, and the subacromial bursa have also been associated with loss of shoulder motion.[24-26,29,36] Adaptive muscle shortening due to the pattern of restricted motion and the commonly observed patient posture, which includes the shoulder being held in an adducted and internally rotated position,[37] may contribute to the stiffness associated with frozen shoulder. Physical examination findings often include tightness of the shoulder internal rotator and adductor muscle groups, with particular involvement of the pectoralis major, the latissimus dorsi, and the teres major. Stretch weakness of the scapular musculature such as the middle and lower trapezius and the rhomboids is also often found. The protracted shoulder girdle posture often assumed by these patients and the increased scapulothoracic joint motion often observed may account for the stretch weakness. These muscle imbalances may contribute to the altered glenohumeral joint mechanics, adding additional abnormal stresses to the capsule and associated structures such as the rotator cuff muscles and the subacromial bursa.

Physical therapy treatment must address these imbalances in order to maximize shoulder function during the rehabilitation process. Differentiation between muscle and capsular tightness is important, since the two tissues respond to different types of manual stretching. The end-feel detected during assessment of passive physiologic and accessory movements at the glenohumeral joint will help the therapist determine the nature of the restriction. Seldom will a patient with frozen shoulder not require both joint and soft tissue mobilization and muscle stretching techniques for improving shoulder range of motion. The brachial plexus is another important structure to be screened in patients presenting with shoulder pain and stiffness. Elvey[38] described methods for placing different components of the brachial plexus and associated peripheral nerves under a tensile load. Adhesions or obstructions restricting the nerve tissue's mobility during cervical or upper extremity movements may result in pain and stiffness in the shoulder area.

Besides assessing the nature of the shoulder dysfunction, the therapist must determine if the shoulder symptoms are local or referred. There are numerous local structures that could be the source of the patient's pain, including bone, joint capsule, ligaments, myofascial units, or bursa. An examination scheme based on Cyriax's theory of diagnosis by selective tension[30] plus the accessory movement techniques and special tests already described should help the therapist determine which structure(s) are involved.

Assessment of patients with frozen shoulder requires examination of numerous anatomic regions. If these different areas are not at least screened, the source of the patient's symptoms and dysfunction directly related to the symptoms could be missed completely, making treatment success unlikely.

Management

Ultimately, decreasing pain and shoulder stiffness is the treatment goal for this patient population. The treatment modalities used depend on which stage of the frozen shoulder cycle the patient is in: early (acute) or late (chronic). In the early stage, decreasing the inflammation and the associated pain and muscle guarding is the primary goal. Numerous modalities are suggested for relief of acute pain and muscle guarding, including transcutaneous electrical nerve stimulation (TENS),[39] cryotherapy, phonophoresis, and iontophoresis.[40] Active-assisted, active, and passive exercises also play an important role in the early rehabilitation of these patients. Increasing local blood flow by exercising the shoulder to the patient's tolerance may decrease local edema and congestion. These events may assist with removal of metabolic waste products, which may be responsible for the stimulation of local nociceptors. A decrease in nociceptor activity may lessen pain perception and muscle guarding. These forms of exercise may also achieve the goal of neuromodulation of the nociceptive input due to stimulation of type I or II mechanoreceptors.[41] Pendulum exercises can be very effective active-assisted home exercises for muscle relaxation, and they are safe as the patient has complete control over how vigorously the upper extremity is exercised. Besides the immediate glenohumeral joint area, muscle guarding is often detected in the cervical and shoulder girdle regions. Therefore, an exercise that incorporates gentle movement throughout these regions can be very effective for muscle relaxation.

Feldenkrais[42] described several such exercises for the entire body. An example of an exercise that may benefit the frozen shoulder patient follows. The patient lies on the uninvolved side with the involved upper extremity supported by the patient's body. Visualizing a clock dial painted on the lateral surface of the involved shoulder, the patient gently oscillates the shoulder toward the ear (12 o'clock) and then toward the hip (6 o'clock) within the pain-free range of motion. Movement between any pair of numbers on the clock can be attempted. At the clinic this exercise can be active-assisted or passive in nature, with the therapist guiding the limb and shoulder girdle through the range. Passive shoulder movements, either physiologic or accessory as listed previously in the examination scheme, should be of the grade I or II range as described by Maitland.[43] These techniques can be very effective in decreasing pain and muscle guarding. Constant reassessment of the patient's symptoms and objective findings is essential to prevent overtreatment or inappropriate treatment. Reassessment of muscle tone, tissue temperature, and selected active and passive movements, paying particular attention to the passive end-feel, can alert the therapist to an adverse reaction to the treatment being performed. Any increase in the cardinal signs of inflammation, spasm end-feel, or pain occurring earlier in the passive range-of-motion is a warning sign that the treatment was or is too vigorous.

Patient education is also an important part of early-phase rehabilitation. The patient must understand the warning signs of being too vigorous with his home exercises to prevent a flare-up of symptoms. The patient also needs to understand the importance of proper posture to help reduce stress on the entire involved upper quarter. In the early stages, improved head-neck, shoulder girdle, and truck positions may decrease activity in the cervical and scapular muscles, which are trying to support these regions. This decreased muscle activity may help relieve local symptoms while also allowing for more normal shoulder motion. In the later, chronic stage of frozen shoulder, the patient should be aware of how the commonly seen forward head posture, with the upper extremity internally rotated and adducted, can propagate muscle tightness and weakness, resulting in abnormal glenohumeral joint mechanics. Postural re-education and rehabilitation may include use of a lumbar pillow and thora-columbar mobility treatment techniques to facilitate the assumption of a less physically stressful posture. All of the above treatment ideas are designed to enhance the wound healing process and decrease the physical stress on all the tissues in the shoulder region. If successful, the pain and muscle guarding will be decreased to a level at which the specific dysfunction can begin to be treated.

The primary goal during the late stage of frozen shoulder is to normalize shoulder movement. Improving soft tissue mobility throughout the glenohumeral joint and shoulder girdle region; joint mobility at the glenohumeral, acromioclavicular, and sternoclavicular joints; and muscle strength and coordination throughout the glenohumeral joint and shoulder girdle regions are all important treatment considerations. The objective examination findings will reveal the specific treatment needs of each individual patient. See Chapter 12 for joint mobilization techniques that may be useful with the frozen shoulder patient. Movement grades III and IV as described by Maitland[43] for accessory and physiologic movements should be used to stretch the involved tissue. High-velocity thrust techniques can also be a useful tool, in the hands of a skilled clinician, to restore glenohumeral joint motion (Fig. 7-11). Because of the adaptive shortening of other soft tissue structures, muscle stretching and soft tissue mobilization techniques are essential for restoration of motion. Soft tissue restrictions are commonly found in the anterior glenohumeral joint and shoulder girdle regions, the inferior glenohumeral joint and the ipsilateral cervical spine areas as a result of the poor posture commonly seen. As previously stated, rotator cuff adhesions are common, and stretching of these muscles may be important for restoration of motion. An excellent reference for muscle stretching techniques is that by Evjenth and Hamberg.[44] Modalities such as ultrasound to facilitate a stretch of tissue and heat to promote relaxation are useful adjuncts to manual stretching techniques.[40] Muscle strengthening and coordination exercises are also necessary for normalizing shoulder motion. Stretch weakness and disuse atrophy are often found throughout the glenohumeral joint and scapular regions.

Feldenkrais and proprioceptive neuromuscular facilitation (PNF) exercises are extremely useful for

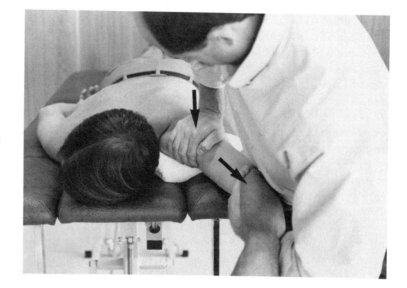

Fig. 7-11. Example of a grade V technique for increasing end-range elevation.

restoring coordination and motor control to the involved areas, a necessary adjunct to strengthening exercises. The therapist should consider Janda's[45] theory that attempting to strengthen weak muscles without stretching tight antagonistic muscle groups could result in an enhancement of the imbalance.

There are few controlled studies in the literature investigating treatment for frozen shoulder, and often no mention is made of whether the patients were in the early or late stages. Hamer and Kirk[46] compared the results of cryotherapy and ultrasound, with both patient groups also receiving active and passive exercises. Both patient groups demonstrated improved shoulder range of motion and decreased pain, but there was not a significant difference between the two groups. Bulgen et al.[47] investigated four patient groups, all of whom used pendulum exercises. Each group also received either no additional treatment, ice packs and PNF techniques, joint mobilization, or intra-articular steroids. All four groups noted decreased pain, and after 6 months of treatment there was no significant difference between the groups. Other studies demonstrate similar findings where various modalities or combinations of therapeutic interventions relieve pain and improve shoulder mobility.[48-50] Treating patients with frozen shoulder can be a long, complicated process because of the nature of the pathology and the intricate relationships among the shoulder and (other) upper quarter structures. Therapists should base their choice of treatment on the specific examination findings and on the techniques that they have found to be most useful to address the individual patient's needs.

ROTATOR CUFF INJURIES

The rotator cuff performs many functions. Passively, the muscles of the rotator cuff lend stability to the glenohumeral articulation; actively, they are a dynamic stabilizer, firmly seating the humeral head within the glenoid fossa so that more superficial muscles, such as the deltoid, can move the glenohumeral joint optimally.[51] Along with this function, studies have suggested that the rotator cuff contributes between one-third and one-half of the power of the shoulder in abduction and at least 80 percent of the power in external rotation.[52,53]

As we have seen, the glenohumeral joint is an extremely mobile articulation. Unfortunately, it has long been recognized that to have great mobility one must sacrifice stability, and contributions toward both functions are demanded of the rotator cuff. This fact alone makes it more prone to injury. Injury to the musculotendinous cuff is quite common and occurs with one or more of the following: (1) trauma, (2) overuse, (3) attrition or aging.[53-55] It is important to be aware of which of these may be involved, since this information will impact on later treatment and prognosis.

Trauma can be differentiated according to the type of forces involved, either tension or compression. A forceful and usually sudden contraction of the rotator cuff is an example of a tensile stress. The major component of tendon is the fibrous protein collagen. In mature tendon completely acellular areas are common. To achieve the high tensile strength necessary to transmit muscular force efficiently, the collagen is arranged into parallel arrays of fiber bundles oriented along its lines of stress. Tendon of any kind has the most tensile stress applied to it when its associated muscle contracts,[56] especially when the contraction is of the lengthening or eccentric type.[57] When tendon is extended beyond its point of elasticity, which is at approximately 8 percent extension of total length, overstretching and rupture of some collagen fibers occur. This type of injury to the rotator cuff is not unusual given its important function as a stabilizer of the glenohumeral articulation.

Compressive trauma is most commonly seen as a fall on an outstretched arm, driving the humerus and cuff up into the coracoacromial arch. The resultant bruising and inflammatory response will compromise the function of the involved muscle-tendon unit. In general, rotator cuff injuries are seen arthroscopically as incomplete tears showing on the undersurface of the muscle-tendon unit. There is minimal to no well-defined demarcation between the supraspinatus, infraspinatus, and teres minor muscles to allow easy identification.[54]

The act of throwing has been shown to be one of the movements that most consistently produce rotator cuff tears with and without other, associated pathologic conditions. In a study of the throwing motion in athletes, out of 178 baseball players reviewed, 122 (68 percent) had rotator cuff tears. Of that number, 100 (82 percent) had supraspinatus muscle involvement; 75 (61 percent) of these injuries were limited to the supraspinatus muscle alone, and 25 (20 percent) were combined supraspinatus and infraspinatus muscle injuries.[58] The deceleration phase of the throwing motion seems to be the causative factor when the rotator cuff is attempting to stabilize the glenohumeral joint.

A second and quite common type of rotator cuff pathology is the overuse or impingement syndrome. This involves impingement upon the rotator cuff and overlying subacromial bursa against the anterior edge of the acromion and its associated coracoacromial arch. Neer[59,60] described three progressive stages of impingement. Stage I usually occurs in individuals younger than 25 years of age but may occur at any age in those who are engaged in excessive overhead use of the arm. The pathologic changes seen are edema and hemorrhaging of the subacromial bursa. If impingement continues, the condition becomes chronic, producing thickening and fibrosis of the bursa and tendinitis of the cuff. Stage II disease is commonly seen in patients 25 to 40 years of age. Stage III disease results from further impingement, producing degeneration or complete or incomplete tears of the rotator cuff. Quite often, this impingement of the cuff is a result of poor shoulder girdle mechanics. It may be due to hypomobility (shortening of soft tissues), hypermobility (lengthening of soft tissues, damage to glenoid labrum), or a strength imbalance of one or more muscles about the shoulder girdle.

The supraspinatus tendon is the most susceptible, because of its location and the fact that there is an area of relative avascularity close to its insertion. Microangiographic studies have revealed a profuse blood supply to the rotator cuff tendons except for a portion of the supraspinatus. This tendon has a so-called critical zone: an area of hypovascularity near its humeral insertion not unlike many tendons with a circular cross section elsewhere in the body. It has been hypothesized that the relative ischemia in this zone can produce changes mimicking tendon degeneration.[53]

The effect of aging on the rotator cuff is one of progressive degeneration of all elements. The attachment to bone and the tendon fibers exhibit disorganization with fragmentation action, and in addition to decreased vascularity there is a loss of tendon cellularity.[55] This limits the ability of the tendon to adapt to stresses, and decreases its ability to heal after injury. Tensile strength is decreased with age, and calcification at the bony insertion is quite common.

Variations in the anatomy of the subacromial region may render some individuals even more prone to degenerative cuff disease. Soon after injury, a vicious cycle begins. Damage to the cuff leads to impairment of its normal function; it can no longer provide the normal glenohumeral fulcrum, and abnormal upward displacement of the humeral head occurs, which results in further impingement, with capillary compression and additional tendon damage.[51] It has also been postulated that acromioclavicular joint disease plays a role in initiating the impingement process and that disease in this joint in conjunction with rotator cuff tears may have an incidence of well over 50 percent.[60] A gradually enlarging osteophyte from a post-traumatic or degenerative acromioclavicular joint, or an extracapsular mechanical erosion of the inferior joint capsule, may also lead to subacromial impingement and rotator cuff pathology.[61]

Examination

Clinical findings at the shoulder for a patient with a rotator cuff problem can vary greatly. There is no list of positive findings that one will always see when the rotator cuff is involved. There are some things that are common among many patients with rotator cuff problems, and we will discuss those findings and their treatment, but we will also mention other possible findings.

We mentioned earlier that the infraspinatus and the supraspinatus are most commonly involved. Active elevation can be painful near end-range secondary to a lack of motion and pinching, or secondary to hypermobility, or there can be an arc of pain between 70 and 120 degrees secondary to mid-range compression under the coracoacromial arch.

Poor-quality movement between the scapula and the humerus is also quite common, especially during the lowering or eccentric phase of elevation, when increased stress is placed on the tendon. The scapula tries to compensate for this with increased movement to take the force off of the rotator cuff. This may take place because of pain and/or weakness.

More often than not, the patient complains of a single, fairly consistent location of pain, but many times the pain moves from a lateral site anteriorly or posteriorly. This change in location may suggest a combination of a cuff problem with instability of the glenohumeral articulation, most commonly anteriorly.[62,63]

Classically, passive movements that stretch or compress the involved tendon also provoke the symptoms. Compression injuries as well as overuse (impingement) syndromes weaken the tendon and usually lead to thickening and increased scarring of the cuff secondary to a chronic inflammatory reaction.

Many times tension forces alone do not provoke a patient's symptoms, but compression of the tendon will give rise to pain. Tension forces include passive stretch of a tendon or contraction isometrically of the associated muscle. Compression forces include weightbearing on the extremity or movements that compress the involved tendons.

Isometric muscle testing of abduction and/or external rotation often reproduces pain and more often shows weakness. It is important to note the position of the shoulder at the moment of resisted muscle testing. If the humerus is placed in a position of 90 degrees of abduction, and the cuff is made to contract and hold there, it is now receiving both compressive and tensile forces under the coracoacromial arch.

Passive accessory movement testing of the glenohumeral joint may reproduce pain as well as demonstrate hypo- or hypermobility. Movements such as cephalic glide of the humerus compress the rotator cuff; inferior glide and lateral distraction stretch the supraspinatus; posterior glide stretches the infraspinatus and teres minor portions of the cuff.

The more chronic the problem, the more likely one is to find dysfunction at the acromioclavicular and sternoclavicular joints as well (Table 7-1).

Treatment

Treatment of rotator cuff injuries depends upon the type and severity of clinical signs. Treatment can be divided into conservative and surgical care.

Conservative treatment is indicated in cuff tendinitis as well as partial-thickness tears. Depending on the severity of signs and symptoms, rest in one form or another is indicated. This consists of an immediate avoidance of all aggravating positions and movements. It may include the use of a sling to immobilize the shoulder for a few days if any use of the arm produces symptoms. At this stage the use of ice, nonsteroidal anti-inflammatory drugs, and/or local steroid injection may also be indicated.[51,53]

It is important to determine early on if the shoulder has an acute or a chronic inflammatory reaction. Acute inflammation is marked by primarily fluid changes (i.e., edema or bleeding) and a stimulus of brief duration. A chronic inflammatory response is marked by fibrous changes with little fluid and a stimulus that persists.[64] For the rotator cuff this is usually some abnormality of shoulder movement or an irritating activity. The prognosis for a quick and full recovery with conservative care is not as good for a large tear, a chronic condition, and an older individual. After cuff injury, rupture of some collagen fibers occurs, accompanied by cell damage. Healing is initiated by the invasion of the area by cells that remove debris and synthesize a new connective tissue matrix. Tendon is a dense regular connective tissue and is therefore mechanically well suited to transmit tensile loads, but it has a low cell count and poor vascular supply and therefore is not a quick healer. Increased tensile strength during healing is enhanced by controlled passive motion; the strength (ultimate load) increases to 35 percent of the value for intact tendons after 84 days, whereas complete immobilization results in an increase to only 21 percent.[65] The greatest amount of tensile force put upon tendon is derived from contraction of its associated muscle. Therefore active and re-sisted movements should be withheld until the tendon is strong enough.

Besides rest and medication, there are obviously a great many modalities within physical therapy (e.g., ice, heat, ultrasound, high-voltage galvanic stimulation, TENS) that can control inflammation and decrease swelling, edema, and pain. These are definitely indicated during the course of rehabilitation of the shoulder, with the eventual goal of normal strength, movement, and function.

Hypomobility or a lack of normal motion at the glenohumeral joint is a common problem. If the joint is not free to move passively, the rotator cuff cannot be expected to perform its normal dynamic function. It is important to determine whether the restrictions are secondary to muscle or inert tissues about the joint (capsule, ligaments, labrum, etc.). This information should be obtained from palpation and by looking at the pattern of restricted movement, as well as from the end-feel upon passive testing. The rotator cuff may be stretched locally at the joint with accessory movement treatment techniques, or the muscle-tendon unit may be lengthened with soft tissue stretching techniques. These may include various forms of massage as well as physiologic muscle stretching techniques (Figs. 7-12, 7-13). In either case, active-resisted exercise utilizing the muscles that maintain the newly gained range should follow immediately, and a home program should be designed to do the same. This

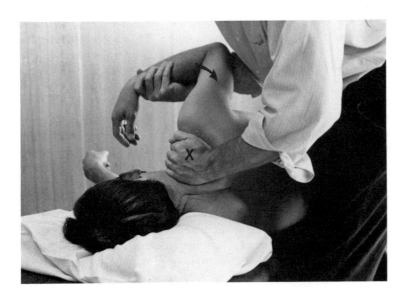

Fig. 7-12. Pump massage (local stretching combined with humeral abduction/adduction) of the supraspinatus.

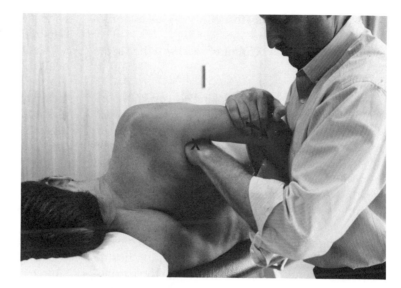

Fig. 7-13. Muscle stretching of the supraspinatus.

should be true both for single movements (i.e., flexion-extension) and more functional motions such as reaching behind the back. This motion commonly tends to be limited especially when the supraspinatus is involved. Reaching behind the back both elongates the muscle-tendon unit and compresses it as it is pulled under the coracoacromial arch with internal rotation. A combination of an accessory and a physiologic muscle stretch for this movement is shown in Figure 7-14. Pain and limitation upon horizontal flexion are also common when the infraspinatus is involved, for similar reasons.

Probably more common than stiffness is hypermobility at the glenohumeral joint with involvement of the rotator cuff. It is with this type of problem that treatment becomes more difficult and progress slower. Treatment is now aimed at muscle re-education and strengthening of the entire shoulder girdle. For the rotator cuff, this type of treatment should be based on the following:

1. Type of tissue (tendon)
2. Function (stabilization and movement of the humerus)

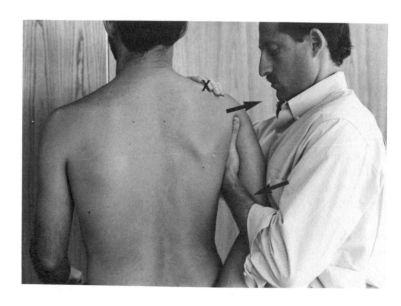

Fig. 7-14. Combining lateral distraction at the glenohumeral joint with physiological stretching with the hand beind the back in sitting.

3. Type of dysfunction (instability versus hypomobility).
4. Severity of lesion (extent of tear, whether acute or chronic)

Once active movement is painfree, resistive concentric exercise is indicated. Isometric "holds" should be incorporated at various points of the range as progress warrants. Movement should be slow so that the cuff can control the motion. This is then followed by slow eccentric exercise,[66] incorporating rotation into the movements whenever possible (e.g., PNF diagonals). As the patient progresses, faster speeds are incorporated into the exercise program. It is very important that constant tension be kept on the muscle and tendon during each set of exercises and that the axis for the particular movement be located at the individual's own joint. Examples of this kind of exercise include manual resistance, dumbbells, cables, and Theraband. This automatically limits the use of machines with fixed axes of motion (e.g., Cybex, Universal, Nautilus). All human joints have a changing axis during motion, and the glenohumeral joint is no exception. Again, the problem here is unstable motion, and movement *must* take place about the normal physiologic axis. A later progression should also include weightbearing exercise (push-ups; modified dips, and so on).

Surgery

When conservative care fails to produce the desired result, surgical intervention may be indicated. This is usually the case with complete cuff tears or chronic persistent problems in an active individual.[51,53]

The most minor and least involved procedure is arthroscopy and shaving of any small defects in the cuff. Anterior acromioplasty (removal of a portion of the anterior and inferior acromium) with limited detachment of the deltoid presently appears to be the most direct, least potentially harmful, and perhaps most effective procedure for persistent rotator cuff tendinitis. This decompressive procedure offers the possibility of satisfactory pain relief and return to normal daily function.[54,67] Neer[59] reported satisfactory results in 15 of 16 shoulders treated by anterior acromioplasty. Results do not seem to be as good for competitive athletes. Tibone et al.[54] reported that 76 percent of the patients studied could not return to their preinjury throwing status or overhead sport following surgery.

A variety of procedures have been advocated to close large defects in the rotator cuff and restore function. Grafting methods include the use of a free biceps tendon, the coracoacromial ligament, freeze-dried cadaver rotator cuff, bovine tendon or ligament tissue, and a variety of synthetic materials.[53,68,69] Any of these requires more extensive surgery and usually offers a less optimistic prognosis than the procedures mentioned previously. Any surgical procedure of course should be followed up with extensive rehabilitation.

Rotator cuff disease is a common and important source of shoulder symptoms. The cuff mechanism functions not only to stabilize the shoulder but also to provide power for movement. The pathogenesis of rotator cuff disease is associated with trauma, overuse, and attrition or aging. The supraspinatus and the infraspinatus are most commonly involved, and their treatment consists usually of graded rest as well as eventually a comprehensive exercise program to restore strength and stability to the area.

ANTERIOR GLENOHUMERAL INSTABILITY

Instability at the shoulder is a common clinical problem, with anterior instability seen most often. The relatively small size and shallowness of the glenoid cavity, and position of the glenoid fossa (facing laterally and forward), and the advantage of the external rotators over the subscapularis combine to make the shoulder susceptible to dislocations in the forward, medial, and inferior directions.[4,5,13] Anterior instability can be subdivided into two groups: acute traumatic anterior dislocation and recurrent anterior dislocation or subluxation.

Acute traumatic anterior dislocation is an injury predominantly of young adults, particularly athletes. It is usually caused by forced external rotation and extension of the shoulder; the humeral head is driven forward and frequently avulses the cartilaginous glenoid labrum and capsule from the anterior aspect of the glenoid cavity.[61] The association between acute traumatic anterior shoulder dislocations and lesions of the rotator cuff has long been recognized. The exact incidence of cuff ruptures is unknown, but McLaughlin has suggested that the incidence may be as high as 70 percent in patients over 40 years of age.[70] A single episode of anterior dislocation is relatively more common in the older patient population. This group is more likely to suffer injury secondary to a fall on an outstretched arm, with the dominant arm involved twice as often as the nondominant arm. The older population also has a higher risk of nerve and vascular injury.[62]

Recurrent anterior dislocation or subluxation is much more common in the younger population, for several possible reasons. The underlying mechanism seems to be either an anterior one, consisting of stretching of the anterior capsule or avulsion of the glenoid labrum (usually occurring in the younger patient), or a posterior one occurring in older patients, consisting of tendon rupture of the rotator cuff.[61] Since rotator cuff tears associated with anterior dislocation are more common in older patients, they tend to give way first, possibly sparing the anterior structures (capsule, labrum, glenohumeral ligaments). In the younger patient, an anterior intracapsular pouch is formed, and healing is generally poor. This is also true for the labrum. It may be supposed as well that older patients are less prone to encounter situations that provoke anterior dislocation than are younger patients, and therefore have a lower incidence.[61,62,71]

Clinical Examination

In the acute traumatic situation, the patient will have a history of a specific activity or event that caused the dislocation, usually involving a fall on an outstretched arm or forced movements of abduction, extension, and external rotation. The patient will be unable to use the arm and often will support it with the opposite extremity. In the situation of recurrent dislocation or subluxation, the patient will report sudden attacks of shoulder pain that occur with certain movements. He may state that he feels a clicking sensation, that the shoulder "pops out," and that these episodes have been more frequent lately. The objective examination will usually show some general atrophy around the involved shoulder girdle. Passive physiologic and accessory movement testing most often reveals hypermobility

or instability about the glenohumeral joint, especially with external rotation and anterior glide testing. It is important to remember in assessing accessory movements in these patients to start with the humeral head in a neutral position, for often it will rest somewhat anterior to the glenoid fossa. This may give false information and confuse the diagnosis. The apprehension test at the shoulder often reveals a painful, hypermobile shoulder and may reproduce the patient's symptoms. It is important to remember the incidence of rotator cuff injury in the patient with anterior shoulder instability, especially in the older population. Resisted testing at the shoulder may show signs of a rotator cuff tear. It is not uncommon for a stretch injury of the axillary nerve to occur after an acute episode of anterior dislocation. Deltoid weakness as well as altered sensation in a small area of skin over the lateral shoulder are to be expected. Clinically we find this also true for patients with recurrent anterior dislocation, although the findings are more subtle.

Roentgenographic evaluation will help to provide additional objective information of anterior shoulder instability. The Hill-Sachs lesion is a posterolateral notch defect (compression fracture) in the humeral head that is created by impingement of the articular surface of the humeral head against the anteroinferior rim of the glenoid fossa. It is the most common radiographic finding in the patient with recurrent anterior dislocation.[72]

The Bankart lesion is a cartilaginous or osseous defect in the anterior margin of the glenoid rim or ectopic bone formation at this site produced by an anterior or inferior translation of the humeral head against the glenoid rim.[72]

Treatment

Conservative treatment should be the first choice in most cases of anterior shoulder instability. This may be subdivided into four basic areas:

1. Address signs of inflammation
2. Normalize the **quality of motion** at the glenohumeral joint
3. Normalize the **quantity of motion** at surrounding joints
4. Strengthen the shoulder girdle and related musculature.

Once the acute signs of irritation (heat, swelling, spasm, pain) have decreased, intervention to help restore the quality of movement at the glenohumeral joint should begin. Passive movements through a normal range of motion without pushing end-range are incorporated first. Also at this time, assessment and normalization of the quantity of movement at the surrounding joints (the acromioclavicular, sternoclavicular, and scapulothoracic joints and the cervical and thoracic spine) are begun, to help decrease abnormal stresses applied to the glenohumeral joint. Shortened musculature also needs to be lengthened. Often the patient with chronic involvement will demonstrate tight anterior chest musculature secondary to a forward shoulder posture.

A good strengthening program should start with slow controlled movements and isometrics, working later into more eccentric contractions, and finally higher speed activities if needed, depending on the individual patient. Ideally we strive for strong and well-balanced musculature throughout the upper quarter. There are, however, some areas that often require special attention.

It is important that the posterior scapular musculature be strong and well coordinated with the rest of the shoulder girdle. In order to maintain good joint congruency, the scapula must be able to elevate and rotate with the humerus, and must not be allowed to overly protract, especially with abduction, extension, and external rotation.

A second important muscle group to strengthen is the rotator cuff. We have already mentioned the high incidence of cuff injury involved with anterior shoulder instability. The external rotation component of the cuff (supraspinatus, infraspinatus, teres minor) helps to keep the humerus posterior in the glenoid upon contraction. It also helps to maintain joint congruency by compressing the humerus into the glenoid.

The third muscle involved is the subscapularis. It may control anterior instability at the shoulder by passively acting as an anterior barrier to the humeral head, as well as a dynamic stabilizer to control external rotation.

When conservative care has failed to give the desired outcome, or if the extent of tissue damage is severe, there are several surgical procedures that may be utilized for anterior instability at the shoulder. In the Putti-Platt procedure, the capsule and the subscapularis muscle are divided and then overlapped. The Bankart procedure deals with repairing and shortening the anterior capsule at the glenoid. Both procedures are designed to leave the patient with some limitation of external rotation, thereby maintaining anterior stability.[70,73]

In the Bristow procedure, a block of bone taken from the tip of the coracoid process, with its attached tendons, reinforces the anterior part of the joint. The bone block is placed near the front of the glenoid at the anterior neck of the scapula with screw fixation. It provides an anterior block and produces a dynamic musculotendinous sling, holding the humeral head posteriorly with the arm in abduction and external rotation. This procedure allows for a quicker return of range of motion and has a low redislocation rate.[68,73] For any of the following procedures to be successful, a comprehensive rehabilitation program must follow. For the most part, the program should include the same treatment guidelines as outlined for conservative care.

Anterior instability at the shoulder, whether a primary acute dislocation or recurrent episodes of anterior dislocation of the humerus, is a common clinical problem. It usually involves both the rotator cuff (primarily in the older patient) and the anterior joint structures (primarily in the younger population). Conservative treatment resolves around passive motion and eventual strengthening of the posterior scapular muscles and the rotator cuff. Surgical intervention primarily involves tightening of anterior joint structures.

SUMMARY

Physical therapists see a great number of patients presenting with shoulder pain and dysfunction. To evaluate and treat these patients adequately, the clinician must not isolate the shoulder from the rest of the upper quarter. Therefore, performing an upper quarter screening examination before performing a detailed assessment of the shoulder region may be beneficial to the clinician. Three common shoulder pathologies seen by physical therapists — frozen shoulder, rotator cuff pathology, and anterior dislocations — were presented in this chapter. This information is important for the therapist because the nature of the pathology may influence treatment planning and goals. Ultimately, however, the signs and symptoms obtained during the evaluation will dictate the specific treatment techniques chosen for each individual patient. If the examination scheme presented in this chapter is carried out carefully, the clinician should have all the information needed to initiate a proper treatment program.

REFERENCES

1. Allender E: Prevalence, incidence, and remission rates of some common rheumatic diseases or syndromes. Scand J Rheumatol 3:145, 1974
2. Westerling C, Jousson BG: Pain from neck-shoulder region and sick leave. Scand J Soc Med 8:131, 1980
3. Maeda K: Occupational cervicobrachial disorder and its causative factors. J Hum Ergol 6:193, 1977
4. Inman V, Saunders M, Abbott L: Observations of the function of the shoulder joint. J Bone Joint Surg 26A:1, 1944
5. Sarrafian S: Gross and functional anatomy of the shoulder. Clin Orthop Rel Res 173:11, 1983
6. Saha AK: Dynamic stability of the glenohumeral joints. Acta Orthop Scand 42:491, 1971
7. Basmajian J, Bazmant F: Factors preventing downward dislocation of the adducted shoulder joint. J Bone Joint Surg 41A:1182, 1959
8. Dempster W: Mechanism of shoulder movement. Arch Phys Med Rehab 46A:49, 1965
9. Turkel S, Panio M, Marshall J, Girgis F: Stabilization mechanisms preventing anterior dislocation of the glenohumeral joint. J Bone Joint Surg 63A:1208, 1981
10. Kent B: Functional anatomy of the shoulder complex: a review. Phys Ther 51:867, 1971
11. Kessel L, Watson M: The painful arc syndrome. J Bone Joint Surg 59B:166, 1977
12. Basmajian JV: The surgical anatomy and function of the arm-trunk mechanism. Surg Clin North Am 43:1475, 1963
13. Last RJ (ed): Anatomy: Regional and Applied. 6th Ed. Churchill Livingstone, New York, 1977
14. Poppen NK, Walker PS: Normal and abnormal motion of the shoulder. J Bone Joint Surg 58A:195, 1976
15. Cailliet R: Shoulder Pain. FA Davis, Philadelphia, 1966
16. Lucas DB: Biomechanics of the shoulder joint. Arch Surg 107:425, 1973
17. Bechtol C: Biomechanics of the shoulder. Clin Orthop Rel Res 146:37, 1980
18. Saha AK: Theory of Shoulder Mechanism: Descriptive and Applied. Charles C Thomas, Springfield IL, 1961
19. Blakely RL, Palmer ML: Analysis of rotation accompanying shoulder flexion. Phys Ther 64(8):1214, 1984
20. Kellgren J: On the distribution of pain arising from deep somatic structures with charts of segmental pain areas. Clin Sci 4:35, 1939
21. Campbell D, Parsons C: Referred head pain and its concomitants. J Nerv Ment Dis 99:544, 1944
22. Maitland GD: Peripheral Manipulation. 2nd Ed. Butterworths, Boston, 1977
23. Loyd JA, Loyd HM: Adhesive capsulitis of the shoulder. Arthrographic diagnosis and treatment. South Med J 76:879, 1983
24. Turek S: Orthopaedics, Principles and Their Application. JB Lippincott, Philadelphia, 1977
25. Lippmann RK: Frozen shoulder; periarthritis, bicipital tenosynovitis. Arch Surg 47:283, 1943
26. Macnab I: Rotator cuff tendinitis. Ann R Coll Surg Engl 53:271, 1973
27. Simmonds FA: Shoulder pain with particular reference to the "frozen" shoulder. J Bone Joint Surg 31B:426, 1949
28. Neviaser JS: Adhesive capsulitis of the shoulder: study of pathological findings in periarthritis of the shoulder. J Bone Joint Surg 27:211, 1945
29. DePalma AF: Surgery of the Shoulder. JB Lippincott, Philadelphia, 1983
30. Cyriax J: Textbook of Orthopaedic Medicine. 7th Ed. Vol 1. Bailliere Tindall, London, 1978
31. Reeves B: Arthrographic changes in frozen shoulder and post traumatic stiff shoulders. Proc R Soc Med 59:827, 1966
32. Akeson WH, Amiel D, Woo S: Immobility effects of synovial joints: the pathomechanics of joint contracture. Biorheology 17:95, 1980
33. LaVigne A, Watkins R: Preliminary results on immobilization: induced stiffness of monkey knee joints and posterior capsule. Perspectives in Biomedical Engineering. Proceedings of a Symposium of the Biological Engineering Society, University of Strathclyde, Glasgow, June 1972. University Park Press, Baltimore, 1973
34. Enneking W, Horowitz M: The intra-articular effects of immobilization on the human knee. J Bone Joint Surg 54A:973, 1972
35. Kapandji IA: The Physiology of the Joints. Vol. 1. Upper Limb. Churchill Livingstone, Edinburgh, 1982
36. McLaughlin HG: The "frozen shoulder." Clin Orthop 20:126, 1961

37. Murray W: The chronic frozen shoulder. Phys Ther Rev 40:866, 1960

38. Elvey R: Treatment of conditions accompanied by signs of abnormal brachial plexus tension. Presented at the Neck and Shoulder Symposium: Manipulative Therapy, Australia, 1983

39. Mannheimer J, Lampe G: Clinical Transcutaneous Electrical Nerve Stimulation. FA Davis, Philadelphia, 1984

40. Santiesteban AJ: Physical agents and musculoskeletal pain. p. 199. In Gould JA, Davies GH (eds): Orthopaedic and Sports Physical Therapy. CV Mosby, St. Louis, 1985

41. Wyke BH. Articular neurology—a review. Physiotherapy 58:94, 1972

42. Feldenkrais M: Awareness Through Movement. Harper & Row, New York, 1972

43. Maitland GD: Vertebral Manipulation. 5th Ed. Butterworths, London, 1986

44. Evjenth O, Hamberg J: Muscle Stretching in Manual Therapy. Vols. I and II. Scand Book AB Alfta, Sweden, 1984

45. Janda V: Central nervous motor regulation and back problems. p. 27. In IM Korr (ed): The Neurobiologic Mechanisms in Manipulative Therapy. Plenum Press, New York, 1978

46. Hamer J, Kirk JA: Physiotherapy and the frozen shoulder: A comparative trial of ice and ultrasonic therapy. NZ Med J 83:191, 1976

47. Bulgen DY, Binder AL, Hazleman BL, et al: Frozen shoulder: prospective clinical study with an evaluation of three treatment regimens. Ann Rheum Dis 43:353, 1984

48. Nicholson GG: The effects of passive joint mobilization on pain and hypomobility associated with adhesive capsulitis of the shoulder. J Orthop Sports Phys Ther 6:238, 1985

49. Lee M, Haq AM, Wright V, et al: Periarthritis of the shoulder: a controlled trial of physiotherapy. Physiotherapy 59:312, 1973

50. Rizk TE, Christopher RP, Pinals RS, et al: Adhesive capsulitis (frozen shoulder): a new approach to its management. Arch Phys Med Rehab 64:29, 1983

51. Gross TP: Rotator cuff injuries. Orthop Rev 15(8):33, 1986

52. Poppen NK, Walker TS: Forces at the glenohumeral joint in abduction. Clin Orthop Rel Res 135:165, 1978

53. Cofield RH: Rotator cuff disease of the shoulder. J Bone Joint Surg 67A:974, 1985

54. Tibone J, Jobe F, Kerland R, et al: Shoulder impingement syndrome in athletes treated by an anterior acromioplasty. Clin Orthop Rel Res 198:134, 1985

55. Brewer B: Aging of the rotator cuff. Am J Sports Med 7(2):102, 1979

56. Weiner DS, McNab I: Superior migration of the humeral head: a radiological aid in the diagnosis of tears in the rotator cuff. J Bone Joint Surg 52B:524, 1970

57. Komi PV: Neuromuscular performance; factors influencing force and speed production. Scand J Sports Sci 1:2, 1979

58. McLeod WD, Andrews JR: Mechanism of shoulder injuries. Phys Ther 66:12, 1986

59. Neer CS II: Anterior acromioplasty for the chronic impingement syndrome in the shoulder. J Bone Joint Surg 54A:41, 1972

60. Neer CS II: Impingement lesions. Clin Orthop 173:70, 1983

61. Craig EV: The geyser sign and torn rotator cuff: clinical significance and pathomechanics. Clin Orthop 191:213, 1984

62. Craig EV: The posterior mechanism of acute anterior shoulder dislocations. Clin Orthop 190:212, 1984

63. Hawkins RJ, Bell RH, Hawkins RH, Koppert GJ: Anterior dislocation of the shoulder in the older patient. Clin Orthop 206:192, 1986

64. Robbins SL, Angell M: Basic Pathology. WB Saunders, Philadelphia, 1976

65. Frank C, Wood SLY, Amiel D, et al: Am J Sports Med 11:379, 1983

66. Standish W, Rabinovich R, Curwin L: Eccentric exercise in chronic tendinitis. Clin Orthop Rel Res 208:65, 1986

67. Post M, Cohen J: Impingement syndrome. Clin Orthop Rel Res 207:126, 1986

68. Post M: Rotator cuff repair with carbon filament. Clin Orthop Rel Res 196:154, 1985

69. Ozaki J, Fujimoto S, Masuhara K, et al: Reconstruction of chronic massive rotator cuff tears with synthetic materials. Clin Orthop Rel Res 202:173, 1986

70. McLaughlin HL, MacLellan DI: Recurrent anterior dislocation of the shoulder. II. A comparative study, J Trauma 7:191, 1967

71. Kummel B: Spectrum of lesions of the anterior capsular mechanism of the shoulder. Am J Sports Med 7:111, 1979

72. Pavlov H, Warren R, Weiss C, Dines D: The roentgenographic evaluation of anterior shoulder instability. Clin Orthop Rel Res 194:153, 1985

73. Ha'Eri GB: Boytchev procedure for the treatment of anterior shoulder instability. Clin Orthop Rel Res 206:196, 1986

8
Arthroscopic Surgery of the Shoulder

RICK K. ST. PIERRE

Arthroscopic surgery of the shoulder is a new and exciting technique. Shoulder arthroscopy is the direct viewing of the glenohumeral joint with a videoscope.[1] Johnson[2] stated that the advent of shoulder arthroscopy has furthered diagnostic accuracy by allowing direct visualization of the pathologic lesions, applying to the shoulder joint the surgical techniques developed for the knee. Caspari et al.[3] noted that, over the past 10 years, developments in arthroscopic techniques in the shoulder have paralleled those in the knee, providing excellent visualization of the joint with minimal morbidity. Andrews et al.[4] found that although the usual diagnostic modalities of radiography, arthrography, radioactive scanning, and magnetic resonance imaging increased their knowledge of the shoulder, they did not compare to the understanding of the intra-articular anatomy and pathology that they acquired with the use of the arthroscope. Shoulder arthroscopy facilitates the diagnosis and treatment of pathologic intra-articular conditions.

The indications for shoulder arthroscopy have been expanding in the past few years with the evolution of new techniques. Andrews et al.,[4] Snyder and Pattee,[5] and Johnson[2] have described the following indications: rotator cuff lesions, glenoid labrum tears, biceps tendon tears, synovitis, loose bodies, shoulder instability, and chronic shoulder pain refractory to conservative treatment. This chapter describes the operative technique, arthroscopic anatomy, and surgical treatment of pathologic lesions of the shoulder.

SURGICAL TECHNIQUE

The procedure is performed on an outpatient basis under sterile conditions in the operating room. General anesthesia is used with endotracheal intubation. The patient is placed in a lateral decubitus position with the chest and pelvis stabilized with a bean bag. The involved arm is suspended in an abducted and forward-flexed position using a traction glove with 10 to 15 pounds of traction weight. The arm is abducted 70 degrees and forward-flexed 20 degrees. The shoulder is then prepped and draped in a sterile manner.

The bony landmarks are used to localize the posterior arthroscopic portal, located 3 cm inferior and 1 cm medial to the posterior tip of the acromion. An 18-gauge needle is used to distend the shoulder joint with saline. The spinal needle is then removed, and a 1-cm skin puncture is made at the insertion point. With a blunt trochar the arthroscopic cannula is inserted into the shoulder joint. The arthroscope is then inserted through the posterior portal into the shoulder joint, with the inflow connected to the arthroscope sheath to maintain distension of the shoulder joint.

Accessory portals are made anteriorly for the introduction of operative instruments. The anterior portal is established under direct visualization after localization with an 18-gauge spinal needle directed between the coracoid process and the acromion. Placement of the portal is verified by direct intra-articular visualization with the arthroscope in

173

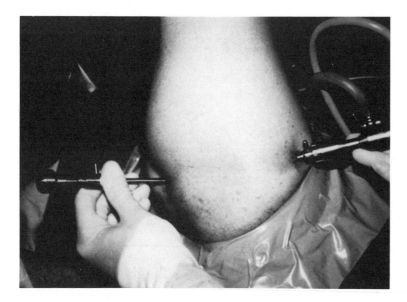

Fig. 8-1. The location of the anterior portal is established under direct visualization with the arthroscope.

the posterior portal. The inflow cannula is then inserted through the anterior portal for maximum distension and better visualization of the shoulder joint (Fig. 8-1). A second anterior portal may be placed adjacent to the first for the insertion of operative instruments (Fig. 8-2). At the end of the procedure the shoulder joint is copiously irrigated and then injected with a local anesthetic. Sterile dressings are applied, and the extremity is placed in a sling for 1 to 2 days.

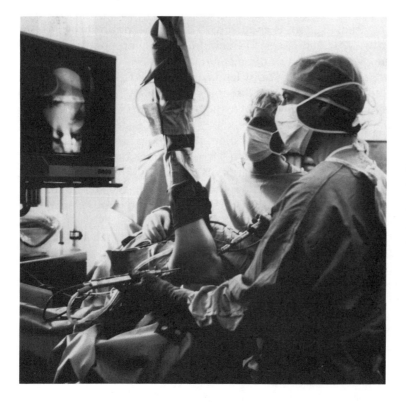

Fig. 8-2. Operative arthroscopy is performed with the arthroscope in the posterior portal and the inflow cannula and motorized shaver in anterior portals. The surgical procedure is performed with the surgeon viewing the video monitor.

ARTHROSCOPIC ANATOMY

Arthroscopic anatomy of the shoulder has been described by numerous authors.[2,4,6-8] They agree that the shoulder joint must be thoroughly and systematically examined. The biceps tendon is the orienting structure that must be traced from its origin on the superior aspect of the glenoid to its exit at the bicipital groove (Fig. 8-3).[7] The articular surface of the humeral head and the glenoid fossa are then inspected for areas of chondromalacia. Attention is then focused on the glenoid labrum, a cartilaginous structure forming the border of the glenoid fossa.[6] The glenohumeral ligaments are next visualized. They are thickenings of the anterior capsule and provide stability to the anterior inferior capsule.[8] The subscapularis tendon and bursae are then visualized between the superior and middle glenohumeral ligaments. Next is the evaluation of the rotator cuff. The supraspinatus component of the rotator cuff is seen superior to the biceps tendon. The infraspinatus and teres minor components of the rotator cuff can be seen by directing the arthroscope posteriorly and superiorly.[4]

SURGICAL TREATMENT OF PATHOLOGIC LESIONS

Resection of glenoid labrum tears, débridement of rotator cuff tears and biceps tendon tears, removal of loose bodies, chondroplasties of the humeral head and glenoid fossa, and synovectomies can all be performed using the three-portal technique.

The most common pathologic lesion is a torn glenoid labrum. The labrum may be injured by impingement between the humeral head and the glenoid.[7] Andrews and Carson[9] noted that all of 73 throwing athletes who underwent arthroscopic examination of the shoulder demonstrated tears of the glenoid labrum. Glenoid labrum tears are resected with intra-articular knives, punches, and motorized shavers. The labrum is visualized with the arthroscope in the posterior portal, and the tear is excised through an anterior portal. The mobile fragment is resected and a contoured rim established[3] (Fig. 8-4).

The next most common pathologic lesion is a partial-thickness rotator cuff tear. The arthroscope is used to inspect the undersurface of the tear (Fig.

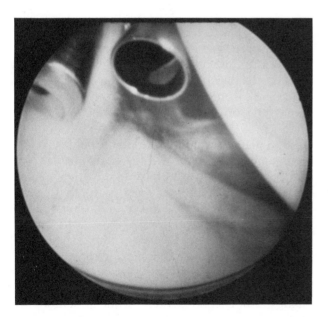

Fig. 8-3. Arthroscopic anatomy of the shoulder joint. The biceps tendon, the humeral head, and the glenoid can be seen.

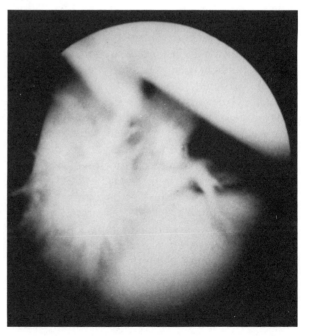

Fig. 8-4. Complex glenoid labrum tear with fragmentation.

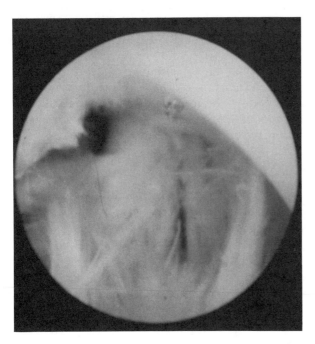

Fig. 8-5. Rotator cuff tear with partial- and full-thickness components.

Two recent advances in arthroscopic shoulder surgery are the treatment of anterior instability and of impingement syndrome. Anterior glenohumeral instability may now be treated arthroscopically. Johnson[2] has developed an arthroscopic operative procedure to grasp, advance, and secure the anterior inferior glenohumeral ligament to the glenoid with a small metal staple, thus correcting the pathologic defect.[2] Snyder and Pattee[5] have described a method for arthroscopically treating impingement syndrome. They use a large motorized burr to perform an acromioplasty as well as resect the coracoacromial ligament.

After arthroscopic shoulder surgery, the extremity is placed in a sling for 1 to 2 days. At 48 hours postoperatively, range-of-motion exercises are initiated. Once the patient has full range of motion, progressive strengthening exercises are begun with light weights and multiple repetitions. When maximum strength and endurance have been achieved, the patient is allowed to return to a normal activity level.

8-5). The loose fragments of rotator cuff are débrided with a motorized resector down to healthy, bleeding tissue. Caspari et al.[3] noted that arthroscopic débridement may result in dramatic relief of pain. Andrews et al.[10] demonstrated that 85 percent of the patients in their series returned to their preoperative athletic activities after arthroscopic débridement of an incomplete rotator cuff tear.

Removal of loose bodies from the shoulder is performed using the same techniques as in the knee. The arthroscope is inserted posteriorly, with the loose bodies removed anteriorly with a grasping clamp. Smaller loose bodies may be removed with the motorized shaver. In addition, partial and complete synovectomies may be performed with the motorized shaver system. Similarly, degenerative and rheumatoid arthritis can be treated with arthroscopic débridement using the motorized synovial resector. Chrondroplasties of the humeral head and glenoid fossa reduce pain, catching, and swelling in the shoulder joint. Caspari et al.[3] demonstrated that the technique is more effective in the shoulder than in the knee, since the shoulder is not a weightbearing joint.

DISCUSSION

Although arthroscopy of the shoulder is a relatively new technique, it is an effective means of diagnosing and treating common shoulder disorders. It is technically more difficult than knee arthroscopy because of the difficulty of entering the glenohumeral joint and avoiding nearby neurovascular structures.[4,8] However, with experience and meticulous attention to detail, arthroscopic techniques can be used to diagnose and treat several shoulder conditions including rotator cuff tears, glenoid labrum tears, biceps tendon tears, loose bodies, rheumatoid and degenerative arthritis, anterior instability, and impingement syndrome. In the short term, the results are comparable to those obtained with extensive open procedures.[2] However, the technique is still in its early stages and needs further research and refinement. With the development of more sophisticated arthroscopic equipment and techniques, arthroscopic surgery of the shoulder will become as universal as arthroscopic surgery of the knee.

REFERENCES

1. Zarins B: Arthroscopy of the shoulder: technique. p. 76. In Zarins B, Andrews JR, Carson WG (eds): Injuries to the Throwing Arm. WB Saunders, Philadelphia, 1985

2. Johnson L: The shoulder joint: an arthroscopist's perspective of anatomy and pathology. Clin Orthop 223:113, 1987

3. Caspari RB, Whipple TL, Meyers JF: Shoulder arthroscopy. p. 87. In Grana WA (ed): Update in Arthroscopic Techniques. Aspen Publishers, Rockville, Maryland, 1984

4. Andrews JR, Carson WG, Ortega K: Arthroscopy of the shoulder: technique and normal anatomy. Am J Sports Med 12:1, 1984

5. Snyder SJ, Pattee GA: Shoulder arthroscopy in the evaluation and treatment of rotator cuff lesions. p. 47. In Paulos LE (ed): Techniques in Orthopaedics. Aspen Publishers, Rockville, Maryland, 1988

6. Carson WG: Arthroscopy of the shoulder: normal anatomy. p. 83. In Zarins B, Andrews JR, Carson WB (eds): Injuries to the Throwing Arm. WB Saunders, Philadelphia, 1985

7. Neviaser TJ: Arthroscopy of the shoulder. Orthop Clin North Am 18:361, 1987

8. Pettrone FA: Shoulder arthroscopy. p. 300. In Pettrone FA (ed): AAOS Symposium on Upper Extremity Injuries in Athletes. CV Mosby, St. Louis, 1986

9. Andrews JR, Carson WG: Operative arthroscopy in the throwing athlete. p. 89. In Zarins B, Andrews JR, Carson WB (eds): Injuries to the Throwing Arm. WB Saunders, Philadelphia, 1985

10. Andrews JR, Broussard TS, Carson WG: Arthroscopy of the shoulder in the management of partial tears of the rotator cuff: a preliminary report. Arthroscopy 1:117, 1985

9

The Elbow Region

DAVID C. REID
SHIRLEY KUSHNER

ANATOMY

The elbow joint is a unique, multifaceted articulation between the capitellum and trochlea of the distal end of the humerus and the radial head and olecranon of the proximal radius and ulna. Nevertheless, it is classically described as a uniaxial hinge joint. This belies the complexity of the anatomy, which is, additionally, closely related to the superior radio-ulnar joint. Both articulations share the same joint capsule, and the joint spaces are continuous.[1] If one appreciates this unusual arrangement of three articulations within one joint space, it is easier to understand why the response of the elbow joint to trauma, exercise, heat, and massage is sometimes surprising, often unusual, and unfortunately, not always good.[1-3]

Capsule and Ligaments

The capsule is a thin structure, reinforced and thickened by the lateral (radial) and medial (ulnar) collateral ligaments, which resist and prevent excessive abduction and adduction stresses and movements (Fig. 9-1). These ligaments do not, however, impede pronation and supination, and some abduction of the ulna always accompanies pronation.

Valgus stability is provided equally by the medial collateral ligament, by the anterior capsule, and by the bony configuration in extension, whereas at 90 degrees of flexion the contribution of the anterior capsule is assumed mainly by the medial collateral ligament.[4] Varus stress is resisted primarily by the

anterior capsule and bony articulation, with only a minor contribution from the radial collateral ligament; this arrangement changes very little throughout the range.[4]

Distraction stresses, which are most significant in high-velocity throwing maneuvers, are resisted primarily by the anterior capsule in extension and the ulnar collateral ligament in flexion[4] (Table 9-1). This information, obtained by necessity from cadaver studies, underscores the considerable contribution to stability made by muscle in the living state.[5] Furthermore, careful dissection reveals that many of the fibers of the so-called collateral ligaments of the elbow are continuous with the collagenous septa of the muscles crossing the joint. Indeed, relatively few ligamentous fibers go directly from bone to bone. The collagen of the radial collateral ligament, for example, belongs to the septa within and around the muscles of the anterolateral muscle group, and the annular ligament to the sheath around the muscle fasciculi of the supinator muscle.[5] A comparable relationship is seen between the muscle fasciculi and the collagenous connective tissue of the ulnar collateral ligament and the common flexor origin. It is the intimate association of the connective tissue of ligament and overlying muscle at the elbow that makes pathology at the site of the muscle insertion sometimes difficult to isolate from the noncontractile portion of the joint. This important concept of muscle fasciculi connected in series with collagenous fibrous strands, blending into the ligament, gives a basis for considering a single musculoligamentous unit as contributing to the dynamic stability of many joints.[5,6]

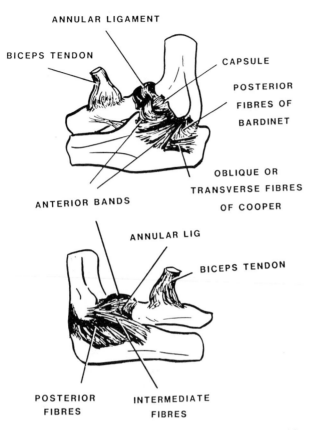

Fig. 9-1. (A) The medial (ulnar collateral) ligament. The very strong anterior fibers are in two bundles, reinforcing the annular ligament. **(B)** Similarly, the lateral (radial collateral) ligament reinforces the annular ligament. Although shown as discrete fibers, in reality the collagenous connections with the overlying intermuscular septa form a musculotendinous unit (Redrawn from Kapandji,[6] with permission.)

Arthrology

Classification

The elbow joint is a compound paracondylar joint in that one bone, the humerus, articulates with two others that lie side by side, by way of two distinct facets. The humero-ulnar component is a modified sellar articulation (convex in one direction and concave at right angles to this first plane). The humeroradial component is an unmodified ovoid (convex or concave in all planes). The proximal radio-ulnar articulation, by contrast, is a modified ovoid.[7]

Resting and Closed-Packed Positions

The resting position of a joint is defined as that position in which the joint capsule is most relaxed and the greatest amount of joint play is possible. The resting position is central to the concept of joint mobilization procedures. In pathologic states, it actually represents the position of maximum intra-articular volume, and hence, the position adapted to minimize capsular tension with effusion and thus reduce pain.

In the humero-ulnar joint, the resting position is with the elbow flexed to 70 degrees and the forearm supinated 10 degrees; this position is most frequently adopted with capsulitis of the elbow. The resting position of the humeroradial joint is in elbow extension and forearm supination. In the superior radio-ulnar joint, the resting position is 35 degrees of supination and 70 degrees of elbow flexion. The position for mobilization of joint play movements is therefore specific for the individual articulation within the elbow joint, although pathology seldom isolates the joint so specifically.

The closed-packed position is the position of the

Table 9-1. Percentage Resistance to Applied Stress

Structure	Valgus Stress		Varus Stress		Distraction	
	Extension	90° Flexion	Extension	90° Flexion	Extension	90° Flexion
MCL	31	54			6	78
LCL			14	9	5	10
Capsule	38	10	32	13	85	8
Osseous	31	33	55	75		

MCL, medial collateral ligament; LCL, lateral collateral ligament.
(Data from Morrey and Kai-Nan[4])

joint in which the capsule and ligaments are tight or maximally tensed; there is maximal contact between articular surfaces, and the surfaces cannot be separated by distractive forces. Testing and mobilization cannot be performed in this position.[8,9]

In the humero-ulnar joint, the closed-packed position is with the elbow extended and the forearm supinated. In the humeroradial joint, the closed-packed position is at 90 degrees of flexion and 5 degrees of supination. In the superior radio-ulnar joint this position is 5 degrees of supination, where the interosseous membrane is tightest.[8]

The capsular pattern is a proportional pattern of limitation of movement at a joint. Initially triggered by pain, effusion, and synovial irritation, and subsequently reinforced and established by capsular shortening and contractures, it is usually accepted as an indication of capsular or intra-articular disease. In the elbow, flexion is usually more restricted than extension, but with time they may become equal. Once marked limitation of flexion and extension is present, pronation and supination may become equally restricted. There are many extrinsic factors, which make a very significant degree of individual variation common at the elbow.

Movement and Joint Play

Joint play or accessory movements are essential for normal function and full range of motion. There is a small amount of side-to-side movement of the ulna on the trochlea of the humerus in flexion and extension. Abduction of the forearm occurs as a conjunct motion with extension and pronation and, conversely, adduction with flexion and supination. There is as well a forward and backward movement of the head of the radius on the capitellum.

Supination and pronation occur at both the radio-humeral joint and the proximal radio-ulnar joint. A backward and forward accessory movement occurs as the radial head moves on the radial notch of the ulna, and the ulna moves forward and backward on the radius.[7,9]

Range of Motion

The lower end of the humerus is offset in two planes. The angulation in the coronal plane, the carrying angle, alters the axis of flexion and exten-

sion so that the forearm sweeps through an arc, facilitating hand-to-mouth movement (Fig. 9-2). The humeral trochlea groove is spiral and is the main factor that dictates the arthrokinematics.[6] Anteriorly, the groove is vertical and parallel to the longitudinal humeral axis, and posteriorly the groove runs obliquely, forming the carrying angle of between 5 and 20 degrees.[9]

Flexion and extension is an impure swing. Flexion is associated with conjunct humeroulnar adduction, whereas extension is of necessity associated with conjunct humeroulnar abduction.

The capitelloradial articulation is an unmodified ovoid, but the degrees of freedom are limited by the ligamentous attachment of the radius to the ulna, and hence the radiohumeral articular pathway follows the axis dictated by the anatomy of the humero-ulnar joint. Restoration of these angles following fracture allows resumption of normal range of motion. Fortunately, fractures in this area occur

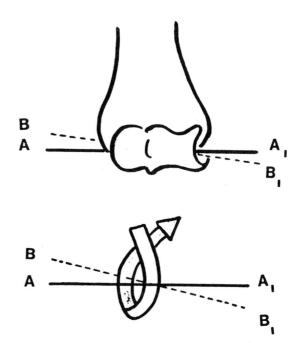

Fig. 9-2. Because of the configuration of the trochlea, the axis of movement changes progressively from horizontal (A–A$_1$) in flexion to oblique (B–B$_1$) in extension. This results in midline movement in flexion and the carrying angle in extension in most individuals. (Redrawn from Kapandji,[6] with permission.)

most frequently in children; although presenting the potential problem of injury to the growth plates, these fractures usually resolve by restoration of the delicate anatomy by remodeling, provided adequate initial reduction is achieved.

The normal range of flexion-extension is approximately 150 to 160 degrees, with about 10 degrees of hyperextension commonly present, particularly in women. Active flexion is usually limited by opposition of the soft parts, but occasionally by bone on bone. Passive flexion is limited by tension of the posterior capsule and passive tension of the triceps. Extension is limited by contact of the tip of the olecranon in its contiguous fossa in the posterior lower humerus. At about the time of apposition, the anterior capsule tightens and tension develops in the elbow flexors so that bony impact is attenuated. If extension continues, ligament rupture must occur, or the olecranon may fracture, leading to a posterior dislocation.[6]

When elbow pathology is treated with splinting, flexion is usually chosen as the resting position; therefore, loss of extension is a common feature following immobilization. The anterior band of the ulnar collateral ligament has been implicated as one of the prime limiting factors in humero-ulnar motion.[10,11] More recently, plication of the anterior band of the ulnar ligament in cadaver studies has failed to support this concept, and it is more likely, particularly in pathologic states, that adhesions and adaptive shortening of the adjacent anterior capsule are more important.[12] Although joint mobilization techniques to the hypomobile humero-ulnar articulation may help restore normal arthrokinematics, it is probably through the influence on the joint capsule as well as the collateral ligament.[9,12,13] Where normal range is possible, the position of active extension is some 5 to 10 degrees short of that obtainable by forced extension. This reflects the contribution of the muscle, as demonstrated by experiments using myoneural blocking agents.[14] The unwillingness of living subjects to allow terminal extension reflects MacConaill's statements that, in living subjects, positions just short of the closed-packed state are used rather than the full closed-packed position.[9]

The superior radio-ulnar joint again highlights the subtle differences in anatomy that make the elbow joint difficult to treat. In this case, 80 percent of the articular surface is made up by the annular ligament as opposed to articular cartilage. This ligament is tough and cone-shaped and will usually prevent dislocation in the adult. The imperfectly formed radial head of the very young child, in contrast, may be easily dislocated by excessive traction with rotation.

The axis for pronation and supination passes from the center of the radial head to the pit adjacent to the styloid process of the ulna distally. This compound movement, involving the three articulations at the elbow as well as the distal radio-ulnar joint and the radiocarpal articulation, can obviously be compromised by pathology at any of these joints. Normal range encompasses 90 degrees of both pronation and supination.

The elbow is a highly congruous joint, which nevertheless depends significantly on its soft tissue restraints during its complex motions. Indeed, the ligaments of the elbow have to resist considerable valgus and, to a lesser degree, varus stresses that accompany rapid flexion and extension. In many throwing activities, for instance, elbow motion exceeds 300 degrees per second, and it is of little wonder that chronic overuse syndromes manifest themselves at this joint.[15]

Muscle Action

During flexion, there is considerable interplay between the biceps, brachialis, and brachioradialis muscles, with all three working to various degrees at different ranges and speeds and between individuals. Hence, it is not surprising that many studies on their actions appear at first glance contradictory.[1,2] The following main points emerge:

1. The biceps and the brachialis are both muscles of considerable bulk, which add power and are the prime movers of flexion.[15,16]
2. The body tends toward economy; therefore slow movements, without added resistance, may be performed by one or the other of these muscles, or by a diminished amount of work by both.
3. The biceps may actively supinate the arm while flexion is taking place, unless this is counteracted.[16,17]
4. In rapid movements the brachioradialis may act in two ways, initially as a shunt muscle, overcom-

ing centrifugal forces acting at the elbow, and then by adding power to increase the speed of flexion. It does this most efficiently in the mid-prone position.[2,16]

5. The common flexor mass from the medial epicondyle may weakly assist the prime movers, or become hypertrophied to assist in flexion in cases of paralysis of the proximal muscles.[1]

Of the three heads of the triceps, the medial head seems to be the most consistent in its action over the extensor mechanism of the elbow.[2,16] The long and lateral heads provide extra strength for this motion but may be relatively electrically silent for slow, low-power movements.[2,16] The triceps is most powerful when the elbow and shoulder are simultaneously extended. Deep extensions from the triceps insert into the capsule of the posterior recess of the joint and help pull the redundant synovium away during extension, thus avoiding impingement.[1] This is similar to the articularis genu mechanism over the suprapatellar pouch at the knee.

The pronator quadratus needs the power offered by the pronator teres for most everyday and all resisted pronation activities.[1] Similarly, the biceps, in most actions, supplements the power of the supinator.[16,17] This is particularly true of high-speed motion.[2]

ASSESSMENT

An adequate history and examination to rule out cervical spine and shoulder pathology is mandatory (Fig. 9-3). Specific points in the history such as age, occupation, pastime, pattern of pain, and functional difficulties should be used to focus the examination on the probable diagnoses. Examples include the complaint of intermittent locking with loose bodies and dislocation of the radial head in children under the age of 6 years. After the history has been obtained, examination of the elbow is performed.

Observation

The patient's elbow is observed for swelling, contours, color, and carrying angle. The carrying angle is normally 5 to 10 degrees in men and 10 to 15 degrees in women. Also, have the patient place the arms at 90 degrees of forward flexion at the shoulder and observe the elbow-wrist relationship in pronation and supination. These relationships may be altered following abduction and adduction lesions.

Range of Motion

Active

Flexion is tested in supination and is normally 150 degrees. Extension is normally to 0 degrees in men and up to 5 degrees in women, but 15 degrees of hyperextension in women or children is not uncommon. Supination and pronation are tested with the shoulder adducted and the elbow held against the trunk to rule out shoulder rotation. These movements range from 0 degrees at the neutral position to 80 or 90 degrees.

Passive

The movements are tested with particular attention to the end-feel. The flexion end-feel is one of soft tissue approximation, whereas that of extension is bone to bone; the end-feel of pronation and supination is one of soft tissue stretch. The forearm should be held proximal to the wrist to rule out movement in this joint.

Muscle Tests

Resisted movements are tested isometrically in a neutral position. The test is repeated for five contractions in order to uncover subtle weaknesses in neurologic conditions, such as nerve root palsies. Minimal to maximal resistance is given. Minimal resistance causing pain is indicative of a contractile lesion, whereas if pain is elicited only with maximal resistance, one must also consider inert structures due to increased articular pressure.

Primary selective tissue tension tests will determine which muscle group is involved. Secondary tests will assist in pointing to the specific muscle involved. For example, if resisted elbow flexion is painful, the biceps, brachioradialis, or brachialis muscle may be involved. Now if pain is elicited on pronation to neutral from full supination, the brachioradialis is likely at fault. If resisted supination from neutral increases the pain, it is likely that the biceps is involved.

Wrist flexion and extension strength tests must be included, along with all elbow motions, because of the proximal insertions of the forearm musculature on the epicondyles and supracondylar ridges.

Ligamentous Tests

The collateral ligaments should be tested 15 to 30 degrees short of full extension and may also be tested in midflexion, since with moderate pathology there may only be signs in selected positions where tension is maximal.

Accessory Movement Tests

The suspect elbow is compared to the normal one with attention to end-feel. The following tests are performed:[8,13]

1. Lateral and medial glide of the ulna on the humerus is tested just short of full extension (Fig. 9-4A).
2. Distraction of the ulna on the humerus is carried out with 70 degrees flexion and 35 degrees supination (Fig. 9-4B).
3. Flexion and extension of the radial head on humerus are performed while passively flexing and extending the elbow by the movement of the therapist's body (Fig. 9-4C).
4. Dorsal and ventral glide of the radial head on the ulna is performed in 70 degrees elbow flexion and 35 degrees supination (Fig. 9-4D).
5. Distraction of the radial head on the humerus is performed in 70 degrees flexion and 35 degrees supination (Fig. 9-4E).
6. Compression of the radial head on the humerus is performed in 70 degrees flexion and 35 degrees supination (Fig. 9-4F).
7. Extension adduction quadrant 10 degrees from full extension (Fig. 9-5A).
8. Extension abduction quadrant 10 degrees from full extension (Fig. 9-5B).
9. Flexion abduction quadrant 10 degrees from full flexion and supination (Fig. 9-5C).
10. Flexion adduction quadrant 10 degrees from full flexion and pronation (Fig. 9-5D).

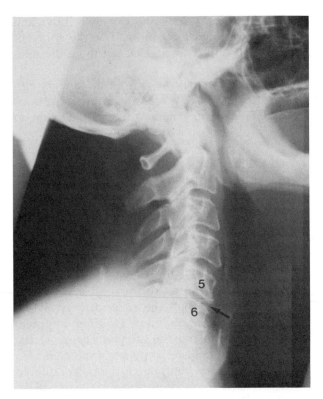

Fig. 9-3. This patient complained of symptoms compatible with lateral epicondylitis. Further interrogation and examination unmasked cervical pathology. The radiograph confirmed C5–C6 degenerative changes. Although local injection settled the elbow problem, recurrence is likely unless the neck dysfunction is also attended to.

Palpation

Palpation should be systematic and include all bony points, tendons, and ligaments with attention to crepitus, pain, boggy edematous changes, and abnormal contours.

Other Tests

Reflexes will have been tested during the cervical scan and include the biceps (C5), brachioradialis (C6), and triceps (C7). These reflexes are compared to those on the opposite side and noted as either hyperreflexic, normal, hyporeflexic, or absent. Dermatomes are also tested with the cervical scan. Generally the lateral elbow is C5, the anterior

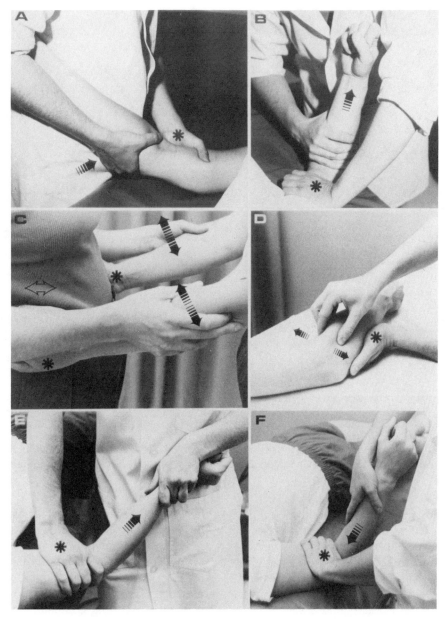

Fig. 9-4. Tests for accessory movements. Asterisks indicate the fixed point, and the arrow indicates direction of movement. **(A)** Lateral and medial ulnar glide; **(B)** ulnar distraction; **(C)** flexion and extension of the radial head; while the patient's hands are fixed on the therapist's hips, forward and backward motion helps produce flexion and extension at the patient's elbows; **(D)** dorsal and ventral glide of the radial head; **(E)** distraction of the radial head; **(F)** compression of the radial head.

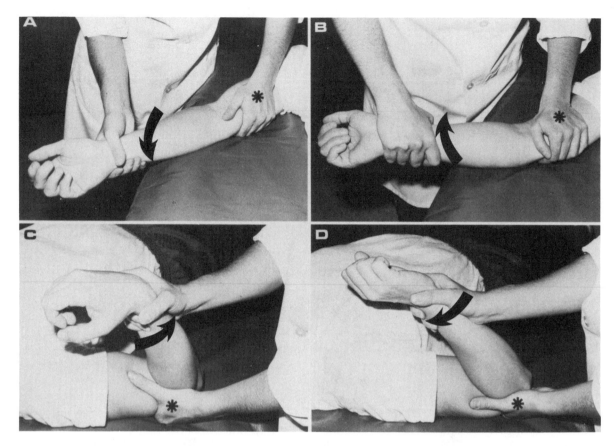

Fig. 9-5. Accessory movement tests. Asterisks indicate the fixed point. **(A)** Extension adduction quadrant; **(B)** extension abduction quadrant; **(C)** flexion abduction quadrant; **(D)** flexion adduction quadrant.

elbow C6, the posterior elbow C7, and the medial elbow T1 and T2. The dermatomes at the elbow, however, are nonspecific, and there is considerable individual variation and overlap.

Special tests for specific pathologic entities conclude the examination and are discussed below in the context of the appropriate conditions.

CONDITIONS

Tennis Elbow Syndrome

Definition

By definition, tennis elbow (lateral epicondylitis, lateral elbow stress syndrome) is a lesion affecting the origin of the tendons of the muscles that extend the wrist. Like many medical terms, its usage is often ill-defined, and the term tends to mean different things to different people (Table 9-2). The term *tennis elbow* has been loosely used to encompass posterior and medial symptoms, which have been referred to as posterior and medial tennis elbow, respectively, adding confusion to an already complicated topic.[18-21] Tennis elbow will here refer only to lateral epicondylitis and associated common extensor origin tendinitis.

Pathology and Symptoms

The exact nature of the pathology at the common extensor origin is open to question, and it is likely that several basic etiologic entities giving rise to slightly different pathologic changes in the tissue

Table 9-2. Pathology of Lateral Tennis Elbow[a]

Region	Possible Pathology
Proximal	Periostitis
	Common extensor origin
	Tendinitis
	Microtearing with painful granulation
	Degenerative changes in tendon
Joint	Lateral ligament strain
	Radiohumeral bursitis
	Inflammation of annular ligament
	Hypertrophic synovial fringe
	Degenerative changes in the radial head cartilage
	Extension/abduction ulnohumeral lesions
Neural	Cervical radiculopathy
	Posterior interosseous nerve entrapment

[a] These causes of elbow pain have all been implicated in the tennis elbow syndrome.

may present a fairly similar clinical picture[23,24] (Table 9-2). The three major sites of pathology are, however, the common extensor origin, the radiocapitellar joint, and the radio-ulnar joint, with fibrillation and chondromalacic changes. Furthermore, neurogenic causes such as C6 radiculopathy and, more locally, radial tunnel entrapment of the posterior interosseous nerve must be considered. With C6 root involvement secondary to dysfunction at the C5–C6 segment, weakness results at the radial wrist extensors, leaving them prone to injury. The patient's clinical picture resembles that of a true tennis elbow that is resistant to treatment. While the elbow is treated, simultaneous attention must be given to the cervical spine (Fig. 9-3). Only then will the patient respond.[24] The "culprit" must be treated and not only the "victim." In view of the high success rate of local limited release of the common extensor origin, and the recovery at surgery of granulation tissue and scar from this area, this site of pathology probably accounts for the majority of cases.

Whatever the etiology, there is generally an element of overuse or overstress; 45 percent of tennis players who practice or play daily experience problems.[25] Tennis elbow syndrome is also a frequent occupational hazard in individuals who frequently perform forceful pronation and supination motions, heavy lifting, or repetitive hammering activities.

There is a local tenderness on the outside of the elbow at the common extensor origin, with aching and pain in the back of the forearm; the condition is aggravated by continual use. Special tests include resisted wrist extension, which precipitates pain at the extensor origin (Fig. 9-6). Performing the test in full elbow extension will decrease the number of false negative results. Painful resisted extension of the middle and ring fingers implicates the extensor digitorum communis, and painful resistance of wrist extension and radial deviation points to the extensor carpi radialis longus and brevis. A further test for tennis elbow is to stretch the insertion by holding the elbow in extension and performing passive wrist flexion and pronation. A positive test is one that elicits pain at the common origin.

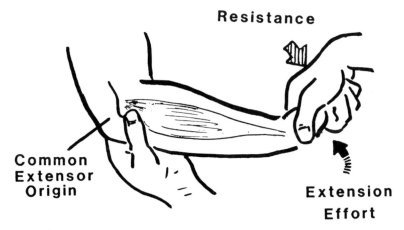

Resistance

Common Extensor Origin

Extension Effort

Fig. 9-6. Palpation over the common extensor origin while resisting extension elicits the patient's symptoms in lateral epicondylitis. The test may be even more sensitive when done in full extension.

The treatment will be outlined in detail for the tennis player, but many of the principles may be extrapolated to other situations. Both sexes are affected equally, and the condition rarely occurs before the age of 20 years. Less experienced players with poor stroke technique, but who play frequently, are the group at risk. The average age of players developing tennis elbow is 40 years. This reflects, first, the typical microcirculatory changes in the blood supply at the myotendinous junction of the extensor muscles at the elbow, and second, an increasing number of joint symptoms occurring with age and not true tennis elbow.

Etiology and Treatment

The etiology and treatment of tennis elbow can be considered under three headings: playing style, anatomic factors, and equipment. An understanding of these etiologic features suggests a logical approach to therapy.

Playing Style

A poorly executed backhand is mainly implicated. The forearm is used as the power source rather than the kinetics of the body and weight transfer from the body to the shoulder.

A typical faulty backhand has no forward weight transfer, and the front shoulder is usually elevated. The trunk leans away from the net at the time of impact, and the racket head is down. The elbow and wrist extend prior to impact, and the power source is forearm extension in the pronated position. The stroke is usually a nonrhythmic, jerky movement, with sharp pronation in the follow-through. When the ball is hit incorrectly, the forces are transmitted as an acute strain up and along the muscle mass to the extensor origin at the elbow.[21] Repetitive stresses may eventually cause the small tears and inflammation that are reflected in the pain associated with tennis elbow.

Anatomic studies confirm that the extensor carpi radialis brevis (ECRB) is under maximum tension when contracting while the forearm is pronated, the wrist flexed, and the ulna deviated.[23] The head of the radius rotates anteriorly against the ECRB during pronation, where a bursa is frequently located,

and this may explain why some individuals experience pain at the head of the radius, perhaps secondarily to inflammation of the bursa.[23]

In the serve, there is usually slightly less stress on the lateral side of the elbow than with the backhand. First, the use of a backhand grip forces the arm into a hyperpronated position, thereby stressing the extensor origin. Second, some tennis players who have played seriously for many years have increased the bulk of their extensor muscles considerably but may have lost full flexibility. Therefore, they experience increased stresses at the completion of the stroke.[23]

A frequent error is an exaggerated effort to hit the ball hard. Maximum speed is imparted to the ball by good style, keeping the eye on the ball and hitting it on the "sweet spot" in the center of the racket. Very little is to be gained by sacrificing style for power. Usually the result of overpowering the stroke is failure to transfer the body weight, thus relying on the forearm as the main source of strength, often aggravating a pre-existing condition further.

As far as technique is concerned, then, the stroke most implicated in tennis elbow is firmly established as the backhand. Investment in a few tennis lessons to improve technique should be considered. The development of a two-handed backhand may also alleviate the problem for some players with chronic repetitive symptoms.

Many more experienced players run into trouble with their forehand and top spin. The common fault is to roll the racket head over the ball in an attempt to produce top spin. This motion produces excessive strain, since the impact is sustained in the hyperpronated position. Supination follows, with the ball in contact with the strings for only 0.004 second. This is not long enough to impart adequate top spin. The more correct long stroking maneuver, starting low and ending high, with a good follow through, is more effective and produces less stress.

During the serve, the racket head travels at 300 to 350 mph before ball impact, at which time it abruptly slows to about 150 mph. With poor use of the trunk and legs, the forearm once again absorbs too much stress.[25]

When recovering from tennis elbow, the patient should commence with the easiest strokes, try not to be too competitive, and only play with people who are willing to have an easy game.

Anatomy

Many individuals play tennis with less than optimal grip strength. Indeed, the average woman has a forearm girth of 9 inches and a grip strength of about 50 pounds, whereas the average man has a forearm girth of 11 inches and a grip strength of approximately 80 pounds. By contrast, the professional tennis player usually has a forearm girth of about 12 inches and a grip strength of 105 pounds.[21] The strength of the normal wrist extensors should be about 50 percent of the flexor strength.[22] The wrist flexors have been found to be the strongest, followed by the radial deviators, the ulnar deviators, and then the extensors. The supinators are normally stronger than the pronators.[9] In regular tennis players, the extensor muscles should be strengthened, so that they are at least 50 percent and probably closer to 75 percent of flexor strength. An even grip, taking care not to allow the thumb to be placed along the axis of the shaft, will assist in even distribution of forces.

Equipment

In individuals with incipient or established symptoms, the racket should only be strung to 52 to 55 pounds.[25] This will allow the impact to be spread over slightly more time and decrease the forces transmitted to the forearm muscles.[26] Sixteen gauge catgut is more resilient than nylon and has the ability to lessen the shock of the impact of the ball. However, gut is expensive and loses resilience quickly; probably 16 gauge nylon is the best compromise.

A racket handle that is too large or too small may produce an uneven force distribution across the hand and hence to the muscles. This may be particularly applicable to women, whose average hand size is about 4⅛ inches. A measurement taken from the proximal hand crease to the tip of the ring finger along its radial border gives an indication of grip size.[21]

Heavy-duty or rubber-centered balls impart more concentrated moments of force and may aggravate the symptoms. Regular-duty balls are recommended. Playing with balls soaked from landing in puddles may also trigger problems.[25]

It is hard to give advice in regard to the racket itself. Both wooden and metal rackets have their merits and disadvantages. The very heavy wooden rackets should be avoided by all but the most experienced players. Nirschl advises a midsize graphite racket weighing only 12 to 12.5 oz. The graphite absorbs the shock of ball impact better than wood, and the midsize racket has a larger "benevolent" or "sweet" zone, the area on the strings where minimal torque is produced on impact.[25] The lighter racket allows players to position more quickly and lessens the chance of hitting late.[27] However, balanced weight, hand size, and stringing are all more significant factors. Most of all, good style, hitting the ball in the sweet spot in the center of the racket, can do more to reduce stresses on the forearm than any change of racket can.

General Treatment

Treatment is aimed at relief of inflammation, promotion of healing, reducing the overload forces, and increasing upper extremity strength, endurance, and flexibility.[21,25] The following are some important points in preventing and treating tennis elbow.

Before practicing, warm up slowly and perform adequate stretching exercises to the forearm and hand. Sometimes rubbing ice onto the common extensor origin before playing may help.

Wearing a tennis arm band (epicondylar splint) of nonelastic fabric, lined with foam rubber to prevent slipping, may reduce the stresses on the common extensor origin. By limiting muscle expansion, the contraction force is reduced, decreasing irritation of the muscle. This band must be wide enough (3 to 3.5 inches); the narrower widths are usually not as effective.[28] The band should be applied tightly while tensing the muscles of the arm. If the elbow band is applied while the muscles are relaxed, it may cut off the circulation. The band should be comfortable with the forearm relaxed. The band should not be applied too far proximally, but rather over the major muscle belly about two fingers' breadth distal to the elbow flexor crease. The efficacy of these bands in decreasing pain during numerous activities has been well documented.[29,30]

Occasionally, a wrist resting splint can be made and adapted for whatever the occupation or sport of the individual entails. This moderate defunctioning of some of the wrist extensor contraction may allow a resistant clinical problem to resolve slowly with considerable comfort during the activities of daily living.

Physiotherapy treatment will initially consist of assessment, modification of activity, ice, and electrical stimulation.[24]

To objectively assess the severity of a clinical complaint, keep in mind that grip strength correlates very well with a visual pain scale and functional incapacity. Even measuring grip strength with the aid of a simple sphygmomanometer cuff, preinflated to 20 mm Hg, can give a reasonable assessment of the pain threshold and progress of treatment.[31-33] Electrotherapeutic modalities such as laser, ultrasound phonophoresis with 10 percent hydrocortisone, interferential therapy, high-voltage galvanic stimulation, and transcutaneous electrical nerve stimulation (TENS) have all been advocated to relieve pain and inflammation. Cure rates from 55 to 90 percent have been reported.[31] Topical application of dimethyl sulfoxide has also been suggested.[32,33] Manual therapy techniques such as transverse frictions, joint mobilization and manipulation, myofascial release, and strain and counterstrain techniques may be used[34,35] (Table 9-3). Mobilization techniques are covered in Chapter 12.

Whatever the treatment employed, as resolution occurs and the patient returns to his sport or occupation, exercise will form a mainstay of treatment, as complete rest is seldom indicated. Reduced physical activity leads to reduction in strength, so that on resuming the activity, a recurrence of the injury could be precipitated by stresses of a lesser magnitude than those that caused the initial insult.[36]

Isometric exercises for the wrist extensors, with the elbow in flexion, moving closer to extension as pain permits, can be used in the acute phase.[35] As pain permits, concentric and then eccentric strengthening using free weights or surgical tubing will be performed. Isokinetic strengthening eccentrically and concentrically may also be used. Not only are the flexors and extensors strengthened, but also the radial and ulnar deviators, pronators, and supinators.

Curwin and Stanish have developed a program to combine stretching and eccentric strengthening of the wrist extensors.[36] Exercising the muscle eccentrically allows it to withstand greater resistance and prevent injury, which occurs by eccentrically loading an inflexible muscle. The patient warms up with local heat or general exercise. The wrist extensors are stretched passively three times, for 30 seconds. Three sets of 10 eccentric contractions are performed with a weight of 1 to 5 pounds; surgical tubing may also be used as an effective way of applying resistance. The stretches are repeated and ice is then applied. This 20-minute session is repeated daily for about 3 weeks.

Before returning to the sport or occupation, the patient mimics the backhand, forehand, and serve, or the specific tasks of the occupation, using surgical tubing or pulleys for resistance. Throughout the physiotherapy treatment, shoulder and trunk strength and range of motion are maintained, as is the patient's cardiovascular fitness, if applicable.

Injection of a steroid preparation can be very effective, provided the lesion is well localized.[31] This treatment is best supplemented with oral anti-inflammatory medication and may be repeated at 1-month intervals for up to 3 months or until the patient is asymptomatic. Considerable care is needed with the injection technique to avoid skin atrophy. It must be stressed that simply injecting the patient with steroids does not constitute complete treatment. Assessment and modification of precipitating factors, as well as exercise therapy, are usually necessary.

When nonoperative management fails, release of the fascia and part of the common extensor origin may be considered. Variations of the procedure involve increasingly radical releases, to include part of the annular ligament of the superior radio-ulnar joint, and the ECRB or the fascial band at the proximal edge of the supinator.[37] These variations in the extent of the procedure reflect confusion as to the exact site of the pathology.[38]

Postoperative rehabilitation involves a short period of gentle active motion and, at 3 weeks, increasing range of motion, strengthening, and stretching exercises.

Table 9-3. Comparison of Manipulation Techniques

	Mills	Cyriax I	Cyriax II (Mills)	Kaltenborn	Mennell	Stoddard
				Author		
Lesion	Frayed or detached orbicular ligament in acute cases. Adhesions in chronic cases.	Partial tear at tenoperiosteal junction of extensor carpi radialis brevis.	Inadequate healing. Scar in extensor carpi radialis brevis at tenoperiosteal junction.	Lateral epicondylitis.	Painful scar in common extensor tendon.	Adhesions binding origin of extensor digitorum communis to radial collateral ligament.
Position	Lying. General anesthetic	Sitting. No anesthetic. Following 5–10 minutes of deep friction.	Sitting. Following 10–15 minutes deep friction.	Sitting or supine. No esthetic.	Standing. Prior injection of local esthetic.	Supine.
Manipulation	Forced extension of elbow. Wrist and fingers fixed. Forearm pronated.	Elbow fully extended. Forearm supinated. Fixation at medial elbow. Varus thrust at lateral wrist.	Shoulder abducted and medially rotated. Forearm pronated, wrist flexed. Fixated at wrist. Extensor thrust at elbow.	Fixation at wrist. Varus thrust at extended elbow.	Fully flexed and pronated wrist and elbow. Elbow extension with forced over pressure.	Shoulder abducted 90° Pronate and supinate to identify maximum tension in extensor digitorum communis. Varus thrust at elbow by forearm adduction.
Indication	Minimal loss of range of motion of elbow extension. Tested with full wrist and finger flexion in pronation. Local epicondylar or radiohumeral joint tenderness.	Pain over the lateral epicondyle or common extensor tendon origin.	Tenoperiosteal variety. Pain on resisted wrist extension and radial deviation.	Lateral epicondylitis. Restricted movement of the radial head.	Painful area at common extensor origin on palpation.	Chronic cases. No response to hydrocortisone injection. Pain on gripping.
Contraindication	Gross limitation of extension. Full range of motion.		Loss of full elbow extension. Osteoarthrosis. Loose bodies, traumatic arthritis.	Inability to fully extend.		Acute condition. Rest pain. Restriction of elbow extension.
Frequency	Usually one manipulation.	Three times per week. Average of four treatments. Range: 1–9 treatments.	2–3 times per week until cure. Range: 4–12 sessions.			

(From Kushner and Reid,[35] with permission.)

Medial Epicondylitis

Etiology

Medial epicondylitis (epitrochleitis, golfer's elbow, medial tennis elbow) is probably a tendinopathy of the common flexor origin including the pronator teres. Pain is located over the medial epicondyle and is exacerbated by resisted wrist flexion and pronation. Pain is also elicited on passive wrist extension and supination. It is an overuse syndrome related to throwing sports, golf, or occupations such as carpentry that involve repetitive hammering or screwing. Chronic symptoms may eventually lead to contractures, with inability to fully extend or supinate.[39]

Treatment

Prevention and restoration of lost range of motion are an important part of the treatment. In the acute phase, ice, ultrasound, and other physical modalities may be used in conjunction with anti-inflammatory medication. Any course of treatment must culminate in a strengthening program. The stretching and strengthening routine described for tennis elbow is used, but the direction of motion is reversed.[36] Injection of a steroid preparation into the area is done with care because of the propensity for skin atrophy in this area as well as the proximity of the ulnar nerve. In recalcitrant cases, a release of the common origin is possible with surprisingly little measurable loss of functional strength.

Injuries to the Throwing Arm (Medial Tension Overload Syndrome)

Throwing Action

The throwing mechanisms used in various sports have more biomechanical similarities than differences, and baseball pitching is frequently used to demonstrate these principles and their effect on the supporting anatomy. Three stages are defined,

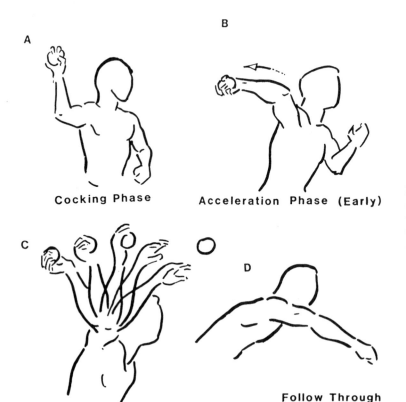

Cocking Phase   Acceleration Phase (Early)

Acceleration Phase (Late)   Follow Through

Fig. 9-7. The throwing mechanism is common to many sports. Stress is initially put on the shoulder and elbow, with a final distraction force largely damped by muscle and ligamentous structures at the elbow.

namely, the cocking phase or windup, the acceleration phase (better considered as divided into early and late), and the follow-through[40,41] (Fig. 9-7).

Cocking Phase

The shoulder is abducted to around 90 degrees and simultaneously taken into extreme external rotation with extension. The elbow is flexed to approximately 45 degrees and the wrist extended.

Early Acceleration

The trunk and shoulder are brought rapidly forward, leaving the forearm and hand behind, prestressing all the structures at the elbow, and in particular the ulnar collateral ligament.

Late Acceleration

As vigorous contraction of the shoulder flexors and internal rotators, with early co-contraction of the elbow extensors and wrist flexors, takes place, the forearm and wrist are accelerated to add speed to the throw. The maneuver results in a whipping action, throwing significant additional stress onto the medial elbow (Fig. 9-7).

Follow-Through

Follow-through begins with the missile release and varies somewhat with the type of throw, but it is characterized by stress on the structures around the olecranon.

Injuries

The sequence of events described, when repeated many times, may result in a series of pathologic changes, best considered under the headings of acute and chronic (Table 9-4). The lateral joint line experiences compressive forces during throwing, while shear forces are generated posteriorly in the olecranon fossa, and tensile forces develop along the medial joint line.[15]

Acute Injuries

Muscular Strains Minor muscular strains are common, presenting with point tenderness to palpation and pain with resisted contraction. These injuries, usually to the common flexor group, are frequently self-limiting, requiring only modified rest, ice, and treatment by electrical modalities and gentle stretching. With healing, progressive strengthening is added to ensure adequate ability to return to function without reinjury. Flexion contractures, which predispose to muscle strains, are present in more than half of all adult professional pitchers.[15]

Major tears or ruptures, usually of the forearm flexors, must be recognized since surgery may be required (Fig. 9-8). Usually deformity and a palpable defect, as well as considerable ecchymosis, will alert the clinician to the correct diagnosis. In the muscular individual, a transverse sulcus may be present at the anterior border of the lacertus fibrosus (bicipital aponeurosis), and this normal groove should not be confused with a rupture of the pronator teres or common flexor muscle belly. Very rarely, the biceps tendon may rupture distally, and this is compatible with acceptable function in the noncompetitive individual. However, surgical repair gives the best results in the heavy manual laborer and the athlete.

Medial Collateral Ligament Sprains Repetitive valgus stress in pitchers and javelin throwers may produce acute inflammation of the medial collateral ligament. Point tenderness over the medial joint

Table 9-4. Throwing Injuries of the Elbow

Type of Injury	Possible Pathology
Medial tension overload	Muscular 　Overuse 　Fascial compression syndrome
	Ligamentous and capsular 　Ulnar traction spur 　Loose bodies 　Medial epicondylitis 　Joint degeneration
Lateral compression injuries	Osteochondritis dissecans Capitellar fractures Loose bodies Lateral epicondylitis Joint degeneration
Extensor overload	Acute 　Triceps strain 　Olecranon fracture
	Chronic 　Bony hypertrophy 　Stress fracture 　Olecranon fossa loose bodies 　Joint degeneration

(Modified from Slocum,[41] with permission.)

line and an absence of instability help to make this diagnosis. Treatment is the same as for muscular strains.

Avulsion of the Medial Epicondyle Prior to epiphyseal closure, rapid strong contraction of the forearm flexors is capable of avulsing the medial epicondyle (Fig. 9-8). Tenderness in the region of the medial condyle in an adolescent should arouse suspicion of this injury. Failure to detect it may lead to increasing varus deformity. When there is extreme tenderness, prophylactic splinting of the elbow for 2 weeks is a safe precaution. A repeat x-ray at this time may show callus. A widely displaced fragment may require surgical reattachment.

Chronic Injuries

The effects of repeated valgus stress of the elbow are most pronounced in the professional pitcher, particularly if the individual began his career at an early age. Clinically, elbow flexion contractures occur in up to 50 percent of professional pitchers, and an increased carrying angle is seen in about 3 percent.[40-42] Repeated stresses result in attenuation of the medial collateral ligament with laxity (Fig. 9-9). Pain and swelling, catching, and locking are often manifestations of additional bony and joint surface changes. X-ray examination may reveal loose bodies, particularly in the olecranon fossa; hyperostotic changes and osteophytes around the posteromedial olecranon process; and traction spurs at the attachment of the medial collateral ligament to the ulna. Oblique views and tomograms may be necessary to elucidate all these changes. Occasionally the joint symptoms are accompanied by ulnar nerve neuritis or neuropathy secondary to repeated minor traction stresses or chronic scarring. Surgical excision of osteophytes and removal of loose fragments may be necessary to restore range of motion and a fully functional elbow.

Little Leaguer's Elbow

The young pitcher is exposed to the risks already outlined, as well as the additional risk of epiphyseal injury. Originally, "little leaguer's elbow" referred to an epiphysitis of the medial epicondylar epiphysis related to the repeated trauma of pitching. This stress is greatly increased by throwing curve balls and other breaking pitches, which require more forceful pronation of the wrist. The clinical features of little leaguer's elbow include pain and tenderness with loss of full extension. Characteristic changes are accelerated growth of the medial side as well as fragmentation of the medial epicondylar epiphysis.[42,43] The term "little leaguer's elbow" has since come to encompass all of the stress changes involved in pitching in the skeletally immature individual. These changes include compression of the lateral joint, which may trigger changes of osteochondritis dissecans of both the capitellum and the radial head. It is important to recognize this condition early, since adequate rest from repeated

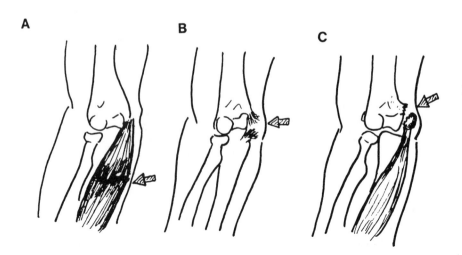

A   **B**   **C**

Fig. 9-8. Acute stress to the medial elbow may result in **(A)** a muscle belly tear, **(B)** a ligament sprain, or **(C)** an avulsion fracture, which, in the skeletally immature, may be an epiphyseal injury.

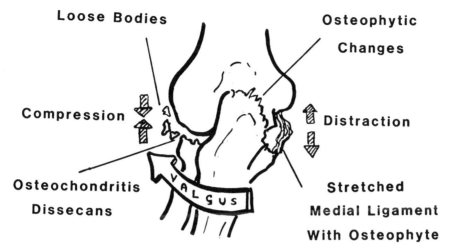

Fig. 9-9. Repetitive valgus stresses associated with throwing produce stretching and instability on the medial side, with shearing forces on the olecranon. The result is growth defects in the young, and degenerative changes in the adult.

stresses may allow resolution of the problems. Failure to protect the joint may result in the formation of loose fragments, pain, deformity, and possibly arthrosis.

The incidence of this problem is unknown and varies widely in reported series.[44] In 1972, before major rule changes were adopted to protect the youngsters, accelerated growth and separation of the medial epicondylar epiphysis were present in up to 90 percent of little league pitchers between the ages of 9 and 14 in Southern California. These same changes were seen in fewer than 10 percent of children of the same age who did not play baseball.[44]

Osteochondritis dissecans, particularly of the capitellum, is reported in other sports, notably gymnastics, where the arms frequently function as weightbearing extremities under stress.[44,45]

Treatment

Treatment is initially aimed at decreasing inflammation with ice and rest, as dictated by the signs and symptoms. Electrical modalities to decrease pain and inflammation are used. These may include TENS, high-voltage galvanic stimulation, ultrasound, interferential, current and laser.

If the patient is partially immobilized, active range-of-motion therapy commences in the whirl-pool. Gentle resisted isometric exercises to pain are started. Once immobilization is discontinued, strengthening with surgical tubing or free weights is begun, progressing to isokinetic strengthening, push-ups, and pull-ups. Shoulder range-of-motion and isometric exercises are performed throughout the rehabilitation period.

Injuries in throwing sports are decreased and prevented by attention to flexibility, decreasing muscle imbalances, and correcting the throwing technique. Proper use of body mechanics will alter the stress on the elbow. Overhead rather than sidearm and curve ball throws should be taught. Whipping and snapping of the elbow should be discouraged. The frequency and length of time each player is allowed to pitch should be decreased. Javelin throwers may have to change their technique or hold in order to reduce the stresses on the medial joint.[46] Prophylactic taping to prevent hyperextension and decrease valgus stresses may be appropriate when the individual returns to practice.

Care of the throwing arm includes:[46]

1. Gently stretching and massaging the elbow and shoulder before throwing
2. Performing throwing actions without the ball
3. Commencing with gentle throwing while wearing a warm-up jacket

4. Gradually increasing the velocity of the throw
5. After throwing, replacing the warm-up jacket, performing gentle stretching, and allowing a period of time to cool down
6. Applying ice after each throwing session

Osteochondrosis of the Capitellum

Etiology

Osteochondrosis of the capitellum (Panner's disease, osteochondrosis deformans, osteochondritis) may be directly related to trauma or to changes in the circulation; this is the so-called Panner's disease of aseptic or avascular necrosis.[47,48] There has been much debate as to the etiology of this condition; cartilage rests, bacterial infection, vascular insufficiency, primary fracture with separation, and hereditary factors have all been espoused.[45–49] However, the evidence always seems to lead back to some form of disordered endochondral ossification in association with trauma or vascular impairment. Certain common features prevail. Over 90 percent of the lesions occur in males, fewer than 5 percent are bilateral, and the dominant arm is virtually always involved in unilateral cases. In children below the age of 8 years, the lesions are similar to those described by Panner, with changes in density and fragmentation of the capitellum, whereas in older children and adolescents loose bodies are more frequent.

Osteochondritis is rarely seen before the age of 5 years, when the chondroepiphysis of the capitellum has an abundant nutrient vascular supply.[48] The lesion usually becomes manifest clinically when the capitellar nucleus is supplied only by one or two discrete vessels with no obvious anastomosis.[44] The path of these vessels from the posterior surface of the chondroepiphysis is through unossified epiphyseal cartilage to the capitellum, and they are therefore situated, at least part of the way, in compressible cartilage.

There exists a vulnerable period as far as the circulation is concerned until fusion of the ossific nucleus in the late teens. Repeated minor trauma may damage the tenuous vasculature and may account for the prevalence of this condition in young baseball pitchers, gymnasts, and javelin throwers. Whatever the underlying etiology, the ultimate outcome may be healing, nonhealing, or loose body formation.

The major presenting symptoms are usually pain, swelling, limitation of range of motion in a noncapsular pattern, and sometimes clicking and locking. Interestingly, the patient may display a soft end-feel when extension is blocked by the displaced fragment, and a hard end-feel when flexion is limited.[34] The diagnosis can usually be made from plain radiographs.

Treatment

Nonoperative treatment requires rest from stress and very rarely a short period of immobilization with a splint. Treatment is the same as outlined for throwing injuries. The indications for surgery include a locked elbow, loose fragments, or failure of conservative therapy to relieve symptoms. Surgical treatment may include removal of loose fragments, excision of the capitellar lesions, and curettage to bleeding bone.[50] Usually, joint motion is restored or improved with manual therapy, a graduated strengthening and stretching program, and adequate therapy. A return to organized competitive sport is possible, provided there have not been excessive joint changes.[50]

Ligament Ruptures and Dislocations

Acute Ligament Tears

Acute ligament tears without dislocation are relatively rare but occasionally result from valgus or varus stresses in sport or recreation. The medial collateral ligament appears to be more vulnerable, and this injury is surprisingly easy to overlook in the acute stage unless there is an index of suspicion and careful valgus and varus stressing is carried out with the elbow flexed at 15 degrees[51] (Fig. 9-10). Often, acute medial collateral ruptures are associated with some ulnar nerve paresthesias. Disability and restriction of range of motion can be prevented and minimizing of adhesion achieved by early protected range-of-motion exercises in minor cases; surgical repair may be considered in more significant tears.

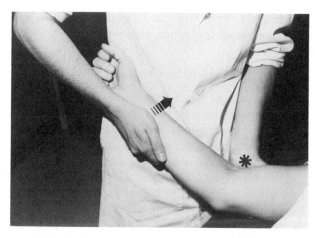

Fig. 9-10. Elbow abduction or valgus stress performed at 15 to 20 degrees of flexion to test the integrity of the ulnar collateral ligament.

For some individuals, a functional brace eliminating valgus or varus stress allows resumption of quite strenuous activities moderately early.

Lee[24] has described Fryette's abduction ulnohumeral lesion secondary to a fall on an outstretched hand, in which the ulna is forced into extension and abduction, increasing the carrying angle. Subsequently the radius glides distally at the radio-ulnar joints, increasing tension on the radio-ulnar ligaments and the interosseous membrane. The radius carries the hand distally with it, increasing tension on the ulnar collateral ligament at the wrist. The wrist is held in an ulnarly deviated position (Fig. 9-11). The radial wrist extensors attempt to pull the hand into functional alignment, and the overuse of these muscles results in tennis elbow-like symptoms. Although these symptoms may be a direct result of the trauma to the elbow, in the above circumstances they represent a dysfunction from a concomitantly sustained lesion to the wrist. The wrist lesion may be related to the well-described carpal shift and carpal collapse subsequent to ligament damage from a fall on the outstretched hand. This lesion must also be distinguished from the well-recognized congenital ulnar negative variance, which may lead to wrist and sometimes elbow pain. The appropriate examination for this condition is observation of the elbow-wrist relationship in pronation. The third digit and metacarpal are held at an

angle of 5 to 15 degrees to the axis of rotation of the forearm. Tests for accessory movements at the wrist and elbow will confirm the findings. Radial deviation is restricted at the radiocarpal joint, as is adduction at the ulnohumeral joint.

The articular dysfunction should be treated first with manual therapy restoring ulnohumeral adduction; the ulnar collateral ligaments and radial wrist extensors should be addressed as well.

Dislocations

Radius and Ulna

A fall on the outstretched hand may result in elbow dislocation, frequently associated with fracture of the olecranon or the coronoid process. After reduction, careful examination of the ulnar nerve is nec-

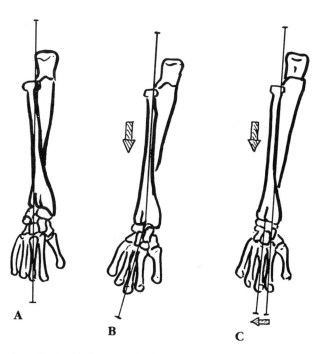

Fig. 9-11. Abduction ulnohumeral lesion. **(A)** The normal functional axis of rotation is disrupted; **(B)** initial adaptation to an abduction ulnar lesion, by distal movement of the radius, forces the carpus into 5 to 15 degrees of ulnar deviation; **(C)** secondary compensation incurs a carpal shift, producing chronic elbow and possible wrist symptoms. This is best demonstrated by examining the outstretched pronated hand.

essary, and then immobilization in a sling for about 3 weeks. At this time gentle range-of-motion exercises can be begun.

Radial Head

In the adult, dislocation of the radial head has a significant tendency to recur. Careful scrutiny of the lateral and anteroposterior films after reduction is mandatory. Immobilization for 3 to 6 weeks in flexion is usually necessary. Any evidence of imperfect reduction is an indication for operative intervention.

Radial Head in Children

The imperfectly formed radial head may allow subluxation or dislocation in association with damage and unfolding of the immature annular ligament (pulled elbow, nursemaid's elbow; Fig. 9-12). Distraction with rotation of the radius caused by swinging the child by the arms gives rise to one of the names for this condition. Reduction is usually easily accomplished by elbow flexion and rotation of the forearm, or may even occur spontaneously. The major features of successful treatment are demonstration of reduction by normal x-ray and restoration of range of motion and prompt resolution of pain. An inadequately reduced radial head will go on to

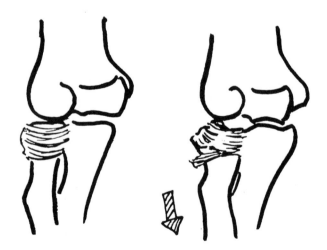

Fig. 9-12. The pulled elbow produced by distraction-rotation forces damages the annular ligament, allowing all or part of it to be carried into the joint.

significant overgrowth and deformity, culminating in serious disability of the elbow joint.

Myositis Ossificans

The proximity of attachment of the fleshy brachialis and triceps to the joint, and the complex nature of the three articulations in one capsule, give the elbow a propensity for stiffness and myositis ossificans after trauma. Usually a fracture or dislocation is involved, but occasionally direct contusion is the precipitating factor. The therapist must constantly be aware of the syndrome of increasing pain and decreasing range during rehabilitation of elbow trauma. The therapist may frequently be the first to recognize the evolution of this condition by detecting a subtle difference in the feel of the motion or an increasing firm mass in the muscle. At the first sign of this problem, soft tissue x-rays should be taken as a baseline and repeated at 2-week intervals if the elbow fails to improve. Heat should be discontinued, anti-inflammatory medication begun, and rest with the exception of gentle active range-of-motion exercises instituted. No resisted exercises should be performed. With stabilization of the condition, as evidenced by decreasing inflammation, bone mass, and pain, gentle therapy is reinstituted and plays an important role in safely pacing the return to full activity. More often, with fractures around the elbow, the myositic ectopic bone is present upon removal of the cast after 3 to 6 weeks of immobilization. With maturity of the ectopic bone, as evidenced by bone scan, surgical excision may be the best treatment to restore a significant loss of range of motion.

Nerve Entrapment, Neuritis, and Neuropathies

Ulnar Nerve

The ulnar nerve is well protected by the bulk of the medial head of the triceps above the elbow and is rarely involved in humeral shaft fractures. However, it is more susceptible to damage in connection with supracondylar and epicondylar fractures (Table 9-5). In passing from the anterior to the posterior compartment of the arm, the ulnar nerve may be

Table 9-5. Factors Contributing to Ulnar Nerve Decompression

Etiology	Pathophysiology
Neuritis	Tension through repetitive elbow flexion
	Subluxating nerve
Neural pressure	Perineural adhesions
	Congenital variations (e.g., bifid nerve)
	Exostosis and osteophytes
	Medial intermuscular septum
	Flexor carpi ulnaris, superficial and deep aponeurosis
Trauma	Fractures
	Dislocations
	Callus
	Progressive valgus deformity
	Prolonged bed rest
	Leaning on elbow (repetitive minor trauma)
	Saturday night palsy (traction or pressure)
Predisposing conditions	Peripheral neuritis
	Anatomy
	Rheumatoid arthritis
	Osteoarthritis

involved in fibrous compression or adhesion to the medial intermuscular septum. This septum slopes from a wide base at the medial epicondyle, where it is thick and unyielding, to a weak thin edge, at varying distances more proximally on the humeral shaft. If the nerve is rerouted by surgery to the anterior aspect of the elbow, it may be drawn across or compressed on the firm edge of the septum unless mobilized sufficiently proximally. This may explain some surgical failures with anterior transposition of the ulnar nerve.[52]

Behind the epicondyle the ulnar nerve is superficial and is particularly vulnerable to direct injury. Dislocations, contusions, traction injuries, fractures of the epicondyle, callus, osteophytes from the radiocapitellar articulation and olecranon, and subluxation of the nerve with flexion and extension may all contribute to neuritis or neuropathy.[53] Simple ganglia and benign tumors such as lipomas have also been implicated in neural compression.

The cubital tunnel as traditionally described by Feindel and Stratford is an osseoaponeuritic canal behind the medial epicondyle.[54] It is formed by the epicondyle, the olecranon, the medial collateral ligament, and an aponeuritic arch giving origin to, and

formed by, the two heads of the flexor carpi ulnaris. This tunnel may be considered to extend distally to varying degrees between the two heads of the flexor carpi ulnaris and may have a superficial and a deep component to the arch, both of which must be released to ensure adequate surgical decompression in resistant cases of tardy ulnar palsy.[1,53,55] This osseoaponeuritic canal has a varying lumen, being wide in extension and narrow during flexion of the elbow. Prolonged flexion, with the associated mild traction on the nerve, may cause sufficient pressure to result in transient paresis in the absence of external pressure, as can repeated rapid movements of the elbow as seen in pitching or serving in volleyball. Contraction of the flexor carpi ulnaris may narrow the tunnel by pulling on the aponeuritic portion and narrowing the interval between the two heads.[1,53]

In sport the commonest malady involving the nerve at the elbow is a frictional neuritis with mainly sensory symptoms of pain and numbness in the classic ulnar distribution of the little finger and the contiguous side of the ring finger. The nerve may be hypersensitive to tapping behind the elbow, exacerbating the distal symptoms. Untreated, the symptoms may progress, and there may be signs of wasting of the intrinsic muscles of the hand, often most noticeable as atrophy of the first dorsal interosseous muscle, reducing the bulk of the web space. Soon weakness of grip starts to accompany the increasing clumsiness in fine prehension, which was initially due to poor stereognosis. Sensation is decreased at the palmar and dorsal surfaces of the little finger and the ulnar half of the ring finger. Two-point discrimination can be measured and recorded and will deteriorate with increasing pathology. In the normal hand, compass points set 3 to 4 mm apart are clearly distinguished as separate stimuli (Fig. 9-13). Testing of the adductor pollicis reveals weakness, a positive Froment's sign. Weakness of the interossei results in inability to squeeze the little finger to the rest of the hand, a positive Wartenburg's sign (Fig. 9-13).

Treatment will depend on the frequency, duration, intensity, magnitude, and etiology of the symptoms. If the neuritis is secondary to repeated blows as in wrestling, or to pressure as with a student studying and writing, a well-constructed pad

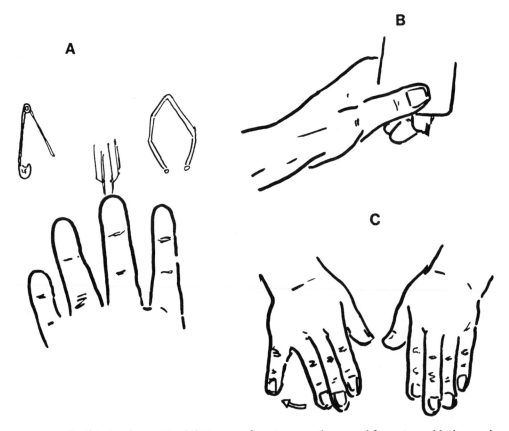

Fig. 9-13. Tests for frictional neuritis. **(A)** Sensory function may be tested for pain and light touch using a safety pin, and two-point discrimination (normal is 3 to 4 mm at the fingertip) with calipers or paper clip; **(B)** weakness of the adductor pollicis is detected by Froment's sign and is compensated for by flexing the thumbtip as the paper is pulled away; **(C)** a positive Wartenburg's sign with inability to obtain close adduction of all fingers.

may help. If the neuritis is frictional, it may be sufficient to block terminal extension for a period of time by initially taping the elbow. Persistent symptoms should not be allowed to continue or progress. Complete rest from the offending activity supplemented by anti-inflammatory medication will usually help the acute case. In more chronic situations the diagnosis and exact location are confirmed by x-ray, and nerve conduction studies and surgical treatment are considered.

Decompression and transposition of the ulnar nerve are the major alternatives, and exact knowledge of the anatomy is needed if success is to be achieved.[56] With tumors or stenosis of the cubital tunnel, decompression is usually adequate; however, sufficient distal release is mandatory to ensure division of both the superficial and the deep aponeurosis.[55] If there are large osteophytes, callus, a subluxating nerve, significant nerve changes and severe clinical signs, or a situation of repeated local trauma, transposition may be a better alternative to ensure minimal continued tension on the nerve. Adequate proximal release is necessary to avoid tension across the medial intermuscular septum.[55] If transposition is desirable but would entail devascularization of too great a section of nerve, medial epicondylectomy with nerve decompression may be the most suitable alternative.[54] This is a particularly useful technique in athletes with large arm girths and in whom over 20 cm of nerve would have to be mobilized for adequate transposition.[53,57] Removal of the condyle does not alter grip strength or elbow flexor power after adequate rehabilitation.[53,54]

Median Nerve

Median nerve entrapment about the elbow is a rare phenomenon, although cases have been reported following posterior dislocation. When it does occur it is usually in children, and recognition of the problem is usually delayed.[58] Progressive involvement of the nerve in developing callus following distal humeral fractures has also been recorded.[58] Rarely the nerve may become compressed above the elbow as it passes under the anomalous ligament of Struthers, which attaches to a spur in the lower third of the humerus. Because of its anterior location, the median nerve may be subjected to direct blows, particularly in some sports. However, the result is generally neuropraxia and infrequently axonotmesis, and patients usually recover without surgical intervention.

There may be decreased sensation to the lateral three digits and the palm, or decreased motor and sensory conduction. Awareness of the potentially more serious injury, with careful initial neurologic assessment and meticulous assessment of pinch and grip strength and two-point discrimination during the early rehabilitation phase, will allow diagnosis of a persistent defect or progressive median nerve function deterioration and point to the need for electromyographic evaluation and potential nerve exploration. In severe nerve injury, a functional splint may be required until recovery is achieved. Active range of motion must be maintained.

Anterior Interosseous Nerve

Entrapment or damage of the anterior interosseous branch of the median nerve is more frequent than injury to the main nerve. It may be involved in scar following trauma or fracture, usually as the nerve passes between the two heads of the pronator teres. Fractures and dislocation of the radius and ulna may also precipitate injury. Infrequently, ganglia or soft tissue tumors such as lipomas may compress the nerve. The deficit is purely motor, involving the flexor pollicis longus and the flexor digitorum profundus to the index and middle fingers and the pronator quadratus. The inability to carry out a tip-to-tip pinch is the diagnostic sign. Attempts at pinching a sheet of paper or a card between the thumb and index finger result in pulp-to-pulp apposition. The patient may also have some difficulty pronating with a flexed elbow. Recovery after release or spontaneously after trauma is to be anticipated. Rehabilitation is directed at strengthening the grip.[59]

Radial and Posterior Interosseous Nerves

The radial nerve is most vulnerable in the spiral groove of the humerus. Midshaft humeral fractures always jeopardize the nerve during both the initial trauma and subsequent callus production. Less frequently the nerve is damaged by direct blows to the lateral aspect of the distal arm just as it dives into the bulk of the brachioradialis and the extensor carpi radialis longus. The most common site of pathology in the forearm is at the point at which the main motor branches of the radial nerve continue as the posterior interosseous nerve (Fig. 9-14). Just before entering the plane between the deep and superficial heads of the supinator muscle, the nerve may be involved in the so-called arcade of Frohse.[60] This is probably a fairly rare syndrome. During extension and pronation, the ECRB and the fibrous edge of the superficial part of the supinator are seen to tighten around the nerve. The resulting entrapment has been referred to as the radial tunnel syndrome and is felt to be important in the differential diagnosis of a tennis elbow that is resistant to treatment (Fig. 9-14).

In a series reported by Roles, clinical findings were fairly uniform.[60] At the onset the patient usually complained of the classic signs and symptoms of lateral epicondylitis, namely, tenderness over the common extensor origin, pain on passive stretching of the extensor muscles, and pain on resisted extension of the wrist and fingers. After all the usual therapies, these patients are often left with pain radiating up and down the arm, weakness of grip, tenderness over the radial nerve, and pain on re-

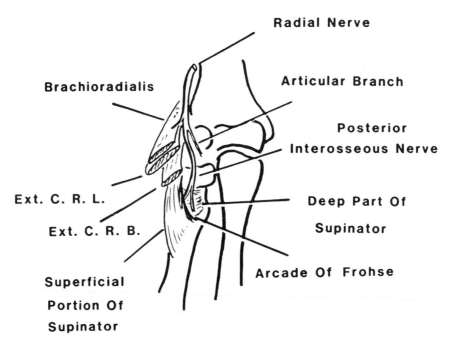

Fig. 9-14. Possible site of entrapment of the posterior interosseous nerve at the level of the arcade of Frohse. Ext.C.R.B., extensor carpi radialis brevis; Ext.C.R.L., extensor carpi radialis longus.

sisted extension of the middle finger, which tightens the fascial origin of the ECRB[60,61] (Fig. 9-14). It has also been suggested that resisted supination is generally much more painful than resisted wrist extension because of the contraction of the supinator muscle.[24] Nerve conduction studies should show significant delay in motor latencies measured from the spiral groove to the medial portion of the extensor digitorum communis. Recognition of the few but significant resistant cases of tennis elbow allows prompt, effective treatment by surgical release of the entrapment.

Olecranon Pathology

Olecranon Bursitis

The olecranon bursa, lying as it does superficial to the insertion of the triceps tendon, can be irritated either by a single episode of trauma such as a fall on the point of the elbow, or by repetitive grazing and weightbearing as is often seen in students or in wrestling. The acute bursitis may present as a swell-ing over the olecranon process, varying in size from a slight distention to a swelling that could be the size of a small chicken's egg. Depending on the acuteness of the inflammatory reaction, there is a variable amount of heat and redness associated with this swelling.

The important diagnostic differential here is between a simple post-traumatic bursitis and an infected olecranon bursa. The former may be treated with ice and elastic wrap and various forms of well-fitting protective pads and will usually, with time, disappear by itself. The infected bursa, however, must be brought to prompt medical attention so that appropriate antibiotic therapy can be started and drainage instituted if necessary. Failure to do this may lead to a spreading cellulitis and an infection involving a large part of the forearm or the upper arm. The proximity of the bursa to the elbow joint itself actually makes treatment all the more urgent. Repeated post-traumatic bursitis may lead to fibrin deposits in the bursa. These may eventually metaplase into a cartilage-like material and form tiny seeds within the bursa itself. These then form a source of aggravation even with minor friction, and a perpetual painful bursitis may be set up. In these instances, conservative treatment is no longer warranted, and surgical excision of the bursa should be considered.

Stress Fractures of the Olecranon

The valgus and varus overload during forceful throwing action has been dealt with in the section on "Injuries to the Throwing Arm." However, stress fractures of the olecranon, while uncommon, must be borne in mind as part of the differential diagnosis.[62] Individuals usually experience pain in the elbow of the throwing arm for some weeks or months before the lesion is obvious on radiography. The etiology is linked to the explosive forces applied to the olecranon during the final phases of delivery, and perhaps the impingement of the olecranon process against the base and medial wall of the olecranon fossa.[63] These injuries are disastrous for competitive athletes, since if ignored they may complete themselves during a throw, and if the fracture line is sufficiently distal, dislocation may occur. Complete cessation of throwing is usually necessary. If the lesion is treated very early, throwing may be resumed in 8 to 12 weeks. However, significant stress fractures or complete fractures may take up to 4 months to heal sufficiently for resumption of throwing if internal fixation is used. Splinting or casting is usually not required. Excision of a very proximal stress fracture of the tip of the olecranon, the most frequent site, allows resumption of throwing at 8 weeks. Fractures treated conservatively may take up to 18 months before throwing is resumed successfully if the lesion is well established.[58]

A similar lesion is a fracture separation of the olecranon epiphysis in children, and an even more rare situation is fracture separation of an incompletely fused olecranon physis in adults.[64] The proximal ulnar ossification center appears at age 8 years in girls and 10 years in boys and usually unites with the ulnar shaft at ages 14 and 16 years, respectively. The size of the olecranon ossification center varies from a small flake to up to 25 percent of the olecranon.[65] The secondary ossification center may also be bipartite. Usually the physis closes from deep to superficial, with rarely a deep posterior cleft persisting. It is this cleft that may form the start of a stress fracture or a weakened area, which may give secondary to a direct blow. The etiology is usually a direct blow from a fall, frequently in a football player. These are difficult injuries to treat, frequently requiring bone grafting as well as open reduction and internal fixation, since there is a propensity to fibrous union.[64]

Tendon Avulsions and Ruptures

Triceps

Injuries involving avulsion or rupture of the triceps tendon are among the least frequent of tendon injuries, and major ruptures of the belly of triceps are even more uncommon.[66,67] The mechanism is essentially the same for both sites, namely, a decelerating stress superimposed upon the contracting triceps muscle either through a fall on the outstretched hand or due to sudden contact during an extension maneuver such as a karate chop. Significant tears of the tendon must be recognized immediately, since a successful functional outcome depends on early surgical repair. Delayed repair is possible but technically more difficult and with less chance of an excellent result. Recognition is through loss of active extension, a palpable gap, pain, and a large hematoma going on to diffuse swelling and ecchymosis.[68] In the case of tendon avulsion, a small fleck of olecranon is often seen on the plain radiograph, and where there is doubt as to the diagnosis, computed tomography accurately visualizes the pathology. Muscle belly tears usually involve only the medial head, and usually nonoperative treatment produces a satisfactory outcome.[66]

It is well to recall that a normal tendon must sustain considerable force before it will rupture; hence avulsion of the insertion is an expected event when the trauma is sufficient. For this reason, rupture of the substance of the tendon should lead to a search for associated pathology. Conditions such as rheumatoid arthritis, systemic lupus erythematosus, hyperparathyroidism, xanthomatous degeneration, and hemangioepithelioma as well as systemic steroids and local steroid injections may all predispose the tendon to rupture.

Biceps

Biceps ruptures at the elbow are extremely rare, and while they are compatible with normal function in a relatively sedentary individual, surgical repair is probably best carried out early in young or very active patients. The diagnosis is made by an inability to palpate the tendon and by altered muscle delineation. Hemorrhage is often considerable and may obscure the diagnosis unless an adequate index of suspicion is maintained. This injury is sometimes associated with a radial head dislocation, and both injuries need therapy.

Brachialis

Most tears of the brachialis are partial, but isolated complete tears may infrequently occur. Dislocation of the elbow is the most common associated injury. The major significance of brachialis rupture is the propensity to myositis ossificans or delayed instability of an associated unrecognized elbow dislocation.

Extensor or Flexor Muscle Mass

Rapid violent contraction in association with a blow to the forearm may lead to rupture of the flexor or extensor muscle mass. Usually this injury is compatible with return to excellent function when treated nonoperatively. Treatment includes splinting and gentle range-of-motion, muscle strengthening, and functional exercises. Avulsion of the muscles from their tendons at the musculotendinous junction should be repaired operatively, and these injuries are usually associated with an excellent surgical outcome. Early mobilization and therapy are the keys to success.

Compartment Syndromes

Volkmann's Ischemic Contracture

Classic Volkmann's ischemic contracture is associated with supracondylar fractures in children, and this entity is discussed in Chapter 10. It is useful to recall, however, that it may also occur with severe bleeding from trauma to the forearm, with crushing injuries, or from a tight cast or bandage for any reason. Awareness of the impending disastrous situation and prompt attention to complaints of numb-ness, swelling, and discoloration of the fingers with increasing pain will avert a very unhappy outcome.

Other Compartment Syndromes

Traditionally, compartment syndromes of the forearm have been synonymous with the more dramatic Volkmann's ischemic contracture secondary to dislocation of the elbow or supracondylar fractures. However, in 1959 Bennett described a fascial compartment compression syndrome secondary to overuse.[66] Repetitive pitching, for example, can lead to a syndrome of medial elbow and forearm pain secondary to swelling and edema within the tight forearm fascial compartments. Recognition of the problem, with adequate rest, sufficient warm-up, and carefully spaced intervals between activity, is usually successful, but in recalcitrant cases fasciotomy may be required.[39]

Systemic Conditions

A selection of systemic conditions are mentioned to emphasize the need for constant awareness of the broad differential diagnosis of elbow pain; treatment for these conditions will not be outlined.

Mainly Monoarticular Conditions

Osteoarthrosis

Osteoarthrosis of the elbow may be the result of repeated minor trauma in such occupations as mining, working with compressed air hammers, and through recreation and sport with repetitive throwing. Mild osteoarthrosis may be relatively painless, although it may be accompanied by loss of extension and occasionally ulnar nerve symptoms.

Chrondromatosis

The elbow, along with the knee and shoulder, is the site of predilection for chondromatosis. The presentation may be pain, limitation of motion, or more usually catching and locking. Synovectomy may be necessary to restore function to the joint.

Pigmented Villinodular Synovitis

Although this uncommon disease of the synovium occurs primarily at the knee, the elbows and ankles are the next most frequent joints involved. Repeated hemarthrosis may be the presenting sign. Treatment may involve synovectomy with very persistent therapy postoperatively if joint range is to be maintained.

Diseases of the Blood and Arthropathies

With the exception of the knee, the elbow is probably the joint most frequently involved in hemophiliacs.[69] Repeated joint bleeds destroy the synovium and joint surface. Normal growth is disturbed with marginal overgrowth of the radial head; early loss of joint range, deformity, and sometimes ankylosis are all possible sequelae of the disease.[68] Similarly, although less commonly, the elbow may be involved in hemaglobinopathies such as sickle cell anemia and thalassemia. In contrast to most elbow pathology, contractures due to severe, advanced hemophilia may respond to prolonged stretching techniques using slings and pulleys or spring-loaded splints. For these specialized techniques, the reader is referred to the classic articles by Duthie et al. and Dixon.[69,70]

Mainly Polyarticular Conditions

Rheumatoid Arthritis

In only about 3 percent of cases does rheumatoid arthritis present for the first time with elbow symptoms. However, after 3 years of disease, almost 50 percent of patients have elbow involvement, and this proportion increases with time. These prevalence figures also probably hold for juvenile chronic arthritis. About 20 percent of rheumatoid patients have rheumatoid nodules, which classically develop on the extensor surface of the olecranon and the proximal ulna. Nodules in association with seropositive disease often indicate a bad clinical course.[68] Whereas the adult disease is characterized by severe painful synovitis and ultimately much joint destruction, bony ankylosis is more common in children with juvenile chronic arthritis.

Seronegative Arthropathies

The seronegative arthropathies include ankylosing spondylitis, Reiter's syndrome, and the reactive arthropathies. In this seronegative group are the arthropathy complicating Crohn's disease and ulcerative colitis, Behçet's syndrome, and Whipple's disease. Generally, the elbow is only involved in patients in whom the disease is widespread and chronic, and usually only one side is affected. The exception is the very destructive psoriatic arthropathy, in which the elbow is frequently involved.[68]

Gout

It is rare for gout to present initially with elbow involvement, but in severe gout almost one-third of patients have involvement of the joint and of the extensor surface of the forearm, and the olecranon is the most common site of gouty tophi.

Chondrocalcinosis

Chondrocalcinosis is an x-ray diagnosis based on visualization of calcification in the joint capsule or cartilage. Chondrocalcinosis of the elbow joint is frequently indicative of hyperparathyroidism but may occur in ochronosis, hemochromatosis, gout, and Wilson's disease. Elbow involvement is seen in approximately one-third of patients with calcium pyrophosphate deposition disease, or pseudogout, where the deposit is mainly in the capsule.

Tumors and Infections

Neoplasms around the elbow, whether primary or metastatic, are rare. Nevertheless, they are an important part of the differential diagnosis in situations where the pain and swelling do not resolve in response to normal treatment regimes or when the radiologic appearance is abnormal. Similarly, although infection is rare, local extension of infection from intravenous therapy may involve the elbow.

SUMMARY

A superficial discussion of the elbow joint necessarily understates the complexity of the anatomy. Arising out of the subtle biomechanics, the proximity of muscle belly attachments, and the multiple articulations is the propensity for loss of range and myositis ossificans. Loss of function at this joint seriously impairs the versatility of the hand and compromises the useful range of the whole upper limb segment, since, unlike in the shoulder, wrist, and fingers, very little in the way of compensatory adjustment is possible. For this reason, early diagnosis and very careful, well-planned, and meticulous therapy are essential to successful treatment. Failure to pick up subtleties of diagnosis or of the changing pathologic state and the institution of mistimed or inappropriate therapy have the potential to result in permanent significant disability. The exclusion of pathology in C5, C6, and C7 must always be kept in mind with elbow pain syndromes. This chapter has been aimed at explaining the more commonly seen conditions, with a guide to treatment approaches.

ACKNOWLEDGMENTS

The authors would like to thank Jim Meadows for his advice and assistance.

REFERENCES

1. Reid DC: Functional Anatomy and Joint Mobilization. 2nd Ed. University of Alberta Press, Edmonton, 1975
2. Basmajian JV: Muscles Alive: Their Function Revealed by Electromyography. 2nd Ed. Williams & Wilkins, Baltimore, 1967
3. Thompson HC, Garcia A: Myositis ossificans: aftermath of elbow injuries. Clin Orthop Rel Res 50:129, 1967
4. Morrey BF, Kai-Nan A: Articular and ligamentous contributions to the stability of the elbow joint. Am J Sports Med 11(5):315, 1983
5. VanMameren H, Drukker J: A functional anatomical basis of injuries to the ligamentum and other soft tissues around the elbow joint. Transmission of tensile and compressive loads. Int J Sports Med, suppl., 5:88, 1984
6. Kapandji, IA: The Physiology of the Joints. 5th Ed. Vol. 1. Churchill Livingstone, Edinburgh, 1982
7. MacConaill MA: A structurofunctional classification of articular units. Ir J Med Sci 142:19, 1973
8. Kaltenborn F: Mobilization of the Extremity Joints. 3rd Ed. Olaf Norlis Bokhandel, Oslo, 1980
9. MacConaill MA: Arthrology. In Warwick R, Williams PL (eds): Gray's Anatomy. 35th Ed. WB Saunders, Philadelphia, 1975
10. Schwab G, Bennett J, Woods G, Tullos H: Biomechanics of elbow instability; the role of the medial collateral ligament. Clin Orthop Rel Res 146:42, 1980
11. Gutieriez L: A contribution to the study of limiting factors of elbow extension. Acta Anat 56:145, 1964
12. Schuit D, McPoil TG, Knecht HG: Effect of tightened anterior band of the ulnar collateral ligament on arthrokinematics at the humeroulnar joint. J Orthop Sports Phys Ther 8(3):123, 1986
13. Maitland G: Peripheral Manipulation. 2nd Ed. Butterworth Publishers, Boston, 1977
14. Cummings GS: Comparison of muscle to other soft tissue in limiting elbow extension. J Orthop Sports Phys Ther 5(4):170, 1984
15. Jobe FW, Nuber G: Throwing injuries of the elbow. Clin Sports Med 5:621, 1986
16. Pauly JE, Rushing JL, Schering LE: An electromyographic study of some muscles crossing the elbow joint. Anat Rec 1:42, 1967
17. Rasch PI: Effect of position of the forearm on strength of elbow flexion. Res Q Am Assoc Health Phys Educ 27:333, 1956
18. Runge F: Zur Genese und Behandlung des Schreibekrampfes. Berl Lin Wochenschr 10:245, 1973
19. Morris H: The rider's sprain. Lancet 133:29, July, 1882
20. Innes CA: Letter to the editor. Lancet 210:5, August, 1882
21. Nirschl RP: Muscle and tendon trauma: tennis elbow. In Morrey BF (ed): The Elbow and Its Disorders. WB Saunders, Philadelphia, 1985
22. Van Swearingen JM: Measuring wrist muscle strength. J Orthop Sports Phys Ther 4:217, 1983
23. Briggs CA, Elliott BG: Lateral epicondylitis. A review of structures associated with tennis elbow. Anat Clin 7:149, 1985
24. Lee DG: Tennis elbow: a manual therapist's perspective. J Orthop Sports Phys Ther 8(3):134, 1986
25. Legwold G: Tennis elbow: joint resolution by conservative treatment and improved technique. Phys Sports Med 12(6):168, 1984
26. Liu YK: Mechanical analysis of racquet and ball during impact. Med Sci Sports Exerc 15(5):388, 1983
27. Elliot BC: Tennis: the influence of grip tightness on reaction impulse and rebound velocity. Med Sci Sports Exerc 14(5):348, 1982
28. Froimson AI: Treatment of tennis elbow with forearm support band. J Bone Joint Surg 53A(1):183, 1971
29. Burton AK: Grip strength and forearm straps in tennis elbow. Br J Sports Med 19(1):37, 1985
30. Burton AK, Edwards VA: Electromyography and tennis elbow straps. Br Osteopath J 14:83, 1982
31. Halle JS, Franklin RJ, Karalfa BL: Comparison of four treatment approaches for lateral epicondylitis of the elbow. J Orthop Sports Phys Ther 8(2):62, 1986
32. Percy EC, Carson JD: The use of DMSO in tennis elbow and rotator cuff tendinitis: a double blind study. Med Sci Sports Exerc 13:215, 1981
33. Burton K: Grip strength as an objective clinical assessment in tennis elbow. Br Osteopath J 16:6, 1984

34. Cyriax J: Textbook of Orthopaedic Medicine. 5th Ed. Vol. 1. Diagnosis of Soft Tissue Lesions. Williams & Wilkins, Baltimore, 1970

35. Kushner S, Reid DC: Manipulation in the treatment of tennis elbow. J Orthop Sports Phys Ther 7(5):264, 1986

36. Curwin S, Stanish WD: Tendinitis: Its Etiology and Treatment. Collamore Press, Lexington, Massachusetts, 1984

37. Ingham B: Transverse friction massage for relief of tennis elbow. Physician Sportsweek 9(10):116, 1981

38. Boyd HB, McLeod AC: Tennis elbow. J Bone Joint Surg 55A:1183, 1973

39. Cabrera JM, McCue FC: Non-osseous athletic injuries of the elbow, forearm and hand. Clin Sports Med 5(4):681, 1986

40. Woods GW, Tullos HS, King JW: The throwing arm: elbow injuries. J Sports Med 1(4):43, 1973

41. Slocum DB: Classification of the elbow injuries from baseball pitching. Tex Med 64:48, 1968

42. Wilson FD, Andrews JR, Blackburn TA, McCluskey G: Valgus extension overload in the pitching elbow. Am J Sports Med 11(2):83, 1983

43. Adams JE: Injuries to the throwing arm—a study of traumatic changes in the elbow joints of boy baseball pitchers. Calif Med 102:127, 1965

44. DeHaven KE, Evarts CM: Throwing injuries of the elbow in athletes. Orthop Clin N Am 4(3):801, 1973

45. Singer KM, Roy SP: Osteochondrosis of the humeral capitellum. Am J Sports Med 12(5):351, 1984

46. Roy S, Irvin R: Sports Medicine Prevention Evaluation, Management and Rehabilitation. Prentice-Hall, Englewood Cliffs, NJ, 1983

47. Panner HJ: A peculiar affection of the capitellum humeri resembling Calve-Perthes' disease of the hip. Acta Radiol 10:234, 1929

48. Haraldsson S: On osteochondrosis deformans juvenilis capituli including investigation of intraosseous vasculature in distal humerus. Acta Orthop Scand, suppl. 38, 1959

49. Lindholm TS, Osterman K, Vankka E: Osteochondritis dissecans of the elbow, ankle and hip: a comparative survey. Clin Orthop 148:245, 1980

50. McManama GB, Micheli LT, Berry MV, et al: The surgical treatment of osteochondritis of the capitellum. Am J Sports Med 13(1):11, 1985

51. Norwood LA, Shook JA, Andrews JR: Acute medial elbow ruptures. Am J Sports Med 9(1):16, 1981

52. Carpendale MT: The localization of ulnar nerve compression in the hand and arm—an improved method of electromyography. Arch Phys Med Rehab 47(6):325, 1966

53. Dangles CJ, Bibs JZ: Ulnar nerve neuritis in a world champion weightlifter. Am J Sports Med 8(6):443, 1980

54. Feindel W, Stratford J: The role of the cubital tunnel in tardy ulnar palsy. Can J Surg 1:287, 1958

55. Wojtys EM, Smith PA, Hankin FM: A cause of neuropathy in a baseball pitcher. Am J Sports Med 14(5):422, 1986

56. Broudy A, Leffert R, Smith R: Technical problems with ulnar nerve transposition at the elbow: findings and results of re-operation. J Hand Surg 3:85, 1978

57. Neblett C, Elini G: Medial epicondylectomy for ulnar nerve palsy. J Neurosurg 32:55, 1970

58. Rappaport NH, Clark GL, Bara WF: Median nerve entrapment about the elbow. Adv Orthop Surg 8:270, 1985

59. Van Der Wuff P, Hagmeyer RH, Rijnders W: Case study: isolated anterior interosseous nerve paralysis: the Kiloh-Nevin syndrome. J Orthop Sports Phys Ther 6:178, 1984

60. Roles NC, Maudsley RH: Radial tunnel syndrome. J Bone Joint Surg 54B(3):499, 1972

61. Spinner M: The arcade of Frohse and its relationship to posterior interosseous nerve paralysis. J Bone Joint Surg 50B(4):809, 1968

62. Hulkko A, Orava S, Nikula P: Stress fractures of the olecranon in javelin throwers. Int J Sports Med 7:210, 1968

63. London JT: Kinematics of the elbow. J Bone Joint Surg 63A(4):529, 1981

64. Kovac J, Baker BE, Mosher JF: Fracture separation of the olecranon ossification centre in adults. Am J Sports Med 13(2):105, 1985

65. Kohler A: Roentgenology: The Borderlands of the Normal and Early Pathology in the Skeleton. William Wood, New York, 1928

66. Kunichi A, Torisu T: Muscle belly tear of the triceps. Am J Sports Med 12(6):485, 1984

67. Sherman O, Snyder ST, Fox JM: Triceps tendon avulsion in a professional body builder. Am J Sports Med 12(4):328, 1984

68. Bach BR, Warren RF, Wickiewicz TL: Triceps rupture—a case report and literature review. Am J Sports Med 15(3):285, 1987

69. Duthie RB, Matthews JM, Rizza CR, Steele WM: The Management of Musculoskeletal Problems in Haemophiliacs. Blackwell Scientific Publications, Oxford, 1972

70. Dickson RA: Reversed dynamic slings—a new concept in the treatment of post-traumatic elbow flexion contractures. Injury 8:35, 1976

10

Dysfunction, Evaluation, and Treatment of the Wrist and Hand

CHRISTINE A. MORAN

Dysfunction in the wrist and hand is often related to trauma or disease. The cause is clear, as is the appropriate treatment. However, mechanical factors can also impose unusual stresses upon the hand and wrist, causing injury. Overuse syndrome is not a common diagnosis in the wrist and hand; therefore, these patients often report pain and dysfunction for long periods before an appropriate treatment is applied—one that addresses the dysfunction and not just the sprain or strain. In some states, overuse syndromes are not reported as such to the worker's compensation board, so the actual incidence of these injuries is not always known.

This chapter reviews the pathology and treatment of overuse syndromes in the hand and wrist. Proper evaluation can make distinctions that will allow the therapist to offer these patients specific treatment and, more importantly to assist them in preventive measures to alleviate the overuse that provoked the original problem.

CAUSES OF OVERUSE SYNDROMES

The scientific and lay press abounds with descriptions of cumulative trauma, repetitive motion disorders, or overuse syndromes. Most often these disorders occur in persons who regularly use industrial machines or computers in such a way as to expose the wrist and hand to constant singular stress. Overuse syndromes include peripheral nerve compressions (radial, ulnar, and median nerves), tenosynovitis, tendinitis, intersection syndrome, synovitis, bursitis, ganglion cysts, strains, sprains, certain forms of arthritis, and myofascial pain syndromes.[1-4]

Occupational stress can occur on the stage as well as in the factory setting. Many articles have cited the frequency of overuse syndromes in musicians. Competition for high levels of production weighs upon these workers, who then push themselves past the point of pain. Likewise, the sports arena provides a situation of constant overstress to the hand and wrist joints.

Although we are more familiar with the overuse stresses of athletics, occupational, industrial, and musical overuse dysfunctions are not new entities. As early as 1717, Ramazinni described mechanical overuse syndromes.[5] Likewise, Bunnell in 1944 acknowledged that trauma, overuse, and unaccustomed work are the chief causes of tenosynovitis.[6]

Musical overuse syndromes may be a popular topic in the scientific community now, but it has been noted that Schumann and Paganini also suffered from overuse dysfunction.[7]

EVALUATION

This chapter addresses the identification and treatment of overuse syndrome in the wrist and hand. Pertinent anatomic knowledge and careful evaluation are needed for successful treatment. Since the structures are small, care is needed in delivering treatment. Excessive treatment is not appropriate. The same goal exists for all overuse problems: to avoid recurrence. Therefore teaching the patient to avoid recurrence is as important as the treatment.

The clinician must take a detailed history, looking for causative factors or specific stressful movement patterns. Often a description of the overuse activity is not enough to indicate the causative factor. Actual simulation of the task may be necessary. As Armstrong reported,[8] the following factors should be identified: repeated exertion to specific soft tissues, increasing repetitiveness while the movement remains the same, unusual amount of force applied to the hand, abnormal posture of the hand and wrist, inclusion of vibration, any temperature variance, use of gloves.[8-12] Most important is the role repetitive use or stress has played in affecting the tissues, the pattern of use, and the resultant overuse of the wrist and hand.[9]

An example of the importance of detailed analysis is the case of a 54-year-old woman seen in treatment for a Colles' fracture, who reported persistent ulnar wrist pain. Local palpation about the ulnar head revealed some tenderness, but local treatment with transcutaneous nerve stimulation (TNS) did not relieve her pain. Observation of the patient's home exercises revealed that wrist extension was performed mainly by the extensor carpi ulnaris (ECU) muscle. A trigger point in the proximal muscle belly was identified and treated. The pain was resolved, and the patient was reinstructed in home exercises to avoid overuse of the muscle (Figs. 10-1 and 10-2).

OVERVIEW OF ANATOMY

It is helpful to review those structures most often implicated in overuse syndromes. Careful palpation and identification of these structures greatly facilitate specific treatment and allow the patient to identify the overuse site and take future preventive measures.

Forearm Musculature

The forearm musculature is divided into volar and dorsal compartments (Table 10-1). The volar muscle compartment is comprised of superficial, middle, and deep layers, whereas the dorsal compartment is comprised of a superficial and a deep layer.[13] Each muscle should be identified through palpation and manual muscle testing.[14,15] In evaluating patients with overuse dysfunction, it is imperative to discretely palpate the muscle belly or the tendon. For example, the therapist must be able to

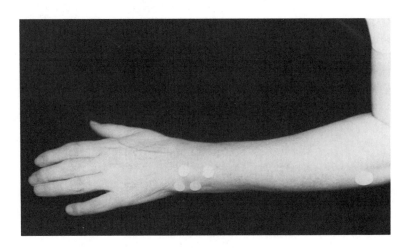

Fig. 10-1. Patient's mapping of referred pain from a trigger point in the extensor carpi ulnaris muscle.

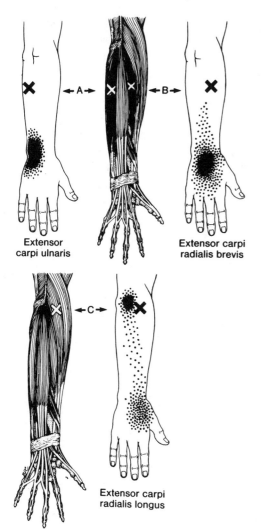

Fig. 10-2. Mapping of ECU muscle. (From Travell et al.,[38] with permission.)

Table 10-1. Muscles of the Forearm

Volar musculature
    Superficial
        Pronator teres
        Flexor carpi radialis
        Palmaris longus
        Flexor carpi ulnaris
    Middle
        Flexor digitorum sublimis
    Deep
        Flexor digitorum profundus
        Flexor pollicis longus
        Pronator quadratus
Dorsal musculature
    Superficial
        Brachioradialis
        Extensor carpi radialis longus
        Extensor carpi radialis brevis
        Extensor digitorum communis
        Extensor digiti minimi
        Extensor carpi ulnaris
        Anconeus
    Deep
        Supinator
        Abductor pollicis longus
        Extensor pollicis brevis
        Extensor pollicis longus
        Extensor indicis

the distinction should be made that overuse compressions are progressive. In the early stages of compression, the patient will have symptoms only during the activity, and so the initial evaluation might not reveal compression. In the later stages, however, nerve compression is constant, with symptoms often present.[17] The nerve compressions most often seen in overuse syndromes are carpal tunnel syndrome (median nerve), pronator teres syndrome (median nerve), cubital tunnel syn-

Table 10-2. Sites of Peripheral Nerve Compressions in Forearm and Hand Overuse Syndromes

Nerve	Site of Compression
Radial	Arcade of Froshe
	Supinator muscle
	Compartment entrapment: posterior interosseous nerve
Median	Pronator teres muscle
	Compartment entrapment: anterior interosseous nerve
	Carpal tunnel
	Digital nerve level
Ulnar	Flexor carpi ulnaris muscle
	Guyon's canal
	Digital nerve level

isolate the extensor carpi radialis brevis (ECRB) muscle from the extensor digiti communis (EDC) muscle. It is not sufficient simply to note that the pain arises in the extensor muscle mass.

Peripheral Nerves

All three peripheral nerves of the forearm are subject to compression.[16–18] As shown in Table 10-2, a variety of causes provoke the nerve compression, including overuse and repetitive stress. However, drome (ulnar nerve), and Guyon's tunnel compression (ulnar nerve). The case example that follows illustrates this point.

A 27-year-old shoe factory worker presented with transient numbness and pain along the right ulnar aspect of her hand. She noted that numbness and tingling were persistent but more apparent at work. Work simulation revealed that the right hand moved into ulnar deviation and maintained that position to steady the shoe while the machine applied a heel. The machine force would kick the shoe back into the patient's hand while she steadied the shoe. Electromyographic testing, sensory testing, and physical examination revealed ulnar nerve compression through the flexor carpi ulnaris (FCU) muscle and at Guyon's canal.

Wrist and Forearm Tendons

Crossing the wrist are seven dorsal tendon compartments and four volar tendon compartments or sections. (Table 10-3).[19] Tendinitis or tenosynovitis can occur at this level as a result of repetitive use.[20,21] Likewise, repetitive stress can cause insertional tendinitis, particularly of the ECRB tendon. Proximally, intersection syndrome frequently occurs when the thumb and wrist are constantly used during extension and deviation motions.[22] This syndrome occurs at the point where the extensor pollicis longus (EPL) tendon lies superficial to the ECRB and ECRL tendons. Patients that perform repetitive thumb and wrist movements develop this tendinitis.

Table 10-3. Tendon Compartments at the Wrist Level

Compartment	Tendon(s) in Compartment
Dorsal	
1	Abductor pollicis longus
	Extensor pollicis brevis
2	Extensor carpi radialis longus
	Extensor carpi radialis brevis
3	Extensor pollicis longus
4	Extensor digitorum communis
5	Extensor digiti quinti
6	Extensor carpi ulnaris
Volar	
1	Flexor carpi radialis
2	Flexor pollicis longus
3	Flexor digitorum sublimis
	Flexor digitorum profundus
4	Flexor carpi ulnaris

The incidence of de Quervain's syndrome, or tenosynovitis of the first dorsal compartment, has risen dramatically. Here the thumb is used repetitively alone or with deviation motions of the wrist.[20] The tendons involved are the extensor pollicis brevis (EPB) and the abductor pollicis longus (APL). An interesting study by Kauer[21] offers a probable explanation for this syndrome. In an electromyographic study, using needle electrodes in normal subjects, he noted that the EPB, APL, and ECU muscles isometrically contracted throughout pronated and supinated dorsiflexion and palmar flexion. This finding led Kauer to conclude that these tendons might serve as dynamic collateral ligaments, supplying further strength to the medial and lateral aspects of the wrist.

The ligamentous support of the carpus follows these guidelines of form and function. The volar carpal ligaments are thicker than their dorsal counterparts. They function to restrain volar carpal glide and resultant wrist extension by becoming taut during this motion. In radial and ulnar deviation, the volar ligaments on the opposite side tighten to restrain these deviating glides. The majority of the volar ligament fibers are oriented toward the capitate. In this fashion, they serve to support the center of rotation (capitate) of all four wrist motions in the proximal end of the capitate.

Biomechanically, it has been noted that individual carpals move during flexion and extension and during radial and ulnar deviation in addition to the proximal and distal rows gliding independently. This individual carpal rotation is necessary to avoid carpal impingement (i.e., of the scaphoid in radial deviation) and allow full osteokinematic movement (i.e., the scaphoid-lunate component motion in flexion-extension).

The ulnar aspect of the wrist presents a unique situation. The ulnar complex or triangular fibrocartilage complex (TFCC) serves several functions, as Palmer and Werner noted. Identified between the articular lip of the radius and the ulnar styloid, this complex serves as an articular surface of the lunate and triquetrum and as a weight-bearing surface (absorbing 40 percent of the distal load when intact verus 60 percent by the radius) and maintains the articulation of the distal radioulnar joint.[22] Palmer and Werner demonstrated that if this tissue complex is removed, the weight-bearing shifted to the radius (95 percent) from the ulna (5 percent) and that the distal radioulnar joint became unstable.

Hand Anatomy

Important anatomic considerations in the hand include the ligamentous configuration and the intrinsic muscles. One often forgets the impact of ligamentous strains and intrinsic tendinitis upon hand function. Very often overuse can occur in these structures, only to be identified as "arthritis."

Ligamentous support of the digital joints is often minimized. The collateral ligaments of the thumb carpometacarpal (CMC) joint, the digital metacarpophalangeal (MCP) joints, and the interphalangeal (IP) joints resist the deforming forces placed on the hand.[23-28] The collateral ligaments of the thumb CMC joint are obliquely arranged, thus becoming maximally taut in CMC joint rotation and thumb opposition.[23] At the level of the digital MCP joints, the radial collateral ligament is as much as 2 to 4 mm longer than the ulnar collateral ligament.[27] This permits ulnar deviation and supination of the phalanx on the metacarpal head during grip and prehension. The collateral ligaments of the IP joints, however, are of equal length and resist mediolateral forces during hand movements.[26] Repetitive use does affect these joints, in the form of both osteoarthritic joint changes and ligamentous strain and pain. The following example illustrates this concept.

A 19-year-old percussion major was referred for persistent hand pain. Upon evaluation, ulnar collateral ligaments the (UCL) of the right hand (proximal interphalangeal (PIP) joints II, III, and IV) were painful as well as the UCL of the left hand (PIP joints II and III). Prior to ligamentous palpation, grip strength, pinch strength, and active range of motion had been measured. Laxity of all PIP joints was noted in extension. Simulation of percussion playing revealed overstresses of the PIP joint ligaments caused by his handhold on the drumsticks.

The intrinsic hand muscles are divided into those used for prehension and those used for grasping, depending on the activity. Since the prehension patterns require a rotatory component, the intrinsic muscle-tendon units are often injured in this fashion.

A frequent cause of injury is car accidents. The patient injures or strains the intrinsic musculature by grabbing the steering wheel or the doorknob to resist the impact forces. As a result, the digits are forcibly rotated, straining the intrinsic muscles. These injuries are usually overlooked until other major injuries are treated, thus increasing the delay before treatment.

TREATMENT OF HAND OVERUSE SYNDROMES

Initially, treatment should focus on reducing irritation of the traumatized tissue by static splinting or taping. The decision to tape or splint is based on the length of time since injury and the patient's activity level. If the injury is recent or mild or the patient is moderately active, taping is preferred. Elastic tape, such as Coban ©*, allows for some movement and prevents rigid fixation. Since this tape is nonadhesive and self-adherent, the patient can retape with ease, and skin irritation is kept to a minimum (Figs. 10-3, 10-4).

However, if the injury is long-standing or severe, or the patient's activity level is high, static splinting is effective. Thumb CMC joint splints or web space splints provide needed rest for the joint's ligaments or the thenar musculature. The PIP joint can be effectively immobilized using a volar gutter splint.

Splints and tape are worn continuously at first. As the pain subsides, the splint is removed for brief periods of inactivity and light exercises. As muscular support and strength recover, the splint is removed for increasing periods of time. The weaning process for taping is slightly different. The layers of taping are gradually decreased until the patient is using a single wrap of tape for brief intervals.

During the initial phase, treatment focuses on pain relief. The use of interferential current, TNS or a TNS probe is particularly helpful (Fig. 10-5). In cases of prolonged stress, phonophoresis provides

---

* © 3m, Minneapolis, Minnesota.

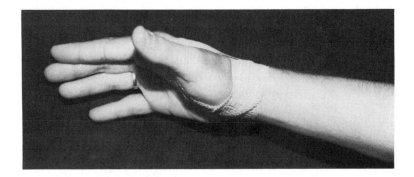

Fig. 10-3. Taping with elastic wrap (Coban) for flexible support following thumb CMC joint sprain.

additional relief and local medication. As soon as the patient is free of pain, resistive strengthening commences. Light putty exercises, wrist curls, weight well strengthening, and work simulation all assist in recovering function.

Of particular importance is work hardening or work simulation. Here the patient has the opportunity to perform each job task in a controlled and graded fashion for strengthening and improved endurance. The therapist can observe how the patient performs each job task with no resistance, with minimal resistance, and under timed conditions. These

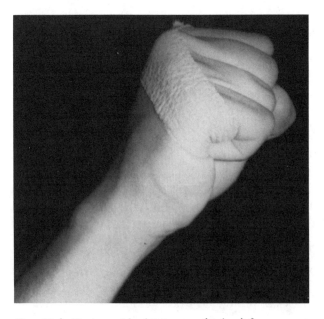

Fig. 10-4. Taping with elastic wrap (Coban) for support following intermetacarpal ligament sprain and/or intrinsic tendinitis.

treatment factors depend upon the job requirements.

While the patient is strengthening, both patient and therapist can spot potentially stressful movements. This can result in strengthening other muscles or changing the patient's upper extremity posture.

WRIST LIGAMENTOUS INJURIES

Repetitive stress of the wrist ligaments is a frequent cause of wrist pain and weakness. Unless there is a tear or ligamentous avulsion that would show on arthrography, arthroscopy, or radiography, these injuries are missed. Usually one can suspect this type of overuse dysfunction in the factory worker or athlete who repetitively performs the same motion under high-impact forces.

These ligamentous overuse injuries can be classified as scaphoid impaction syndrome, triquetrohamate impingement, (midcarpal ulnar instability), scapholunate ligament tear, lunotriquetral tear, distal radioulnar joint dysfunction, and pisotriquetral chondromalacia.[29-35] This is not a complete list, but is rather representative of the literature.

The mechanism of injury is most often repetitive loading of the carpus over a period of time. Machine operators, assembly line workers, and shipment loaders frequently fall into this classification; those athletes who participate in gymnastics, riflery, baseball, weightlifting, football, cycling, and tennis most often are found in this group.

The optimal treatment of these individuals depends on identification of the stress injury. Local palpation, joint play maneuvers, TNS probe, arthros-

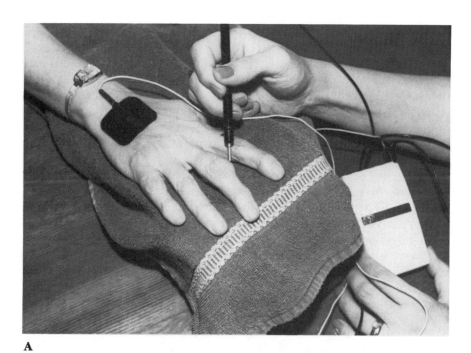

A

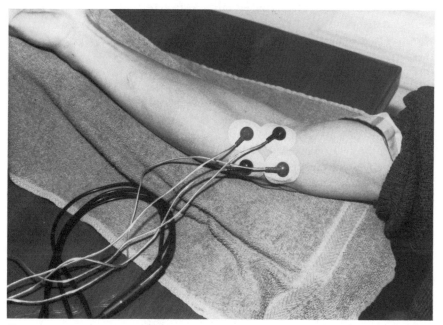

B

Fig. 10-5. Treatment of pain relief in hand overuse syndrome. **(A)** TNS probe treatment for sprain of the long digit radial collateral ligament. **(B)** Interferential current treatment for overuse syndrome and medical epicondylitis.

copy, and arthrography provide the necessary information.[35] Following diagnosis, the options in physical therapy treatment are phonophoresis, interferential current, TNS probe, ice, and static splinting or taping. In addition to a pain-relieving modality, a static splint may be necessary to support the wrist. The splint reduces continued stressing of the ligament.

After the patient is free of pain and the joint is stable, strengthening can begin. At this point in rehabilitation, work simulation and work hardening are extremely beneficial.[36] The therapist can observe the patient and make suggestions for altering damaging forces, possible joint taping, changing positions, or performing special strengthening exercises for additional support to the stressed joint.

An 18-year-old collegiate gymnast was referred for evaluation and splint fabrication following radiographic diagnosis of right midcarpal ulnar stability. Upon stress testing, the midcarpal joint was shown to subluxate. The patient observed that during his gymnastic career the right wrist had become painful and "clicked" more often. His main gymnastic event was the rings.

Upon examination, midcarpal stability testing revealed discomfort and subluxation. Motion measurements revealed decreased active range, since the patient subluxated in positions of extension and ulnar deviation with diminshed grip strength.

The patient decided not to have a partial fusion for pain relief or increased stability since the wrist only bothered him during sports activities. He also decided not to pursue Olympic or collegiate gymnastic competition. However, he did wish to continue racquetball and weightlifting. A single hinge dynamic wrist splint was fabricated. The splint allowed the patient motion in the flexion-extension plane only.

MYOFASCIAL PAIN SYNDROME AND OVERUSE

Equally evasive of diagnosis as an overuse syndrome is the myofascial pain syndrome (MFP). Again, MFP is not often considered in treating wrist and hand injuries. By definition, MFP is a syndrome of specific pain patterns and autonomic symptoms that are caused by a local irritation of muscle, fascia, tendon, or ligament.[37-40] These symptoms are pain patterns that are easily reproducible, are specific to the tissue, and usually refer distally. The one exception in the hand is the adductor pollicis.[37] The difference in treatment of these patients is that the clinician must be able to identify the locus of the patient's pain, not the location of the pain perception.[41]

Evaluation of these patients is guided by body mapping of their pain, first by the patient and then by the therapist during the actual examination (Fig. 10-6). Once the trigger points or actual loci of irritation are identified, treatment of the trigger points begins. Often the patient's diagnosis is misleading, since myofascial pain syndrome is still gaining acceptance. It is not uncommon to receive diagnoses of hand pain, hand arthritis, or even carpal tunnel syndrome when in actuality only the patient's pain pattern is being recognized and not the pain locus.[42]

Many authors have detailed the etiologies of myo-

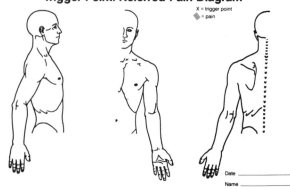

Fig. 10-6. Body mapping form for patient and therapist use during evaluation of myofascial pain complaints.

fascial pain and have mentioned these specific trigger point mappings.[37,39,40] The important factors in the patient's evaluation are whether the therapist can reproduce the symptoms and whether the patient actually hurts where the pain is perceived.

Treatment ranges from direct trigger point injection with lidocaine or a corticosteroid to stretch and spray/fluoromethane spray to a composite of several physical therapy techniques.[37,38,43-47] The success of treatment is based on comparison of initial symptoms and body mapping to subsequent body mappings.[41]

A professional violist reported persistent hand pain after receiving cortisone injections into the left third palmar interosseous muscle for pain due to a rotational injury. The patient noted that he continued to have flareups and was having difficulty playing. He had been told to soak his hand and refrain from playing.

Grip strength was decreased, as was active motion of the fourth and fifth digits. The span of the transverse intermetacarpal ligament was also decreased. Body charting revealed pain in the palm and referred pain into the third web space and the medial aspect of the fourth digit. While playing his instrument, the patient displayed an abducted and hyperextended posture of the fifth digit. He noted that he had assumed the posture 10 months earlier after the first injection.

Myofascial pain treatment consisted of ultrasound to the interosseous muscle trigger point, friction massage, ischemic pressure technique,[37] intermetacarpal ligament stressing, and local icing. When not in therapy, the patient wore a Coban wrap at the distal transverse arch level for support. As the pain subsided, he began a graded program of stretching, strengthening, and practicing. He removed the wrap in increasing frequency as strength increased. He was discharged to resume full-time playing and teaching. When contacted 2 years later, he had had only one recurrence.

MUSICIAN OVERUSE SYNDROMES

Before the 1980s, little information was published regarding overuse syndromes in musicians. Most musicians felt that, as part of their profession, they must bear the pain or leave the profession.[48] However, musicians can be classified as "upper extremity athletes" and need our attention so that they can continue to perform. Unfortunately, they do not have the luxury of rest after injury, for they might lose their position in the orchestra or simply may not have the funds necessary for protracted medical care.

The same tissues are overstressed in musicians as in athletes, but in a different fashion and the syndromes are called by different names.[49-55] These include clarinetist's thumb, lutist's wrist, viola paresthesia, and flutist's neuropathy. During evaluation, the patient is requested to play the instrument. As the patient plays, the therapist can observe how the patient holds and fingers the instrument, positions the upper extremity, and positions the rest of the body. This information is compared to the chief complaint, and objective measurements are recorded.

Again, emphasis on the actual playing component of the evaluation is key to successful treatment. The therapist can monitor the impact of treatment and offer positioning suggestions as the patient continues practive. This also allows the patient to remain active. When the patient is free of pain, having responded to either interferential current, TNS, or phonophoresis, strengthening begins. The injured muscle and its antagonist muscle are strenthened using eccentric and concentric exercises. Positional and postured changes are gradually introduced so as not to insult the professional musician's playing style. During treatment, the patient needs to continue playing for brief controlled periods daily. Finally, the patient must be discharged with positive suggestions on posture changes (if applicable) and self-stretching.

SUMMARY

Overuse syndromes or dysfunctions in the hand and wrist are broadly divided into three areas: industrial/occupational, athletic, and musical. In all three areas, knowledge of how the stress was created is imperative to successful treatment. Frequently these patients need discharge stretching instructions according to the tissue involved and the stress encountered to minimize recurrence.

REFERENCES

1. Louis DS: Cumulative trauma disorders. J Hand Surg 12A:823, 1987

2. Armstrong TJ, Foulke JH, Joseph BS, Galdstein SA: Investigation of cumulative trauma disorders in a poultry processing plant. Ind Hyg Assoc J 43:103, 1982

3. Silverstein BS, Fine L, Stetson D: Hand-wrist disorders among investment casting plant workers. J Hand Surg 12A:838, 1987

4. Lutz G, Hemsford T: Cumulative trauma disorder controls: the ergonomics program at Ethicon, Inc. J Hand Surg 12A:863, 1987

5. Ramazinni B: The Diseases of Workers (Wright W, transl.). University of Chicago Press, Chicago, 1940 (originally published 1717)

6. Bunnell S: Surgery of the Hand. 5th Ed. JB Lippincott, Philadelphia, 1944

7. Henson RA, Urich H: Schumann's hand injury. Br Med J 1:900, 1978

8. Armstrong TJ: Ergonomics and cumulative trauma disordrs. Hand Clin 2:553, 1986

9. Halder NM, Gillings DB, Imbus HR: Hand structure and function in an industrial setting. Arthritis Rheum 21:210, 1978

10. Tichauer ER: Some aspects of stress on forearm and hand in industry. J Occup Med 8:63, 1966

11. Mackworth N: Finger numbness in very cold winds. J Appl Physiol 5:533, 1953

12. Meagher SW: Tool design for prevention of hand and wrist injuries. J Hand Surg 12A:855, 1987

13. Gardner ED, Gray DJ, O'Railly R: Anatomy: Regional Study of Human Structure. 4th Ed. WB Saunders, Philadelphia, 1975

14. Hoppenfeld S: Physical Examination of the Spine and Extremities. Appleton-Century-Crofts, New York, 1976

15. Kendall HO, Kendall FP, Wadsworth GE:Muscles — Testing and Function. 2nd Ed. Williams & Wilkins, Baltimore, 1971

16. Wood MD, Linscheid RL: Abductor pollicis longus bursitis. Clin Orthop 83:293, 1973

17. Spinner M, Spencer P: Nerve compression lesions of the upper extremity. Clin Orthop 104:46, 1974

18. Tanzer RC: The carpal tunnel syndrome. J Bone Joint Surg 41A:626, 1959

19. Lampe E: Surgical Anatomy of the Hand. Clin Symp 21:1, 1969

20. Thompson AR, Plewes LW, Shaw EG: Peritendinitis crepitus and simple tenosynovitis: a clinical study of 544 cases in industry. Br J Ind Med 8:150, 1951

21. Kauer J: Functional anatomy of the wrist. Clin Orthop 149:9, 1980

22. Palmer A, Werner F: The triangular fibrocartilage complex of the wrist — anatomy and function. J Hand Surg 6:153, 1981

23. Phalen GS: Spontaneous compression of the median nerve at the wrist. JAMA 145:1128, 1951

24. Bojsen-Moller, F: Osteoligamentous guidance of movements of the human hand. Am J Anat 147:71, 1976

25. Pagalidis T, Kuczynski K, Lamb D: Ligamentous stability at the base of the thumb. Hand 13:29, 1981

26. Pieron A: The mechanism of the first carpo-metacarpal joint. Acta Orthop Scand (Suppl.)148, 1973

27. Kuczynski K: The proximal interphalangeal joint. J Bone Joint Surg 50B: 656, 1968

28. Hakistan R, Tubiana R: Ulnar deviation of the fingers. J Bone Joint Surg 49A:299, 1967

29. Bowers WH: Sprains and joint injuries in the hand. Hand Clin 2:93, 1986

30. Linscheid RL, Dobyns JH: Athletic injuries of the wrist. Clin Orthop 198:141, 1985

31. Linscheid RL, Dobyns JH: Wrist sprains. p. 970. In Tubiana R (ed): Surgery of the Hand. Vol. 2. WB Saunders, Philadelphia, 1985

32. Taleisnik J: Post traumatic carpal instability. Clin Orthop 149:73, 1980

33. Dobyns JH, Sim FH, Linscheid RL: Sports stress syndromes of the hand and wrist. Am J Sport Med 6:236, 1978

34. Reagan DS, Dobyns JH: Lunotriquetral sprains. J Hand Surg 9A:502, 1984

35. Snook GA, Chrisman OD, Wilson TC, Wietsma RD: Subluxation of the distal radioulnar joint by hyperpronation. J Bone Joint Surg 51A:1315, 1969

36. Levinsohn EM, Palmer AK: Arthrography of the traumatized wrist. Radiology 146:647, 1983

37. Baxter PL: Physical capacity evaluation and work therapy for industrial hand injuries. Clin Phys Ther 9:137, 1986

38. Travell J, Simons DG: Myofascial Pain and Dysfunction. The Trigger Point Manual. Williams & Wilkins, Baltimore, 1983

39. Travell J, Rinzler SH: The myofascial genesis of pain. Post-grad Med 11:425, 1952

40. Kellegran JH: Observation on referred pain arising from muscles. Clin Sci 3:175, 1938

41. Inman V, Saunders J: Referred pain from skeletal structures. J Nerve Ment. Dis 99:660, 1944

42. Moran CA, Saunders SR, Tribuzi ST: Myofascial pain syndrome in the wrist and hand. In Hunter JM, Schneider L, Mackin EJ, Callahan A (eds:) Rehabilita-

tion of the Hand. 3rd Ed. CV Mosby, St. Louis, 1988

43. Moran CA, Saunders SR: Referred pain in the wrist and hand, research in progress

44. Travell J: Ethyl chloride spray for painful muscle spasm. Arch Phys Med Rehabil 291, 1952

45. Melzack R: Prolonged relief of pain by brief, intense transcutaneous somatic stimulation. Pain 1:357, 1975

46. Lewit K: The needle effect in the relief of myofascial pain. Pain 6:83, 1979

47. Antich T: Phonophoresis: the principles of the ultrasonic driving force and efficacy in treatment of common orthopaedic diagnosis. J Orthop Sports Phys Ther 4:99, 1982

48. Chamberlin GJ: Cyriax's friction massage: a review. J Orthop Sports Phys Ther 4:16, 1982

49. Ziporyn T: Medical news-pianists cramp to stage fright: the medical side of music making. JAMA 252:985, 1984

50. Hiner SL, Brandt KD, Katz BP, French RN, Beczkie-wicz TJ: Performance-related medical problems among premier violinists. Med Prob Performing Artists 2:67, 1987

51. Caldron PH, Calabrese LH, Clough JD, et al: A survey of musculoskeletal problems encountered in high level musicians. Med Probl of Performing Artists 1:136, 1986

52. Fry HJH: Incidence of overuse injury syndrome in the symphony orchestra. Med Prob Performing Artists 1:51, 1986

53. Fry HJH: Overuse syndrome of the upper limb in musicians. Med J Aust 144:182, 1986

54. Lederman RJ, Calabrese LH: Overuse syndromes in instrumentalists. Med Probl Performing Artists 1:7, 1986

55. Newmark J, Hockberg FH: "Doctor, it hurts when I play." Painful disorders among innstrumental musicians. Med Probl Performing Artists 2:93, 1987

11

Reconstructive Surgery of the Wrist and Hand

JOSEPH S. WILKES

The hand is the main manipulative organ of the human body and performs many different types of functions, ranging from lifting very heavy objects to repairing objects with microscopic instruments. Reconstructive surgical considerations for acquired and congenital problems of the hand and wrist pose challenges of considerable magnitude for both the surgeon and the physical therapist. Attempts to correct these problems can be very satisfying to all involved; they can also prove frustrating if problems arise either in the surgical procedure or in the rehabilitation. To overcome these potential problems a separate specialty dedicated to hand and wrist problems has been formed among both surgeons and therapists. These professionals are trained to examine all aspects of the hand as well as to consider the life-style and occupation of the patient. Two patients with similar severe impairments but with different life-styles may require different surgical procedures to restore function and to allow them to use the hand in their chosen life-style or occupation. Hand injuries alone, however slight, render the patient completely unemployable in his normal occupation. Therefore, care of hand injuries, for patients and for workers' compensation boards, can be among the most costly areas of medical care in our modern technical world.[1]

EXAMINATION

A good history should accompany any physical examination, but especially one involving the hand. Specific areas to define are (1) the onset of the problem, whether acute or insidious; (2) the length of time the problem has been present; (3) the types of movements that exacerbate the problem as well as what seems to make the problem better; (4) associated manifestations relating either to the arm or to other parts of the body. The examination itself should include both active and passive motion of all joints along with palpation of the joints as indicated by swelling or history of pain.

Any deformity of the hand should be noted in detail. The tendons about the wrist as well as the fingers should be palpated through the skin and their excursion appreciated on active movement. The bony prominences that may be involved should be palpated, and the clinician should note whether they are in their normal position and whether there is any swelling or tenderness. The tendons and muscles should be tested separately for the wrist as well as for each finger, and each tendon or muscle for the fingers (Fig. 11-1). There can be some trick movements with intrinsic and extrinsic muscles, and therefore specific testing is necessary.[2] Specific testing for the radial, ulnar, and median nerves is necessary. These peripheral nerves innervate the hand; there is also occasional innervation of the dorsum of the wrist by the musculocutaneous nerve.

Once a thorough physical examination and history have been taken, further studies may be necessary. Radiographs certainly are valuable in evaluating the bony structures and joint spaces. Other tests for problems more difficult to diagnose may include bone scans, arthrograms, nerve conduction testing, tomograms, and electromyographic testing.

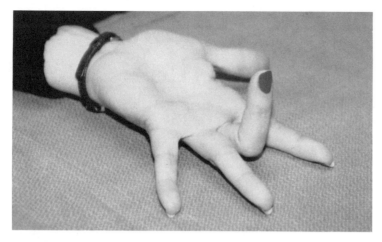

Fig. 11-1. Inability to flex the DIP joint indicates that the flexor digitorum profundus to the finger is not functioning.

TRAUMATIC INJURIES

Traumatic injuries account for the largest number of problems of the hand and wrist.[3] The injuries can range from simple sprains or contusions to major disruptions of hand function including amputation. Traumatic injuries can occur in any setting including work, home, or recreational activities. Traumatic injuries frequently seen by the hand surgeon include fractures, sprains, tendon injuries, and nerve injuries (Fig. 11-2).

Fractures

Fractures occur when the hand or wrist is struck by a force of such magnitude that the osseous structure is interrupted, causing a bone to separate into two or more fragments. Treatment of displaced fractures includes a general realignment of the part so that, when healing takes place, the part will function in an essentially normal manner. In the hand and fingers close anatomic approximation of the fracture surfaces is generally required to achieve this level of function.

External support, such as a cast, is usually necessary for stable fractures for several weeks to allow bony union to occur. If the fracture is not immobilized long enough to allow healing to occur, nonunion may result, or malunion if the fracture should displace during the healing process. The soft tissue structures should be tested at the time of initial examination to be sure that the neurovascular and muscular structures of the area are intact. If they are found to be involved, treatment of the fracture may be altered.

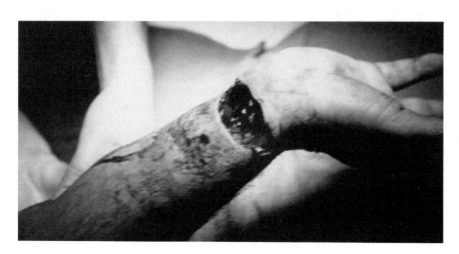

Fig. 11-2. Severe laceration to the wrist disrupts the tendons and major nerves and arteries to the hand.

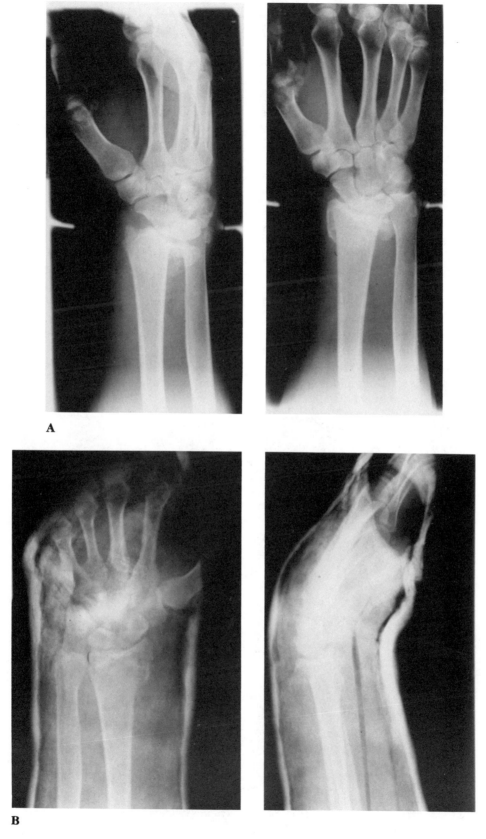

Fig. 11-3. Distal radius fracture. **(A)** Radiograph shows mild displacement; **(B)** after closed reduction and casting acceptable alignment is seen.

The distal radius fracture or Colles' fracture is one of the most common fractures of the wrist and hand. It can occur in any age group but appears to be more prevalent in older patients in whom osteoporosis is a factor. This injury generally occurs, as do a large proportion of hand injuries, when the patient falls on an outstretched hand. Depending on the magnitude of the force and the direction in which it is applied, the fracture pattern may vary, but most commonly the fracture occurs within 1 inch of the articular surface, causing a dorsal angulation of the distal fragment in the metaphyseal area of the distal radius, with or without a fracture of the ulnar styloid (Fig. 11-3A). In most cases this fracture can be treated by closed reduction with appropriate anesthesia to allow relaxation of the muscles. The type of cast varies from a short arm splint to a long arm cast, depending upon the fracture pattern and whether there is comminution. In older individuals the cast is retained for 3 to 4 weeks until early healing is accomplished. In younger patients a longer period,

closer to 6 to 8 weeks, is required for sufficient stability to start early motion. After the cast is removed, a removable splint is used to protect the fracture while early motion and strength of the healing bone are restored (Fig. 11-3B). If the fracture involves the articular surface or cannot be maintained by an external support such as a cast, then some type of fixation of the fracture will be necessary.

There are many methods of fixation of a Colles' fracture. They include simple closed reduction, a pin or a rod across the fracture surface, plates and screws, or a metallic external fixator. The metallic external fixator is held in place by pins placed in the bone proximal and distal to the fracture site, holding the fracture in a reduced position (Figs. 11-4, 11-5). Generally, if this fracture can be reduced to even a marginally acceptable position, good function will be regained after the fracture heals and appropriate therapy is concluded.

Another very common fracture of the wrist and hand is navicular fracture (Fig. 11-6A). The navicu-

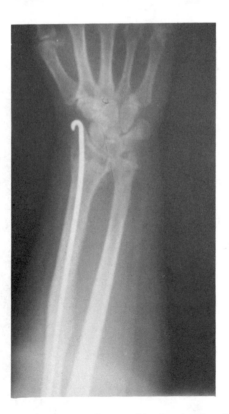 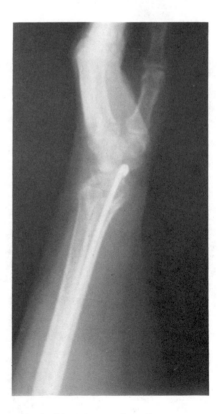

Fig. 11-4. Unstable distal radius fracture is held with a Rush rod.

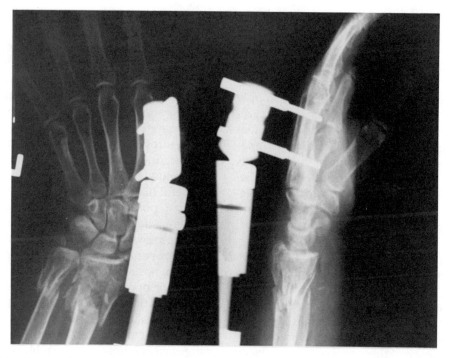

Fig. 11-5. Extremely comminuted distal radius fracture held in alignment with an external fixator.

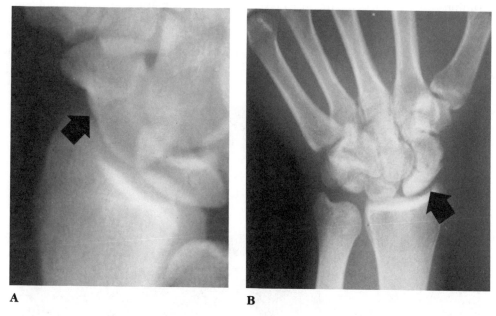

A

B

Fig. 11-6. Navicular fracture. **(A)** A hairline navicular fracture; **(B)** a navicular fracture that progressed to avascular necrosis and nonunion.

lar bone has an unusual blood supply, entering from the distal pole and proceeding retrograde into the proximal pole.[4] Fractures may occur at any level in the navicular, but the more proximal the fracture, the greater the chance of avascular necrosis of the proximal fragment because of loss of blood supply and nonunion of the fracture site (Fig. 11-6B). Frequently these fractures are hard to see on the initial radiograph because they have a hairline component. Also, because of the anatomy of the bone it is very difficult to get straight anteroposterior and lateral views of the bone. The result is that these fractures are frequently missed. In this situation, when a patient has wrist trauma and pain in the anatomical snuffbox on the radial aspect of the wrist, the thumb, wrist, and forearm should be at least splinted for 10 to 14 days, after which a re-examination is done to determine if a fracture has in fact occurred. This protects the patient and should decrease the incidence of nonunion and avascular necrosis. Early immobilization is essential in this type of fracture to reduce the incidence of these problems. Displaced fractures of the navicular may require open reduction and internal fixation either with crossed Kirschner wires or with a special screw made particularly for the navicular called the Herbert screw.[5] Also, delayed union or nonunion of the fracture may require a subsequent surgical procedure for bone grafting and/or fixation of the fracture to stimulate healing.[6]

The length of time necessary for a navicular fracture to heal is variable, from a minimum of 6 weeks to as long as 9 months. This fracture is treated with a thumb-spica cast, holding the thumb in the palmar abducted position; the wrist is generally kept in a neutral position or some other position that will maintain reduction of the fracture; and either a short or long arm cast is used, depending upon the surgeon's preference.

Fractures or dislocations of the other carpal bones may occur, and a high index of suspicion is generally needed to diagnose these problems (Fig. 11-7). A careful history and physical examination are necessary to point the clinician to the appropriate area for consideration. Frequently, multiple radiographic views and/or follow-up studies with tomograms or bone scans may be necessary for a definitive diagnosis. Treatment of these fractures is by closed or open reduction as necessary, including the dislocations, and then splinting for an appropriate period of time to allow healing. Fractures of the nonarticular portions of the metacarpals and phalanges most frequently are stable injuries, and close anatomic alignment with external support will generally suffice for these injuries.

Intra-articular fractures involving the wrist or hand require anatomic alignment of the articular surfaces. The articular surface is a smooth gliding surface on which movement occurs in the wrist and fingers. If there is a step-off or a significant gap in this smooth surface, deterioration of the joint can occur very quickly. If the fracture is displaced and

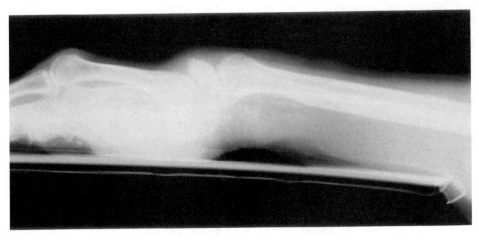

Fig. 11-7. Volar perilunate dislocation of the wrist and hand on the arm.

cannot be reduced, open reduction and internal fixation must be considered to provide close to normal function when the fracture heals (Fig. 11-8). Also, fractures that are in close association with the insertion of a tendon, whether in the wrist or the fingers, are frequently unstable because of the muscle pull, which cannot be completely neutralized. If the fractures cannot be brought into a stable, reduced position by closed technique, open reduction and internal fixation are frequently needed to immobilize the fracture against the pull of the muscle and tendon in order for alignment to be maintained.

Fractures associated with injuries to adjacent structures, such as tendon ruptures or nerve lacerations, may require more aggressive treatment such as open reduction and internal fixation to allow for appropriate repair and rehabilitation of the tendons and nerves.[7] This can allow for an earlier introduction of therapy for range of motion and gentle use of the hand for rehabilitation.

Tendon Injuries

Tendinitis is an inflammation of the tendon unit. It can be associated with either an overuse syndrome or a sprain of the muscle-tendon unit resulting from a traumatic episode. Tendinitis can generally be treated with a period of immobilization to allow the initial inflammation to settle down, followed by gentle stretching and toning exercises with local therapy such as ultrasound, ice, heat, and friction massage to allow the tendinitis to subside.

More serious tendon injuries include ruptures and lacerations. These injuries generally are treated by open repair, since approximation of the tendon ends is very difficult with closed methods of treatment, and therefore loss of function is likely. One condition in which rupture of a tendon can be frequently treated satisfactorily by closed methods is mallet finger.[8] In this injury the extensor tendon is avulsed at the level of the distal interphalangeal joint, causing lack of extension of the joint (Fig. 11-9). Splinting in a hyperextended position generally allows for healing of the tendon and excellent function subsequently.

Most other tendon injuries are approached surgically for open repair. A tendon that does not require significant excursion with motion, such as most extensor tendons, especially the wrist extensors or the abductor of the thumb, can be treated after open repair with casting for 4 to 6 weeks and then gentle mobilization. Adhesions in extensor tendon areas generally are not severe, and near-normal function is usually achieved. In the flexor tendons of the fingers and thumb the excursion is much greater, and therefore adhesions can significantly inhibit the regaining of normal function. The repair of these tendons is very delicate, and an atraumatic method of repair is used to secure the tendon and ensure a smooth surface at the level of the cut (Fig. 11-10A). Repair of flexor tendons in "no-man's-land," the area in the digits where the flexor superficialis and the flexor profundus glide against one another in

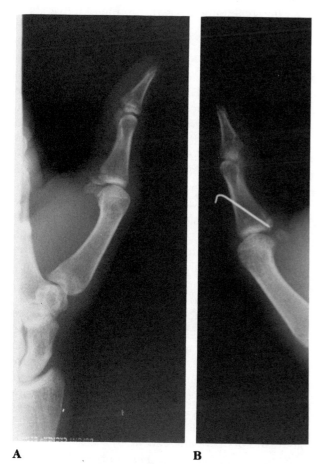

A   **B**

Fig. 11-8. Intra-articular fracture. **(A)** Displaced intra-articular fracture of the thumb metacarpophalangeal joint; **(B)** after open reduction and pin fixation.

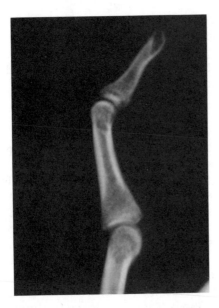

Fig. 11-9. Abnormal flexion of the DIP joint after disruption of the extensor tendon distal to the PIP joint, typical of a mallet deformity.

the fibro-osseous tunnel, is the hardest area in which to gain good function. Repair of both tendons at this level is generally recommended, as with all flexor tendon lacerations of the digits. Additionally, early motion with a dynamic splint as recommended by Kleinert and Lister allows for early function and decreased problems with adhesions[9] (Fig. 11-10B).

Repair of the pulley system of the fibro-osseous tunnel is very important in decreasing the incidence of serious adhesions to a lacerated flexor tendon.[10] If adhesions do limit the range of motion and function of the finger, a tenolysis should be performed no earlier than 6 months after the original repair. This allows for settling down of the original scar tissue so that scar is not reactivated and only the reaction to the new surgery becomes an inhibitor. With tenolysis the fibro-osseous tunnel should be repaired if possible to allow for good nourishment of the tendon, decrease of adhesions, and better mechanical function of the tendon. After tenolysis, active and active-assisted range of motion exercises are initiated unless there has been a violation of the tendon itself. Late repairs of tendon ruptures may require insertion of a Silastic rod to re-establish the

synovial space in the sheath and allow for reconstruction of the pulley system before introduction of a graft tendon. Once the pulley system has been established and full passive motion is achieved in all joints, a tendon graft can be inserted from the distal stump usually proximal to the carpal tunnel.[11] Passive range of motion is performed over approximately 6 weeks to achieve full range. Again, early motion with a dynamic splint is recommended with a prolonged rehabilitation time to allow for vascularization of the grafted tendon.

Nerve Injuries

Nerve injuries may occur anytime a nerve undergoes trauma. The injury may be a simple contusion, a stretch-type injury, or a disruption of nerve fibers secondary to a laceration. Nerve injuries are also frequently associated with fractures and particularly flexor tendon injuries, where the nerves run in close proximity to the flexor tendons not only at the wrist but in the fingers. Three types of nerve injuries can cause nerve dysfunction. Neurapraxia occurs when an injury such as a contusion causes electrical interruption of the conduction of the nerve but without disruption of the nerve itself and without degeneration of the axons. Recovery is generally expected within days to several weeks. The next, more serious type of injury, axonotmesis, occurs when the nerve is injured to such an extent that, although the nerve appears intact when inspected, degeneration occurs from the point of injury distally. Healing requires regrowth of the axons from the point of injury to the area of innervation. This can cause a prolonged period of nonfunction of the nerve but generally results in excellent return of function once the axons have regenerated. The most serious type of injury to the nerve is neurotmesis, in which the nerve is actually severed. Because there is disruption of the nerve bundles, even with surgical repair these bundles are very crudely realigned and return of function is variable, although with microsurgical techniques the return of function is generally fair to good and occasionally excellent.[12]

In the rehabilitation of these nerve injuries, it is very important to educate the patient as to the type of nerve injury suspected or known and the length of time that dysfunction of the nerve is expected to

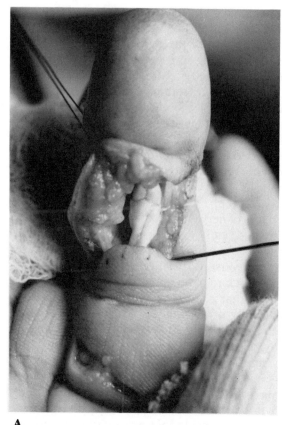

Fig. 11-10. Tendon repair. **(A)** Suture of the flexor digitorum profundus after laceration; **(B)** immediate dynamic splinting mobilization for early rehabilitation.

A

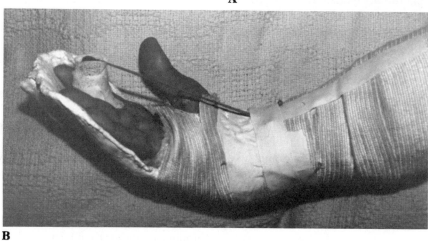

B

persist. This allows the patient to adjust his daily life-style around the dysfunction and to protect any areas of lost sensation from injury.[13]

If nerves to muscle groups are involved, splinting may be necessary to avoid contractures of joints and loss of function secondary to the temporary loss of muscle function. Nerve regeneration from axonotmesis or neurotmesis occurs at a rate of approximately 1 mm/day; thus the length of time before return of function can be estimated by the distance from the nerve injury to the most proximal innervation site. Depending on the nature of the injury, the healing response of the particular individual, the amount of scarring in the area of injury, and the surgical technique used for repair, this return of sensation can range from only protective sensation (against sharp objects, heat, and cold) to almost normal sensation. Muscle groups are generally the most difficult to restore to function because of the time needed for return of the axon to the muscle; during this time atrophy and fibrosis can occur in the muscle.

Carpal tunnel syndrome is a very common acquired loss of nerve function, which if encountered and treated early, whether conservatively with splinting and medication or surgically with release of the transverse carpal ligament, results in early functional return of the nerve, because the injury is only neurapraxic. Prolonged carpal tunnel disease with atrophy of the thenar muscles is associated with an axonotmesis, and occasionally scarring has already occurred in the area of compression. In these cases functional return is sometimes incomplete even after release and neurolysis. With severe chronic carpal tunnel syndrome some return of sensation is typically achieved, but motor return is poor. Both in carpal tunnel syndrome with atrophy of the thenar muscles and in neurotmesis injuries of motor nerves about the wrist, muscle transfers can be performed using muscles innervated by a different nerve to substitute for the muscles no longer functioning from the injured nerve. This naturally requires a period of rehabilitation for re-education of the muscle tendon unit as well as for mobilization of the joints that were immobilized to allow for healing of the transferred muscle-tendon unit. Loss of the nerve supply without full return can also cause hypersensitivity to cold weather. Therefore repair of major nerves about the wrist and the fingers is indicated to restore satisfactory function of the hand.

Wrist Sprains

Sprains of the wrist are very common and generally mild. A sprained wrist that presents with moderate to large amounts of swelling or pain inappropriate to the level of suspected injury should indicate to the clinician that a more serious injury may have occurred.[14] One such injury is hairline fracture of the navicular bone, which frequently cannot be picked up on initial radiographs.

Other injuries associated with a wrist sprain that could be of clinical importance include tears of the intercarpal ligaments or of the triangular fibrocartilage complex. These injuries can be seriously debilitating and can over time cause degeneration of the wrist joints, further limiting function of the wrist and requiring more extensive and radical surgical correction. A tear of the scapholunate ligament is probably the most common symptomatic ligament tear of the wrist area. A tear of this ligament severs the connection between the proximal row of carpal bones, which includes the proximal half of the navicular, the lunate, and the triquetrum, from the distal row (Fig. 11-11). The scaphoid is the interconnecting link that coordinates not only flexion and extension movements but also radial and ulnar deviation between the two rows of carpal bones. When the scapholunate ligament is ruptured, the scaphoid generally falls into a plantar flexed position, and the proximal row is then an unconnected middle segment between the distal forearm and the more stable distal carpal row and the hand. This allows for subluxation in either a dorsal or a volar direction, depending upon the forces transmitted, as well as any other ligamentous stretching that might have occurred at the time of the injury. Thus a painful, weak wrist results, which does not respond to conservative treatment. The wrist may get over the initial soreness, but when normal use is attempted soreness and weakness are noted.

With a high index of suspicion, the ligament tear can be diagnosed by the history and physical examination, noting tenderness and swelling dorsally over the junction of the scaphoid and the lunate; on x-ray examination a widened space between scaphoid and lunate is observed. On the anteroposterior x-ray the scaphoid may have the appearance of a signet ring rather than its normal oblong shape. The ligament sometimes can be repaired acutely, but it is a very short ligament, and frequently it is difficult to get adequate sutures to repair this ligament. In this situation or in the case of chronic scapholunate dissociation, a limited intercarpal fusion such as a triscaphi fusion can stabilize the carpus. This proce-

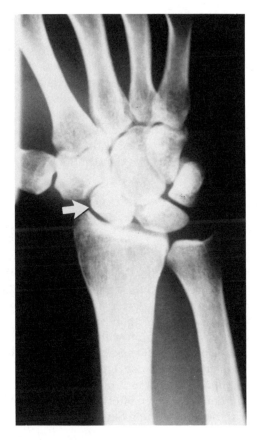

Fig. 11-11. The space between the scaphoid and lunate indicates scapholunate dissociation. Signet ring formation of the scaphoid indicates volar rotation of the scaphoid.

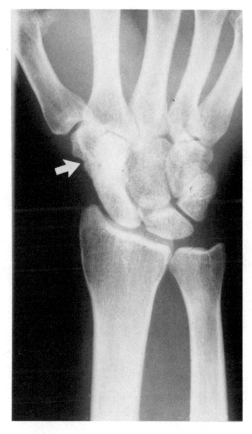

Fig. 11-12. Treatment of scapholunate dissociation by triscaphi fusion.

dure fuses the scaphoid to the trapezium and the trapezoid so that it maintains a reduced position in its normal dorsiflexed attitude rather than the plantar flexed attitude associated with the ligament tear (Fig. 11-12). Minimal loss of motion in the wrist is associated with this limited fusion, but pain is generally relieved, advancement of degeneration can be slowed down or stopped, and strength returns.

On occasion an intercarpal ligament tear or a tear of the triangular fibrocartilage cannot be diagnosed on clinical examination and plain radiography alone. In this situation the patient generally presents with a prolonged history, usually of several months after a traumatic episode, complaining of persistent pain, occasional swelling, and popping or clicking in the wrist. A wrist arthrogram may be able

to elucidate the torn ligament or triangular fibrocartilage (Fig. 11-13). Once the diagnosis of intercarpal ligament tear is made, a limited intercarpal fusion may solve the problem, and if a torn triangular fibrocartilage is found it should be repaired if possible. An arthroscopic partial débridement of the triangular fibrocartilage may be sufficient. With advanced degenerative changes from old trauma, either Silastic replacement with limited intercarpal fusion to unload the Silastic prosthesis or a wrist fusion may be necessary to restore satisfactory function of the hand.

After repair of an intercarpal ligament or an intercarpal fusion, immobilization is necessary for a sufficient length of time to allow the ligament to heal or the fusion to become solid. Immobilization frequently will need to include one or several fingers in addition to the wrist and forearm. The time in the

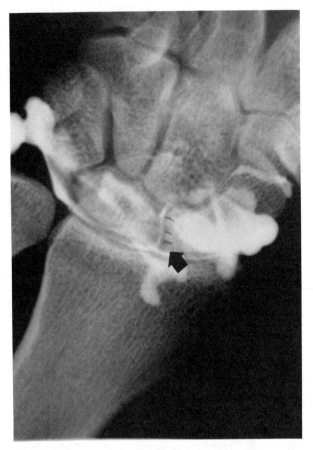

Fig. 11-13. An arthrogram of the wrist showing dye leakage through the scapholunate space into the distal carpal row, indicating a disruption of the scapholunate ligament.

case is usually no less than 6 weeks, and the wrist and hand can be very stiff once the cast is removed. Physical therapy is generally indicated to increase the range of motion both passively and actively as well as to strengthen the wrist. Methods for reduction of swelling along with heat and ultrasound can be useful to decrease the likelihood of tendinitis associated with the prolonged immobilization.

WRIST ARTHROSCOPY

Wrist arthroscopy has become available in recent years and is being perfected. Currently the indications for wrist arthroscopy are the following: identification of problems that may be associated with

unresolved wrist pain; removal of loose bodies; débridement of the triangular fibrocartilage, as mentioned above; synovectomy for a chronic synovitis or associated with rheumatoid arthritis; visualization of depressed intra-articular wrist fractures during limited open reduction and internal fixation. This approach can limit the amount of scarring associated with this procedure and allow for more normal return of function and a more adequate reduction of the fracture under visualization.

Technique

Wrist arthroscopy is a surgical procedure that is performed in the surgical suite. The patient undergoes either a regional or a general anesthetic, and the shoulder is abducted 90 degrees and the elbow flexed 90 degrees with the fingers suspended, usually from a finger-trap device, to distract the wrist. The wrist and hand are then prepared for surgery. Arthroscopic visualization with a 3-mm or smaller arthroscope provides the best overall view and is the least traumatic to the wrist (Fig. 11-14). The arthroscope is introduced between the third and fourth extensor compartments, after insufflating the wrist joint with normal saline by injection needle.

Working instruments can be brought in either between the first and second dorsal compartment groups or more laterally between the fourth and fifth or just lateral to the sixth compartment. Visualization of the articular surfaces is usually very good, and the intercarpal ligaments between the scapholunate and lunotriquetral articulations can be evaluated (Fig. 11-15). The triangular fibrocartilage and the fossa of the ulnar styloid are also visualized through the arthroscope. The midcarpal joint can also be entered between the lunate and the capitate, visualizing these surfaces for occult chondromalacia and loose bodies.

Assuming no open procedure is necessary in association with the arthroscopy, the patient is usually allowed to go home the same day with a light dressing on the wrist, and gentle range-of-motion exercises are started immediately. After the initial soreness settles down in 2 to 5 days, physical therapy can be started to increase mobility and regain strength about the wrist. When the procedure is performed under appropriate conditions, patients are gener-

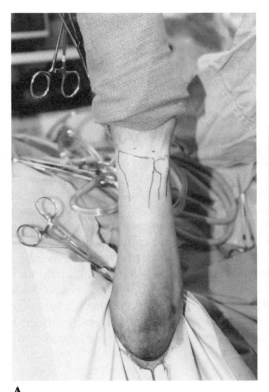

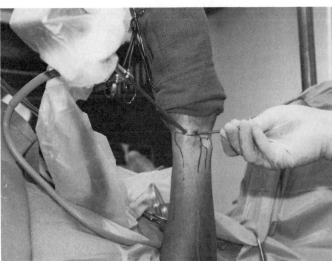

Fig. 11-14. Technique of wrist arthroscopy. **(A)** Primary portals for arthroscope and working instruments are between dorsal compartments 3 and 4 and 4 and 5; **(B)** setup for wrist arthroscopy, with the arthroscope in the entrance portal between the second and third extensor groups.

A   **B**

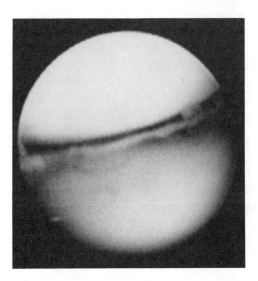

Fig. 11-15. Intra-articular view of the wrist. The lunate is over the triangular fibrocartilage. A motorized instrument is trimming the torn triangular fibrocartilage.

ally functioning at a normal level within at least a few weeks, and return to normal activities is much faster than when an open procedure is used.

ARTHRITIS

Arthritis by definition means inflammation of a joint, but the term generally refers to a pathologic process involving inflammation that causes destruction of the joint. Many processes can cause arthritis, such as general wear and tear producing osteoarthritis; metabolic abnormalities, such as that which causes gouty arthritis; immune abnormalities resulting in rheumatoid arthritis or lupus arthritis; infections can cause septic arthritis; and traumatic injuries that result in damage or unevenness of the joint surfaces, causing traumatic arthritis.

Osteoarthritis of the wrist and hand occurs mostly in the wrist, the distal interphalangeal joints of the fingers, and the carpometacarpal joint of the thumb (Fig. 11-16A). Control of the inflammation may be accomplished conservatively by using nonsteroidal antiinflammatory medications, heat, and maintenance of motion in the joints. Developing deformities may be controlled by intermittent splinting, although this is necessary only in a small proportion of patients with osteoarthritis. Surgical procedures for severe arthritis, in which there is uncontrolled pain, destruction of the joint on x-ray examination, or deformity with loss of function, may include simple débridement of the joint with removal of osteophytes or bone spurs and débridement of abnormal cartilage in the joint. Capsular reinforcement may also be necessary to control deformities. For more involved destruction, fusion of the joint may be necessary or, specifically in the case of the basilar thumb joint and the wrist, a Silastic prosthesis may be useful to retain function after removing the abnormal joint (Fig. 11-16B). Physical therapy is occasionally necessary with conservative treatment for

maintenance of range of motion in acutely inflamed joints, by use of gentle range-of-motion exercises as well as heat, paraffin baths, and massage. Again, intermittent splinting may be necessary for some patients. After surgical procedures immobilization is usually needed for a period of time, after which return of function is achieved through exercise and strengthening.

Rheumatoid arthritis is particularly debilitating to the hand, and treatment can be very involved (Fig. 11-17A). Briefly, rheumatoid arthritis not only affects the articular surfaces but also involves the soft tissues to a large extent, including the ligamentous structures as well as the tendinous structures about the wrist and hand. The cartilage surfaces are destroyed, and the soft tissue structures are weakened by degradation of the collagen and infiltration with the rheumatoid process. The joints most often involved are the wrist, the carpometacarpal joint of the thumb, and the metacarpophalangeal joints of the fingers. Deformity can occur simply by collapse of

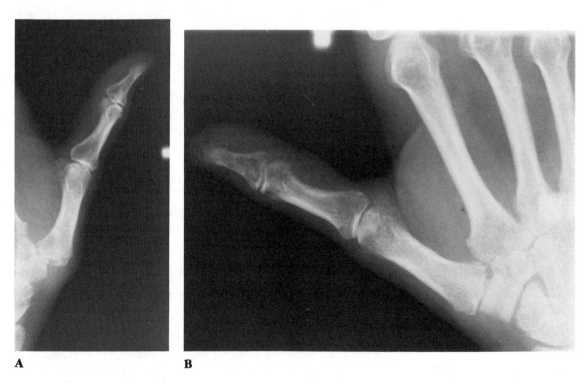

A   **B**

Fig. 11-16. Osteoarthritis. **(A)** Degeneration and subluxation of the carpometacarpal joint of the thumb; **(B)** carpometacarpal joint of the thumb after prosthetic replacement.

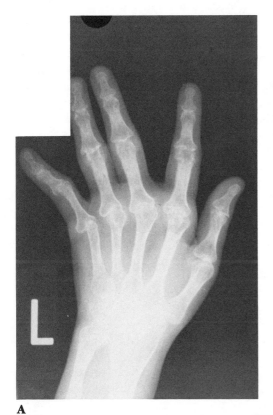
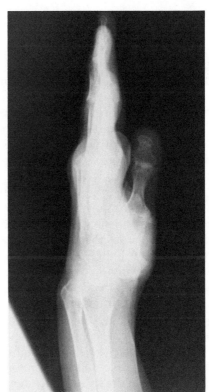

Fig. 11-17. Rheumatoid arthritis. **(A)** Severely degenerative rheumatoid hand showing degeneration and subluxation of the metacarpophalangeal joints as well as severe degeneration of the wrist. **(B)** Postoperative view with Silastic metacarpophalangeal joints in place.

A

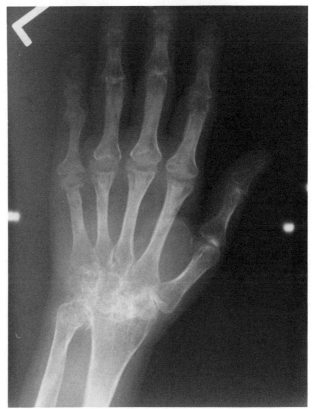

B

the joint surfaces or in combination with laxity of the surrounding capsular and ligamentous structures, causing subluxation and subsequent abnormal pull of the muscle-tendon units, resulting in grossly abnormal function of the hand. The tendons can also become involved, particularly the flexor tendons, and chronic uncontrolled inflammation can cause rupture of the tendons.

Treatment is by controlling the disease process with medication, splinting to prevent stretching of the soft tissue structures and subsequent subluxation of the joints, and vigorous therapy to maintain strength and motion in the digits and the wrist. Surgical treatment in cases of minimal involvement of the articular surfaces can be accomplished by synovectomy and soft tissue reconstruction as necessary, and then rehabilitation once healing of the reconstructions has occurred. In cases of more advanced destruction of the joints along with subluxation, soft tissue releases of the tight structures and reinforcement and reconstruction of the loose structures are necessary. Silastic joint replacement, particularly for the metacarpophalangeal joints, the basilar joint of the thumb, and the wrist may be indicated, or fusion of the joints, especially the basilar thumb joint or the wrist joint, if stability is needed because of severe involvement of the soft tissues (Fig. 11-17B). Reconstruction of ruptured tendons is necessary to regain function but will fail if control of the disease by medication or synovectomy is not achieved. Prolonged dynamic splinting after reconstruction is generally necessary, with slow return of function, but because of the severe deformities, reconstructions of rheumatoid hands are generally very satisfying.

Septic arthritis can occur either through direct introduction of bacteria into the joint from a puncture wound or surgical procedure or via the bloodstream through hematogenous seeding of the joint with bacteria. Sepsis in a joint that is not treated early will result in destruction of the articular surfaces of the joint and cause septic arthritis.[15] Initially, control of the infection is necessary, and if arthritis sets in from the septic process, a fusion or resection arthroplasty may be indicated, depending upon the joint involved. It is only with hesitation that a Silastic or artificial joint would be placed in a previously septic joint.

Traumatic arthritis can occur when any traumatic episode results in injury to the articular surface and damage to the cartilage covering or to the ligamentous stability of the joint that causes abnormal mechanics and motion about the joint. Once the arthritis has set in it is approached much like osteoarthritis, with control by nonsteroidal anti-inflammatory medications. Maintenance of joint mobility and function is important. Once the disease process has advanced past the point of control by conservative methods, arthrodesis or replacement of the joint may be indicated.

AMPUTATION

Amputations may be present for many reasons; trauma, vascular disease, surgical resection of tumors, and uncontrolled infections are some of the possible causes. Traumatic amputations or near-amputations that have, because of the mechanism of injury, maintained satisfactory tissue on either side of the amputation may lend themselves to reimplantation. This has become a specialized area within hand surgery. The reimplantation surgeon must consider many complex problems when anticipating reimplantation of a digit or hand. The length of ischemia time and the temperature of the divided part during that time can play a very important role in whether the tissue of the amputated part will survive. Also, with longer periods of ischemia the arterial and venous anastomoses have a lower incidence of patency after repair. The coordination of the several procedures—fixation of the skeletal structure, repair of the muscle-tendon units, as well as repair of the arteries, veins, and nerves that supply the part—must be taken into account. This is very tedious work, and frequently failure of one or more of these areas can cause subsequent loss of the digit. Reimplantations of digits distal to the distal interphalangeal joint are rarely considered except on the thumb, and reimplantation of amputations proximal to the wrist becomes much more complicated because of the amount of muscle tissue involved and the amount of myoglobin produced due to muscle necrosis, which can cause systemic complications, particularly in the kidneys.[16]

After loss of a part of the hand, if digits remain, it is very important to provide some type of pincer mechanism for grasping. Therefore, if the thumb has been lost, one of the other digits will need to be transferred into an opposing position to the other one or two digits to produce the pincer motion.

Loss of a single digit distal to the distal interphalangeal joint does not appear to be a serious impairment for most individuals. Loss of a single digit proximal to the proximal interphalangeal joint, particularly the long or the ring finger, can cause dysfunction when trying to hold fairly small objects such as coins, which can fall through the gap in the fingers. In these cases ray amputation is frequently indicated to allow for more normal hand function. A hand with three fingers and one thumb does seem to work very satisfactorily and almost as well as a regular hand. Occasionally in a heavy laborer, maintenance of the partially amputated digit rather than ray amputation may be desirable to maintain the breadth of the hand and allow for greater grip strength. When the thumb has been amputated, or when all the digits have been amputated with maintenance of some function of the thumb, a toe-to-hand transfer using free-tissue technique can restore for pincer movement of the hand. Amputation proximal to the base of the metacarpals is very difficult to reconstruct, and a prosthetic replacement may provide satisfactory function.

Rehabilitation when only a single digit is involved can be as simple as re-educating the individual in use of the hand without the amputated digit. If, to replace the thumb, transfer of digits within the same hand or toe-to-hand transfer is performed, the rehabilitation and re-education in use of the hand can be very complex. Therapy after reimplantation is very prolonged because of the scarring through the area of the amputation and repair. Consideration must be given to bone healing, the sliding and gliding motions of the tendons, and protection of the digit until sensation returns.

REFERENCES

1. Flynn JE: Disability evaluations. p. 635. In Flynn JE (ed): Hand Surgery. 2nd Ed. Williams & Wilkins, Baltimore, 1975
2. Lee M: Tendon injuries. p. 150. In Crenshaw AH (ed): Campbell's Operative Orthopaedics. 7th Ed. Vol. 1. CV Mosby, St Louis, 1987
3. Nichols HM: Manual of Hand Injuries. Year Book Medical Publishers, Chicago, 1957
4. Taleisnik J, Kelly PJ: The extraosseous and intraosseous blood supply of the scaphoid bone. J Bone Joint Surg 48A:1125, 1966
5. Herbert TJ: Use of the Herbert bone screw in surgery of the wrist. Clin Orthop 202:79, 1986
6. Cooney WP, Dobyns JH, Linscheid RL: Fractures of the scaphoid: a rational approach to management. Clin Orthop 149:90, 1980
7. Lee M: Fractures. p. 186. In Crenshaw AH (ed): Campbell's Operative Orthopaedics. 7th Ed. Vol. 1. CV Mosby, St Louis, 1987
8. Abouna JM, Brown H: The treatment of mallet finger: the results in a series of 148 consecutive cases and a review of the literature. Br J Surg 55:653, 1968
9. Lister GD, Kleinert HE, Kutz JE, et al: Primary flexor tendon repair followed by immediate controlled mobilization. J Hand Surg 2:441, 1977
10. Pennington DG: The influence of tendon sheath integrity and vincular blood supply on adhesion formation following tendon repair in hens. Br J Plast Surg 32:302, 1979
11. Schneider LH, Hunter JM: Flexor tendons—late reconstruction. p. 1969. In Green DP (ed): Operative Hand Surgery. 2nd Ed., Vol. 3. Churchill Livingstone, New York, 1988
12. Poppen NK: Recovery of sensibility after suture of digital nerves. J Hand Surg 4:212, 1979
13. Frykman GK, Waylett J: Rehabilitation of peripheral nerve injuries. Orthop Clin North Am 12:361, 1981
14. Johnson RP: The acutely injured wrist and its residuals. Clin Orthop 149:33, 1980
15. Neviaser RJ: Infections. p. 1027. In Green DP (ed): Operative Hand Surgery. 2nd Ed., Vol. 2. Churchill Livingstone, New York, 1988
16. Urbaniak JR: Replantation of amputated parts—technique, results, and indications. p. 64. In AAOS Surgical Symposium on Microsurgery: Practical Use in Orthopaedics. CV Mosby, St Louis, 1979

12
Mobilization of the Upper Extremity

MICHAEL J. WOODEN

Joint mobilization has become an increasingly popular and important physical therapy tool. As recently as twenty years ago, "manipulation" was a controversial topic, considered off-limits to any practitioners other than chiropractors or osteopaths. Thanks, however, to the dedication of many pioneers in this field, peripheral and vertebral joint mobilization has become standard fare in most physical therapy curricula.

In particular, the profession is indebted to such teachers as Paris, Maitland, and Kaltenborn, themselves physical therapists, and to such physicians as Mennell, Cyriax, and Stoddard, who were willing to share their knowledge. Their efforts have mushroomed into such developments as continuing education courses as well as graduate programs in "manual therapy" and orthopaedics. These programs have stimulated an increase in graduate-level research, both basic science and clinical. Indeed, interest in joint mobilization was the major factor leading to creation of the American Physical Therapy Association's Orthopedic Section, which has paved the way for specialization in physical therapy.

An additional benefit has been the publication of some excellent books dealing with assessment and treatment including joint mobilization. Many are cited in the references and suggested readings of this chapter and Chapter 25. The purpose of these two chapters is to briefly summarize the information contained in the various texts and to describe the peripheral joint techniques with which I have had the most success.

GENERAL PRINCIPLES

In general terms, mobilization is defined as restoration of joint motion,[1] which can be accomplished by various forms of active or passive exercise, or by such mechanical means as continuous passive motion (CPM) machines. In the context of manual therapy, however, mobilization is passive range-of-motion (ROM) exercise applied to the joint *surfaces*, as opposed to the physiologic, cardinal plane movement of the joint as a whole. Passive movement of the joint surfaces requires a knowledge of arthrokinematics, first described by MacConail and Basmajian[2] as such intimate movements as roll, spin, glide, compression, and distraction. These movements occur between the joint surfaces (hence the term *arthrokinematic*) and are necessary for normal, physiologic, or *osteokinematic* movement of bones.

To illustrate, MacConail and Basmajian described movement of a convex joint surface on a concave surface (e.g., the head of the humerus in the glenoid cavity). As the convex bone rolls in any direction, it must simultaneously slide (minutely) in the opposite direction on the concave bone to keep the two surfaces approximated. Conversely, when a concave bone surface moves on a convex one (e.g., the tibia on the femur), the glide of the concave surface will occur in the same direction.

Mennell[3] elaborated on these arthrokinematic movements, labeling them as "joint play": move-

239

ments that are small but precise, which cannot be reproduced by voluntary muscle control, but which are necessary for full, painless range of motion. An example is the downward movement of the humeral head in the glenoid cavity during shoulder flexion and abduction. Similarly, Paris[4] classified these movements as *accessory* movements, either joint play or component. He stressed that these movements occur not only during physiologic movement, but also at end-range to protect the joint from external forces. End-range joint play is assessed by applying overpressure at end-range to determine end-feel and the presence of pain. Kaltenborn's[5] system uses similar arthrokinematic principles.

The techniques to be described later in this chapter are based on accessory motion concepts and are primarily osteopathic in nature. Where possible, they are linked with the physiologic movements that they theoretically enhance.

THEORIES OF MOBILIZATION

In the periphery, mobilization is used either for its effect on reducing joint restrictions (mechanical) or to relieve pain or muscle guarding (neurophysiologic). This section reviews the theoretical bases for each.

Joint Restrictions

Loss of range of motion can be caused by trauma or immobilization or, most often, a combination of the two. Picture a contracted elbow joint that has been immobilized for 6 to 8 weeks following a supracondylar fracture. Experience tells us that this elbow, despite weeks of aggressive therapy, may never regain full mobility. What are the reasons for this? The effects of trauma and immobilization on joint-related structures are discussed in detail in Chapter 1. To summarize, the most significant range-limiting effects are:

1. Loss of extensibility of periarticular connective tissue structures: ligaments, capsule, fascia, and tendons[6-9]
2. Deposition of fibrofatty infiltrates acting as intra-articular "glue"[10]

3. Adaptive shortening of muscles[11,12]
4. Breakdown of articular cartilage[13]

All of the above could contribute to abnormal limitation of movement and must be dealt with in treatment.

Muscle has been shown to be an incredibly plastic tissue, with the ability to regenerate and return to normal length even after prolonged immobilization.[11,12] However, there is little research to show the direct effects of mobilization techniques per se on immobilized connective tissue. It has been demonstrated that passive movement does seem to maintain distance, lubrication, and mobility between collagen fibers.[6,14] During the healing of traumatized connective tissue, passive movement restores the ability of collagen fibers to glide on one another as scar tissue matures.[15] Stress to this healing connective tissue, applied as early as 3 weeks but no later than 3 to 4 months after injury, appears to reduce the formation of cross-links between and within collagen fibers.[16,17] Therefore, the scar is allowed to lengthen in the direction of the stress applied as its tensile strength increases. Thus, joint contracturing is reduced.[16,17] Finally, forceful passive movement has been shown to rupture intra-articular adhesions that form during immobilization.[10,18]

Pain and Muscle Guarding

Wyke[19] has identified receptor nerve endings in various periarticular structures. These nerve endings have been shown to influence pain, proprioception, and muscle relaxation.

Type I (postural) and type II (dynamic) mechanoreceptors are located in joint capsules. They have a low threshold and are excited by repetitive movements including oscillations. Type III mechanoreceptors are found in joint capsules and extracapsular ligaments; they are similar to Golgi tendon organs in that they are excited by stretching and, perhaps, thrusting maneuvers. Pain receptors, or type IV nociceptors, are found in capsules, ligaments, fat pads, and blood vessel walls. These receptors are fired by noxious stimuli as in trauma and have a relatively high threshold.

Pain impulses from type IV nociceptors are conducted slowly. Impulses from the type I and II mechanoreceptors are fast, conducting at a much lower threshold. The differences between types I and II and type IV conductivity may explain why oscillating a joint relieves pain. Theoretically, the faster mechanical impulses overwhelm the slower pain impulses. Whether this is achieved by "closing the gate" [20] or, perhaps, by release of endorphins in the central nervous system is still under investigation.

Muscle relaxation is an additional benefit of passive movement. One theory is that causing type III joint receptors and Golgi tendon organs to fire by stretching or thrusting a joint results in temporary inhibition or relaxation of muscles crossing the joint.[4,19] This in itself may cause an increase in range of motion and helps prepare the joint for further stretching and mobilization.

APPLICATION

There are many schools of thought regarding the hands-on approach to manual therapy. Mobilization can be applied with osteopathic articulations, distraction of joint surfaces, oscillations, stretching, and thrust manipulations. When using stretching and oscillations, I favor those techniques that stress accessory motion based on arthrokinematics. These are primarily glides, distractions, and capsular stretches. Except for gentle stretching one should avoid mobilizing, especially thrusting, in physiologic movements. Ultimately, which techniques are chosen should not matter as long as the therapist is well trained and follows a few guidelines. Most importantly, the therapist should follow Paris' [4] simple but critical rules *before* mobilizing:

1. Identify the location and direction of the limitation; for example, in a stiff ankle, is it posterior glide of the talus that is restricted?
2. Prepare the soft tissues; that is, first decrease swelling, pain, muscle guarding or tightness, and so on.
3. Protect neighboring hypermobilities. This is particularly important in spinal mobilization but could apply, for example, to a shoulder dislocation that has resulted in anterior capsule laxity. In mobilizing to increase abduction and rotation,

one would want to avoid anterior glide or other maneuvers that would stress the anterior capsule.

A fourth rule, really an extension of the above, applies to postsurgical cases.

4. Communicate with the surgeon. Find out which tissues have been cut or sacrificed, and what motions to avoid at least initially.

Maitland's [21] description of the grades of joint movement has been a major contribution to manual therapy. He uses oscillatory movements of various amplitudes applied at different parts of the range of motion, either accessory or physiologic. Grade I oscillations are of very small amplitude at the beginning of the range, whereas grade II oscillations are large-amplitude oscillations from near the beginning to midrange. No tissue resistance is encountered with grade I or II movements, and so they do not "mobilize" to increase range. However, they do reduce pain and induce relaxation through the mechanoreceptor mechanisms already described. The actual mobilization movements, those which are taken into tissue resistance, are grades III, IV, and V. A grade III movement uses large amplitudes from mid- to end-range, hitting at end-range rather abruptly. A grade IV movement also goes to end-range, but is of very small amplitude. Because it may be less painful and less likely to traumatize a joint, grade IV movements should be used before grade IIIs, the latter being more useful as the joint becomes less acute. A grade V movement is a small-amplitude thrust beyond end-range, a so-called "manipulation."

Figure 12-1A depicts Maitland's grades of movement in a normal joint, whereas Figure 12-1B shows movements applied to a restricted joint. Note that in the latter the end-range (limited) will gradually approach end-range (normal) as treatment progresses.

Often a restricted joint is also a painful joint, and the therapist must decide whether to treat the pain or the stiffness. One advantage of the Maitland system is that grades of movement provide the tools for either.

To generalize, grades I and II oscillations are used for pain; grades III, IV, and V are for stiffness. The therapist must now decide when to use them.

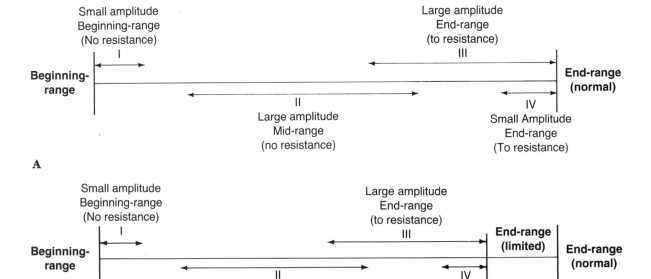

Fig. 12-1. Grades of movement. **(A)** In a normal joint; **(B)** in a stiff joint. (Adapted from Maitland,[21] with permission.)

INDICATIONS FOR MOBILIZATION

Following trauma, surgery, and immobilization there are no predetermined schedules that state when mobilization can begin. The severity of trauma, extent of surgery, complications, and length of time since onset all need to be considered. Even when the patient has been "cleared" for rehabilitation, including passive exercise, experience tells us there is great variability regarding safety and tolerance.

To reduce the chances of being too aggressive, the therapist should try to determine what stage of the healing process the injured joint is in: acute with extravasation, fibroplasia, or scar maturation (see Chapter 1). At best this is an educated guess, but certain steps in the subjective and objective evaluation will increase accuracy.

Subjectively, one must determine the irritability[21] of the joint, that is, how much of a particular activity increases the pain and to what extent. Take, for ex-

ample, a post-traumatic knee. At one extreme is the patient who experiences severe pain and effusion for several days after mowing his lawn. Compare him to the patient who reports moderate soreness for a few hours after playing two sets of tennis. Obviously, the first patient's joint is highly irritable, that of the tennis player much less so.

Subjective responses can be reinforced by assessing objectively the level of reactivity.[4] By carefully taking the joint through its passive range the sequence of pain versus resistance[4,22] is monitored. If the patient reports pain before tissue resistance (not muscle guarding) is felt by the therapist, the joint is highly reactive and, theoretically, is in an acute, inflammatory stage. Therefore, the joint should remain protected and splinted. If necessary, the therapist can apply grade I oscillations to reduce pain.

Moderate reactivity is assumed when pain and tissue resistance are simultaneous. The joint is now subacute, perhaps indicating that fibroplasia and early scar formation are under way. The patient will tolerate careful active range-of-motion exercises as

Table 12-1. Objective Reactivity Levels

Reactivity Level	Sequence	Stage of Healing	Treatment
High	Pain before resistance	Acute, inflammatory	Immobilize Grade I oscillations for pain
Moderate	Pain and resistance simultaneous	Fibroblastic activity	Active ROM Grade II oscillations for pain
Low	Resistance before pain	Scar maturation and remodeling	Passive ROM Grade III, IV, and V movements as indicated

ROM, range of motion.

well as grade I and II oscillations to decrease pain. Actual mobilization (grades III and IV) should be delayed, however, to avoid disturbing the immature scar.

If significant tissue resistance is felt before (or in the absence of) pain, then low reactivity is assumed. By now the collagen matrix has matured, and so mobilization is needed to stress and remodel the scar. At this time grade III, IV, and V movements are indicated (Table 12-1). If these more aggressive maneuvers induce soreness, the therapist can fall back on grade I and II movements to ease off the pain.[21] The key to preventing overaggressiveness is to assess the patient's response to treatment and reactivity for each restriction at every session.

Some conditions that require precautions before mobilization in the periphery are moderate reactivity, osteoporosis, and recent fractures. Choose techniques that will minimize stress to a fracture site while mobilizing an adjacent joint. Also beware of the patient with poor tolerance to treatment, that is, when mobilization sessions consistently increase pain and reactivity.

A few contraindications should also be considered: high reactivity, indicating the presence of acute inflammation; active inflammatory disease; malignancy; and hypermobility from trauma or disease (e.g., rheumatoid arthritis).[4,21]

TECHNIQUES

It is always difficult to determine which techniques are the most effective. The references and suggested readings list volumes in which literally hundreds of techniques are described. One cannot state which are the best for every clinician, but those discussed here are, in the author's experience, safe, easy to apply, and effective. Each technique is either an accessory motion or a specific capsular stretch, and can be applied with any grade of movement. However, grade V thrust maneuvers are not discussed and should not be used without appropriate hands-on training.

The reader must realize that these are also evaluative techniques. They should first be used to determine reactivity and the need for mobilization. In addition to goniometric measurement of physiologic range of motion, accessory movement testing is done using the mobilization positions. To assess the quality and quantity of movement, the accessory motions are usually compared to those in the contralateral limb. This passive movement testing is somewhat out of context in this chapter, since it is actually part of the evaluation process. The reader is referred to Chapters 7 through 11, which review other evaluation procedures for each joint. These chapters also contain information pertaining to anatomy, mechanics, and pathology.

Mobilization is difficult to teach on paper without the benefit of laboratory sessions. However, those experienced in basic manual therapy will be able to follow the figures. For each technique the patient's position, the therapist's hand contacts, and the direction of movement are described. Table 12-2 is for reference, listing each technique with the physiologic movement it theoretically enhances.

Table 12-2. Summary of Upper Extremity Techniques

Joint	Mobilization Technique	Movement Promoted	Figure
Sternoclavicular	Superior glide	Elevation	12-2
	Inferior glide	Depression	12-3
	Posterior glide	General	12-4
Acromioclavicular	Anteroposterior glides	General	12-5,12-6
Scapulothoracic	Distraction	General	12-7, 12-8, 12-9
	Superior glide	Elevation	12-10B
	Inferior glide	Depression	12-10C
	Upward and downward rotation	Rotation	12-11A,B
Glenohumeral	Anteroposterior glides in neutral, flexion, abduction	Flexion, abduction	12-12, 12-13, 12-14, 12-15
	Inferior glide	Flexion, abduction	12-16, 12-17
	Lateral glide	General	12-18
	Long axis distraction	General	12-19
	Distraction with rotation	Internal and external rotation	12-20
	Distraction in flexion	Flexion	12-21
	Anterior capsule stretch	External rotation	12-22
	Anterior capsule stretch	Horizontal abduction	12-23, 12-24
	Inferior capsule stretch	Abduction	12-25
	Inferior capsule stretch	Flexion	12-26
	Posterior capsule stretch	Horizontal adduction	12-27
Humero-ulnar	Abduction	Extension	12-28
	Adduction	Flexion	12-29
	Distraction	General	12-30
Radiohumeral and Radioulnar	Distraction	General	12-31
	Upward and downward glides	Radial and ulnar deviation	12-32
Distal radio-ulnar	Inward and outward roll	Pronation, supination	12-33
	Anteroposterior glides	General	12-34
Radiocarpal	Glides	Flexion, extension, deviation	12-35A,B
	Distraction	General	12-36
	Scaphoid glide	General	12-37
	Lunate glide	General	12-38
Ulnomeniscotriquetral	Glide	General	12-39
Intercarpal and carpometacarpal	Specific carpal movements	Hand and wrist mobility	12-40, 12-41, 12-42 Table 12-3
Metacarpophalangeal	Distraction	General	12-44
	Anteroposterior glide	Flexion, extension	12-45
	Mediolateral glide	Adduction, abduction	12-46
	Mediolateral tilt	Adduction, abduction	12-47
	Rotations	Rotation, grasp	12-48
Interphalangeal	Distraction	General	12-49
	Anteroposterior glides	Flexion, extension	12-49
	Mediolateral glide and tilt	Adduction, abduction	12-50

THE SHOULDER
The Sternoclavicular Joint

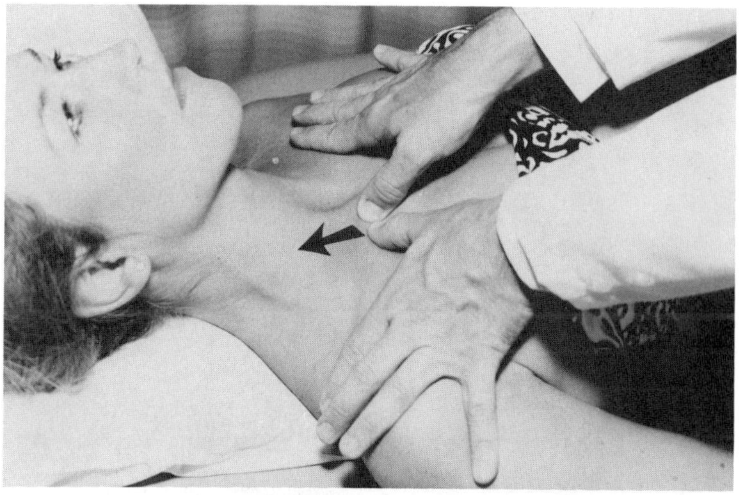

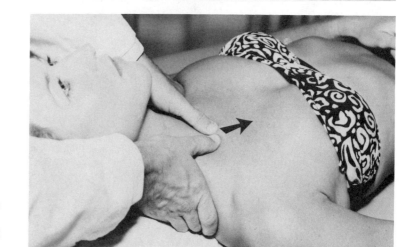

Fig. 12-2. Superior glide.
Patient position: supine.
Contacts: both thumbs inferior to the proximal end of the clavicle.
Direction of movement: push cephalad.

Fig. 12-3. Inferior glide.
Patient position: supine.
Contacts: both thumbs superior to the proximal end of the clavicle.
Direction of movement: push caudally and slightly laterally.

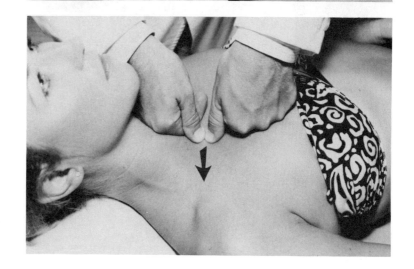

Fig. 12-4. Posterior glide.
Patient position: supine.
Contacts: both thumbs anterior to the proximal end of the clavicle.
Direction of movement: push posteriorly.

The Acromioclavicular Joint

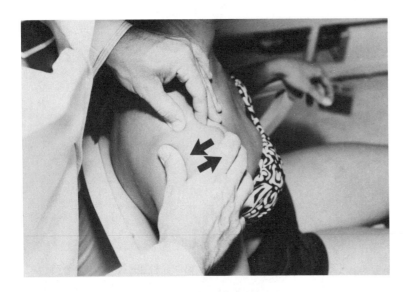

Fig. 12-5. Anteroposterior glide.
Patient position: sitting.
Contacts: grasp the distal end of the clavicle with the thumb and forefinger of one hand; the other hand grasps the acromion process.
Direction of movement: glide the acromion anteriorly and posteriorly.

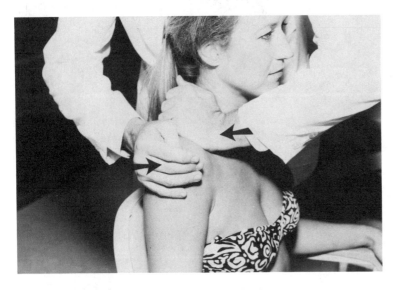

Fig. 12-6. Anteroposterior glide.
Patient position: sitting.
Contacts: the pisiform of one hand contacts the anterior aspect of the distal end of the clavicle; the carpal tunnel of the other hand contacts the posterior aspect of the acromion.
Direction of movement: hands push in opposite directions.

The Scapulothoracic Joint

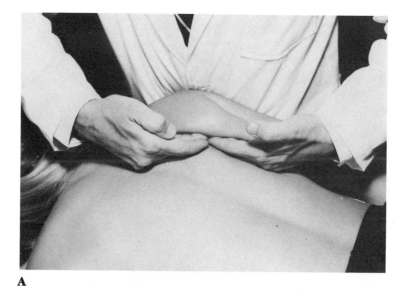

A

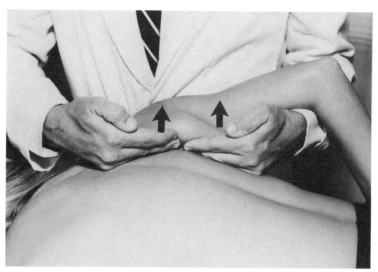

B

Fig. 12-7. Scapular distraction.
Patient position: prone, arm at side.
Contacts: ulnar fingers of both hands under the medial scapular border **(A).**
Direction of movement: the scapula is distracted or "lifted" away from the thorax **(B).**

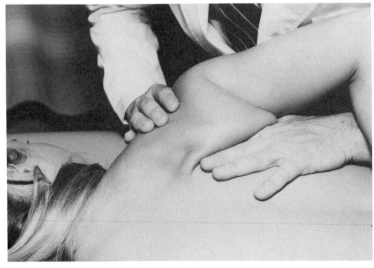

A

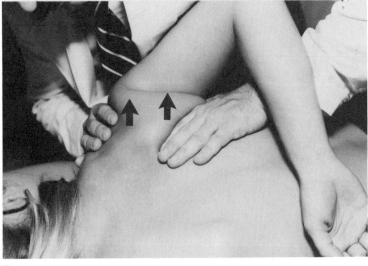

B

Fig. 12-8. Scapular distraction.
Patient position: prone, forearm behind back (if patient is able).
Contacts: index finger of one hand under the medial scapular border; the other hand grasps the superior border **(A).**
Direction of movement: the scapula is distracted from the thorax **(B).**

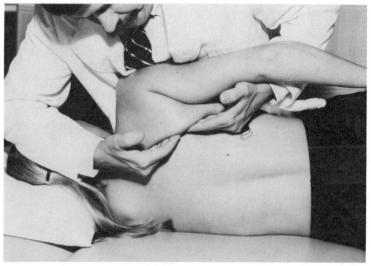

A

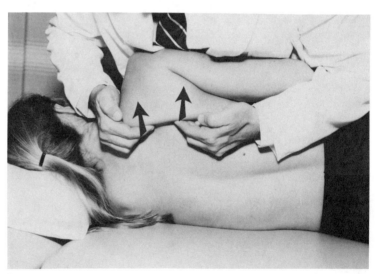

B

Fig. 12-9. Scapular distraction.
Patient position: side-lying, arm at side.
Contacts: ulnar fingers under the medial
scapular border **(A).**
Direction of movement: distract the scap-
ula from the thorax **(B).**

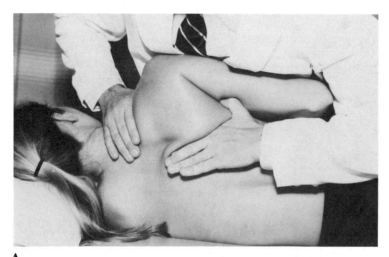

A

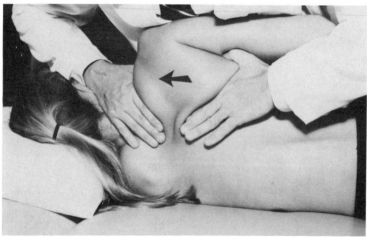

B

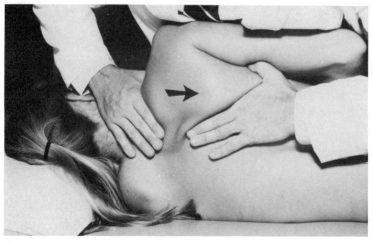

C

Fig. 12-10. Superior and inferior glide.
Patient position: side-lying, arm at side.
Contacts: index finger of one hand under
the medial scapular border; the other
hand grasps the superior border **(A).**
Direction of movement: under slight dis-
traction the scapula is moved superiorly
(B) and inferiorly **(C).**

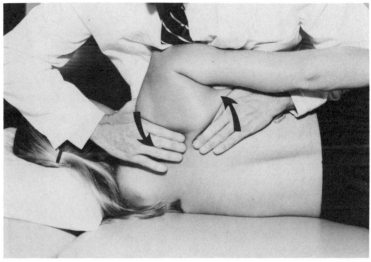

A

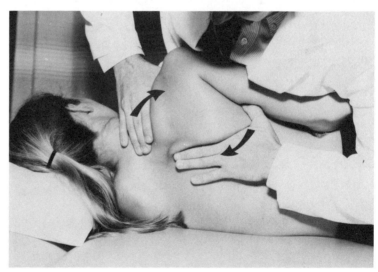

B

Fig. 12-11. Rotation.
Patient position: side-lying, arm at side.
Contacts: same as in Fig. 12-10A.
Direction of movement: under slight dis-
traction rotate the scapula upward **(A)**
and downward **(B)**.

The Glenohumeral Joint

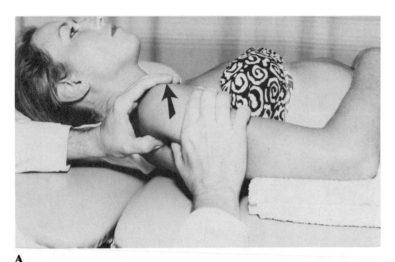

A

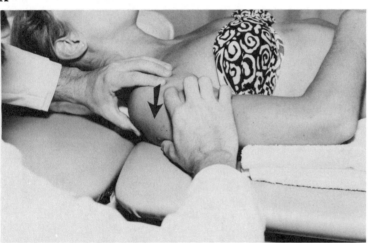

B

Fig. 12-12. Anteroposterior glide.
Patient position: supine, arm at side, elbow propped.
Contacts: hands grasp the humeral head; thumbs posterior, fingers anterior.
Direction of movement: glide the humeral head anterior (**A**) and posteriorly (**B**).

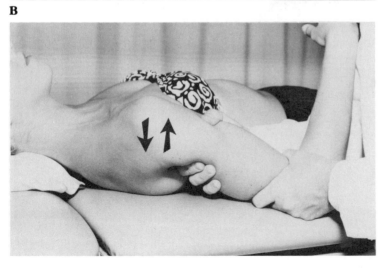

Fig. 12-13. Anteroposterior glide.
Patient position: supine, arm at side.
Contacts: one hand stabilizes at the lateral aspect of the elbow; the other hand grasps the humerus near the axilla.
Direction of movement: glide the humeral head anteriorly and posteriorly.

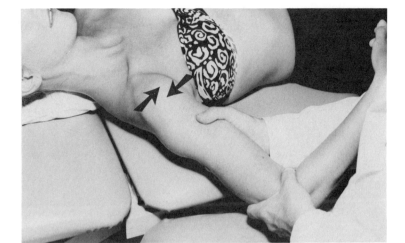

Fig. 12-14. Anteroposterior glide at 45 degrees.

Patient position: supine, arm in 45 degrees abduction.

Contacts: one hand stabilizes the lateral aspect of the elbow; the other hand grasps the humerus near the axilla.

Direction of movement: glide anterior and posterior while maintaining abduction.

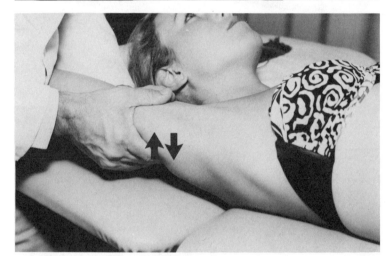

Fig. 12-15. Anteroposterior glide in full flexion.

Patient position: supine, arm at end-range flexion.

Contacts: both hands grasp the proximal humerus with thumbs near the axilla.

Direction of movement: glide anteriorly and posteriorly.

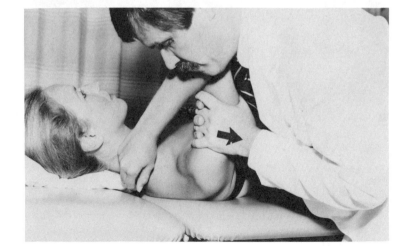

Fig. 12-16. Inferior glide (depression) in flexion.

Patient position: supine, shoulder flexed to 90 degrees.

Contacts: the patient's elbow is stabilized by the therapist's shoulder; hands grasp the proximal humerus with fingers interlocked.

Direction of movement: pull the humeral head inferiorly.

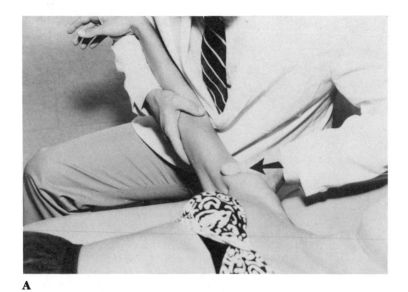

A

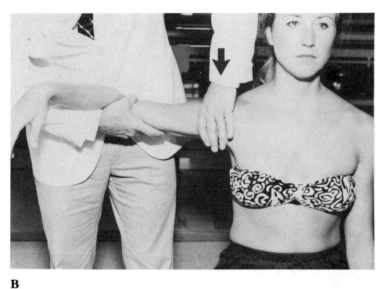

B

Fig. 12-17. Inferior glide (depression) in abduction.

Patient position: supine **(A)** or sitting **(B).**

Contacts: grasp the arm near the elbow to stabilize in 90 degrees abduction; the first web space of the other hand contacts the head of the humerus.

Direction of movement: depress the head of the humerus (inferiorly).

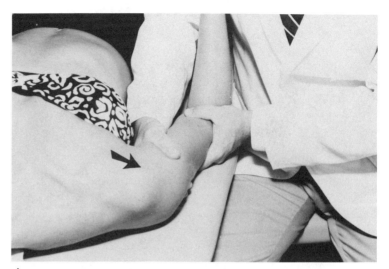

A

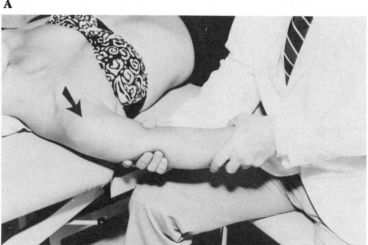

B

Fig. 12-18. Lateral glide (distraction).
Patient position: supine, arm at side **(A)**;
   supine, arm in 45 degrees abduction
   (B); supine, arm in 90 degrees flexion **(C).**
Contacts: grasp near the elbow to stabilize;
   the other hand grasps the proximal humerus at the axilla.
Direction of movement: distract the humeral head laterally.

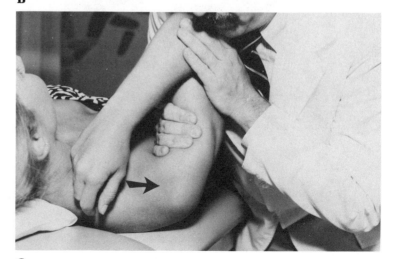

C

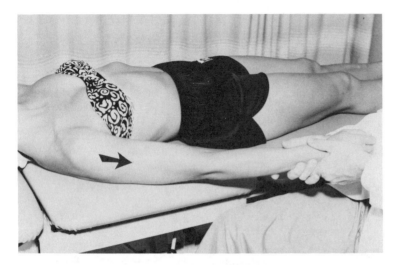

Fig. 12-19. Long axis distraction.
Patient position: supine.
Contacts: hands grasp the forearm above the wrist.
Direction of movement: pull along the long axis of the arm.

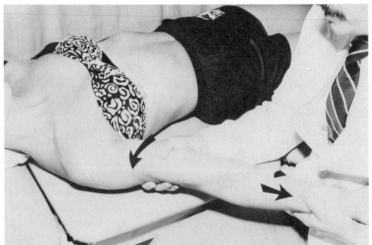

A

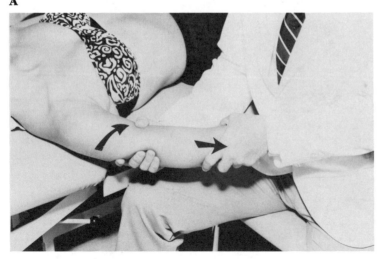

B

Fig. 12-20. Long axis distraction with rotation.
Patient position: supine.
Contacts: one hand grasps the forearm to distract; the other hand grasps the proximal humerus medially.
Direction of movement: while distracting, rotate externally **(A)** or internally **(B)**.

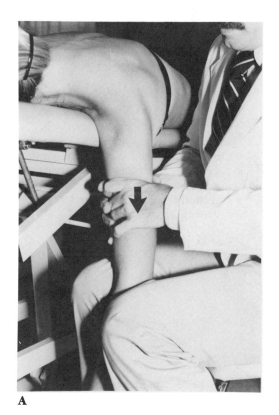

A

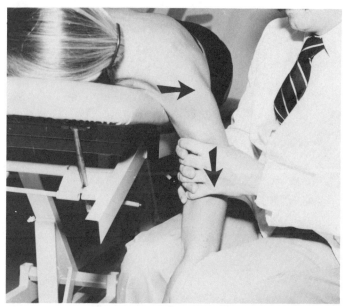

B

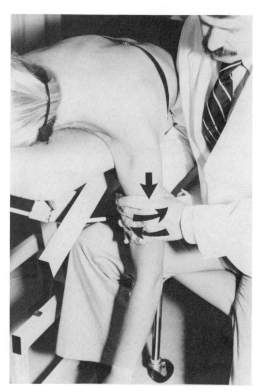

C

Fig. 12-21. Distraction in flexion.
Patient position: prone, arm in 90 degrees flexion off the
edge of the table.
Contacts: hands grasp the midshaft of the humerus with
fingers interlocked.
Direction of movement: distract along the long axis of the
arm **(A)**; while distracting, glide laterally **(B)** or rotate
(C).

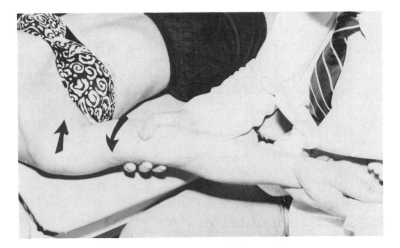

Fig. 12-22. Anterior capsule stretch.
Patient position: supine, arm abducted.
Contacts: one hand grasps the forearm to stabilize; the other hand grasps the proximal humerus medially.
Direction of movement: externally rotate while gliding anteriorly.

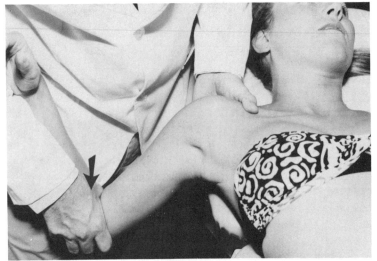

Fig. 12-23. Anterior capsule stretch.
Patient position: supine, near the edge of the table.
Contacts: one hand stabilizes the posterior aspect of the shoulder; the other hand grasps the humerus above the elbow.
Direction of movement: stretch into horizontal abduction.

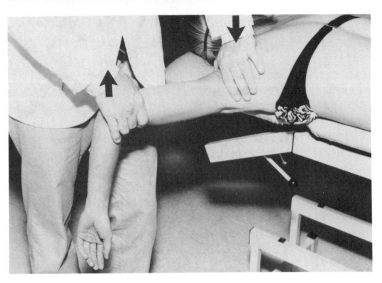

Fig. 12-24. Anterior capsule stretch.
Patient position: prone, near the edge of the table.
Contacts: the palm of one hand stabilizes the posterior aspect of the shoulder; the other hand grasps the humerus above the elbow.
Direction of movement: stretch into horizontal abduction.

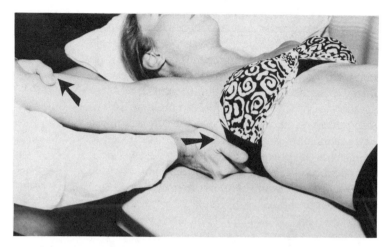

Fig. 12-25. Inferior capsule stretch.
Patient position: supine, arm in end-range abduction.
Contacts: carpal tunnel contact of one hand stabilizes the lateral border of the scapula; the other hand grasps the humerus above the elbow.
Direction of movement: stretch into abduction.

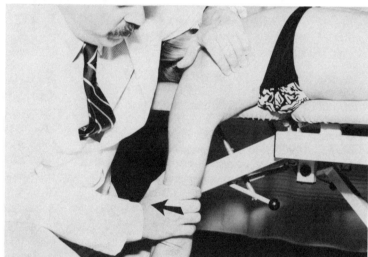

Fig. 12-26. Inferior capsule stretch.
Patient position: prone, arm in flexion off the edge of the table.
Contacts: the fingertips of one hand stabilize the lateral scapular border; the other hand grasps the humerus above the elbow.
Direction of movement: stretch into flexion.

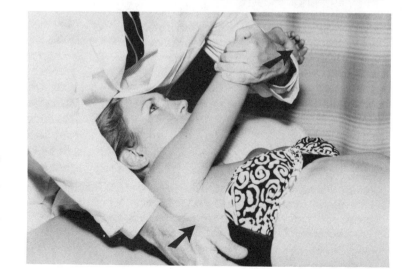

Fig. 12-27. Posterior capsule stretch.
Patient position: supine, arm in 90 degrees flexion, elbow flexed.
Contacts: stabilize the lateral scapular border with carpal tunnel contact; the other hand grasps the elbow and cradles the forearm.
Direction of movement: stretch into horizontal adduction.

THE ELBOW
The Humeroulnar Joint

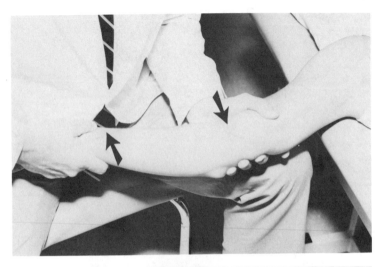

Fig. 12-28. Abduction.
Patient position: supine.
Contacts: stabilize the distal humerus laterally; the other hand grasps the ulnar aspect of the forearm above the wrist.
Direction of movement: the forearm is abducted on the humerus.

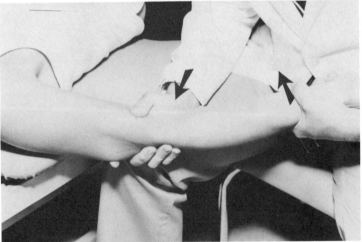

Fig. 12-29. Adduction.
Patient position: supine.
Contacts: stabilize the distal humerus medially; the other hand grasps the radial aspect of the forearm above the wrist.
Direction of movement: the forearm is adducted on the humerus.

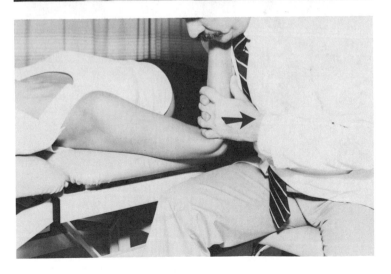

Fig. 12-30. Distraction.
Patient position: supine, elbow flexed to 90 degrees.
Contacts: the patient's forearm is stabilized against the therapist's shoulder; the therapist's hands grasp the proximal aspect of the forearm with fingers interlocked.
Direction of movement: distract the forearm from the humerus.

The Radiohumeral and Proximal Radioulnar Joints

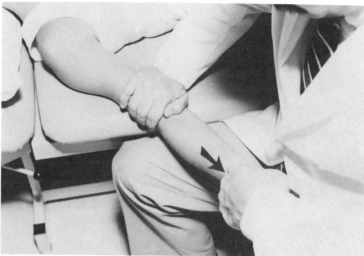

A

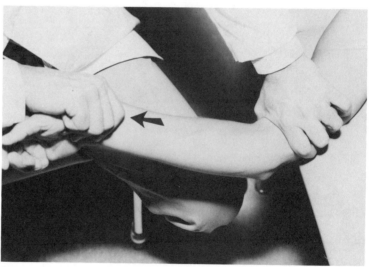

B

Fig. 12-31. Radial distraction.
Patient position: supine, arm abducted.
Contacts: stabilize by holding the elbow on the treatment table; the other hand grasps the radius above the wrist.
Direction of movement: pull the radius distally.

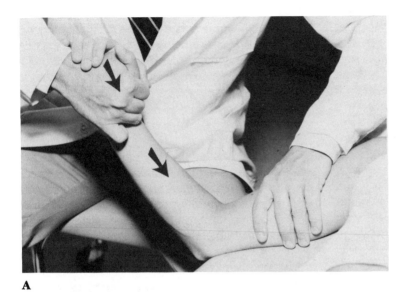

A

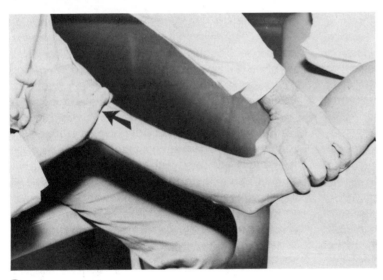

B

Fig. 12-32. Upward and downward glide. Patient position: supine.

Contacts: stabilize by holding the arm on the table; grasp the thenar eminence with a "handshake" grip.

Direction of movement: glide the radius upward by pushing the wrist into radial deviation **(A)**; glide the radius downward by pulling the wrist into ulnar deviation **(B)**.

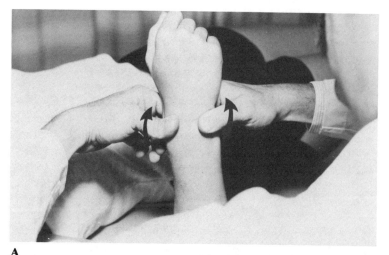

A

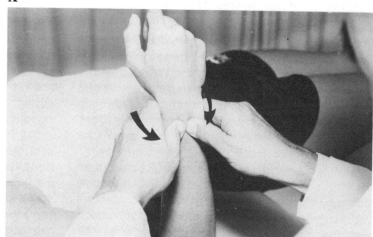

Fig. 12-33. Inward and outward roll.
Patient position: supine or sitting.
Contacts: Grasp the distal aspects of the radius and ulna with thumbs dorsal and fingertips volar.
Direction of movement: roll the radius and ulna inward (**A**) and outward (**B**) on one another.

B

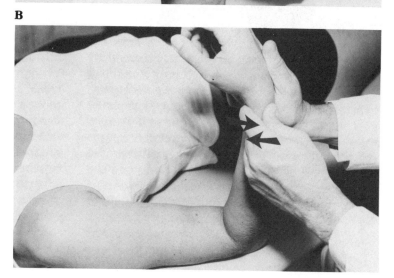

Fig. 12-34. Anteroposterior glide.
Patient position: sitting or supine, elbow flexed.
Contacts: stabilize the ulna with thenar grasp; the other hand grasps the radius with thumb and forefinger.
Direction of movement: glide the radius anteriorly and posteriorly.

The Radiocarpal Joints

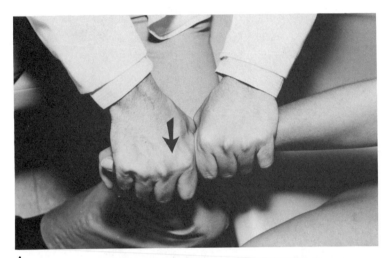

A

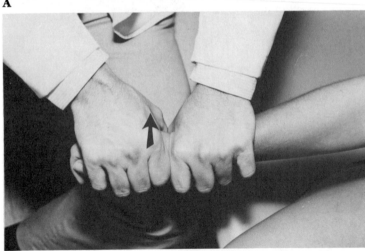

B

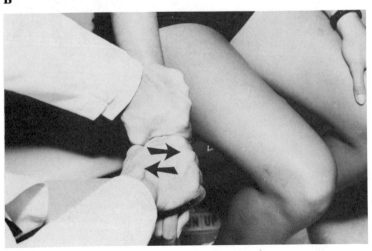

C

Fig. 12-35. Radiocarpal glides.
Patient position: supine or sitting.
Contacts: with the thumb, index finger, and first web space stabilize the radius and ulna dorsally; the other hand grasps the proximal row of carpal bones.
Direction of movement: glide the carpal bones anteriorly **(A)**, posteriorly **(B)**, medially, and laterally **(C).**

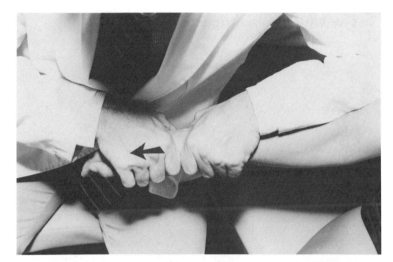

Fig. 12-36. Distraction.
Patient position: supine or sitting.
Contacts: same as in Figure 12-35.
Direction of movement: distract the carpal
  bones distally.

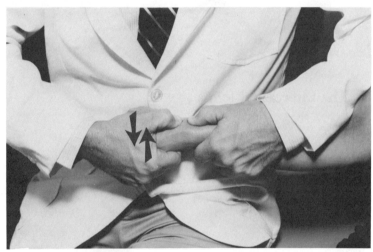

Fig. 12-37. Scaphoid on radius.
Patient position: supine or sitting.
Contacts: using the thumbs and forefingers, stabilize the radius and grasp the
  scaphoid.
Direction of movement: glide the scaphoid anteriorly and posteriorly on the
  radius.

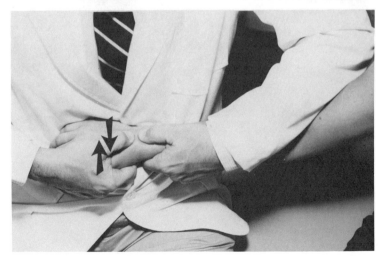

Fig. 12-38. Lunate on radius.
Patient position: supine or sitting.
Contacts: stabilize the radius; grasp the lunate.
Direction of movement: glide the lunate
  anteriorly and posteriorly on the radius.

The Ulnomeniscotriquetral Joint

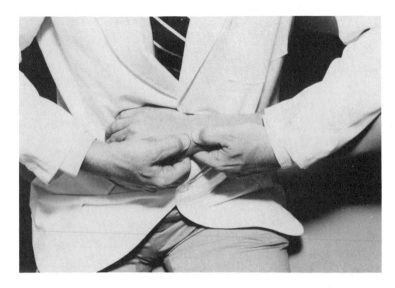

Fig. 12-39. Ulnomeniscotriquetral glide.
Patient position: supine or sitting.
Contacts: stabilize the ulna, grasp the triquetrum.
Direction of movement: glide the triquetrum anteriorly and posteriorly on the ulna.

The Intercarpal Joints

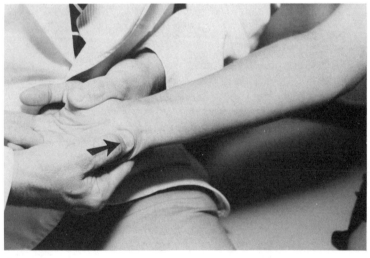

A

Fig. 12-40. Pisiform glides.
Patient position: supine or sitting.
Contacts: grasp the patient's hand firmly to stabilize; contact the thumbtip against the pisiform bone.
Direction of movement: glide the pisiform cephalad **(A)**, caudally **(B)**, medially **(C)**, and laterally **(D)**.

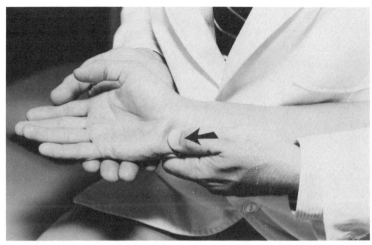

B

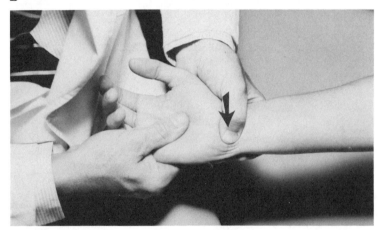

C

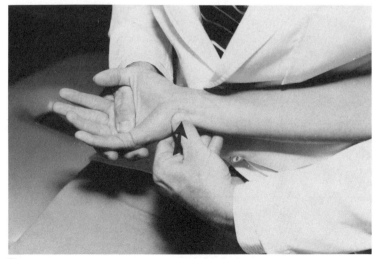

Fig. 12-40 *(continued).*

D

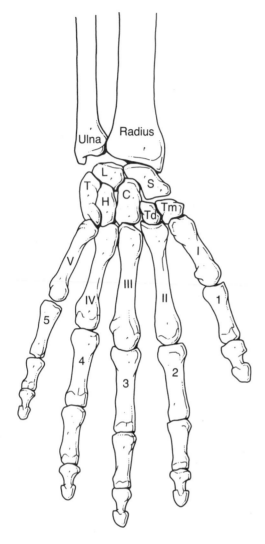

Table 12-3. Specific Intercarpal and Carpometacarpal Glides

Stabilize	Mobilize
Scaphoid	Lunate
	Capitate
	Trapezium
	Trapezoid
Lunate	Capitate
	Triquetrum
	Hamate
Triquetrum	Hamate
Hamate	Capitate
	Base of 5th metacarpal
	Base of 4th metacarpal
Capitate	Base of 3rd metacarpal
	Trapezoid
Trapezium	Base of 1st metacarpal
Trapezoid	Base of 2nd metacarpal

Fig. 12-41. The bones of the wrist, hand, and fingers (dorsal view of right wrist). Key: S, scaphoid; L, lunate; T, triquetrum; Tm, trapezium; Td, trapezoid; C, capitate; H, hamate; I-V, metatarsals; 1-5, proximal phalanges.

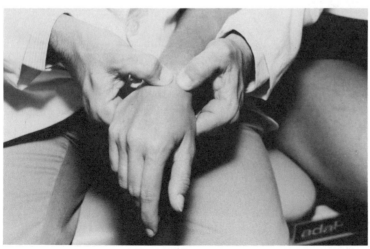

Fig. 12-42. Intercarpal and carpometacarpal glides.

Patient position: supine or sitting.

Contacts: use the thumbs and forefingers of both hands, with the thumbs on the dorsal aspect; grasp the adjacent carpal bones (see Table 12-3).

Direction of movement: glide the carpals anteriorly and posteriorly.

The Intermetacarpal Joints

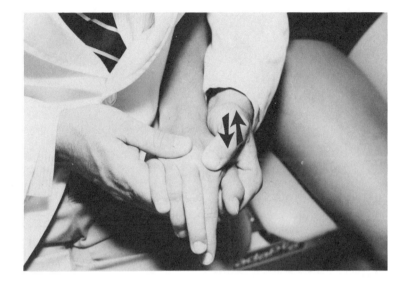

Fig. 12-43. Intermetacarpal glide.

Patient position: supine or sitting.

Contacts: stabilize the head of the third metacarpal with the thumb and forefinger; the other hand grasps the head of the second metacarpal.

Direction of movement: glide the second metacarpal anteriorly and posteriorly; repeat for the third, fourth, and fifth metacarpals.

The Metacarpophalangeal Joints

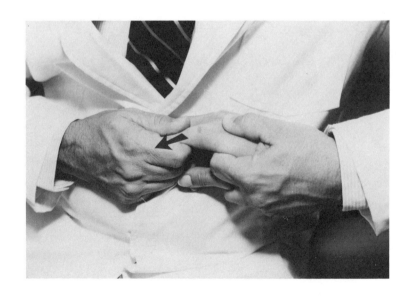

Fig. 12-44. Metacarpophalangeal distraction.

Patient position: supine or sitting.

Contacts: stabilize the shaft of the second metacarpal; the other hand grasps the shaft of the proximal phalanx.

Direction of movement: distract the phalanx from the metacarpal; repeat at each metacarpophalangeal joint.

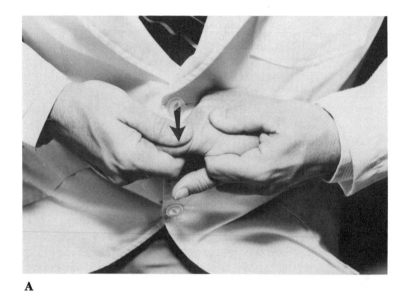

A

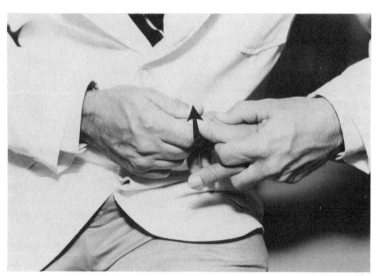

B

Fig. 12-45. Anteroposterior glide.
Patient position: supine or sitting.
Contacts: same as for metacarpophalangeal distraction.
Direction of movement: glide the proximal phalanx anteriorly **(A)** and posteriorly **(B)**; repeat at each joint.

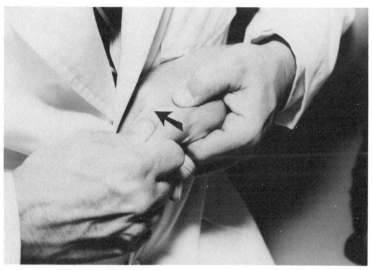

A

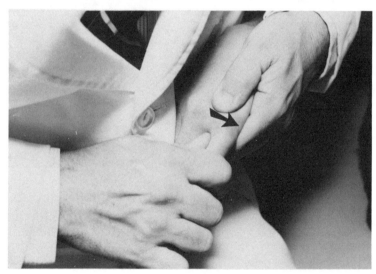

Fig. 12-46. Mediolateral glide.
Patient position: supine or sitting.
Contacts: stabilize the shaft of second metacarpal as above; the proximal phalanx is grasped on the medial and lateral aspects of the shaft.
Direction of movement: glide the phalanx medially **(A)** and laterally **(B)**; repeat at each metacarpophalangeal joint.

B

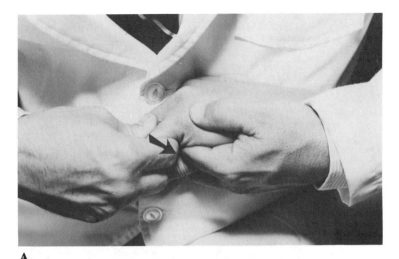

A

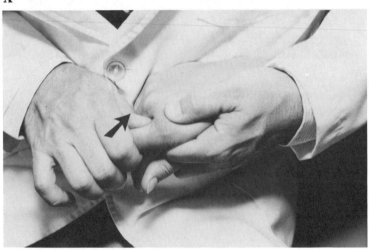

B

Fig. 12-47. Mediolateral tilt.
Patient position: supine or sitting.
Contacts: stabilize the shaft of the second metacarpal; the proximal shaft is grasped the same as for mediolateral glide.
Direction of movement: tilt the phalanx medially **(A)** and laterally **(B)** by using the forefinger or thumb as fulcrum; repeat at each metacarpophalangeal joint.

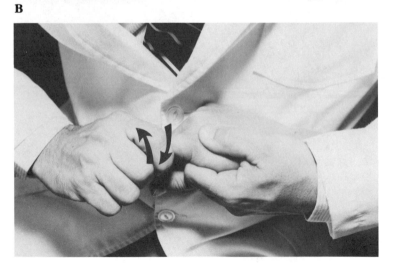

Fig. 12-48. Rotation.
Patient position: supine or sitting.
Contacts: same as for mediolateral tilt.
Direction of movement: rotate the phalanx medially and laterally; repeat at each metacarpophalangeal joint.

The Interphalangeal Joints

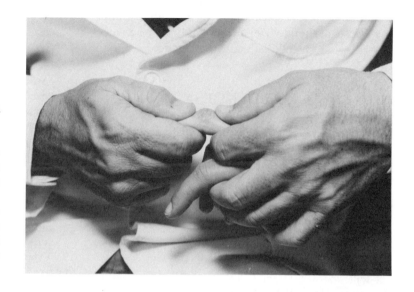

Fig. 12-49. Interphalangeal distraction and anteroposterior glide.

Patient position: supine or sitting.

Contacts: stabilize the shaft of the proximal phalanx; the other hand grasps the anterior and posterior aspects of the middle phalanx.

Direction of movement: the middle phalanx can be distracted or glided in an anterior or posterior direction; repeat for all proximal and distal interphalangeal joints.

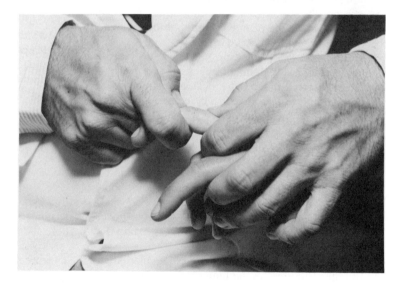

Fig. 12-50. Interphalangeal mediolateral glide and tilt.

Patient position: supine or sitting.

Contacts: stabilize the shaft of the proximal humerus; the other hand grasps the medial and lateral aspects of the shaft of the middle phalanx.

Direction of movement: glide or tilt the middle phalanx in a medial or lateral direction; repeat for all proximal and distal interphalangeal joints.

ACKNOWLEDGMENTS

The author thanks Janie Wise, MMSc, PT (the photographer), Amelia Haselden, PT (the model), and the Physical Therapy Department at Emory University Hospital for their valuable assistance.

REFERENCES

1. Clayton L (ed): Taber's Cyclopedic Medical Dictionary. FA Davis, Philadelphia, 1977
2. Basmajian JV, MacConail C: In Warwick R, Williams P (eds): Gray's Anatomy. 35th British Ed. WB Saunders, Philadelphia, 1973
3. Mennell JM: Joint Pain: Diagnosis and Treatment Using Manipulative Techniques. Little, Brown, Boston, 1964
4. Paris SV: Extremity Dysfunction and Mobilization. Institute Press, Atlanta, 1980
5. Kaltenborn F: Manual Therapy of the Extremity Joints. Olaf Norlis Borkhandel, Olso, 1973
6. Akeson WH, Amiel D, Woo S: Immobility effects of synovial joints: the pathomechanics of joint contractures. Biorheology 17:95, 1980
7. Woo S, Mathews JV, Akeson WH, et al: Connective tissue response to immobility: correlative study of biomechanical and biochemical measurements of normal and immobilized rabbit knees. Arthritis Rheum 18:257, 1975
8. Akeson WH, Amiel D, LaViolette D, Secrist D: The connective tissue response to immobility: an accelerated aging response. Exp Gerontol 3:289, 1968
9. LaVigne A, Watkins R: Preliminary results on immobilization: induced stiffness of monkey knee joints and posterior capsules. In Proceedings of a Symposium of the Biological Engineering Society, University of Strathclyde. University Park Press, Baltimore, 1973
10. Enneking W, Horowitz M: The intra-articular effects of immobilization on the human knee. J Bone Joint Surg 54A:973, 1972
11. Tabary JC, Tabary C, Tardieu C, et al: Physiological and structural changes in cat soleus muscle due to immobilization at different lengths by plaster cast. J Physiol (London) 224:231, 1972
12. Cooper R: Alterations during immobilization and regeneration of skeletal muscle in cats. J Bone Joint Surg 54A:919, 1972
13. Ham A, Cormack D: Histology. 8th Ed. JB Lippincott, Philadelphia, 1979
14. Akeson WH, Amiel D, Mechanic GL, et al: Collagen crosslinking alterations in joint contractures: changes in reducible crosslinks in periarticular connective tissue collagen after 9 weeks of immobilization. Connect Tissue Res 5:5, 1977
15. Peacock E: Wound Repair. 3rd Ed. WB Saunders, Philadelphia, 1984
16. Arem AJ, Madden JW: Effects of stress on healing wounds: intermittent non-cyclical tension. J Surg Res 20:93, 1976
17. Kelly M, Madden JW: Hand surgery and wound healing. In Wolfort FG (ed): Acute Hand Injuries: A Multidisciplinary Approach. Little, Brown, Boston, 1980
18. Evans E, Eggers G, Butler J, Blumel J: Immobilization and remobilization of rats' knee joints. J Bone Joint Surg 42A:737, 1960
19. Wyke B: Articular neurology—a review. Physiotherapy 58(3):94, 1972
20. Melzack R, Torgerson WS: On the language of pain. Anesthesiology 34:50, 1971
21. Maitland G: Peripheral Manipulation. 2nd Ed. Butterworths, London, 1978
22. Magarey ME: The first treatment session. In Grieve G (ed): Modern Manual Therapy of the Vertebral Column. Churchill Livingstone, Edinburgh 1986

SELECTED READINGS

Corrigan B, Maitland G: Practical Orthopaedic Medicine. Butterworths, London, 1985

Cyriax J: Textbook of Orthopaedic Medicine. Vol. I: Diagnosis of Soft Tissue Lesions. Balliere Tindall, London, 1978

Cyriax J: Textbook of Orthopaedic Medicine. Vol. II: Treatment by Manipulation, Massage and Injection. 9th Ed. Balliere Tindall, London, 1977

Cyriax J: Illustrated Manual of Orthopaedic Medicine. Butterworths, London, 1983

Hoppenfeld S: Physical Examination of the Spine and Extremities. Appleton-Century-Crofts, New York, 1976

Kapandji IA: The Physiology of the Joints. Vol. I: The Upper Limb. Churchill Livingstone, Edinburgh, 1982

THE LOWER QUARTER

13

Lower Quarter Evaluation: Structural Relationships and Interdependence

ROBERT DONATELLI
RANDY WALKER

The interrelationships and interdependence of the lower quarter segments are best described by Dempster,[1] who said that, "integrated and harmonious roles of all links are necessary for full normal mobility." The lower quarter is a series of bony segments interconnected and interrelated by soft tissue and muscle. Movement at one segment within the lower quarter influences and is dependent upon movement of the other segments. The lower quarter segments include the lumbar spine, the sacrum, the pelvis, the femur, the tibia, and the foot and ankle complex. These segments make up what is commonly referred to as the lower kinetic chain.

The lower extremity is frequently defined as a closed kinetic chain during the stance phase of gait. Steindler[2] defined a closed kinetic chain as "a combination of several successively arranged joints constituting a complex motor unit, where movement at one joint influences movement at other joints in the chain." The lower quarter functions as a complex organ during ambulation. Proper arthrokinematic and osteokinematic movement influences the ability of the lower quarter to distribute and dissipate forces such as compression, extension, and shear during the gait cycle.[2] Inadequate distribution of forces can lead to abnormal stress and the eventual breakdown of connective tissue and muscle. The harmonious effect of muscle, bone, ligaments, and normal mechanics will result in the most efficient force attenuation.

In addition to normal arthrokinematic and osteokinematic movement, the proper relative arrangement and relationship of each segment to the others is essential for coordinated intersegmental function. Proper arrangement of the lower quarter segments is referred to as *normal posture*. By definition, normal posture is the state of muscular and skeletal balance that protects the supporting structures of the body against injury or progressive deformity.[3] Faulty posture may cause prolonged mechanical deformation of soft tissue and length adaptations of muscle.[3] The maintenance of an erect upright posture and the performance of voluntary movements are highly integrated harmonious functions of muscle, soft tissue, and the central and peripheral nervous systems.[2,3]

This chapter discusses the normal interrelationships and interdependence of the lower quarter structures. The connecting tissues are described in terms of their anatomic relationships and function. The interdependence of the structural links during active movement is emphasized. The functional components of gait are reviewed to demonstrate how the links are interrelated during functional movement. Pathomechanical changes resulting in joint dysfunction and a comprehensive treatment approach are examined in a case study.

277

APPLIED ANATOMY AND MECHANICS OF THE LOWER QUARTER

The lower quarter structures are anatomically interrelated and interdependent. Muscles and connective tissue connect the segments of the lower kinetic chain. Muscles connect the lumbar spine and the sacroiliac joint to the lower extremity. The hip, knee, and ankle are also connected by two-joint muscles.

During normal body motions muscles act in groups, promoting coordinated movements.[4] The interrelationship of muscle movements at the hip, knee, and foot is enhanced by muscles that act over two joints. For example, the sartorius flexes the hip and knee in initiating the forward swing of the lower extremity after push-off.[4] The combined action of a two-joint muscle produces an important coordinated movement of the lower extremity during gait.

A total of 14 muscle groups in the lower quarter are classified as two-joint muscles. They are the iliacus, the psoas major and minor, the gluteus maximus, the piriformis, the rectus femoris, the semitendinosus, the semimembranosus, the biceps femoris, the sartorius, the bracilis, the gastrocnemius, the plantaris, and the tensor fasciae latae-iliotibial band tract. The psoas minor and the plantaris are not present in most individuals.[5] The role of these two muscles as connecting links in the lower quarter is insignificant.

Ligaments and fascia also connect the lumbar spine and pelvic region. The combined effect of muscle, tendon, ligament, and fascia produces coordinated intersegmental movements of the lower quarter.

Two-Joint Muscles of the Lower Quarter and Related Connective Tissue Structures

The psoas muscle requires special consideration as a connection of the femur to the pelvis and the lumbar spine to the innominate bone and femur. The psoas muscle arises from an extensive origin that includes the lower border, anterior surface, and base of the lumbar transverse processes, and the sides of the lumbar vertebral bodies and corresponding intervertebral disks.[5,6] The psoas courses downward into the pelvis where it unites with the iliacus, forming the iliopsoas tendon. The iliopsoas passes beneath the inguinal ligament and in front of the hip capsule, inserting on the lesser trochanter of the femur. The iliacus and the psoas act together as prime flexors of the hip. The psoas muscle may become a hyperextensor of the lumbar spine under certain circumstances. This reversed function is called the psoas paradox.[4] The contraction of the psoas and the iliacus flexes the hip and pulls the lumbar vertebrae in an anterior and inferior direction.[4] Anterior pelvic tilt is counteracted by action of the abdominals. Weak abdominals, therefore, may result in an unstable pelvis, causing an anterior pelvic tilt and resultant hyperlordosis of the lumbar spine. In addition to these actions, the iliopsoas acts as a weak external rotator of the hip, and acting unilaterally it produces lateroflexion of the spine.[5]

The iliac fascia covers the psoas and iliacus. It is connected to the intervertebral disks, the margins of the vertebral bodies, and the upper part of the sacrum.[5] The iliac fascia is continuous with the inguinal ligament and the transversalis fascia (the part of the fascia between the peritoneum and the abdominal walls).[5]

The lumbar spine, pelvis, and femur are interconnected by ligamentous and fascial tissue. One ligament of the pelvic region that connects the pelvis to the lumbar spine is the iliolumbar ligament. The iliolumbar ligament establishes a strong attachment of the transverse processes and bodies of the fourth and fifth lumbar vertebrae to the iliac crest.[5,6] In addition, part of the ligament passes downward into the pelvis to blend with the anterior sacroiliac ligament. The upper part of the iliolumbar ligament attaches to the quadratus lumborum and the lower portion to the lumbodorsal fascia.

The lumbodorsal fascia is an extensive connective tissue organ connecting many tissues within the pelvic region. This massive structure attaches to the transverse processes of the lumbar vertebrae, the iliac crest and the iliolumbar ligament, the twelfth rib, the quadratus lumborum, the lateral portion of the psoas major, and the aponeurotic origin of the transversus abdominis.[5]

The gluteus maximus is not traditionally described as a two-joint muscle. However, close inspection demonstrates that the muscle crosses over the hip and the sacroiliac joint. The muscle originates from the posterior gluteal line of the ilium and the posterior portion of the lower part of the sacrum. It then inserts on the gluteal tuberosity of the femur. A large portion of the muscle inserts into the iliotibial tract of the fascia lata.[3,4]

The piriformis is the most prominent lateral rotator of the hip.[7] It arises from the front of the sacrum between the first, second, third, and fourth anterior sacral foramina.[7] The piriformis passes out of the pelvis through the greater sciatic foramen and attaches to the greater trochanter of the femur. It contributes to extension and abduction of the hip joint. The piriformis is one of ten muscles of the gluteal region that function collectively to stabilize the pelvis, on which the body is supported and balanced.[7] Seven of these muscles are lateral rotators of the thigh (the sartorius, the obturator externus and internus, the superior and inferior gemelli, the piriformis, and the quadratus femoris), and three are medial rotators (the gluteus medius and minimus, and the tensor fasciae latae).[7]

Because the piriformis courses over two joints, the hip and the sacroiliac, movement can occur at either joint. Movement of the sacrum via contraction of the piriformis occurs around the oblique axis of the sacroiliac joint.[8] If the right piriformis muscle contracts, there will be left oblique axis rotation of the sacrum.[8]

The sciatic nerve crosses under the belly of the piriformis. In 15 percent of anatomic dissections studied, the piriformis has two muscle bellies with the sciatic nerve passing between them.[9] Hollinshead[10] noted that in over 10 percent of cases the piriformis is perforated by the sciatic nerve. Therefore, with dysfunction of the piriformis an impingement of the sciatic nerve may develop.[8,9] This may become an important factor in referred pain and impairment of the lower quarter.

The sartorius, as previously noted, is an important muscle, initiating the forward movement of the lower extremity after push-off. The sartorius flexes the hip and knee. The muscle originates from the anterior superior iliac spine and inserts on the proximal part of the medial surface of the tibia.[3,4]

The rectus femoris is the only two-joint muscle of the quadriceps group. The proximal attachment of the rectus femoris is closely related to the iliofemoral ligament of the hip. The posterior head, with

a portion of the fascia lata, blends with the capsule of the hip.[11]

The gracilis is a long, thin muscle arising from the inferior ramus of the pubis and inserting into the tibia. The gracilis is a weak hip flexor and adductor.[11] Deep to the sartoris is the subsartorial fascia, which binds the vastus medialis to the adductor longus and magnus.[11]

The fascia of the thigh is continuous with the fascia of the gluteal region and the leg. It crosses the knee joint, attaching to the patella and the head of the fibula.[11] A portion of the thigh fascia lying over the vastus lateralis forms the iliotibial band. The iliotibial band extends to the lip of the linea aspera and lateral supracondylar line as the lateral intermuscular septum.[11] The band is attached above to the gluteus maximus posteriorly and anteriorly to the tensor fasciae latae.[5,6] These two muscles, the iliotibial band, and the lateral intermuscular septum form a continuous, strong structure that is important in maintaining posture during ambulation.[11] The gluteus maximus, the tensor fasciae latae, and the iliotibial band form a Y-shaped structure designed to act as a lateral stabilizer of the hip and pelvis.[6]

The muscles of the back of the thigh—the semitendinosus, the semimembranosus, and the biceps femoris—are collectively know as the hamstrings. This two-joint muscle group extends the hip and flexes the knee. A part of the adductor magnus aids the hamstrings in extension of the hip.[11] The biceps femoris holds the greatest clinical interest. Although the long head of the biceps attaches to the tuberosity of the ischium, many of its fibers are continuous with the sacrotuberous ligament.[12] Tension of the sacrotuberous ligament may be related to tightness of the hamstrings and contribute to pelvic imbalances and pain.

Finally, the gastrocnemius is the only significant two-joint muscle below the knee. The actions of the gastrocnemius include knee flexion, plantar flexion of the talocrural joint, and supination of the subtalar joint.[13]

Two-joint muscles and connective tissue promote an interdependency of movement and function within the joints of the lower quarter. The connective sheaths between the muscle fibers known as the endomysium, the perimysium surrounding each fasciculus, and the epimysium surrounding the entire muscle connect the muscle to the fascial sheaths. The epimysium is continuous with the perimysial septa and the connective tissue of surrounding structures.[5] Dysfunction of one of the links can augment a breakdown of other links in the chain, producing symptoms throughout the lower quarter.

Action of Two-Joint Muscles

The actions of two-joint muscles are complex. During normal movement, muscles tend to act in groups to produce a coordinated action of several joints. The muscles are selected according to the type of motion desired.[4] The combination of tendinous action and Lombard's paradox reveals the teamwork and versatility of the muscular system. For example, hip flexion is caused by contraction of the iliopsoas. Simultaneously the rectus femoris is slackened, allowing the tightness of the hamstrings to flex the knee by tendinous action. Knee flexion allows the gastrocnemius to slacken, which in turn permits a contraction of the tibialis anterior to dorsiflex the ankle.[4] If the hip, knee, and ankle joint are in a position of flexion, the muscle action changes. The gluteus maximus contracts, extending the hip, and removing the tension on the hamstrings while stretching the rectus femoris. Knee extension is facilitated by this action of the gluteus maximus. Knee extension takes up the slack in the gastrocnemius, causing plantar flexion at the ankle.[4]

The functional activity of rising up from a sitting position describes Lombard's paradox. Palpation of the rectus femoris and the hamstrings reveals a co-contraction of both muscle groups. It may seem contradictory to find both muscle groups active, since the rectus femoris tends to extend the knee and flex the hip, whereas the hamstrings extend the hip and flex the knee.[4] Studies of the action of two-joint muscles in dogs seem to indicate that one part of a two-joint muscle may shorten while the other end lengthens.[4] In humans the action of two-joint muscles occurs at both ends at the same time.

Kinematics of Functional Movement

Functional activities of the lower quarter mainly involve walking and running. The mechanics of the lower quarter during gait, described in that chapter, exemplify the interdependency and interrelationship of function.

Inman et al.[14] described six determinants of gait: pelvic rotation, pelvic list, knee flexion in the stance phase, foot and knee mechanisms, and the lateral displacement of the pelvis. Inman et al. described intersegmental rotation as an important component of the six determinants of gait.[14] Rotation is defined as movement of a body in a circular motion about its center of mass.[14] The axis of rotation is perpendicular to the plane of movement.[14] For example, rotation in the sagittal plane is accomplished by the movements of flexion and extension.

The interrelated movements of the body segments during walking are best exemplified by intersegmental rotations. Inman et al. described rotation in three body planes—coronal, sagittal, and transverse—during walking.

Coronal Plane Rotations

Coronal or frontal plane rotations begin at the hip joint. Hip joint rotation is nearly the same as thigh rotation.[14] In the coronal plane it is influenced by side-to-side motion of the trunk and rotation of the pelvis.[14] Coronal plane rotation of the hip and knee depends on the amount of abduction and adduction, or the side-to-side movement of the trunk. At toe-off, the pelvis is centrally positioned and is moving toward the side of the weightbearing foot.[14,15] The total excursion of hip adduction is approximately 2 cm. Maximum hip adduction is reached shortly after midstance.[14] After midstance the pelvis starts to deviate toward the opposite side. The foot remains stationary on the ground while this side-to-side motion is occurring. The leg segments between the foot and the pelvis accommodate this motion by rotating in the coronal plane.[14,15]

At the knee apparent adduction and abduction movements occur during the first half of the swing phase and the middle of stance, respectively.[14] The coronal plane movement at the knee is measured by observing the combined effect of flexion, extension, adduction, and abduction.[14]

The foot and ankle also accommodate the side-to-side movement of the pelvis by movement in the coronal plane. The long axis of the foot is perpendicular to the long axis of the leg. Therefore, when describing abduction and adduction between the lower leg and the heel, the terms *inversion* and *eversion* apply.[14] Immediately after heel-strike the subtalar joint pronates, producing an everted calcaneus.[13,16] From midstance to toe-off the subtalar joint is supinating, producing inversion of the calcaneus.[13,16] The coronal plane movements of inversion and eversion at the subtalar joint correspond to the side-to-side movements of the pelvis. From heel-strike to toe-off the ankle joint is also moving from adduction to abduction, attempting to accommodate the side-to-side movement of the pelvis. This movement can be observed by movement of the talus. Directly after heel-strike, talus adduction occurs in conjunction with calcaneal eversion. From midstance to toe-off abduction of the talus coincides with inversion of the calcaneus. The movements of the talus and the calcaneus correspond to the transverse rotations of the tibia during the stance phase. Tibial internal rotation, talar adduction, and calcaneal eversion occur simultaneously directly after heel-strike.[13,14] Tibial external rotation, talar abduction, and calcaneal inversion occur from midstance to toe-off.[13,14] Clinically, movement at the ankle joint in the coronal plane can best be observed by the combined movement of the tibia and the talus.

In summary, the side-to-side movement of the pelvis is accommodated throughout the lower quarter during the stance phase of gait. The greater part of this accommodation takes place at the hip, knee, ankle, and subtalar joint. Hip adduction, knee adduction, tibial internal rotation, talus adduction, and calcaneal eversion occur simultaneously to allow proper intersegmental movement and lower extremity function.

Sagittal Plane Rotations

Hip, knee, and ankle movements in the sagittal plane are coordinated throughout the gait cycle. Hip flexion, knee flexion, and ankle joint dorsiflexion are sagittal plane rotations. They occur synchronously for clearance of the nonweightbearing limb as it swings past the weightbearing limb. At the beginning of stance the hip extends and the knee straightens, reaching maximal extension shortly before heel-strike, and the ankle is dorsiflexed.[14] At heel contact the foot rapidly descends to the ground with plantar flexion at the ankle, the knee is imme-

diately flexed, and the hip is maintained in flexion.[14] The shock-absorbing mechanism of hip and knee flexion coinciding with ankle plantar flexion and subtalar pronation. The ankle joint dorsiflexion continues into the stance phase. As toe-off begins, there is a rapid plantar flexion movement that continues until shortly after toe-off.[14] Maximum knee flexion is achieved directly after heel contact. The knee then starts to straighten, reaching maximum extension at midstance.[14] The hip joint is extending through most of the stance phase, supplying the power at push-off.[17]

In summary, the sagittal plane rotations at the hip, knee, and ankle are coordinated to allow for foot clearance and propulsion.

Transverse Plane Rotations

Finally, transverse rotations are the most extensive interconnecting movements in the lower quarter. Gregerson and Lucas[18] studied the transverse rota-

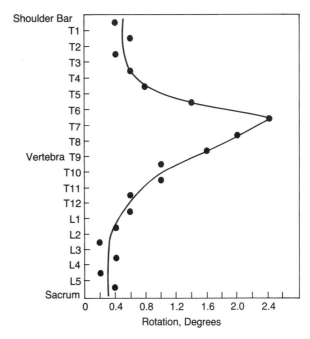

Fig. 13-1. Transverse rotation between adjacent vertebrae. Seven adult males walking at 73 meters/min. (From Inman et al.,[14] with permission.)

tions of the spine during walking. Their studies, conducted on seven males walking at 73 meters/min on a treadmill, indicate that rotation in the transverse plane occurs as high as the first thoracic vertebra.[18] The vertebrae below T7 rotated forward with the pelvis on the side of the swinging leg. Above T7 rotation occurred forward with the shoulder girdle on the side opposite the swinging leg.[18] Maximum rotation occurred between T6 and T7 (Fig. 13-1). Lumbar vertebral rotation was minimal and coincided with pelvic rotations.[18]

From heel-strike to foot-flat the whole lower limb

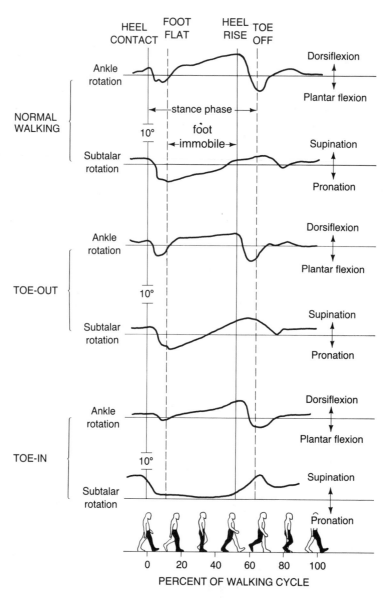

Fig. 13-2. Synchronous motions in the ankle and subtalar joints. Variations in toe-out and toe-in cause variations in the magnitude, phasic action, and angular movement of both ankle and subtalar joints. (From Inman et al.,[14] with permission.)

is internally rotating. From midstance to push-off the lower limb externally rotates.[16] As noted previously, the rotations of the lower limb coincide with the foot's triplane movements of pronation and supination.

The talus, an important component of the subtalar joint, has been described as the torque convertor of the lower limb. Movement of the talus is dictated by the rotation of the tibia. The talus is often referred to as the extension of the tibia into the foot.[14,16] The transverse rotations of the lower limb are converted at the subtalar joint into sagittal plane and transverse plane movements of the talus. Plantar flexion of the talus occurs during pronation, and dorsiflexion during supination (Fig. 13-2).[16]

In conclusion, the kinematics of the lower quarter have been described in terms of the interrelationship of movements throughout the lower kinetic chain. The rotational components of normal ambulation occur in the coronal, sagittal, and transverse planes. The segmental rotations are interdependent and interrelated with each other. Movement at one joint in the chain influences and to some degree dictates movement at other joints within the lower kinetic chain. This interdependence of movement is established by connective tissue and muscle function. It is important in the evaluation of the lower quarter to understand the significance of the integrated and harmonious roles of all its links.

EVALUATION OF THE LOWER QUARTER

Evaluation of the lower quarter should include a combined assessment of muscle and soft tissue flexibility, neurologic impairment and pain, and lower quarter function. This section presents an overview of evaluation of the lower quarter.

Muscle and Soft Tissue Flexibility

It is important to assess the flexibility and function of the interconnecting soft tissue structures and muscles of the lower quarter. There are several tests to determine the flexibility of the two-joint muscles throughout this area.

The Thomas test specifically tests the flexibility of the iliopsoas (Fig. 13-3).[19] Care must be taken to prevent hyperextension of the lumbar spine during the test. The opposite hip is flexed, and pillows are placed under the head and upper trunk area to flex the lumbar spine. The test is traditionally performed on a hard surface such as a treatment table. A modification of the test is to perform it over the edge of a treatment table with the opposite hip flexed and held against the side of the examiner (Fig. 13-4A).

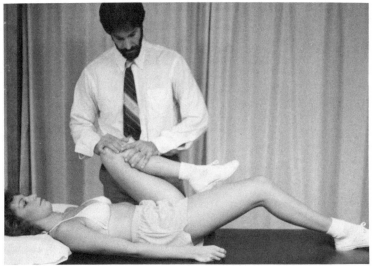

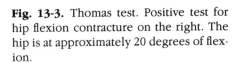

Fig. 13-3. Thomas test. Positive test for hip flexion contracture on the right. The hip is at approximately 20 degrees of flexion.

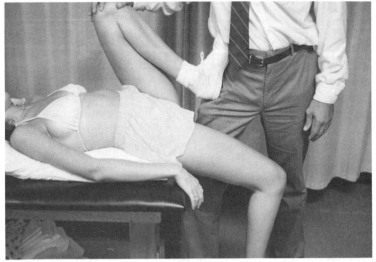

A

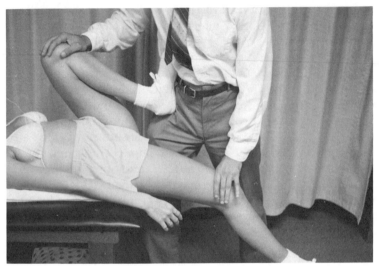

B

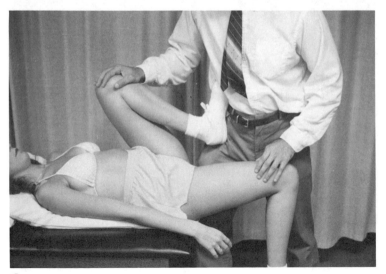

C

Fig. 13-4. (A) Modified Thomas test. The left hip is held in flexion with the foot against the examiner's hip. Pillows are used to reduce the lumbar lordosis. The hip is in extension and the knee is flexed to 90 degrees, demonstrating normal flexibility of the hip flexors and the rectus femoris. **(B)** Modified Thomas test positive for tight rectus femoris. The knee does not fall into 90 degrees of flexion. **(C)** Modified Thomas test positive for tight hip flexors. The hip is flexed approximately 15 degrees.

This modified test can determine rectus femoris flexibility (Fig. 13-4B and C).

The Ober test is used to determine flexibility of the fasciae latae and the iliotibial band. The test is performed with the patient in a side-lying position, the hip held in extension and the knee flexed (Fig. 13-5A and B). Stretching of a tight fasciae latae or iliotibial band from this test position can produce pain at the lateral aspect of the hip or the knee, respectively. Reid et al.[20] demonstrated that iliotibial band tightness is a contributing factor in lateral hip and knee pain. Iliotibial band syndrome, external snapping hip syndrome, and greater trochanteric bursitis are several "friction syndromes" associated with a tight iliotibial band.

Hamstring flexibility is also important to determine in lower quarter assessment. Hamstring flexibility should be tested in the supine position, preventing the contralateral hip from moving into flexion. Flex the hip first to 90 degrees and then straighten the knee (Fig. 13-6). Knee extension will be limited by a tight hamstring muscle group.

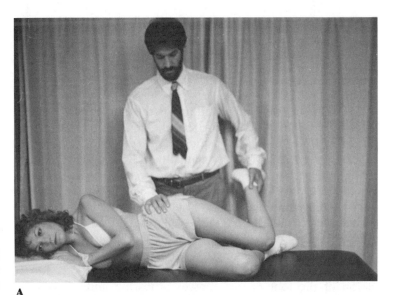

A

Fig 13-5. Ober test. The hip is extended while the ankle is held at the level of the hip. **(A)** Negative test: The knee falls to the table. **(B)** Positive sign for tightness of the iliotibial band: The knee does not drop to the table. The lack of flexibility causes the thigh to be held in abduction without the assistance of the examiner.

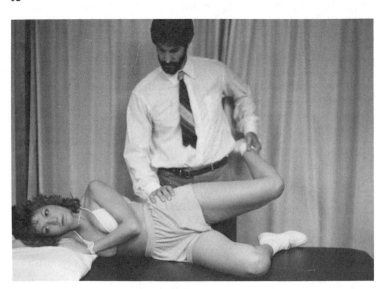

B

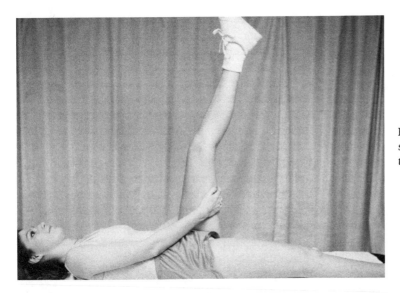

Fig. 13-6. Hamstring flexibility test assesses the ability of the patient to extend the knee with the hip flexed to 90 degrees.

To isolate the two-joint hip adductor, the gracilis, from the one-joint hip adductors, the leg is abducted with the knee in extension and with the knee flexed (Fig. 13-7A and B). By maintaining knee extension the gracilis is put on maximum stretch. The gracilis is a primary hip adductor and secondary knee flexor and internal rotator. Knee flexion places the gracilis on slack, isolating the one-joint hip adductors (pectineus, adductor longus, adductor brevis, and adductor magnus).

Gastrocnemius tightness can be masked by pronation of the foot in the nonweightbearing and weightbearing positions. Open kinetic chain pronation includes dorsiflexion, eversion, and abduction of the foot.[13] If the gastrocnemius muscle group is tight, the patient can compensate by pronating the foot. Dorsiflexion of the ankle joint should be isolated by holding the subtalar joint in a neutral position (Fig. 13-8; Chapter 22 describes the neutral position). The gastrocnemius should also be differentiated from the soleus muscle group by maintaining the knee in extension (Fig. 13-9A and B).

Pain Assessment in the Lower Quarter

The assessment of pain is important in the evaluation of the lower quarter. The clinician must differentiate between local pain and referred pain from the lumbar spine.

Pain following trauma to the musculoskeletal system may be local or referred, immediate or delayed.[21] Local pain of immediate onset may be a result of distortion of the subcutaneous, perivascular, and periarticular nerve plexuses.[21] Delayed local pain usually results from distention of the joint capsule or fascial compartments by blood or tissue fluid transudate.[21] The persistence of pain after the effects of the injury have subsided indicates a continued inflammatory reaction.[21]

Referred pain may be deep or superficial and shows a segmental pattern following the existing sclerotomes, myotomes, or dermatomes. The transference of pain away from the injured area represents an interconnection of the lower quarter structure. Referral pain patterns may extend from the lumbar spine into the foot (Fig. 13-10).

Referred pain patterns may result from myofascial pain. Myofascial pain is associated with trigger points or fibrositis nodules. A trigger point is a hyperirritability in a muscle or its fascia.[22] Compression of the trigger point area gives rise to local tenderness and may also refer pain away from the local trigger point area (Fig. 13-11). For example, pain from a trigger point in the adductor muscle group may refer pain distally into the ankle. A gluteus minimus trigger point may refer pain anteriorly and posteriorly into the thigh, calf, and ankle. Referred pain patterns may be very misleading. The patient's complaint of pain can be unrelated to the location of the trauma.

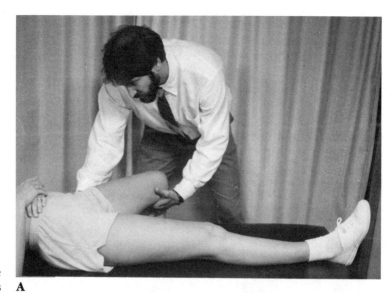

A

Fig. 13-7. **(A)** Test for flexibility of the one-joint hip adductors. The knee is flexed to 90 degrees. **(B)** Test for flexibility of the two-joint hip adductors (gracilis). The knee is extended.

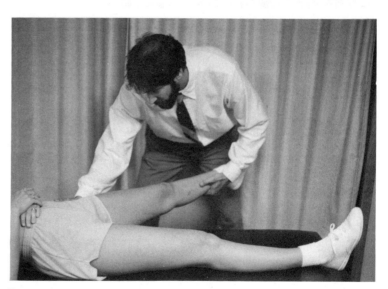

B

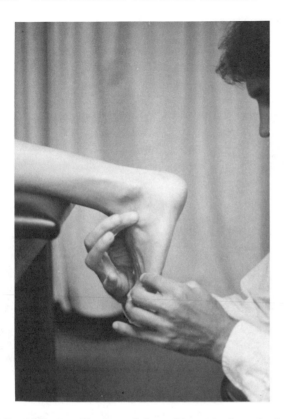

Fig. 13-8. Dorsiflexion of the ankle with the subtalar joint held in the neutral position. The examiner is palpating the head of the talus, while loading the lateral border of the forefoot. Passive dorsiflexion is performed, not allowing the forefoot to evert.

In addition to musculoskeletal pain within the lower quarter, spinal pain must be assessed. Spinal pain may originate from the vertebral column and its related tissues. O'Brien[23] classified three distinct anatomic areas, each with different sensations of pain. The first area, the motion segment, includes the disks, the vertebrae, the facet joints, and their connecting ligaments and muscles. The second anatomic area consists of the superficial tissues surrounding the vertebral column, including the skin, the fascia, the superficial ligaments and muscles, and the tips of the spinous processes. The third category involves the spinal nerve and the sympathetic trunk.

Pain from spinal sources can also be referred into the lower extremity. The referral pain pattern usually follows a dermatome, sclerotome, or myotome (Fig. 13-12A and B). The greater the intensity of the pain, the more distally it is perceived.[21] However, anatomically identifying the source of the pain is difficult because of the overlap of innervation at each level and the overlap of pain patterns.[23] For example, pain arising from root compression or from soft tissue injuries can be felt superficially within the affected dermatome. The referred pain is felt not only within the skin but also within the deeper tissues. The deeper pain will follow sclerotome patterns of the affected tissue.[21]

The final assessment of pain is made by taking a thorough patient history. A careful clinical history will give the examiner useful information about the lesion. The mechanism of injury will often help to determine the general location of the involved tissues and the extent of damage. The immediate response to injury is a useful index of severity. For example, rapid swelling indicates bleeding within the joint. Slow swelling suggests a traumatic synovitis.[21]

The following key questions should be asked as part of the pain assessment and history:[24]

1. Was the onset of pain insidious or sudden?
2. How long have the symptoms persisted?
3. What was the mechanism of injury (twist or strain, lifting or pushing)?
4. Is this the first occurrence of the pain?
5. Is there a history of previous injuries?
6. Where is the location of the worst pain?
7. Where does the pain radiate to?
8. Is there numbness or paresthesia?
9. Is the pain constant or intermittent?
10. What reduces the pain or increases it?

In summary, assessment of the soft tissues of the lower quarter should follow a sequential examination to determine the source of pain and injury. The sequence should include a history, inspection, palpation of soft tissue structures, active and passive range-of-motion testing of the joints, and resisted testing of the surrounding muscles.[25] The active and passive testing will help to distinguish normal from abnormal tissue end-feels, the sequence of pain and limitation, capsular versus noncapsular patterns, ligamentous adhesions, internal derangement, and extra-articular lesions.

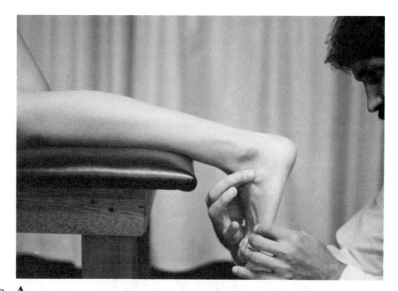

Fig. 13-9. **(A)** Dorsiflexion of the ankle with the knee extended. **(B)** Dorsiflexion of the ankle with the knee flexed.

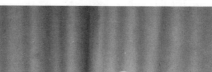

A

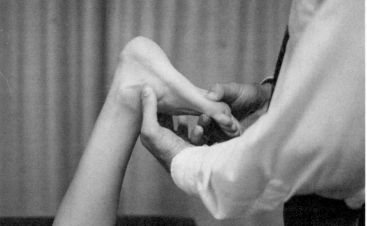

B

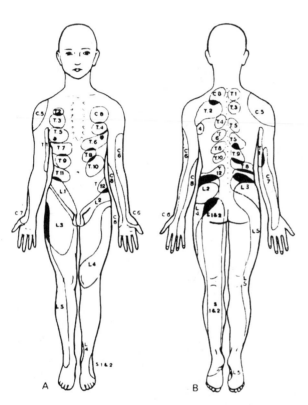

Fig. 13-10. Referral pain pattern may extend from the lumbar spine into the foot.

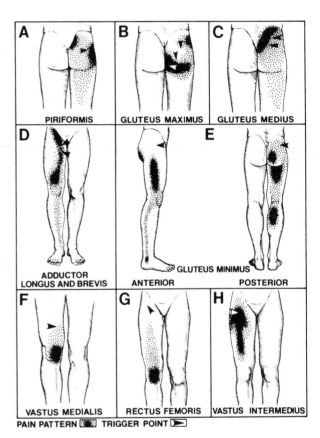

Fig. 13-11. Myofascial referral pain patterns into the lower extremity. (From Simons and Travell,[22] with permission.)

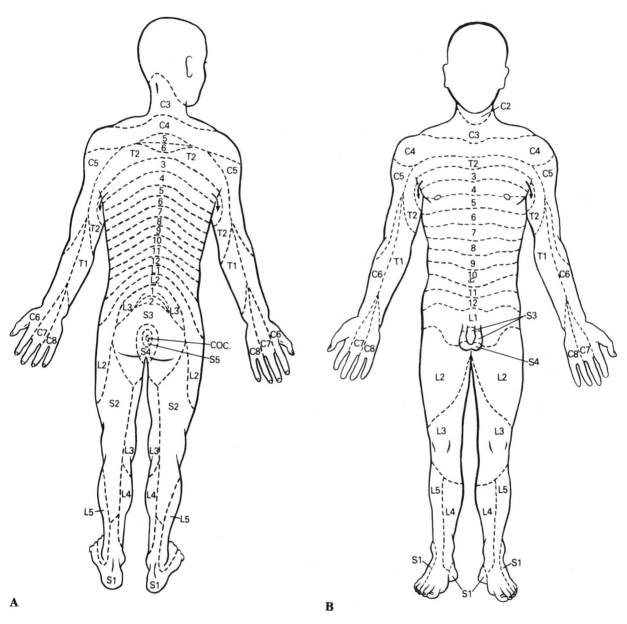

Fig. 13-12. (A,B) Dermatome and **(C,D)** sclerotome charts. (From Devinsky and Feldmann,[43] with permission.) *(Figure continues.)*

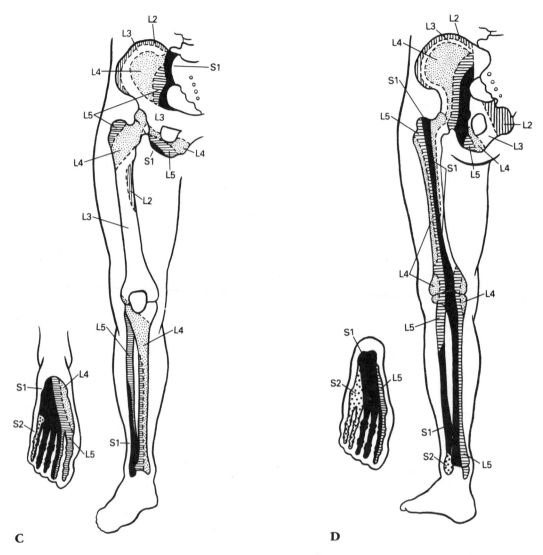

Fig. 13-12 *(continued).* **C, D.**

DYSFUNCTION OF THE LOWER QUARTER

Dysfunction is defined as abnormal, inadequate, or impaired function of an organ or part.[26] Dysfunction in the lower quarter can result from changes in the muscle and connective tissue structures surrounding synovial joints. These changes in soft tissue structures can result from immobilization or trauma. The trauma can be macrotrauma, such as a compound fracture, or microtrauma, in which the per-

sistent irritation of periarticular tissue produces an inflammatory response. Continued irritation can cause scarring, tendinitis, bursitis, capsulitis, and muscular trigger points.[27] The pain associated with microtrauma is of an insidious nature. Usually the patient is unaware of the exact cause of the pain. A sequential evaluation of the soft tissue will assist the clinician in determining the location and cause of the microtrauma.

The following section represents a hypothetical sequence of events leading to dysfunction in the lower quarter. It demonstrates how a change in the normal mechanics and function of one segment can alter the mechanics of other segments in the chain.

Abnormal Pronation

Abnormal pronation of the foot is a common cause of overuse syndromes of the lower quarter.[13] The patient typically reports an insidious onset of pain during and/or after functional activities. Root et al.[13] defined abnormal pronation as a persistent and excessive movement during the stance phase of gait. Excessive pronation usually occurs at the subtalar joint. As previously noted, the talus is considered the extension of the tibia into the foot. The talus thus represents a link between the foot and the lower quarter. Therefore, movement of the talus can influence and even dictate other movements throughout the lower quarter.

A common etiology of excessive pronation is a tight gastrocnemius muscle group.[13,28] A tight gastrocnemius muscle causes restricted dorsiflexion at the ankle joint. The subtalar joint attempts to compensate for this restriction by pronating. If pronation of the subtalar joint is maintained beyond the first 25 percent of the stance phase, the movement of the talus and calcaneus is excessive. During abnormal pronation, plantar flexion and adduction of the talus produce a medial stress to the foot and lower limb. The medial rotation of the talus forces the navicular and cuneiform bones medially and downward, gapping their joints.[29] Increased pressure of the talus on the anterior medial facet of the calcaneus forces the medial side of the calcaneus downward, and the calcaneus assumes a valgus or everted position. The everted position of the calcaneus places the gastrocnemius (lateral two-thirds of the achilles tendon) on slack, while the soleus (medial one-third of the achilles tendon) is stretched.[30] The soleus, attaching to the medial lower third of the tibia, may be traumatized. Microtears of the soleus at its insertion on the tibia can produce an inflammatory response.[30]

The tibia and fibula, as part of the ankle joint, rotate medially with the talus. As previously noted, medial rotation of the lower limb is normal as the foot contacts the ground and immediately after.

However, excessive pronation prolongs medial rotation of the tibia, fibula, and femur. With the foot fixed on the ground, the medial rotation force throws the knee into a valgus position, causing strain on the internal ligaments of the knee. Prolonged internal rotation of the femur and tibia may produce an excessive transverse rotation force to the patellofemoral joint. The patella assumes a more medial position, increasing the stress to the medial facet of the patellofemoral joint. This change in position of the patella can alter the function of the quadriceps muscle group. In addition, the fascia of the thigh crosses the knee joint and attaches to the patella and the head of the fibula. The fascia may become strained by the prolonged internal rotation of the tibia, fibula, and patella.

Internal rotation of the femur is accompanied by rotation of the pelvis and sacrum. As described previously, a number of soft tissue structures interconnect the pelvis, sacrum, and femur.

Internal rotation of the femur can result in a forward and downward tilting of the pelvis. The forward tilt of the pelvis increases the lumbar lordosis and places the iliopsoas muscle in a position of slack. In addition, the resting position of the hamstring muscle group is altered by the superior movement of the ischial tuberosity. The increased stretch position of the hamstrings may contribute to altered knee mechanics and frequent muscle strains. Increased stress on the biceps femoris muscle can produce tension on its attachment to the sacrotuberous ligament, causing pain and pelvic imbalances.[12]

A forward tilt of the pelvis can also increase tension on the iliolumbar ligament. As noted previously, this ligament attaches to the iliac crest and to the transverse processes and bodies of the fourth and fifth vertebrae. This ligament also blends with the anterior sacroiliac ligament, the quadratus lumborum, and the lumbodorsal fascia. Stress to the lumbar spine may become excessive as a result of the increased tension on the above connective tissue structures and muscle.

Reduced tension on the iliopsoas muscle group allows greater medial rotation of the femur. Internal rotation of the femur produces increased tension on the piriformis muscle group. A maintained stretched position of the piriformis can traumatize the muscle, causing local inflammation and muscle guarding. If the piriformis is perforated by the sciatic nerve, trauma to the nerve may also occur.

The patient may have a history of lumbar and pelvic discomfort, medial knee pain, shin splints, and medial foot pain, although at the time of examination medial knee pain may be the only complaint.

The use of foot orthotics to control the abnormal pronation is an important aspect of treatment. However, to place the patient in orthotics without consideration of the soft tissue changes would be detrimental. Mobilization, soft tissue techniques, stretching exercises, strengthening exercises, and treatment of the inflamed tissue together constitute a comprehensive approach. The short-term goal is to relieve the immediate pain. Controlling the excessive foot pronation to reduce the medial forces to the knee is essential. The long-term goals for such a patient should be to restore normal function of the lower quarter by means of treatment techniques designed to restore normal alignment, strength, and flexibility.

Case Study: Lumbar Spine Dysfunction

Dysfunction and pain in the lower quarter can also originate from dysfunction in the lumbar spine and sacroiliac joints. The problem may be as straightforward as an acute strain of the erector spinae muscles from a hyperflexion injury or as complex as an overuse syndrome with a history of repeated injury to structures about the lumbar spine. Patients may simply complain of localized low back pain, or they may complain of bilateral weakness and paresthesias in the lower extremities. The primary task of the clinician is to perform a thorough patient examination, including a relevant history, to identify the tissues involved and develop and implement a treatment program to manage the problems identified. The treatment program should not only address the patient's chief complaint, but also include a total approach to management of dysfunction in the lower quarter. The following case is an example of how low back dysfunction can have an impact upon function in the kinetic chain.

Orthopaedic Assessment

A 35-year-old male office worker with a diagnosis of muscle strain recently presented with a complaint of right hip and buttocks pain, which occasionally radiated down into his calf. The patient's pain was localized to an area extending from the iliac crest superiorly to just above the gluteal fold inferiorly. Anteriorly, the pain extended to within 1 inch of the greater trochanter; the pain did not cross the midline posteriorly. The patient reported that his pain was not constant, but was brought about by standing without walking for approximately 15 minutes. The pain was relieved by walking about for a couple of minutes or by rest in the supine position. The pain felt deep and muscular in origin.

Relevant history revealed that the patient had not experienced any traumatic injury to the area or to his low back. He experienced this pain about four times per year, usually following some outdoor activity such as golf or after playing several games of softball. Previous treatment consisted of muscle relaxers, which gave temporary relief, and ultrasound and stretching exercises, which usually helped relieve the symptoms. The patient now complained that the repetitive episodes of pain were increasing in frequency.

The objective examination revealed that the patient stood erect with a slightly increased lordotic curve at the lumbar spine, and his pelvis was rotated to the left and anteriorly tilted on the right. These signs were consistent with adaptively shortened iliopsoas muscles, with the right side being tighter than the left, and restrictions of the fascia iliaca, which covers the psoas major and iliacus. The patient could bend forward to a point where his fingertips reached midtibia, whereupon he complained of both his buttock pain and posterior leg discomfort bilaterally. Forward bending of the trunk is commonly limited by a combination of adaptively shortened erector spinae and hamstring muscles, and restricted thoracolumbar fascia and deep fascia of the thigh.

Kendall et al.[3] have pointed out that shortened gastrocsoleus muscles also contribute to limitations in forward bending when the knees are extended. Extension in this patient was limited to approximately 40 degrees; sidebending to the left was approximately 30 degrees and caused pain in the right buttocks; sidebending and trunk rotation to the right were moderately limited and did not reproduce any symptoms. The neurologic examination was negative for muscular weakness and altered sensations.

Passive testing of the lumbar spine (central posterior/anterior glides/(PAs) and sidebending) showed mild restrictions throughout the entire lumbar area, with sidebending to the left having a greater restriction than that to the right. Passive straight leg raising was restricted to approximately 60 degrees on the left and 50 degrees on the right, both limited by tight hamstring muscles. Neither the buttock pain nor the radiating leg pain was reproduced during straight leg raising. The Ober test of the tensor fasciae latae was positive on the right only. This positive test was consistent with the continuation of the fascial restrictions located about the right pelvis. The fascia lata is continuous with the pectineal fascia and fascia iliaca. The Thomas test for the iliopsoas was minimally positive bilaterally. Dorsiflexion of the ankle was within the normal range, both passively and actively.

Palpation of the right buttock revealed a tender and tight piriformis; the left side was tight but not tender. A trigger point was present in the right piriformis, which reproduced the referred pain down into the calf. The right iliopsoas muscle was tender and tight to palpation. The erector spinae muscles along the lumbar spine and the thoracolumbar fascia were restricted in mobility and minimally tender to deep palpation.

Treatment Program

Since the patient's primary goal was to be able to participate in sports occasionally without pain and to reduce the episodic periods of pain, the initial treatment program consisted of ultrasound, parallel and perpendicular soft tissue mobilizations, and stretching exercises of the right piriformis muscle and bilateral iliopsoas muscles. The patient was also treated with central PAs, grade III, for his lumbar spine hypomobility.

After six treatments, the patient's goal was achieved, and he could have been discharged with a positive end result. However, because of the generalized restrictions in the muscles of the lower quarter, and because the symptoms were recurrent in nature, this patient was further treated with soft tissue mobilizations, joint mobilizations, and a home exercise program intended to diminish the restrictions in his soft tissues and reverse the adaptive shortening of the involved muscles. The soft tissue techniques used to treat the muscle restrictions included strumming, perpendicular strokes, and parallel strokes to the hamstrings and erector spinae muscles and parallel stroking of the iliotibial band. These techniques are described in detail in the following section. The joint hypomobility in the lumbar spine was treated with accessory and physiologic grade III central PAs as described by Maitland.[31] The patient's home exercise program consisted of sustained stretching and functional activities to encourage lengthening of the back and thigh muscles. After an additional 2-week period of three treatments per week, the patient was discharged with his home program painfree, and his flexibility was greatly improved.

SOFT TISSUE MOBILIZATION

As early as 1917, Mennell[32] stated that massage is a means to the desired end of restoration of function. Massage achieves its mechanical effect "by tension on some structure which we hope to free or stretch." Perhaps this is why many therapists state that soft tissue manipulation is nothing more than massage. However, the techniques employed with soft tissue manipulation differ quite markedly from the traditional massage strokes of effleurage and tapotement. This section describes and illustrates the soft tissue mobilization treatment techniques that are most commonly employed, all of which can be used to treat soft tissue problems in the lower quarter.

Before the techniques can be explained, a brief explanation of the effects of soft tissue manipulation should be presented. As soft tissue mobilization is being implemented, which tissues are being affected, and what is changing in the tissues?

Chapter 1 contains a detailed explanation of the different types of connective tissues found in the body. According to Calliet,[33] connective tissue functions to create "restraining mechanisms of moving parts by the formation of bands, pulleys, and check ligaments," and "furnishes sites for attachment of muscles." The types of connective tissue that Calliet is referring to are regular and irregular dense connective tissues. Examples of regular connective tissue are fascia, ligaments, and tendons; examples of irregular dense connective tissue are perimysium and epimysium, the connective tissue that surrounds the fasciculi and the entire muscle and is continuous with the muscle's tendon. Soft tissue mobilization primarily attempts to influence these tissues to improve their mobility.

Tabary and colleagues[34] demonstrated that muscles respond to external stress by adding sarcomeres, but they did not discuss what happens to the associated connective tissues. Arem and Madden[35] showed that new scar tissue, which is connective tissue, can be remodeled to make the collagenous fibers of the scar become closely aligned and parallel to the direction of external forces. Applying inductive reasoning to these studies, it appears that Gratz[36] was correct in his thinking when he wrote, "Clinically it is believed that impaired functions of the fascial planes of the lower part of the back and thigh may be caused by fascial adhesions interfering with the normal translatory motion of the muscles which the planes enclose and secondarily involving the nerves." Therefore, it seems reasonable that soft tissue mobilization can be beneficial to patients who demonstrate loss of function because of adaptive shortening of muscle or adhesions in any of the tissues associated with movement.

Other possibilities for explaining the effects of soft tissue mobilization include the treatment of trigger points, described by Travell and Simons[27]; myostatic contractures, first described by Ransom and Dixon[37] and expanded by Tardieu et al.[38]; and pseudomyostatic contractures, first explained by Cummings.[39] Since the literature is inconsistent at present, and available research does not clearly explain how connective tissue is changed with soft tissue mobilization, practitioners must rely upon clinical experience until further research is published.

TREATMENT TECHNIQUES

Many of the concepts and treatment techniques described here are the work of Greg Johnson and Vicki Saliba[40] from the Institute of Physical Art, who teach continuing education programs throughout the United States. It is beyond the scope of this chapter to describe in detail the different components of the evaluation process and why each is important to the total evaluation and management of each patient; the chapters on examination of specific upper and lower quarter segments explain evaluation techniques.

General Principles

1. The choice of which soft tissue mobilization treatment technique to employ is based upon a thorough evaluation of the patient to identify restrictions in the soft tissues as well as other problems in the musculoskeletal system.
2. The patient must be comfortably and properly positioned to achieve support for all body parts and general relaxation.

A muscle cannot be mechanically deformed (i.e., by the application of soft tissue mobilization) if it is in an active state of contraction. In addition, muscle tissue cannot be stimulated to add sarcomeres while it is actively contracted. Therefore, proper positioning is a crucial aspect of effective treatment.

3. The tissues being treated must be placed in the desired degree of tension during the application of soft tissue mobilization.

Muscle and connective tissues can be placed in varying degrees of stress or tension. They can be placed in a shortened or slack position, in midposition, or in a lengthened position. Factors that influence the degree of tension include the amount of tenderness that is present during palpation of the tissue, the reactivity of the tissue during and after treatment, and the nature of the tissue dysfunction.

4. The patient's condition must be considered as the treatment program is being devised and implemented.

Patients with recent trauma and an acute dysfunction should be treated less aggressively than patients who have a chronic dysfunction. The depth of the treatment should be less for an acute condition.

Types of Contact

The types of contact or grips that are used with soft tissue mobilization can be classified as either general or specific. General contacts include the therapist's olecranon, the base of the hand, the lateral border of the hand, the dorsum of the proximal interphalangeal or metacarpophalangeal joints, and the lateral crest or flexor surface of the forearm. Specific points of contact include the thumb and the ends of the fingers.

Methods of Application

Techniques can be applied either with oscillations or in a sustained manner. The oscillations are similar to Maitland's[31] grade III or IV treatment techniques. Sustained pressures are low-intensity stretches lasting up to 2 minutes.

Soft tissue mobilization techniques can be applied either parallel or perpendicular to the fibers of the tissue being treated. Muscles that are guarding or splinting seem to respond better to parallel stroking, whereas muscles that have adaptively short-ened or have adhesions respond better to perpendicular strokes.

Techniques can be performed with the therapist either pulling the contact point back toward his or her body or pushing away from his or her body.

Techniques can be performed as the patient is lying quietly and still on the treatment table, or the therapist can passively oscillate the trunk or body part in a slow rhythmic manner as the soft tissue mobilization stroke is being applied. The slow associated oscillations are used to facilitate relaxation by the patient as the treatment is being given. Patients can also be requested to actively contract a muscle while a technique is being applied.

Specific Techniques

Parallel stroking of the body part, as pictured in Figure 13-13, can be performed using any combination of methods of application and types of contact described above. The stroke pictured is a parallel stroke, pushing into a restriction of the gastrocnemius-soleus muscles while the muscles are held in the lengthened position. The depth of this stroke can be increased with each repetition, depending on the response of the patient and whether it is indicated for the dysfunction. This stroke can be applied in the middle of the muscle or along its

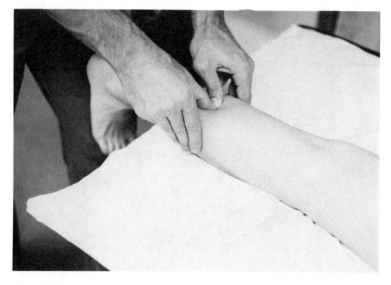

Fig. 13-13. Soft tissue mobilization in which the technique is being applied parallel to the fibers of the muscle. Pressure is applied, pushing into the restriction. The use of a skin lubricant makes this technique much more tolerable for the patient.

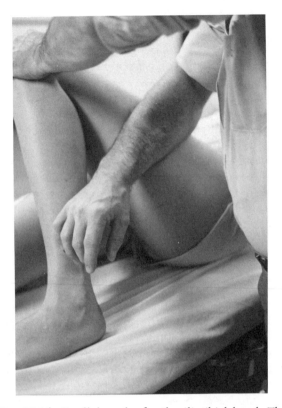

Fig. 13-14. Parallel stroke for the iliotibial band. The flexor surface of the forearm is used to apply pressure and slide from proximal to distal along the length of the iliotibial band while it is held in a position of mild stress.

border to facilitate movement independent of the adjacent structures.

Figure 13-14 demonstrates a parallel stroke, with a general contact approach to a restricted iliotibial band. The flexor surface of the forearm is used to slide down the proximal two-thirds of the band to place a lengthening stress on this dense connective tissue. This stroke is repeated with increasingly deeper pressure for each stroke.

Perpendicular strokes can be performed on fascia or contractile tissue, using any of the methods of application and types of contact described above. Figure 13-15 illustrates a perpendicular stroke being applied to the medial hamstrings. This application would be used to mobilize an intramuscular or intermuscular adhesion. The therapist should work directly over as well above and below the restriction to avoid overstimulation of the problem area.

The J stroke is used primarily to mobilize restrictions in the skin or subcutaneous fascia. Figure 13-16 demonstrates the application of the J stroke over the medial femoral epicondyle to improve skin mobility. In this case, the skin is being stabilized as the fingers are pushed away from the therapist; the technique could be reversed so that the fingers are pulled toward the therapist. The unlocking spiral (i.e., the curve of the J) is important to this stroke because it places a shear force on the restriction to

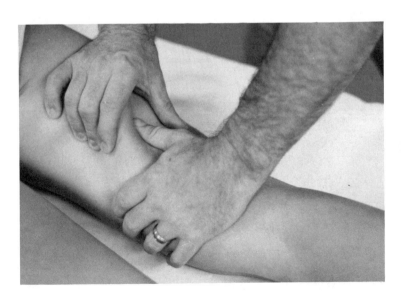

Fig. 13-15. Perpendicular stroke. Techniques that apply a perpendicular stress to the fibers of the tissue being treated are primarily indicated to mobilize an adhesion or restriction.

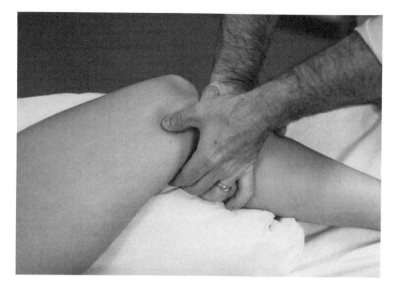

Fig. 13-16. The J stroke, a modified parallel stroke in which a torsional stress is applied over the restriction. The shearing force is directed into the restriction to improve mobility of the skin or superficial fascia.

facilitate its lengthening. This stroke can also be used to treat a restriction on either side of the achilles tendon or anywhere in the lower limb that skin mobility is important.

Skin rolling, as depicted in Figure 13-17, is also a very effective technique to improve skin mobility. To perform this technique, slide the thumbs along over the skin as the fingers are alternately flexed to pick up and push the skin back against the thumbs. The patient may experience some burning discomfort during application of this technique.

Strumming is a very effective technique to encourage lengthening of an adaptively shortened muscle. As demonstrated in Figure 13-18, the fingertips of both hands are moved back and forth across the muscle, the lateral hamstring in this case, to deform it with a perpendicular stress. When the muscle is stressed to its limit, it is allowed to glide under the fingers and "pop" back into its resting position. This technique is performed in a rhythmic oscillation for 1 to 2 minutes, with the points of contact varying up and down the length of the mus-

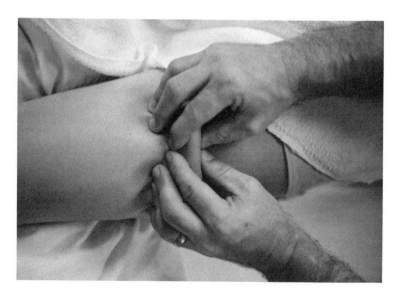

Fig. 13-17. Skin rolling. The thumbs slide along over the skin as the fingers are alternately flexed to lift the skin and push it back toward the thumbs. The end result is an area of skin that is pulled away from the underlying connective tissues.

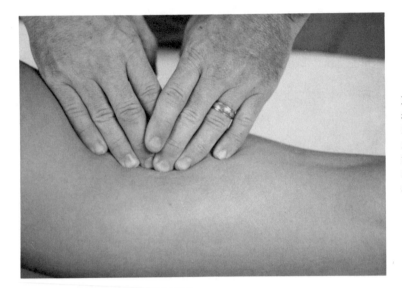

Fig. 13-18. Strumming. Firm pressure is applied perpendicular to a muscle to push it away from its resting position. When the muscle is pushed to its limit, it is allowed to "pop" back under the fingers. The technique is analogous to strumming the strings of a guitar.

cle. The amount of vertical pressure applied to the muscle during this technique should vary according to the tolerance of the patient and the restriction of the muscle. Associated oscillations are commonly superimposed over strumming to facilitate relaxation of the patient.

Another very beneficial technique is what Johnson and Saliba (personal communication, 1985) call clearing around bony landmarks. For the lower quarter, this technique improves the mobility of the superficial and deep tissues surrounding the greater trochanter, the crest of the ilium, the patella, the femoral condyles, and the malleoli of the ankle. Clearing of the bony landmarks is performed using a combination of parallel and perpendicular strokes, which are applied progressively deeper with each repetition.

Cyriax[41] advocated and described the use of deep friction massage to treat isolated painful structures and restrictions. Cummings (personal communication, 1985) described a variation of deep frictions, which he calls traditional frictions and which are very effective for localized, chronic inflammation in dense connective tissues. Traditional frictions, as pictured in Figure 13-19, are performed in much the same manner as Cyriax's[41] deep friction massage in that the exact point of tenderness must be located with palpation, the therapist's point of contact and the patient's skin must move together over the

deeper tissues, and the friction should be applied perpendicular to the fibers of the structure being treated. Once the point of tenderness is located, the therapist applies a graded pressure to the tender spot to stimulate a mild but distinct pain in the tissue. While maintaining this precise pressure, friction is initiated with a back-and-forth movement over the tender spot. The friction is applied only over the tender area; neither the pressure nor the friction should be exerted while moving on and off of the painful structure. Within 15 seconds of initiating the friction, the patient should be asked to describe the pain: "Is the pain changing?" If the pain is getting worse, maintain the constant pressure and continue for up to 1 minute. If the pain continues to worsen during this period, the technique should be discontinued. If the pain diminishes, continue the frictions with the constant pressure until the pain completely subsides. The therapist should ask the patient on a repetitive basis whether the pain is changing. Once the pain has subsided, the therapist should then increase the pressure to again stimulate a mild but distinct pain in the tissue, and continue to apply friction until the pain again subsides. This process is repeated for up to 3 minutes, until additional pressure does not result in a further compression of the tissue. This treatment should be performed daily, and positive results should be attained within three or four treatments. Patients such as

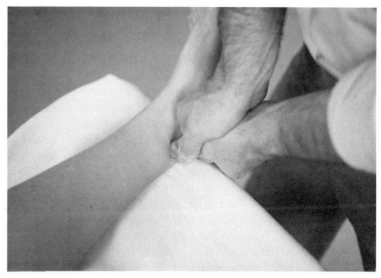

Fig. 13-19. Traditional frictions. Direct, perpendicular pressure is applied to a localized point of tenderness in dense connective tissue. The technique is only effective if the amount of pain perceived by the patient is limited to a minimal level and the frictions are only applied over the affected area.

runners who have chronic overuse syndromes should be instructed to perform the friction technique on themselves.

Another technique described by Cummings (personal communication, 1985) is what he calls "Dutch trigger point massage." This technique combines the concepts of ischemic compression from Travell and Simons,[27] massage of pressure points from Sohier,[42] and strain-counterstrain from osteopathy to create a muscle trigger point massage that is painless and effective. After traditional massage techniques have been employed to facilitate muscle relaxation, palpation is used to isolate the trigger point, which will feel like a small mass within the muscle. The joints associated with the muscle are positioned so that the muscle is placed in a loosened position. Using the ends of the thumbs as the point of contact, light pressure is applied directly over the trigger point until the small mass can be felt by the therapist. The patient should not experience any pain at this point; if pain is present, the pressure is reduced. This technique is completely painless.

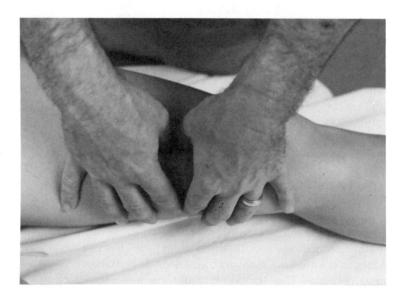

Fig. 13-20. Dutch trigger point massage. Light and painless pressure is applied directly over a muscle trigger point. This pressure is maintained until the trigger point begins to diminish, at which time the pressure is increased to "follow" the trigger point.

The light pressure is maintained over the trigger point, and after a brief period of time the mass will slowly begin to diminish. The pressure should be slowly increased to maintain the light pressure on the trigger point as it decreases in size, but the patient should not experience any pain. After approximately 3 minutes, the small mass initially palpated in the muscle should no longer be present, and the amount of pressure will have increased until the therapist's thumb is deeply depressed in the muscle tissue. The amount of pressure may have slowly increased up to 20 to 30 pounds. The pressure is slowly released, and the trigger point should be gone. If the trigger point is what Travell calls a primary myofascial trigger point, this technique should be very beneficial. If it returns, the technique has not been successful, and the patient will experience some soreness. Most likely the trigger point is not the primary source of the problem. Figure 13-20 illustrates the application of this technique on a trigger point located in the vastus medialis.

All of the soft tissue mobilization techniques described can be applied to most areas of soft tissue dysfunction throughout the body. This list of techniques is not meant to be exhaustive, but to present the more common techniques that can be directly applied to the lower quarter.

SUMMARY

Evaluation of the lower quarter requires examination of all soft tissue structures and involved synovial joints that comprise this complex chain. This chapter has emphasized the importance of recognizing the interrelationships and interdependency of the lower quarter structures. Fourteen two-joint muscles and their related connective tissue structures were reviewed. The combined effect of muscle, tendon, ligaments, fascia, and nerves produces coordinated intersegmental movement of the lower quarter.

The kinematics of the lower quarter was reviewed specific to segmental rotations in the three body planes. Rotations occur throughout the lower quarter during functional activities such as walking and running. The transverse rotations were described as the most extensive interconnecting movements throughout the lower quarter. Studies demonstrate that rotations in the transverse plane during walking start in the upper thoracic spine. The talus has been described as the torque convertor, converting the transverse rotations of the lower quarter into sagittal and frontal plane movements. This conversion of the transverse rotations allows coordinated intersegmental movement during walking and running.

It is important for the clinician to recognize the interrelationships and interdependency of the structures and movements in the lower quarter. Dysfunction of one link in the lower kinetic chain can produce muscle imbalances, altered alignment, and abnormal mechanics throughout the lower quarter. Evaluation and treatment of all the links in the lower quarter are necessary to restore normal function.

REFERENCES

1. Dempster WT: Mechanism of shoulder movement. Arch Phys Med Rehab 46A:49, 1965
2. Steindler A: Kinesiology of the Human Body. Charles C Thomas, Springfield, IL, 1966
3. Kendall HO, Kendal FP, Boynton DA: Posture and Pain. Robert E Krieger, Huntington, NY, 1977
4. Rasch PJ, Burke RK: Kinesiology and Applied Anatomy. Lea & Febiger, Philadelphia, 1974
5. Warwick R, Williams PL (eds): Gray's Anatomy. 35th British Ed. WB Saunders, Philadelphia, 1973
6. Pratt WA: The lumbopelvic torsion syndrome. JAOA 51:335, 1952
7. Tepoorten BA: The piriformis muscle. JAOA 69:126, 1969
8. Retzlaff EW, Berry AH, Haight AS, et al: The piriformis muscle syndrome. JAOA 73:55, 1974
9. Pace JB, Nagle D: Piriform syndrome. West J Med 124:435, 1976
10. Hollinshead WH: Buttock, hip joint and thigh. p. 108. In Hollinshead WH: Anatomy for Surgeons: The Back and Limbs. Hoeber Medical Division, Harper & Row, New York, 1969
11. Gardner E, Gray D, O'Rahilly R: Anatomy: A Regional Study of Human Structure. WB Saunders, Philadelphia, 1967
12. Cathie AG: The influence of the lower extremities upon the structural integrity of the body. JAOA 49:443, 1950

13. Root ML, Orien WP, Weed JN: Clinical Biomechanics. Vol. 11. Normal and Abnormal Function of the Foot. Clinical Biomechanics, Los Angeles, 1977
14. Inman VT, Ralston HJ, Todd F: Human Walking. Williams & Wilkins, Baltimore, 1981
15. Saunders M, Inman VT, Eberhart HD: The major determinants in normal and pathological gait. J Bone Joint Surg 35A:543, 1953
16. Subotnick SI: Podiatric Sports Medicine. Futura, New York, 1979
17. Cavanagh PP: The biomechanics of lower extremity action in distance running. Foot Ankle 7:197, 1987
18. Gregerson GG, Lucas DB: An in vivo study of the axial rotation of the human thoracolumbar spine. J Bone Joint Surg 57A:759, 1975
19. Kendall FP, McCreary EK: Muscles: Testing and Function. Williams & Wilkins, Baltimore, 1983
20. Reid DC, Burnham RC, Saboe LA, Kushner SF: Lower extremity flexibility patterns in classical ballet dancers and their correlation to lateral hip and knee injuries. Am J Sports Med 15:347, 1987
21. Yates A, Smith MA: Musculo-skeletal pain after trauma. In Wall PD, Melzack R (eds): Textbook of Pain. Churchill Livingstone, Edinburgh, 1984
22. Simons DG, Travell FG: Myofascial pain syndrome. In Wall PD, Melzack R (eds): Textbook of Pain. Churchill Livingstone, Edinburgh, 1984
23. O'Brien JP: Mechanisms of spinal pain. In Wall PD, Melzack R (eds): Textbook of Pain. Churchill Livingstone, Edinburgh, 1984
24. McRae R: Clinical Orthopaedic Examination. Churchill Livingstone, Edinburgh, 1983
25. Cyriax J: Textbook of Orthopaedic Medicine. Vol. I. Diagnosis of Soft Tissue Lesions. Williams & Wilkins, Baltimore, 1976
26. Clayton L (ed): Taber's Cyclopedic Medical Dictionary. FA Davis, Philadelphia, 1977
27. Travell JG, Simons DG: Myofascial Pain and Dysfunction. The Trigger Point Manual. Williams & Wilkins, Baltimore, 1983
28. Harris RL, Beath T: Hypermobile flatfoot with short tendo achilles. J Bone Joint Surg 30A:116, 1948
29. Pratt WA: The pronation syndrome. p. 112. In Academy of Applied Osteopathy Yearbook. Edwards Brothers, Ann Arbor, Michigan, 1951
30. Michael R, Holder L: The soleus syndrome: a cause of medial tibial stress (shin splints). Am J Sports Med 13:87, 1985
31. Maitland GD: Vertebral Manipulation. 5th Ed. Butterworths, London, 1986
32. Mennell JB: Physical treatment by movement, manipulation and massage. 3rd Ed. Blakiston, Philadelphia, 1934
33. Cailliet R: Soft tissue pain and disability. FA Davis, Philadelphia, 1977
34. Tabary JC, Tabary C, Tardieu C, et al: Physiological and structural changes in cat's soleus muscle due to immobilization at different lengths by plaster casts. J Physiol 224:231, 1972
35. Arem AJ, Madden JW: Effects of stress on healing wounds: 1. Intermittent noncyclical tension. J Surg Res 20:93, 1976
36. Gratz CM: Biomechanical studies of fibrous tissues applied to fascial surgery. Arch Surg 34(3):461, 1937
37. Ransom SW, Dixon HH: Elasticity and ductility of muscle in myostatic contracture caused by tetanus toxin. Am J Physiol 86:312, 1928
38. Tardieu C, de la Tour CH, Bret MD, Tardieu G: Muscle hypoextensibility in children with cerebral palsy: I. Clinical and experimental observations. Arch Phys Med Rehab 63(3):97, 1982
39. Cummings G: Orthopedics Series. Vol. II. Selection of Treatment of Soft Tissue Contractures. Unpublished manuscript, 1984
40. Johnson G, Saliba V: Functional Orthopedics I & II: Course Notes. The Institute of Physical Art, Fairfax CA, 1984
41. Cyriax J: Textbook of Orthopaedic Medicine. 11th Ed. Vol. II: Treatment by Manipulation, Massage and Injection. Bailliere Tindall, Philadelphia, 1984
42. Sohier R: Kinesitherapy of the Shoulder. John Wright & Sons, Bristol, 1967
43. Devinsky O, Feldmann E: Examination of the Cranial and Peripheral Nerves. Churchill Livingstone, New York, 1988

14

Kinematics and Kinetics During Gait

DAVID TIBERIO
GARY W. GRAY

Human locomotion is an exquisite interaction of the body's neurologic, musculoskeletal, and cardiopulmonary systems. No one has to teach human beings how to walk or run. In fact, the ability to walk is considered by some authorities to be the product of programmed motor responses occurring at the spinal cord level.[1] Once acquired through the "practice" of normal development, human locomotion occurs at a subconscious level. During walking or running, there is no actual volitional activation of muscles. Even adjustments or alterations in our walking pattern, such as stepping off a curb, are responses to visual stimuli that we barely notice.

This lack of conscious learning, although quite amazing, works against the practitioner who tries to evaluate and rehabilitate patients with locomotor dysfunction. Walking is not a product of conscious practice that can be imparted to a patient in the way certain athletic skills can. In order to effectively evaluate and rehabilitate patients with locomotor dysfunction, practitioners must acquire knowledge regarding the joint motions (kinematics) and muscle forces (kinetics) during walking and running.

ENERGY EXPENDITURE

Human locomotion is a very efficient activity. The major energy-expending activities of locomotion relate to the body's center of mass. As the body moves forward, the center of mass moves from side to side and up and down. Because of the force of gravity, most of the energy is spent lifting up the center of mass, and catching it as it falls. Therefore, the efficiency of the human locomotor system lies in the body's abilities to minimize the vertical and horizontal displacements, to smooth the reversal of motion, and to translate as much energy as possible into forward motion.

In an effort to determine what factors contribute to locomotor efficiency, Saunders et al.[2] synthesized the major research findings of a number of studies. Their work produced the six "determinants" of gait: pelvic rotation, pelvic tilt, knee flexion in stance, the foot mechanism, the knee mechanism, and lateral displacement of the pelvis. Collectively, they serve to decrease the arcs through which the center of mass must travel, and to smooth the transition from one direction to another. These determinants are not the only contributors to efficient locomotion, but the clinician should understand that abnormal function at any joint in the lower quarter will disrupt the normal locomotion pattern and increase energy expenditure.

Practitioners must gain knowledge of, and recognize the difference between, joint position and joint motion. Joint motion is the movement of the bones of a joint toward one extreme of the range of motion. For example, dorsiflex*ion* is movement of the dorsum of the foot toward the leg. The suffixes *-ion* and *-ing* denote motion. Position, on the other hand, refers to the alignment of the bones compared to a reference point. The reference point for the ankle is zero (90 degree position). If the bones are aligned on one side of this reference point the ankle is dorsiflex*ed*; if on the other side it is plantar flex*ed*. The suffix -*ed* (or -*us*) infers a joint position at a particular time.

The fact that motion and position are different concepts becomes crystallized when one considers that ankle motion can be one of dorsiflex*ion*, even though the joint at that instant may be in a plantar flex*ed* position. The difference is also important at the subtalar joint when considering the primary functions of the foot. Certain functions are dependent upon subtalar joint position (supinat*ed*, pronat*ed*), whereas other functions are dependent upon motion (supinat*ion*, pronat*ion*).

CLOSED CHAIN MOTION

Joint motion is usually described in the context of open chain motion. Open chain motion occurs when the proximal bone segment of a joint is fixed, and the distal bone segment is free to move. Unfortunately, most clinically significant daily activities that involve the lower extremities occur when the foot is on the ground. Whenever the distal bone segment (in this case the foot) is fixed, closed chain motion occurs. In closed chain motion there is motion on both sides of the joint being evaluated. With open chain motion, the motion occurs distal to the joint being evaluated and studied. Closed chain motion alters the nature of muscle contractions as well as bone motion. An example of this is dorsiflexion of the ankle joint. During open chain dorsiflexion, the dorsum of the foot moves up toward the lower leg. Closed chain dorsiflexion of the ankle during gait occurs when the tibia moves forward while the foot remains stationary on the ground. This motion is not produced by contraction of the dorsiflexor muscles. Rather the dorsiflexion results from forward movement of the lower leg over the foot. The muscles that produce plantar flexion (the calf group) are active during closed chain dorsiflexion in order to eccentrically control this motion.

An understanding of closed chain motion of the subtalar joint is particularly important because of its effect on the proximal bone segments of the lower quarter. In closed chain pronation the calcaneus and the rest of the foot will still evert, abduct, and dorsiflex. As the calcaneus everts, the talus slides in a distal and medial direction; the head of the talus adducts and plantar flexes, with a resultant internal rotation of the body of the talus.[3] Because the ankle joint does not allow a significant amount of rotation in the transverse plane, the rotation of the body of the talus forces the ankle to rotate in the same direction. This creates an obligatory internal rotation of the lower leg whenever subtalar joint pronation occurs.[3-6] Closed chain supination of the subtalar joint produces an obligatory external rotation of the lower leg. These obligatory rotations will become important to appreciate during the discussion of knee motion and hip motion during gait.

It is also important to note the effect that closed chain pronation and supination at the subtalar joint have on arch height. The axis of the subtalar joint can vary significantly. Isman and Inman found that the pitch of axes can range from 20 to 60 degrees up from the horizontal.[7] These differences in the subtalar joint axis correlate with different inclination angles of the calcaneus and produce different arch heights. A higher pitch to the axis produces a high architecture to the foot, whereas a low inclination angle creates a lower architecture. Regardless of the arch height, motion of the subtalar joint creates a dynamic change in arch height. As the head of the talus adducts and plantar flexes during closed chain pronation, the arch height decreases. With closed chain supination, as the head of the talus abducts and dorsiflexes, the arch height relatively increases.[3,8] The practical implication of this motion is that the arch height is a response to motion at the subtalar joint as well as a response to motion at the midtarsal joint, which is influenced by the subtalar joint. Closed chain pronation not only lowers the arch, but also lowers the pelvis by creating a functional decrease in leg length. If subtalar joint motion is asymmetrical, then the motion of the pelvis will be asymmetrical; and must be assessed in all 3 planes of motion.

PRIMARY FOOT FUNCTION

Joint motion and muscle function during human locomotion are much easier to understand in the context of the primary functions of the foot. The foot has three basic functions. First, it must adapt to ground surfaces that may not be level or smooth.

The ability of the foot to perform this function comes from the significant amount of motion in all three body planes that is present in the joints of the rearfoot (ankle and subtalar joint) and the forefoot (oblique and longitudinal axes of the midtarsal joint).

The ability of the forefoot to adapt to the ground depends on the midtarsal joint being mobile. In order for the midtarsal joint to be mobile, the subtalar joint must be in a pronated position. This pronated position alters the position of the talus and the calcaneus, thereby affecting the relative positions of the talonavicular and calcaneocuboid articulations. This pronated position allows for increased mobility or "unlocking" of the midtarsal joint. Therefore the ability of the midtarsal joint and the foot to adequately adapt to their environment is provided by the pronated position of the subtalar joint.

A second major function of the foot is to act as a facilitator of shock absorption as the foot hits the ground. This occurs simultaneously with the surface adaptation. As the advancing leg begins to bear weight, the ground reaction force travels up the musculoskeletal system. In order to absorb a significant portion of this force, the knee must flex. It is this knee flexion, with the concurrent eccentric contraction of the quadriceps, that dampens the ground reaction force as it travels up the musculoskeletal system. The joint mechanics of the knee dictate that when the knee flexes, an internal rotation must occur at the tibia. This component motion of internal rotation with flexion is the reversal of the well-documented external rotation with extension (locking home mechanism). This obligatory rotation of the lower leg that occurs with knee flexion is present during the first 15 to 20 degrees of motion. As was mentioned in the section on closed chain motion, internal rotation occurs with subtalar joint pronation. Therefore it is important for the subtalar joint to pronate when the knee is flexing in order for the lower leg to promote the necessary motion at both the knee and the subtalar joint. This will be discussed further as it relates to human locomotion.

The third major function of the foot is its function as a rigid lever for propulsion. In order for the heel to rise off the ground without the arch of the foot collapsing, the mobility of the midtarsal joint must be reduced. This is described as "locking" of the

midtarsal joint, and it occurs when the subtalar joint moves into a supinated position. This supinated position, by changing the relative alignment of the bones, reduces joint mobility and allows for effective propulsion. A variety of structural changes have been postulated for this reduction in midtarsal joint mobility. When the subtalar joint is in the supinated position, there is more compression and less bony mating of the articular surfaces. There also appears to be capsular and ligamentous tightening, which reduces joint play. Finally, this increased stability has been attributed to alterations in the angle of muscle forces due to increased arch height when the subtalar joint is in a supinated position. The reduction in midtarsal joint mobility, as a result of the supination of the subtalar joint, allows the foot to function as a rigid lever and allows for the propulsive mechanism off that rigid lever to be effective.

KINEMATICS OF LOCOMOTION
Gait Cycle

The basic unit of human locomotion is called the gait cycle. Repetition of this cycle allows the body to move from one place to another. A normal gait (or walking) cycle is defined as from heel-strike of one foot to heel-strike of that same foot again. Studying the component parts of the gait cycle facilitates an understanding of the practical aspects of human locomotion. Figure 14-1 depicts the cycle as divided into the time when the foot is in contact with the ground (stance) and when it is in the air (swing). The stance phase accounts for approximately 61 percent, whereas the swing phase lasts for 39 percent of the cycle.[9] To give some temporal reference to these two phases, it is advantageous to assume that the gait cycle lasts for 1 second. Stance phase then becomes slightly longer than 0.6 seconds, and swing phase lasts just less than 0.4 seconds.

It is important to consider how the motion of the other leg affects the gait cycle. Figure 14-2 shows how the stance and swing phases of each leg overlap. Part of the time both feet are on the ground. This interval is called the period of double limb support and occurs twice in each cycle. Single limb support is created when the opposite leg swings forward to renew ground contact. Each period of double limb

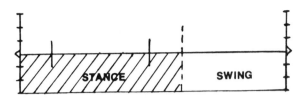

Fig. 14-1. Gait cycle divided into stance phase and swing phase. (Reproduced with permission of On-Site Biomechanical Education and Training, 1988.)

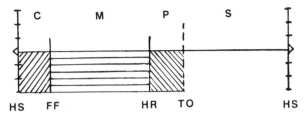

Fig. 14-3. Division of stance phase into contact, midstance, and propulsion. (Reproduced with permission of On-Site Biomechanical Education and Training, 1988.)

support lasts only about 0.11 seconds, whereas each single limb support lasts 0.39 seconds, which corresponds exactly to the swing time of the opposite leg.

Stance phase has three major subdivisions, which are determined by the manner in which the foot contacts the ground.[3,8] The stance phase of one leg is depicted in Figure 14-3. Four different events can be identified by when analyzing the foot-ground interface. These four events — heel-strike, foot-flat, heel-rise, and toe-off — divide the stance phase into three parts or phases. The period from heel-strike until the foot is flat on the surface is the contact phase. The midstance phase extends from foot-flat to heel-rise. The propulsion phase begins with heel-rise and ends with toe-off. By looking at the overlap of both legs (Fig. 14-4), it becomes apparent that as one leg propels the body forward, the other leg is receiving the body weight during contact.

Swing of one leg occurs simultaneously with midstance of the other leg. Swing can also be divided into three sections, although the divisions are more arbitrary. These three sections are most commonly called acceleration, midswing, and deceleration.

Individual Joint Motion

The patterns of limb rotation in all three planes are consistent with the primary functions of the foot and the phases of gait. By studying the joint motions separately and then detailing the kinematic links among the joints, the delicate synchronicity of human locomotion becomes evident.

The motion of the subtalar joint is shown in Figure 14-5. During the stance phase, the motion of the subtalar joint is directly related to the primary functions of the foot. The calcaneus strikes the ground on the lateral aspect, and the subtalar joint begins its pronation from a slightly supinated position. Once the subtalar joint is in a pronated position, the midtarsal joint mobility is increased, and the foot is able to adapt to uneven ground surfaces during contact phase. The closed chain pronation produces obligatory internal rotation of the tibia, which facilitates the knee flexion that is necessary for shock attenuation and smooth weight acceptance.

When the foot is flat on the ground, surface adaptation and shock attenuation are complete. The sub-

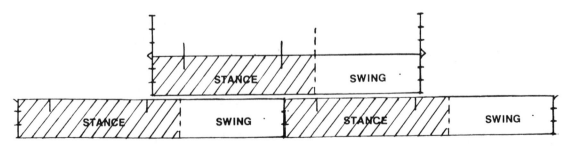

Fig. 14-2. The relationship of the stance and swing phases of each leg. Overlap of stance produces double limb support whereas swing produces single limb support. (Reproduced with permission of On-Site Biomechanical Education and Training, 1988.)

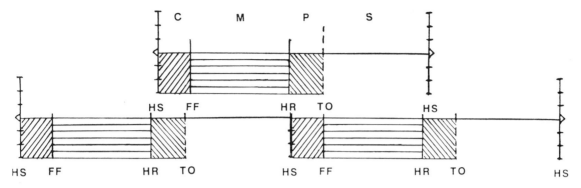

Fig. 14-4. Overlap of two legs, indicating the transfer of body weight from the back leg (propulsion) to the front leg (contact). (Reproduced with permission of On-Site Biomechanical Education and Training, 1988.)

talar joint now enters the midstance (transition) phase in changing from a mobile adaptor to a rigid lever. At foot-flat the subtalar joint is maximally pronated. Subtalar joint supination begins in order to ensure that the joint reaches its neutral position before the heel rises from the ground. As the joint passes from a pronated to a supinated position, the mobility in the midtarsal joint decreases in preparation for propulsion.

Propulsion begins when the heel rises. The transition from mobile adaptor to rigid level has occurred. The foot is now an effective lever for propelling the body forward because of the stability of the midtarsal joint gained from the supinated position of the subtalar joint. The subtalar joint continues to supinate throughout propulsion as the center of mass is accelerated forward and the body weight is transferred to the forward leg.

During swing phase, the subtalar joint moves from its maximally supinated position at toe-off to a position of slight supination just before heel-strike, at which time the cycle repeats itself.[6]

Ankle

Ankle joint motion occurs primarily in the sagittal plane. At heel-strike, the ankle is close to the neutral (or 90 degree) position (Fig. 14-6). As contact phase is initiated with heel-strike, the ankle plantar flexes until the foot is flat on the ground. During midstance phase, the lower leg moves forward over the foot. The average amount of dorsiflexion just before heel rise is 10 degrees. The degree of dorsiflexion needed for normal ambulation will vary depending on the surface inclination and heel height, as well as the forefoot structure.

Ankle dorsiflexion is quickly reversed during the propulsive phase. Plantar flexion reaches a peak at toe-off. Immediately upon toe-off, the ankle dorsiflexes to prevent toe drag. The ankle returns to the

Fig. 14-5. Motion of the subtalar joint. P, pronation; S, supination. (Reproduced with permission of On-Site Biomechanical Education and Training, 1988.)

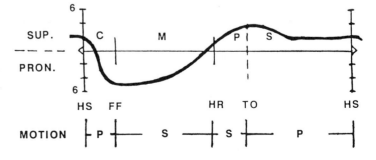

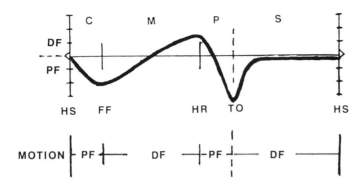

Fig. 14-6. Motion of the ankle joint. PF, plantar flexion; DF, dorsiflexion. (Reproduced with permission of On-Site Biomechanical Education and Training, 1988.)

neutral position, which it maintains until the heel strikes the ground again.[4,9]

Knee

Figure 14-7 depicts the motion of the knee joint during walking. The knee flexes to about 20 degrees during contact phase. This flexion attenuates the shock due to ground contact. Knee flexion and weight acceptance are complete at foot-flat. The knee then begins to extend as a result of the forward movement of the trunk over the foot. The knee almost attains full extension at the time of heel-rise. The knee flexes again during propulsion and continues to flex during the acceleration portion of swing. The knee then quickly extends to a minimally flexed position in preparation for heel-strike and a new cycle.[4,9]

Hip

Hip motion occurs in all three planes during the gait cycle. Figure 14-8 shows the sagittal plane motion. At heel-strike the hip is flexed about 30 degrees.

The hip begins to extend during contact phase, and this extension continues until heel-rise. The hip motion changes when propulsion begins, with flexion occurring throughout the propulsion and swing phases. At heel-strike the hip has returned to 30 degrees of flexion.[4,9]

Motion of the hip in the frontal plane (adduction and abduction) is depicted in Figure 14-9. The position of the hip at heel-strike is dictated by the width of the walking base. In spite of these variations which affect hip position, the direction of joint motion is clear. At heel-strike the pelvis and the center of gravity are moving laterally over the limb that is accepting the body weight. This lateral shift produces closed chain adduction during contact and the first half of midstance phase. Once the lateral shift is decelerated, the motion of the hip changes to abduction for the rest of stance. The path of the hip is variable during swing, but the goal is to bring the foot into proper position for heel-strike.[9]

Hip rotation in the transverse plane is depicted in Figure 14-10. Internal rotation is occurring at the hip as the leg accepts the body weight and adapts to the ground. The motion changes to external rota-

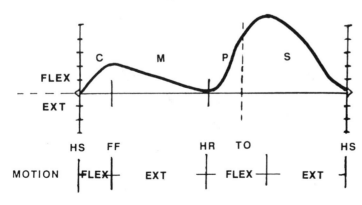

Fig. 14-7. Motion of the knee joint. (Reproduced with permission of On-Site Biomechanical Education and Training, 1988.)

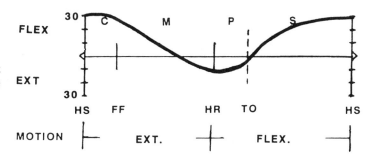

Fig. 14-8. Hip flexion and extension during gait cycle. (Reproduced with permission of On-Site Biomechanical Education and Training, 1988.)

tion during midstance and propulsion. As swing begins, the leg initiates the internal rotation that will continue when ground contact is renewed.[4,10]

Synchronicity

The transverse plane motion of all the bone segments is consistent throughout the phases of the gait cycle.[10] Figure 14-11 shows the motions of the pelvis, femur, and tibia. It is not coincidental that the motions occur in the same direction. The bone segments exhibit an exquisite synchronicity that is essential for normal human locomotion. At the bottom of Figure 14-11 the closed chain motion of the subtalar joint during stance is shown, with the obligatory tibial rotation delineated. This rotation due to subtalar joint motion is consistent with the rotation patterns in the proximal segments and demonstrates the importance of subtalar joint function on lower quarter mechanics.

It is clear that although the segments rotate in the same direction, the amount and rate of the motion are not the same across segments. If they were, there would be no joint motion except at the lumbosacral junction. Because the motions are not equal, a "relative rotation" is produced at the hip and knee joints. An example of this is the fact that the femur is internally rotating faster than the pelvis during contact phase. This produces a "relative" internal rotation at the hip joint. This comparison of the rate of movement between one bone and another is also critical at the knee joint.

Again referring to Figure 14-11, although both the tibia and the femur are internally rotating during contact phase, the tibia is moving faster than the femur. This produces a relative internal rotation at the knee, which is a component motion of knee flexion during the first 15 to 20 degrees. Knee rotation facilitates the knee flexion that is vital for shock attenuation during contact phase. During midstance phase all motions reverse: The subtalar joint supinates (external rotation), the knee extends (external rotation), and all the segments externally rotate while the tibia moves faster than the femur (relative external rotation). The synchronous linkage of the segments continues.

The subtalar joint continues to supinate (external rotation) during propulsion, but the knee flexes (internal rotation). The synchronicity seems to have disappeared, but actually it is still present. During

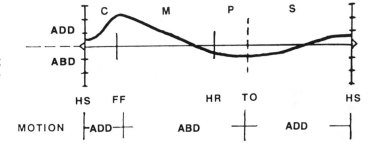

Fig. 14-9. Hip abduction and adduction during gait. (Reproduced with permission of On-Site Biomechanical Education and Training, 1988.)

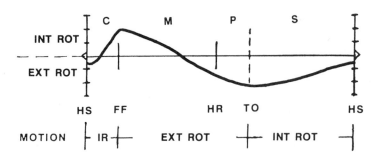

Fig. 14-10. Hip internal and external rotation during gait cycle. (Reproduced with permission of On-Site Biomechanical Education and Training, 1988.)

the beginning of propulsion the pelvis and the femur are externally rotating faster than the tibia. This produces relative internal rotation at the knee, which provides the component motion for knee flexion during the first 15 to 20 degrees of motion. Therefore, it is not biomechanically inconsistent that the subtalar joint can supinate while the knee

flexes, as long as the rate of rotation between the femur and tibia is precise.

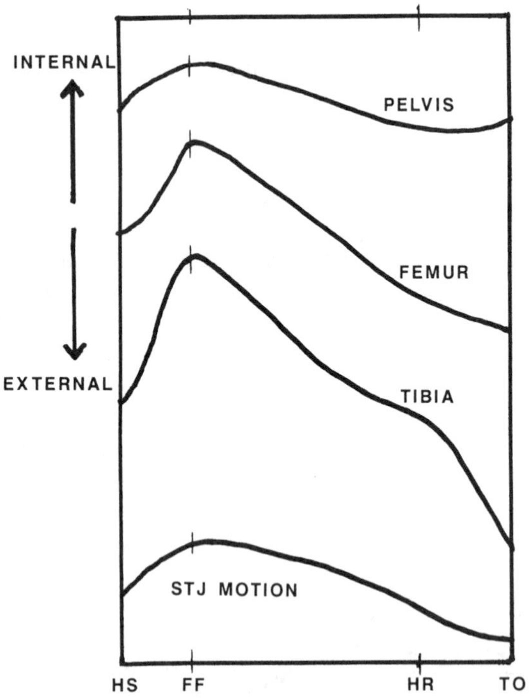

KINETICS OF LOCOMOTION
Muscle Function

The functions of muscles usually are taught on the basis of a concentric contraction when the distal segment is free to move (open chain). For example, this approach applied to the tibialis anterior muscle would describe its function as dorsiflexing the foot (concentric), or as producing the open chain action of moving the dorsum of the foot up toward the leg. Although it is certainly reasonable to learn muscle function from this perspective, it is also very limiting. Muscle function during activities in which the distal segment is fixed, thereby closing the chain, is quite different.[11]

Understanding muscle function during closed chain activities is facilitated by describing the effects of different types of muscle contractions on joint motion. A concentric contraction produces or accelerates joint motion. An eccentric contraction controls or decelerates the motion to which it is antagonistic.

Another important consideration is the function of multi-joint muscles. All of the extrinsic muscles that cross the ankle joint also have functions at the subtalar joint; many cross the midtarsal joint as well. Therefore a muscle will have simultaneous effects on more than one joint unless a synergistic contraction of another muscle neutralizes the muscle's function at one of the joints. These synergistic functions are not well understood. Therefore, the discussion of muscle function in this chapter will focus

Fig. 14-11. Rotation of the bone segments during stance phase. Steepness of slope represents rate of rotation. Motion of subtalar joint as a reference appears at the bottom of the figure. (Reproduced with permission of On-Site Biomechanical Education and Training, 1988.)

on the acceleration and deceleration of joint movement.

Ankle

The specific function of muscles is determined when knowledge of muscle anatomy and joint motion are combined, and then verified whenever possible by electromyographic research.[3,4,12-14] Figure 14-12 shows the activities of the muscles that control ankle function. During contact phase the ankle is plantar flexing, but the muscles that dorsiflex the foot are active. The actual motion is produced by the ground reaction force when the heel strikes the ground. The tibialis anterior works eccentrically to decelerate the foot's movement to the ground. Paralysis of this muscle produces the well-known foot slap.

Once midstance phase begins, the calf group becomes active. These muscles decelerate the forward movement of the tibia over the foot. The activity increases to a peak at heel-rise. At this point the calf muscles shift from an eccentric to a concentric contraction, which plantar flexes the foot. This muscle action initiates the propulsive phase. This manner of muscle function, decelerating the motion before

accelerating in the opposite direction, is frequently seen in human locomotion.

As swing begins, the ankle must dorsiflex to keep the foot from dragging. This acceleration by the anterior tibialis is followed by an isometric contraction to hold the foot in position for heel-strike, when the cycle will begin again. The function of these muscles at the subtalar joint cannot be overlooked. During contact, when the anterior tibialis is decelerating plantar flexion, it can also assist in the deceleration of subtalar joint pronation. The acceleration of supination during midstance and propulsion is assisted by the calf group contraction affecting ankle motion.

Subtalar Joint

It seems appropriate now to consider the extrinsic muscles that function primarily at the subtalar joint. The primary decelerator of pronation during contact is the posterior tibialis (Fig. 14-13). Therefore, an eccentric contraction during contact, decelerating pronation, will transition into a concentric contraction as midstance begins with the acceleration of supination at the subtalar joint.

During propulsion, subtalar joint supination con-

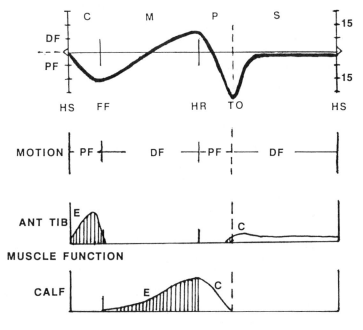

Fig. 14-12. Selected muscle function at the ankle joint. Striped area represents eccentric contraction. Open area represents concentric contraction. (Reproduced with permission of On-Site Biomechanical Education and Training, 1988.)

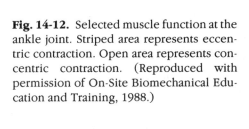

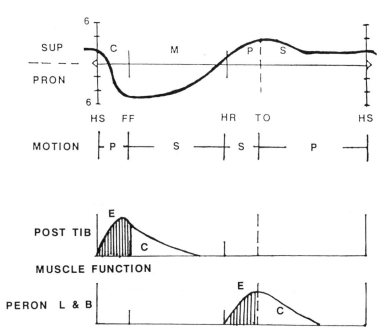

Fig. 14-13. Selected muscle function at the subtalar joint. (Reproduced with permission of On-Site Biomechanical Education and Training, 1988.)

tinues even though the activity of the posterior tibialis has ended. Now the lateral extrinsics need to be active to control and limit the amount of supination. Therefore the peroneus longus and brevis work eccentrically until swing begins, and there will probably be some concentric activity to return the subtalar joint near to its neutral position prior to heel-strike. The peroneus longus also provides important stability to the forefoot during propulsion. It allows the forefoot to maintain ground contact during subtalar joint supination and stabilizes the first metatarsal during propulsion off the hallux.

Knee

Knee flexion for shock absorption requires the quadriceps to contract eccentrically to decelerate this motion during contact phase. The quadriceps works concentrically during the beginning of mid-stance phase as the knee extends. The quadriceps becomes active again during propulsion and early swing as the knee flexes. Because the motion is flexion, this activity of the quadriceps must be eccentric.

Figure 14-14 shows that the hamstrings are active during contact phase at the same time the quadri-

ceps is working. Until now, our description of muscle activity has shown that when one muscle was active, the antagonist was inactive. The hamstrings and quadriceps exhibit a different pattern. It must be remembered that the hamstrings are fairly powerful hip extensors as well as knee flexors. Before heel-strike the hamstrings are contracting strongly to decelerate the hip flexion and knee extension. Once the heel strikes the ground and the forward movement of the leg is slowed, the hamstring activity prevents the trunk from flexing forward at the hip. The hamstrings' ability to prevent hip flexion and then accelerate hip extension is dependent on a stable distal attachment.

Hips

As the knee flexes during contact, the hamstrings' effectiveness is lost and the activity gradually ceases. In order to complete hip extension the body "substitutes" the gluteus maximus for the hamstrings, because the maximus is a single-joint muscle. Figure 14-15 shows how the activity of the gluteus maximus rises correspondingly to the decrease in hamstring activity. One might logically question why the gluteus maximus is not active from the be-

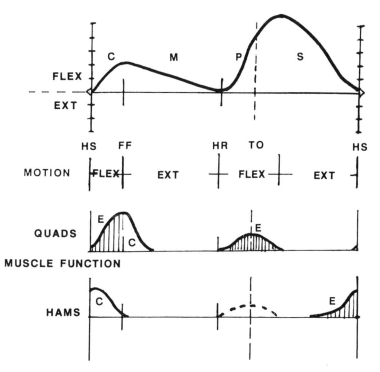

Fig. 14-14. Selected muscle function at the knee joint. (Reproduced with permission of On-Site Biomechanical Education and Training, 1988.)

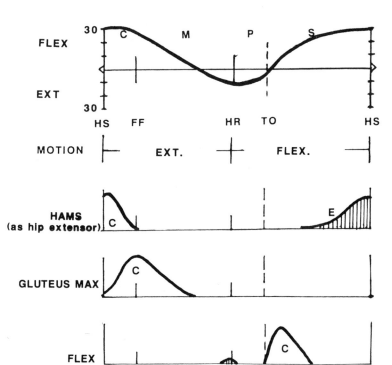

Fig. 14-15. Selected muscle function at the hip joint in the sagittal plane. (Reproduced with permission of On-Site Biomechanical Education and Training, 1988.)

ginning of hip extension. The hamstrings, being decelerators of both knee extension and hip flexion, are already active during the end of swing. It is efficient to use the already active hamstrings as hip extensors by changing to a concentric contraction upon heel-strike. This demonstrates the delicate interplay between joints and muscle that is present during efficient locomotion.

The primary role of the hip flexors is to accelerate the leg forward at toe-off. This concentric activity ceases by midswing. The hip flexors are also active just before heel-rise, apparently to limit the amount of hip extension, which peaks at this time.

The abductors of the hip begin to activate once the heel strikes the ground (Fig. 14-16), and their activity peaks during single limb support. The initial activity is eccentric, as the pelvis is shifting laterally over the stance leg. Once this lateral displacement is decelerated, the abductors accelerate the pelvis back toward the opposite side. The hip adductors function at two times during the cycle. The purpose of these contractions is not clear, but the first may decelerate the abduction occurring as the body weight shifts to the other leg. The second activity during swing may ensure proper foot placement at heel-strike. Figure 14-16 shows the activity of both groups of muscles that control the hip in the frontal plane. It may be imagined as the abductors of each hip playing catch with the center of gravity. One side "catches" the center of gravity eccentrically and then "throws" it back concentrically to the opposite side, which repeats the catch and throw.

There is not a lot known about the hip rotator muscles, but given the anatomic function of these muscles and the joint motions during gait, it would seem logical that the external rotators would work to decelerate the internal limb rotation during contact phase and to accelerate external rotation during midstance.

Ground Reaction Forces

In addition to muscle forces, the ground reaction forces deserve attention. Ground reaction forces are created when gravity (and sometimes muscles) force the body against the ground, and the ground pushes back as predicted by Newton's third law. The "collision" between the foot and the ground produces both translation (linear forces) and rotations (torques). These are measured by force plates over which subjects walk. In this section only the translation or linear forces are presented. Most readers are familiar with the vertical ground reaction force. Figure 14-17 shows a typical vertical ground reaction force pattern for walking.[2,3,15-17] There are two peaks to this force, one at maximum limb loading during weight acceptance and the second during propulsion. The second peak is often higher if the calf contraction at heel-rise is powerful and if the

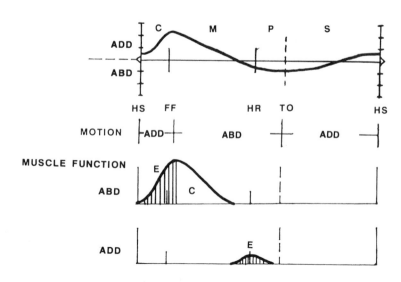

Fig. 14-16. Function of muscle groups at the hip joint in the frontal plane. (Reproduced with permission of On-Site Biomechanical Education and Training, 1988.)

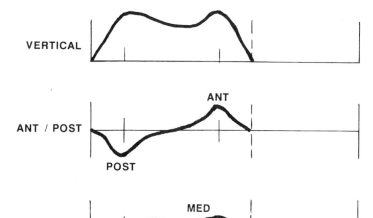

Fig. 14-17. Ground reaction forces in three planes. The forces are equal in magnitude, but opposite in direction to the forces applied by the body to the ground. (Reproduced with permission of On-Site Biomechanical Education and Training, 1988.)

forefoot is stable and the foot is functioning as a rigid lever.

There is also a horizontal ground reaction force that is directed anteroposteriorly (fore and aft). This reaction force (Fig. 14-17) will be posterior when the heel strikes the ground, and anterior during propulsion. A third ground reaction force occurs in a mediolateral direction. As the leg strikes the ground and internally rotates, the reaction force is directed laterally, but during propulsion it shifts to a medial direction. Gravity, the ground reaction forces, and muscle contractions combine to exert large forces on the articular surfaces of the joints. This topic is beyond the scope of this chapter, but the reader should be aware that the majority of these joint compressive forces during dynamic activity are due to muscle contraction. The forces have been calculated to reach 2 to 3 times body weight at the hip and tibiofemoral joint during normal walking.[17]

Running

Running is a natural form of human locomotion. As the speed of walking increases, the time during which both legs are on the ground (double leg support) decreases. As speed of locomotion continues to increase, the stance leg will toe off before the swinging leg contacts the surface. Double leg support is eliminated and an airborne period is created. The locomotion is now running.

As would be expected, as the cycle time decreases, stance time decreases both absolutely and as a percentage of the cycle. The range of motion at the joints increases.[12] The increase in motion combined with a decrease in cycle time means that the speed of the joint motion increases dramatically. The muscles are required to decelerate more motion in a shorter period of time. In some cases the mode of muscle function (eccentric or concentric) changes.

Since the advent of the running boom, running has been studied extensively. Walking was used as a reference for these studies, and emphasis was placed on the differences between walking and running. Although understanding these differences is important, just as crucial is an appreciation of the similarities between these two forms of human locomotion. During running the primary function of the foot and lower leg remains the same. The leg must accept the body weight, the foot must adapt to the ground, and the ground reaction force must be attenuated. Immediately thereafter the body weight moves forward, the knee begins to extend, and the foot propels the body forward. Joint motions consistent with these functions are present in both walking and running.[18] At ground contact the subtalar joint pronates for surface adaption, the knee flexes for shock absorption, and the leg internally rotates to allow synchronous motion from the pelvis down to the foot. The motions reverse during propulsion. The subtalar joint supinates to create the rigid lever, the knee extends to move the body forward, and the leg externally rotates to maintain synchronicity of the joints and to allow the pelvis to rotate with the swing of the opposite leg. The midstance or transition phase occurs rapidly as the stance phase time decreases.

The ground reaction forces are also dramatically increased. Figure 14-17 has shown that the vertical ground reaction force for walking was just in excess of 1 body weight equivalent. Running research has shown that this force increases as the speed of running increases and is in the range of 2 to 3.5 times body weight.[18-20] As in walking, there appear to be two peaks of the ground reaction force in most runners (sprinters may be the exception). The impact peak is gradual in some subjects, but exhibits a sharp spike in others. In addition, during running the anteroposterior shear force increases.

In 1980 Brody[21] described three different styles of running based on how the foot achieves ground contact. The foot can either (1) simulate walking with a heel-to-toe gait, (2) land simultaneously on the heel and the forefoot, or (3) land with a toe-to-heel sequence. This and other articles have associated these different styles with the speed of running. Although there is some correlation, it would be a mistake to assume that a runner uses a particular style based solely on the speed of running.

These different styles necessitate different motions at the ankle joint and therefore different muscle functions.[12] The heel-to-toe runner plantar flexes at the ankle on ground contact, putting more stress on the tibialis anterior. The other two styles dorsiflex upon ground contact, placing more stress on the calf group (eccentrically). The landing pattern is also likely to alter which muscles assist the posterior tibialis in decelerating pronation. It may be that, from a biomechanical and rehabilitation standpoint, the importance of different running styles lies primarily at the ankle joint, which alters the potential for different musculotendinous units to be injured.

The Role of Clinical Analysis

Analysis of human locomotion in the clinical setting is an important evaluative procedure. Identification of gait deviations during walking or running provides information that may help the practitioner determine the cause of the patient's problem and/or decide on a particular course of treatment. Historically, gait evaluations were performed visually by the practitioner. Visual gait examinations provide valuable information when performed by the trained eye. Except for the identification of muscle contractions, visual assessments provide information on the kinematic aspects of human locomotion, information that complements other components of a physical examination.

Visual gait examinations have major limitations. Certain aspects of walking and almost all aspects of running occur too quickly for the human eye and nervous system to consciously detect. Also, the information obtained by visual assessment is very subjective, and no permanent record is available for subsequent analysis. Fortunately, with the development of video cameras and recorders, a readily available, low-cost alternative to visual examination exists. The permanent record created by the videotape combined with the slow motion and freeze-frame capabilities of the videocassette recorder provide excellent clinical assessment of both walking and running.

Unfortunately, at present the standard videotape systems purchased for home use are not able to provide the type of kinematic data required by researchers. These data must be acquired and analyzed using equipment found only in specialized medical centers and research institutions. The data analysis is invariably performed by computer programs, whereas the acquisition systems vary greatly. High-speed film cameras and high-speed videotape and optic-electric systems all provide the more exact measures necessary for scientific studies.

Information about the kinetics of human locomotion (muscle function and ground reaction force) is not commonly analyzed in the clinical environment. Electromyographic and ground reaction data from force plates or multiple tranducer pads, when synchronized with kinematic data, constitute the optimal level of analysis of human locomotion.

Motion can be abnormal if (1) the amount of motion is too much or not enough, (2) it occurs too quickly or too slowly, or (3) it occurs at the wrong time. Too little motion may not allow proper dissipation of forces, which may increase joint compression; too much motion may generate excessive tensile forces on ligaments and muscle-tendon units. Motion that occurs too quickly may tax the ability of the muscle-tendon unit to decelerate the motion. Motion occurring at the wrong time will disrupt not only the primary functions of the foot, but also the synchronous movement of the entire lower quarter.

SUMMARY

Human locomotion is a sequential and synchronous activity, which, when functioning properly, is a marvelous sight to behold. Its complexity becomes apparent when dysfunctions arise which present as gait deviations, and the gait deviations cause tissue symptoms. Determining the cause of the deviation, as well as the proper treatment approach to correct the deviation, is often very difficult. Knowledge of normal human locomotion provides the template against which we compare our visual or videotape analysis. Understanding the sequential and synchronous relationships allows the clinician to find the cause of the patient's symptoms when this cause is not in the same anatomic region as the symptoms.

Abnormal gait kinematics need to be considered from three different perspectives: the amount of motion, the speed and direction (velocity) of that motion, and the sequential timing of the motion in the gait cycle. When gait deviations are discovered, there must be analyzed in reference to (1) their effect on the primary functions of the foot, and (2) the resultant tissue stresses placed on proximal structures, or compensatory motions by the proximal structure to avoid the tissue stress.

It is important for the practitioner who desires to understand and assess gait also to have a comprehensive ability to assess the various segments of the lower quarter independently in both an open chain and a closed chain position. The ability to gain segmented information and then to put this information together as a whole allows the practitioner to begin to understand the causes of the gait deviations visualized and identified. There is much we do not know about human locomotion. The intricacies and the various compensations that occur in allowing an individual to walk are beyond our abilities to effectively measure, observe, or even understand. However, as we continue to strive toward a more comprehensive understanding of the biomechanics of human locomotion, we will be better equipped to offer our patients solutions to the causes of their problems with locomotion.

REFERENCES

1. Schmidt RA: Motor Control and Learning: A Behavioral Emphasis. Human Kinetics, Champaign IL, 1982
2. Saunders JBdeCM, Inman VT, Eberhart HD: The major determinants in normal and pathological gait. J Bone Joint Surg 35A:543, 1953
3. Root ML, Orien WP, Weed JH: Normal and Abnormal Function of the Foot. Clinical Biomechanics Corp, Los Angeles, 1977
4. Inman VT, Ralston HJ, Todd F: Human Walking. Williams & Wilkins, Baltimore, 1981
5. Inman VT: The Joints of the Ankle. Williams & Wilkins, Baltimore, 1976
6. Wright DG, Desai SM, Hengerson WH: Action of the subtalar and ankle complex during the stance phase of walking. J Bone Joint Surg 46A:361, 1964
7. Isman RE, Inman VT: Anthropometric studies of the foot and ankle. Bull Prosthet Res 10–11:97, 1969
8. Sarrafian SK: Anatomy of the Foot and Ankle: Descriptive, Topographic, Functional. JB Lippincott, Philadelphia, 1983
9. Murray MP: Gait as a total pattern of movement. Am J Phys Med 46:290, 1967
10. Levens AS, Inman VT, Blosser JA: Transverse rotation of the segments of the lower extremity in locomotion. J Bone Joint Surg 30A:859, 1948
11. Gray GW: Manual: When the Foot Hits the Ground Everything Changes. Practical Programs for Applied Biomechanics, 1984. Toledo, Ohio
12. Mann RA, Hagy J: Biomechanics of walking, running and sprinting. Med Sci Sports Exerc 8:345, 1980
13. Ericson MO, Nisell R, Ekholm J: Quantified electromyography of lower limb muscles during level walking. Scand J Rehab Med 18:159, 1986
14. Basmajian JV: Muscles Alive: Their Functions Revealed by Electromyography. 3rd Ed. Williams and Wilkins, Baltimore, 1974
15. Cunningham DM: Components of floor reaction during walking. Prosthetic Devices Research Project, University of California at Berkeley, Series II, Issue 14, 1950
16. Perry J: The mechanics of walking: a clinical interpretation. Phys Ther 47:778, 1967
17. Soderburg GL: Kinesiology: Application to Pathological Motion. Williams & Wilkins, Baltimore, 1986
18. Bates BT: Biomechanics of running. Presented at

Medithon — A Multidisciplinary Seminar on Running Injuries, 1985

19. Frederick EC, Hagy JL: Factors influencing ground reaction forces in running. Int J Sport Biomech 2:41, 1986

20. Cavanaugh PR, LaFortune MA: Ground reaction forces in distance running. J Biomech 13:397, 1980

21. Brody DM: Running injuries. Clin Symp 32(4):1, 1980

15
Dysfunction, Evaluation, and Treatment of the Lumbar Spine

PETER I. EDGELOW

This chapter discusses the consequences of dysfunction of the lumbar spine in a manner that will help the physical therapist effectively treat and manage patients with these disorders. The proper role of the physical therapist is to mobilize all positive forces that can improve function. These forces consist of the body's ability to heal itself, and the practitioner's ability to identify through examination the signs, symptoms, and effective treatment methods and to teach patients to become their own therapists by participating in and enhancing the healing process through positive expectations and constructive actions.

The *mobile segment* is the structure that forms the basic anatomic unit of the lumbar spine.[1-4] A brief review of the anatomy of the mobile segment is presented in this chapter, emphasizing those aspects that are relevant to the patient's understanding of the mechanisms of injury to the system and as a rationale for treatment. Methods that can assist the therapist in training the patient to understand the nature of the injury and to assist the healing process are presented throughout this chapter.

Next, the value and limitations of diagnostic labels are discussed. Traditionally, the pathology of a particular body region involves the study of structural and functional changes that occur in disease. Numerous texts effectively describe the pathologic symptoms in the lumbar spine that indicate specific diagnoses.[5-10]

The discussion of pathology here has a twofold purpose: The first is to present some of the features of musculoskeletal disorders of the lumbar spine that a clinician can convey to patients to assist them in approaching the problem from a position of real knowledge. This will assist patients in establishing a positive belief system about getting well.[11] The second purpose is to distinguish between two types of diagnostic labels in physical treatment: those that either contraindicate or indicate the need for caution in applying physical treatment, and those in which the signs and symptoms are what must guide the therapist in treatment, not the labels themselves.

In the discussion of dysfunction, the practitioner is encouraged to look closely at the history of specific signs and symptoms, and then to develop treatment plans that are appropriate to those signs and symptoms. These treatment plans are in turn modified as the patient responds during the healing process.

In treatment as it relates to the diagnostic label, the approach in this chapter is guided by the history of signs and symptoms of the disorder as much as by the knowledge implied in the disorder's diagnostic label. For purposes of this discussion, theories of medical treatment are separated into two broad categories: those that are "pathology-focused" and those that are "signs, symptoms, and patient-focused." Before Hippocrates, the Cnidian school of medicine rested on the notion that for every illness there existed one specific cause and one specific treatment.[12] Present-day medicine, or at least one aspect of it, is very Cnidian in approach. For every infection there is a specific antibiotic for treatment, and for every injury a specific routine of exercises.

One can view this Cnidian approach as a "pathology-focused treatment," in which the medical practitioner focuses on the diagnosis the patient's condition has been given and offers whatever the standard treatment is for this diagnosis.

The problem with the pathology-focused, or one-cause, one-treatment approach is that it fails to appreciate the broader picture of the disorder. This approach also ignores the fact that the physical body that houses the ailment also houses an emotional and intellectual being, the human patient. The injury invariably affects the person intellectually and emotionally as well as physically, and an essential aspect of effective treatment is that the whole person must be acknowledged and ministered to in order for treatment to progress optimally. In short, the foundation of treatment should rest on the "signs, symptoms and patient-focused treatment" model of medicine, the roots of which can be traced to Hippocrates. In this approach, the practitioner looks at the total wellness of the patient and how to strengthen the body's own defenses against illness or injury as well as treating the signs and symptoms with a foreign agent or set of physical treatments.[13]

Since Chapters 16 and 17 discuss surgical and mobilization treatment methods in detail, this chapter will focus on patient handling and home care, paying special attention to the role of walking in the treatment process. The chapter closes with a case study, which illustrates the important concepts presented.

ANATOMY

This section discusses those aspects of the anatomy of the lumbar region that should be communicated to patients so they can take a more active role in the treatment process. In addition, the characteristics of the anatomy of the mobile segment that affect treatment procedures are highlighted.

The vertebral mobile segment is a more complex structure than a peripheral joint, and this complexity and the interrelationships of anatomic, biomechanical, and neurophysiologic factors in the lumbar region have crucial implications for treating injuries or disease in this area. One aspect of the complexity of injuries to the mobile segment is that they almost invariably bring the sympathetic nervous system into play. The sympathetic nervous system, the main vasomotor controlling system in the body, tends to exaggerate the disturbance. This results in an impeding of blood flow; normalizing the sympathetic system thus has a beneficial effect on circulation. When you control the blood flow to a given area, you control its life, its capacity for recovery, and its ability to survive, resist further injury, and maintain its integrity as a tissue.[14]

Another aspect of the complexity of the mobile segment is illustrated by contrasting pathology in a mobile segment with pathology in a peripheral joint such as the hip. When the hip joint becomes osteoarthritic and symptomatic, the muscles that move that joint undergo characteristic changes. In general, one group of muscles becomes tight, with the antagonistic group becoming weak and undergoing atrophy. In the case of the hip, the flexors become tight and the extensors weak.[15] Further, a loss in proprioception in the joint coupled with weakness and poor motor control sets up a perpetuating cycle of further microtrauma.

In injuries of the mobile segment it is more difficult to maximize healing through all stages of recovery than with a peripheral structure such as the hip. To promote healing of an injured body part, one must control the amount of stress placed on the injury. During stages when the hip is in acute inflammation, the patient can still remain functional by using crutches to reduce stress. During subsequent stages in recovery, when passive motion of the hip in a nonweightbearing position will promote further healing,[16] this can again be accomplished fairly easily while still allowing function. Peripheral structures are easier to treat than mobile segments because we have more control over the stresses placed on them. However, since the spine is central to virtually everything we do mechanically, it is much more difficult to isolate and protect any one mobile segment from stresses that do not promote healing or lead to further damage. Once the body part has recovered sufficiently to allow loaded activity to promote healing, resolution of the condition is much more rapid.

The discussion of anatomy in this chapter is divided into the following three sections:

1. A brief description of the mobile segment, as a base for comparison or analogy to a hinge
2. A description of the structures that act as pain generators in the mobile segment (Table 15-1)
3. Discussion of the circulation to the mobile segment and the factors that might interfere with nutrition to the system and lead to degeneration of the segment or interfere with maximum healing of injuries.

All of these topics are covered within the context of how the information can be conveyed to the patient to empower the patient to assist in the healing pro-

Table 15-1. Structures That Act as Pain Generators in the Mobile Segment

1. Vertebral body and epidural veins
2. Intervertebral disk and supporting ligaments
3. Zygapophyseal joints, surrounding capsule, and supporting ligaments
4. Dorsal and ventral ramus and mixed spinal nerve
5. Dorsal root ganglion
6. Muscles
7. Dura mater

cess. What follows is a description of the mobile segment that the therapist can use to assist the pa-

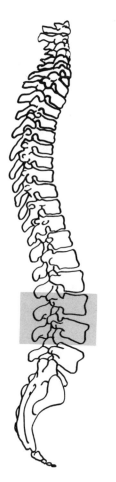 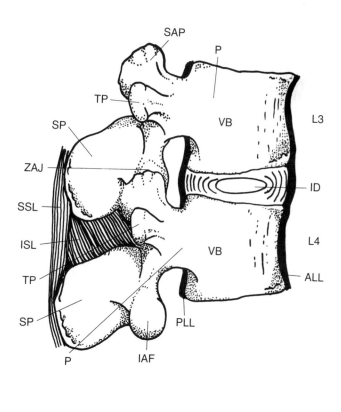

Fig. 15-1. Lumbar 3–4 mobile segment and its relationship to the entire vertebral column. P, pedicle; SAP, superior articular process; VB, vertebral body; ID, intervertebral disk; ALL, anterior longitudinal ligament; PLL, posterior longitudinal ligament; IAF, inferior articulate facet; SP, spinous process; TP, transverse process; ISL, interspinous ligament; SSL, supraspinous ligament; ZAJ, zygapophyseal joint. (Redrawn from Bogduk and Twomey,[4] with permission.)

tient in gaining a better picture of those factors that contribute to an understanding of the injury. It can be helpful for the therapist to draw a picture of the motion segment for the patient, diagrammatically emphasizing its features (Figs. 15-1, 15-2).

The mobile segment consists of two vertebrae with an intervening disk. A bridge of bone connects the left and right sides of the vertebrae. Projections of bone, the facets, jut inferiorly from this bridge to join the other facets from below, overlapping one another like the shingles of a roof. These zygapophyseal joints have ligamentous and capsular support and a synovial membrane lining that provides synovial fluid for lubrication and nutrition.

Other projections of bone, the right and left transverse processes and the spinous process, act as outriggers for the attachment of ligaments and muscles. The ligamentous attachments provide static support, the muscular attachments provide dynamic stability, and together they control and guide movement. As the therapist describes the mobile segment to the patient, it is useful to draw an analogy with the hinges on a door. A hinge consists of the following components: two flanges, a connecting pin, and screws to connect the flange to the frame of the doorway and to the door. Problems in function can be described, such as the door squeaking when moved. The patient can be led through the problem-solving process by considering whether the squeak is due to "loose screws" (problems of instability) or "need for oil" (problems of quality of movement). To carry the hinge analogy further, the therapist can compare a patient's problem involving a mobile segment that is both unstable and lacking in mobility to a hinge that has loose screws and cannot be fully opened or closed. Proper treatment would be to use gentle oscillating midrange movements (oil the hinge) to reduce friction, and then carefully use gentle end-range oscillating movements (open or close the door). Change in pain behavior is used as a guide to whether the structure can withstand the stress of the motion. If the structure cannot withstand the end-range motion, then bracing or surgery (tightening up the screws of the hinge) might be necessary. Such analogies are important methods of translating anatomic knowledge into more familiar language to ensure that the patient's understanding will be a guide in treatment and not a source of confusion.

In discussing the ligaments of the mobile seg-

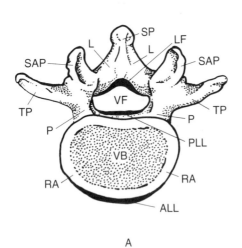

A

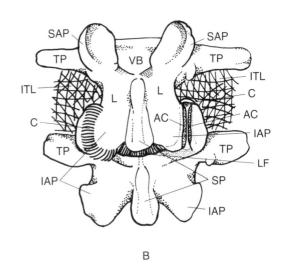

B

Fig. 15-2. Lumbar 3–4 mobile segment viewed from **(A)** above and **(B)** posterior. RA, ring apophysis; P, pedicle; TP, transverse process; SAP, superior articular process; L, lamina; SP, spinous process; LF, ligamentum flavum; VF, vertebral foramen; PLL, posterior longitudinal ligament; VB, vertebral body; ALL, anterior longitudinal ligament; IAP, inferior articular process; C, capsule of the joint; ITL, intertransverse ligament; AC, articular cartilages. (Redrawn from Bogduk and Twomey,[4] with permission.)

Table 15-2. Ligaments of the Mobile Segment

1. Anterior longitudinal ligament
2. Posterior longitudinal ligament
3. Ligamentum flavum
4. Interspinous and supraspinous ligaments
5. Intertransverse ligament
6. Anterior and posterior facet capsular ligaments

ment with the patient, it can be of value to name the ligaments (Table 15-2) and briefly describe their function in providing stability. The ligaments function like the screws that support the hinge. If they are too loose, they will allow excess movement to occur during function (opening the door). If they are too tight, they restrict motion in certain directions.

The Function of the Muscles of the Lumbar Spine

The function of the muscles of the lumbar spine is well described by Macintosh and Bogduk.[17] Of particular importance is their hypothesis that the intertransversarii mediales may act as large proprioceptive transducers. These muscles, together with the multifidus, are innervated by the lumbar dorsal rami of the nerve of that segment. Therefore, injury to that segment can interfere with the muscle activity of the prime proprioceptive muscle and the prime stabilizing muscle of the segment. However, such injuries do not necessarily interfere with the innervation to the multisegmental muscles of the spine such as the latissimus dorsi and the gluteus maximus, which initiate and control movement and function of the extremities, and also the erector spinae, which provides both power and control of movement of the spine as a whole.

Pain arising from one or more of the structures listed in Table 15-1 remains poorly understood, and over time many "stories" have developed to account for pain arising from the back. Bogduk and Twomey discuss two types of classical lumbar pain: (1) pain generated from structures 1, 2, 3, 6, or 7 in Table 15-1, termed *somatic pain,* and (2) pain from disorders of structures 4 or 5 in Table 15-1, termed *radicular pain.*[4]

Bogduk and Twomey cite studies that have clearly incriminated the zygapophyseal joints,[18,19] disks,[20-26] and dura mater[27,28] as possible sources of pain, with only the epidural blood vessels and the vertebral bodies not having been experimentally studied to prove that they can also be a source of pain. Circumstantial evidence points to the epidural blood vessels as a possible source of pain.[29] Only the bone of the vertebral bodies has not been proved to be a pain generator, although it could, wisely or unwisely, be assumed that the pain of osteoporosis is an example of bone as a pain generator.[4] The possible causes, then, of pain arising from any one of the somatic structures are any pathologic processes that stimulate nociceptive nerve endings in any one of the structures named. This stimulation may be due to either chemical or mechanical irritation. The methods by which these processes can cause stimulation are well described,[4,30] and this detailed knowledge is not essential for patients' understanding of why they hurt, although this information can help therapists assist patients in viewing pain as a guide rather than a curse.

To paraphrase Bogduk and Twomey, the somatic referred pain mechanism appears to be the activation by afferent impulses from the mobile segment of neurons in the central nervous system, which also happen to receive afferents from the lower limbs, buttocks, or groin. Stimulation of central system neurons by messages from the mobile segment may cause the perception of pain arising from all of the other tissues innervated by these neurons. Therefore, pain is perceived as arising from a structure in the limbs, even though there is no signal actually coming from this structure. There is some evidence that the distance of referral into the limb is proportional to the intensity of the stimulus of the mobile segment.[4]

The pathology of nerve root compression is a complex issue, and there are conflicting and erroneous explanations in the literature. The reader is encouraged to explore the explanation advanced by Bogduk and Twomey as the most interesting currently available.[4]

The pain generator is unlikely to be one structure. A much more common scenario is the nerve root compression syndrome. In the presence of neurologic changes (e.g., weakness, numbness, decreased reflexes) together with the characteristic lancinating pain of radicular origins, there may be concomitant somatic and somatic referred pain from the structures adjacent to and surrounding the nerve root.

In order for patients to have some understanding of the origin of their complaints, the following factors can be discussed with them: pain generators, somatic as well as radicular referral of pain, and central nervous system modulation of pain.

Circulation and Nutrition of the Mobile Segment

There are five circulatory systems involved in nutrition within the mobile segment: (1) the arterial system, (2) the venous system, (3) the cerebrospinal fluid system, (4) the lymphatic system, and (5) the synovial fluid system. Optimum functioning of all these systems is essential for health. Any factor that interferes with this optimum function will affect the process of injury repair.

It is not the purpose of this chapter to consider the function of these systems in any detail. The reader can obtain this information from numerous sources,[4,31-34] although there is a great deal not yet fully understood. However, from the patient's point of view, the important factors are those which interfere with circulation and nutrition. The disk appears to live and thrive on movement, and change and die slowly through lack of it.[35] The same is true of all structures of the mobile segment. If one considers the negative effects of immobilization on all structures and systems, then the clinician's job in treatment is to sell the patient on the need to move the injured parts.[36-39]

A useful metaphor in assisting the patient's awareness of the importance of adequate circulation is that of a lake. When the flow of water (circulation) in and out of the like (the mobile segment) is impeded by a damming of the exiting tributary (injury), the lake may turn into a swamp (inflammation). Increasing the water flow by removing the dam (mobility) drains the swamp and restores life to the lake.

The normal healing response to injury is as follows: Injury results in an inflammatory process, set off by the enzymes released by the damaged tissue in dead cells. Inflammation is a change in the local network of capillaries that leads to an outpouring of inflammatory exudate, a fluid rich in antibodies that lays down a network of fibrin. Within the exudate, vast numbers of cells enter and begin to clear up the dead cells. The inflammatory exudate may still be growing by the third or fourth day following injury, especially if there is a large amount of damage or more damage from continuous use.[40]

The general method of healing of tissue is by fibrous repair. Repeated damage to fibrous connective tissue will not only mean a thickened and contracted tissue, but also result in extensive loss of proprioceptive nerve endings. The repair process that follows results in an initial consolidation of the injured tissue. This consolidation period is followed by scarring. If the tissue being healed is kept absolutely immobile, the resultant fibrous scarring is weak.

When there are no natural forces on the healing tissue, collagen is laid down haphazardly and, although it may be plentiful, is poorly engineered. Fibrous healing is stronger if natural movements are encouraged. The stress of the natural movements determines the manner in which the collagen fibers are laid down. Gentle, normal movements provide natural tensions in the healing tissue, resulting in much stronger healing. However, if there is continued inflammation, fibrous healing will be poor.

Healing also requires a good blood supply in order to support the phagocytes by supplying oxygen and nutrients to the worker cells, carrying off waste, and preventing further cell death secondary to anoxia and other factors. No injury can be made to heal faster than its natural speed. The tools of healing, the cells getting on with their job, cannot be improved. All that can be done is to make sure that no contrary influences are allowed and that all possible favorable conditions are encouraged.

The important factor that is often forgotten, or at least not stressed in repair, is that there is a remodeling period following cell formation that results in a strengthening and realignment of the scar to the point where the opportunities for reinjury are minimized. It is this remodeling stage that is of critical importance in repair of injury to the mobile segment, and in particular the disk.

After an injury, the healed tissue is never the same as it was before. Fibrous connective tissue, such as ligament or joint capsule, will be repaired, but it will not have the same structure or properties as the original. Moreover, the nerve end organs do not regenerate. Damaged muscles do not regenerate. They heal with a scar of fibrous tissue.[40]

CONSEQUENCES OF DYSFUNCTION IN THE LUMBAR REGION

Pathology is the study of the structural and functional changes that occur in disease. This section expresses some philosophical views on the value of pathologic knowledge and the risks and drawbacks of this knowledge as it relates to treatment, and presents a list of disorders under these broad categories: those in which physical therapy treatment is contraindicated, those which call for certain precautions in treatment, and those in which physical therapy is indicated, guided by the signs and symptoms. Finally, this section presents a method of looking at disorders of the musculoskeletal system that is functionally oriented and designed to assist the therapist in explaining to the patient what is wrong in a manner that facilitates treatment. It is important to stress that when the clinician collects the data base, a methodical, orderly method of establishing a necessary minimum of information is employed. These data are then used to arrive at a presumptive diagnosis, or treatment diagnosis. Tables 15-3 and 15-4 show what types of information gathered in the examination process are associated with a particular pathology and should alert the examiner to the potential risks in treatment. The tables are organized according to the method of examination taught by Maitland.[41,42]

Effective treatment of low back injuries should include a careful musculoskeletal evaluation and careful instructions on which movements risk further injury and which movements enhance healing. The common sense the patient uses instinctively to reduce stress to an injury to a peripheral joint is simply not as useful in the lumbar spine, with its immense backup system of mobile segments. In addition, the patient's knowledge of this region is not as instinctive as with peripheral joints such as the knee or hip.

Thus, the therapist must isolate the particular injured segment through careful methodical examination and then determine which is the appropriate resting position as well as the best functional movement. Since the biomechanics of the spine changes from level to level, the resting positions and positions of stability change also. This helps to explain why in upper lumbar injuries the patient is more comfortable in a semireclined than a fully reclined position. Conversely, in injuries to the lower lumbar region the patient is more comfortable either fully reclined with the hips and knees flexed to allow lumbar flexion, or with a rolled towel to support the low lumbar spine in some degree of extension. After these determinations, the therapist explains to the patient how to best assist the healing process through an appropriate combination of rest and activity.

The value of the pathologic label, or diagnosis, is to provide the therapist with information that may contraindicate certain treatments or indicate caution in treatment. An example of a diagnosis that contraindicates treatment is that of a spinal tumor. In this instance, physical treatment would be useless in correcting the problem. Another example is cauda equina symptoms, such as difficulty in initiating urination and numbness in the perineum. These symptoms indicate the possibility of compression of the sacral nerve roots or cauda equina, which innervates the bladder and provides sensory distribution to the perineum. Any lesion that is gross enough to provide these symptoms requires immediate referral to a physician for emergency evaluation and treatment (Table 15-3).

An example of a disorder that indicates the need for caution in treatment is osteoporosis. (See Table 15-4 for a more detailed account of disorders that indicate a need for caution in treatment.) The diagnostic label itself indicates that there is at least a 35 percent demineralization of the bone, which may be in part responsible for the patient's problem.[31] It is important to understand, however, that there may be a mechanical component in addition to the demineralization. In treatment of the mechanical component, one would be cautious not to apply forces that might fracture a bone weakened by demineralization. Still, the therapist should guide the treatment by assessing changes in the patient's signs

Table 15-3. Disorders in Which Physical Treatment is Contraindicated

Disorder	Subjective Symptoms					Radiographic Evidence	Objective Signs			
	Area	Description	Behavior	History	Special Questions		Observation	Active and Passive Movements	Neurologic Examination	Other Tests
Malignancy (primary or secondary)	Nonspecific	Severe intractable pain	Not always altered by rest or activity; Worse at night, patient wakes and must get up and move around	Onset slow and insidious; may have past history of illness or surgery	General health poor, recent weight loss	Early in disease no changes; later may show loss of spinous process, transverse process or pedicle				
Inflammatory Conditions Tuberculosis Osteomyelitis Paget's Disease		Pain constant and severe	Unaltered by rest or activity; Night sweats		General health poor, possible weight loss					
Spinal cord compression	Bilateral paresthesia of hands and/or feet, stocking/glove, nearly always bilateral						Unsteadiness of gait		Hyperreflexive, hypertonic, ankle clonus, positive plantar response (Babinski)	Incoordination, muscle weakness in lower extremities
Cauda equina disorder	Saddle paresthesia or anesthesia				Bladder retention; possible overflow, incontinence, or bowel retention			Protective spasm	Hyperreflexive, hypertonic, ankle clonus, positive plantar response (Babinski)	

(Adapted from Grieve,[31] with permission.)

and symptoms that may be caused by mechanical problems within the system rather than by the weakened bone structure. Since the diagnosis of osteoporosis is not always clear-cut, the therapist should be particularly careful in the treatment of injuries of postmenopausal women where a minor back injury has produced a severe response, particularly in the presence of involuntary muscle spasm. Routine radiography may miss a minor compression fracture.

Once the clinician has excluded those disorders that contraindicate or indicate caution in physical treatment, treatment of the pathologies that remain should be guided more by the history, signs, and symptoms than by the information inherent in the diagnostic label alone. There is a tendency in some treatment situations to stop once one has a diagnostic label and carry on with treatment based strictly on this label. This should be guarded against, since it is the signs, symptoms, and stage of the pathology that require treatment, not the label.

Some individual pieces of information are pathognomonic, or so specific to one pathologic condition that by themselves they can guide one in treatment. For example, the knowledge that a patient has spondylolisthesis tells the practitioner that a structural weakness exists both with extension movements of the spine and posteroanterior forces on the spine. This does not imply that all extension movements of posteroanterior mobilizations are contraindicated, but rather that the signs and symptoms must be read carefully, as the therapist uses these movements to ensure that functional extension for the patient is restored while respecting the structural weakness.

In contrast, other patients present constellations of signs and symptoms that point in certain treatment directions, but are not as clear-cut. In these more vague cases, the therapist must carefully observe changes in signs and symptoms as the patient responds to a particular treatment plan, refining and altering the treatment plan in response to these changes.

THE EXAMINATION OF THE THORACOLUMBAR SPINE

To make the most use of the signs and symptoms of a disorder or injury, a detailed examination is essential. Once a data base has been gathered by examination, it can be used in assessment and as a guide to treatment, which is one of the cornerstones of the Maitland concept of examination, treatment, and assessment as a continuous loop.[41-44]

The examination process is divided into two sections: the subjective examination, or what the patient reveals about the complaint in response to questioning, and the objective examination, or what the examiner determines based on certain tests and measures.

The subjective examination can be divided into four sections:

1. The area of the symptoms, in which one clarifies the location of the complaint and its distribution and obtains a description of the complaint
2. The behavior of the symptoms, in which one traces the aggravating and easing characteristics of the complaint, based on a functional evaluation over the previous 24-hour period
3. The history of the onset of the complaint and the progress of symptoms and signs from onset until the present, as well as its present stability and any past history of similar complaints that might relate to this problem
4. The patient's response to certain specific questions as they may relate to an understanding of the disorder or of its cause. These questions relate to such factors as general health, relevant change in the patient's weight, whether x-rays have been taken and the findings, and any medically prescribed drugs the patient is using. Of specific significance in the low lumbar spine is the possibility of cauda equina symptoms (numbness in the perineum and difficulty in initiating urination). In the upper lumbar spine, the possibility of a cord lesion with symptoms of bilateral numbness of the feet and unsteadiness of gait is also significant.

The objective examination covers the following factors:

1. Observation of posture and gait
2. Active movements of the spine
3. Passive movements of the spine
4. Accessory movements of the spine

Table 15-4. Disorders in Which Precaution Is Indicated in Applying Physical Treatment

		Subjective Symptoms				Radiographic Evidence	Objective Signs			Other Tests
Disorder	Area	Description	Behavior	History	Special Questions		Observation	Active and Passive Movements	Neurologic Examination	
Recent fracture		Pain may be intermittent, sharp in character, and severe	Severe catches of pain with minimal movement	History indicates possible compression fracture-sudden loading of spine, severe coughing, fall on buttocks		May not be evident on standard x-ray and may require CT scan		Protective spasm		
Osteoporosis	General ache	Persistent pain	Relieved by lying, aggravated by prolonged standing, sitting, or walking	Age-postmenopausal, Sex-female > male, prolonged immobilization, onset may be insidious or sudden and severe from minimal incident	Prolonged steroid therapy	Will require at least 35–50% demineralization before radiologic appearance	May have a degree of kyphosis	Severe protective spasm		

Condition	Pain	Behavior / timing	Onset / history	Systemic	Radiographs	Posture / ROM	Objective testing	Weakness / tension	Special tests
Ankylosing spondylitis, active stage	Severe intractable pain	Worse at night, morning stiffness takes longer than 30 minutes to loosen, (generally 1 hour)		Signs of systemic illness, weight loss			If tests positive, reduces si-debending bilaterally and equal early in disease; reduced chest expansion	General weakness secondary to disease	Sacroiliac tests often positive, raised erythrocyte sedimentation rate
Spondylolisthesis	Pain increases with standing and walking, decreases with sitting				Characteristic "scotty dog" appearance		Extension decreased and painful, passive testing (p/a) produces pain easily. Palpations of "step"; PP-MT test* positive for instability		
Juvenile disk		Often complaints are minimal and yet patient may have difficulty walking	Often onset associated with trauma (e.g., in sports)			Loss of lordosis	Considerable spasm	Pronounced tension signs	
Scheuermann's disease	Often vague pain in lower extremities, nondermatomal; May be described as "like growing pains"	Pain is stress- and time-dependent	Present in adolescents (boys more than girls), onset insidious		Often severe changes, fuzziness of disk/vertebral body interface, may be vertebral wedging	May have thoracic kyphosis			

*PP-MT, passive physiological movement test.
(Adapted from Grieve,[31] with permission.)

5. Tests for muscle function (e.g., weakness, lack of coordination, or muscle pain)
6. Tests of other joints (e.g., sacroiliac, hip, knee, and ankle)
7. Neurologic tests (e.g., reflexes, sensation, and motor power)
8. Dural tension signs tested singly or in combination (e.g., passive neck flexion, straight leg raise, prone knee flexion, and slumped sitting).

The purpose of testing movements is to determine the quantity and quality of the range of motion, the effect of movement on the patient's resting symptoms or on production of symptoms, and the presence of spasm or lack of symmetry during movement. Abnormal movement is a fact to be assessed for relevance to the complaint and as to why the complaint exists. It is also a piece of data to be used in assessing changes during treatment. For example, suppose a patient presents with constant right-sided lumbar pain and intermittent right calf pain. Trunk flexion is limited such that the patient's fingertips reach only to the upper border of the patella, with an increase in lumbar pain and production of calf pain. Upon returning to the erect position, there is a further increase in lumbar pain, and the patient has to assist himself by pushing on his thighs. In this example, the quantity of motion is measured by the position of the fingertips, the quality is characterized by the pain on attempted extension from the flexed position, and the abnormal movement is relevant to the complaint since it alters the symptoms. The quantity and quality of this range of flexion motion will be a useful benchmark in assessing the patient's progress.

Data from the objective examination are very seldom pathognomonic. It is not one piece of information that indicates a specific direction in treatment, but rather how the pieces fall into a pattern. An effective examination process involves gathering one piece of data, interpreting its meaning or relevance, and then reassessing that interpretation as new data are added. It is not poor technique to jump to a conclusion based on one piece of information, provided you confirm this interpretation through other supportive data or form a new interpretation if additional data so indicate. For example, a flattened lumbar spine might indicate a loss of extension mobility, requiring increased extension to restore maximum function. Similarly, a lateral shift with a flattened lumbar spine in the standing position might require restoration of lateral movement and then restoration of extension before the patient can regain maximum function. However, the critical point is that, by itself, lack of extension on observation does not indicate a need for extension. The observed posture together with the effect of movements on the symptoms are factors that direct treatment.

The objective examination is divided into those tests done in standing, sitting, and lying positions, so as to minimize patient movement (Table 15-5). A methodical examination allows for development of the intuitive process, which Erik Berne describes as "knowledge based on experience." Berne believes that the beginning clinician must "resort to a method

Table 15-5. Movements Tested in Standing, Sitting, and Lying Positions

Movements tested in the standing position
Observation of static posture
Observation of gait
Functional test—squatting
Trunk flexion—single and repeated movements
Trunk extension—single and repeated movements
Lateral shift—left and right
Sidebending—left and right
Neurologic tests in standing—gastrocnemius power
Combination of movement—i.e., extension, sidebending, and rotation

Movements tested in the sitting position
Trunk rotation—left and right
Spinal canal movements—slump tests (Ref. 41)

Movements tested in the supine position
Passive neck flexion to assess spinal cord mobility
Passive straight leg raising test to assess sacral plexus mobility
Resisted isometric muscle tests for pain production
Neurologic tests when indicated, tested in the supine position
Sacroiliac joint tests
Other tests—leg length, circumferential tests for muscle wasting

Movements tested in the prone position
Prone knee flexion to assess lumbar plexus mobility
Palpation for:
    Temperature and sweating changes
    Soft tissue tenderness and thickening
    Position and alignment of the vertebrae
    Intervertebral accessory movements
Passive accessory intervertebral movement test

Movements tested in the side-lying position
Passive physiologic intervertebral movement tests
Passive posteroanterior stability tests

of data collection which is additive in nature in order to reach the advanced skills seen in the experienced clinician."[45] As the beginner gains experience through a systematic approach to making diagnoses, he or she gradually rises to a level where diagnostic processes begin to occur at an earlier stage of the examination and on a more subconscious level.

After completing the objective examination, the therapist should ideally have found the specific joint or structures causing the symptoms and have clarified the type of movement disorder present. The type of disorder may be hypermobility or hypomobility, and must be verified by performing a passive physiologic movement test in the side-lying position or a stability test.[46]

After using the data collection process outlined here, the therapist should:

1. Understand the area of pain and be able to "live" the patient's symptoms over a period of 24 hours.
2. Know at least two activities that aggravate or ease the symptoms and that are measurable enough to allow assessment of small increments of change.
3. Have identified at least two objective measures that will cause an increase in the patient's symptoms and can be used to assess small increments of change. Where there is both spinal and dural movement abnormality, an objective measure of each component is required.

With this information, treatment becomes a logical process of action and reaction. As the patient is affected by a treatment technique, the above information is used to measure the change that occurs. The therapist who examines and treats in this manner can only improve as experience teaches him or her how to proceed in assisting the patient to restore maximal function to the musculoskeletal system. In the more acute stage of the condition, if the therapist finds both limitation and pain when examining the tension sign (straight leg raise), this sign may be used to assess the effect of the treatment technique, whereas the distance and frequency of walking can be used to assess progress over time. As the condition improves, other objective factors may be more appropriate to use in assessment, such as trunk mobility, repetitive bending, and lifting of weight.

Assessment

After gathering the data about physical signs and symptoms, the therapist should make a judgment as to whether the intellectual and emotional responses of the patient are not interfering with the patient's problem or are a major component of the problem. One simple way to characterize this judgment is through the use of the PIE notation, which expresses the relationship between the physical (P), intellectual (I), and emotional (E) factors.

If the condition is primarily physical, with intellectual and emotional characteristics not affecting accurate assessment of the physical findings, this is noted as "Pie," with the capital "P" indicating the primacy of the physical factors. However, if it is the practitioner's judgment that the intellectual and emotional factors have equal importance with the physical findings, this can be indicated by the notation "PIE."

In the "PIE" notation, the term *intellectual* applies to the patient's problem-solving or cognitive abilities, whereas *emotional* applies to the patient's feelings. Thus, if a patient is particularly disorganized and unable to follow a treatment routine, the patient's primary obstacle to progress is intellectual, and this is noted as "pIe." If a patient is well organized but prone to assume the worst, the negative emotions that accompany the injury can be an obstacle to effective treatment; this situation is noted as "piE".

The following example illustrates the use of this notation: Assume that during the subjective examination of a patient's complaint, the patient describes the symptoms with general statements such as "I can't do anything" and "I feel terrible." At this point, it would be realistic to note that the intellectual and emotional components of the patient's response to the injury are likely to be important considerations in treating the problem. The clinician's notation of the physical, intellectual, and emotional relationship would be "pIE" to indicate that the intellectual and emotional factors may be interfering with accurate assessment of the physical problem. However, if during the objective examination the patient presents consistent objective data that clarify the physical complaint, the notation at the end of the objective examination would be "PIE," indicating that the physical, intellectual, and emotional characteristics all require consideration in treatment. On the second visit, if the patient responds to the question "How are you?" with "I'm feeling better," and to "How much better?" with "I slept better, only waking up once instead of three or four times," the assessment would be "Pie," indicating that the intellectual and emotional factors of this patient's personality are not interfering with the patient's understanding of the physical problem.

One indication of intellectual or emotional interference is an inability to express clearly what aggravates and what eases the problem. A patient who is unable to give a clear picture of what has happened from the onset of the disorder to the present tends to have intellectual and emotional factors that, while they may not be responsible for the problem, often interfere with adequate recovery and need to be addressed in treating that problem.

The physical, intellectual, and emotional factors form a circle of interrelationships (Fig. 15-3). For example, a physical stimulus (e.g., a slap in the face) elicits a physical response (red face and pain), an intellectual response (wondering why it was done and how to respond), and an emotional response (anger). Similarly, an emotional stimulus such as being ridiculed produces an emotional response (embarrassment), a physical response (blushing), and an intellectual response (why?). To harness the full power of the patient in the recovery process, one wants to have P, I, and E working in concert with one another. One way to assist patients in doing this is to share with them information that will help them get a cognitive grasp of the problem while gathering data during the examination process. As patients become involved intellectually in understanding their problems, they feel more in control, and emotional reactions are diffused.

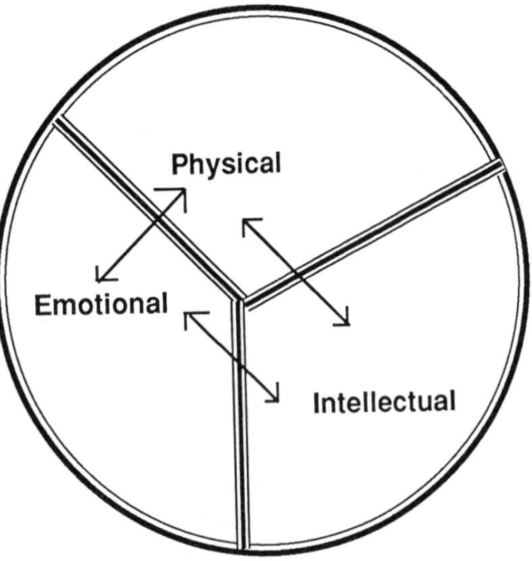

Recent medical studies scientifically demonstrate what has long been common wisdom, namely, that positive emotions maximize the body's healing abilities.[11,47] These studies demonstrate a relationship between positive emotions and increased pituitary gland secretion. The pituitary hormones released in turn stimulate the adrenal cortex to release steroids, which have an anti-inflammatory effect. Positive thinking has also been shown to be related to hypothalamic release of endorphins.[48] Negative emotions, such as fear and anxiety, will not result in production of the same high levels of endorphins and steroids. Therefore, in assessing the intellectual and emotional components of the injury and teaching the patient to have greater access to the positive emotions, the therapist can actually have a constructive impact on the patient's biochemistry.[49]

Fig. 15-3. The interrelationship of physical, intellectual, and emotional factors in treatment.

"No-Name" Disorders and Dysfunctions

The problem with classifying the more common disorders of the lumbar spine is that the injuries are not always severe enough to clearly incriminate one structure rather than another. In a patient with low back injury, although it is clear that the mobile segment is not functioning properly and is responsible for symptoms, what is not as clear is what aspect or part of the mobile segment is the pain generator. Whether it is a simple problem with one structure or a link in a series of interrelated problems requires further clarification. Even in conditions that present with radiographic changes, such as spondylolisthesis, where one might be led to blame the mechanical fault seen on the film for the symptoms, it is not always the spondylolisthesis that is responsible for the symptoms. It may be a segment above or below that segment, and the radiographic findings may in fact be of no value in indicating which level is responsible for the patient's complaint.

Therefore, in discussing the more common disorders that are not illuminated by radiographic findings, electromyographic findings, CT scans, and other standard tests;, the term "no-name disorders" will be used. In theory, the skilled diagnostician considers the initial diagnostic label a treatment diagnosis and a step in a total process. The final step in this process is a definitive differential diagnostic label. In practice, the treatment diagnosis often is the first and last label. Physical therapists are very familiar with diagnoses that do not clearly define what the pathology is, but rather speak in terms of symptoms, for example, low back strain, low back sprain, lumbosacral strain, low back strain with sciatica, sacroiliitis, muscle spasm, muscle strain, degenerative disk disease, spondylitis, and so on.

The difficulty in using these diagnostic labels in treatment is that they never clearly indicate how to treat the problem, since there is no basis for equating two patients with the same diagnostic label. They may in fact have the same label, but the severity and presentation of the problem can differ, and hence the signs and symptoms they present will differ. Similarly, even the same patient during various stages of his condition can present with a different picture of pain, spasm, and disability. Therefore, the signs and symptoms and the functional limitations produced by the disorder have more meaning in terms of understanding the problem and knowing how to treat it than does the label itself.

In short, diagnostic labels in mechanical injuries do more to interfere with effective treatment than to assist it. Hence, in the "no-name disorder" there is no textbook for the patient to use to compare with how his "no-name disorder" behaved. The only textbooks are the patients themselves, and as each patient understands his own textbook — that is, his own signs and symptoms — and the aggravating and easing factors of the problem, he will have a more positive experience in recovering. As the severity of the disorder becomes apparent through CT scans, MRI, and the like, the clinician can be aided in treatment by this kind of knowledge. But those aids are

an assistance in directing treatment; they do not provide a rigid set of directives for a treatment plan.

It has been demonstrated that abnormal CT scans can be found in asymptomatic individuals.[50] Hence, it is imperative to relate these test results with other relevant data such as that provided by movement tests. The findings on passive movement tests indicating a symptomatic motion segment may assist in determining whether the abnormal CT findings are in fact associated with the patient's symptoms. Similarly, other objective tests such as thermograms may also assist in determining whether abnormal CT and MRI scans indicate disorder. Studies that have compared abnormal thermograms and abnormal movement tests before and after treatment have indicated that treatment resulted in normalized thermograms and normalized movements (Ref. 51 and Paul Goodley, personal communication). There is a real need for further clinical research to show the relationship among CT scans, MRI, movement tests, and thermograms.

A more accurate diagnostic label for all the conditions listed under the "no-name disorder" category is "somatic dysfunction of a specific mobile segment."[52] For example, picture a 33-year-old male who has never had symptoms of back pain other than minor stiffness from sitting too long or not getting enough exercise. He now develops acute low back pain after working in the garden over the weekend, lifting, bending, hoeing, and raking. The patient walks into the physician's office with a flattened lumbar spine and obvious muscle spasm and pain in the low back that is greater on the right than on the left. Following the initial examination, the physician might come up with one of five or more different diagnostic labels for the condition, depending on the physician's experience and expertise. Thus, diagnostic labels are not only relatively useless in forming a treatment plan, they are also highly subjective.

If on examining this hypothetical patient one were to find that the L5–S1 mobile segment had the most abnormal movement and was most responsible for the patient's pain, then one could hypothesize that during the activity described the patient injured that mobile segment, resulting in abnormal movement of that segment. If radiographs, CT scans, an MRI, and neurologic findings are all within normal limits, than the label of "somatic dysfunction of the L5–S1 mobile segment secondary to a strain" makes total sense. Such a description has no negative connotations. One would expect that the patient should heal quite well if it is a first injury, and if the patient is an otherwise healthy individual who knows how to deal with a problem. In addition, given the knowledge gained in the treatment process, the patient should be able to prevent a similar occurrence.

If the patient has habit patterns that need to be changed in order to prevent a problem from developing or recurring, those habits will only change if the patient is self-motivated. These patients, who can be looked upon as accidents waiting to happen, will not be motivated to make habit changes based on theory. They will be motivated by compelling emotional forces such as fear, and fear of course is what they experience when they begin to get symptoms and signs of a disabling problem.

The signs and symptoms that are found in patients with somatic dysfunction of a specific mobile segment are illustrated in Tables 15-6 and 15-7. Table 15-6 lists those symptoms that indicate a need to be gentle in applying physical treatment. Table 15-7 lists the symptoms that would not limit treatment prior to its application. In the final analysis, these tables are only an aid in the therapist's learning process. The ultimate guide is the patient and the manner in which the signs and symptoms change as treatment is applied.

TREATMENT

Since Chapters 16 and 17 discuss surgical treatment and mobilization methods of the thoracolumbar spine area in specific detail, comments here will emphasize approaches to patient handling and home care, paying special attention to the role of walking in the healing process.

In treatment, the teaching of the patient is crucial. Many people, even very academically intelligent people, are what one might think of as "physical illiterates." These patients often ignore the symptoms the body presents and stoically go on about their business. Such patients must be taught to pay attention to the signals from the body in order to

maximize recovery. On the other hand, a hypochondriac patient will be so overwhelmed by symptoms as to not known how to cope. In either case, the treatment process becomes more effective as the patient understands which specific mobile segment is injured and how that segment needs to be protected yet still used to promote healing. In addition, we no longer live in a society in which people will blindly follow the suggestions of an authority. Many people will become engaged in their own treatment only if they have a thorough understanding of why they should follow a certain regimen and only if this knowledge fits with their personal beliefs.

Another important aspect of treatment is the role the therapist plays in increasing the patient's commitment to the healing process. A person with a basically healthy mobile segment that is traumatized has a much better chance of recovery than someone with an initially unwell mobile segment. Frequently, however, one is not only treating the injury, but attempting to catalyze a change in the patient's life-style, which is often a life-style that led to the injury in the first place. The essential problem in treating such a patient is determining what changes in life-style need to occur. This process involves problem solving by both patient and therapist, although the ultimate responsibility for change rests with the patient. Still, by acting in the role of educator and coach, the therapist can encourage the patient to make the necessary life-style changes.

Therefore, the beginning of treatment is the time to discuss the need for prevention with the patient. Although the patient has not been able to prevent the first occurrence, preventing recurrence and progressive deterioration of a system is a realistic goal. It is important, then, to recognize the first signs of deterioration of a system and to understand the pattern of behavior that led up to it. At that point, the therapist can assist the patient in making changes that will aim at re-establishing a healthy system and maintaining that system throughout life. It is important not to impose advice on the patient, since this advice comes from the therapist's reality, not the patient's. If you ask the patient, "How can you change?" and leave the patient to come up with the correct answer, you will get a better result. For example, if a patient says he can't remember to exercise and uses this as an excuse for not following a

Table 15-6. Symptoms and Signs Indicating Need for Gentleness in Treatment

Subjective Symptoms					Objective Signs		
Area	Description	Behavior	History	Special Questions	Observation	During Testing of Active or Passive Movements	Neurologic Examination
Distal symptoms more severe than proximal	Constant pain with difficulty finding relief	Irritable: small amount of movement produces severe increase of symptoms requiring a long time to settle	Acute	Frequent medication	Patient appears in acute distress with severe pain and very ill	Pain alters markedly with movement	Positive tension signs
Dermatomal distribution suggesting nerve root	Latent pain	All movements hurt severely	Severity of the incident and degree of disability are not comparable	Anti-inflammatories	Postural spasm or deformity protecting joint	Pain severe	Any evidence of conduction loss
	Paresthesia or anesthesia	All postures, positions painful; difficult to ease	Easily provoked	Steroids for a prolonged period		Pain occurs early in range	Muscle weakness
	Pain severe	Pain at rest	Condition is getting worse	Potent analgesics required		Pain builds quickly	Sensory deficit
	Pain shooting or lancinating	Unable to bear weight or lie on affected side	Suggests any neurological deficit (nerve root, cord, cauda equina)	Poor general health		Pain felt earlier than stiffness	Lost or diminished reflex
	Pain intractable	Unable to sleep well		Recent weight loss or suggestion of systemic illness		Area: spinal movements provoke distal symptoms	
		Unable to find comfortable position		Positive response to cord, cauda equina, vertebral artery		Spread: buildup of pain or spread distally with sustained midrange position	
		Wakes with severe pain forcing patient to move from bed				Latent pain	
		Wakes frequently, requires a long time to return to sleep				Pain through range which builds to an "ache" and may require extended period to settle	
		Coughing and sneezing provoke distal symptoms as related to vertebral column				Spasm provoked with slow, gentle handling	
						Abrupt spasm limits further movement	
						Nature of limit is pain, empty end-feel and boggy	

(Adapted from Grieve,[58] with permission.)

Table 15-7. Symptoms and Signs That Allow Progressive Vigor in Physical Treatment

	Subjective Symptoms				Objective Signs		
Area	Description	Behavior	History	Special Questions	Observation	During Testing of Active or Passive Movements	Neurologic Examination
Proximal symptoms more severe than distal Nondermatomal distribution suggesting somatic referral pain	Not severe Intermittent Occasional Momentary symptoms	Not irritable Pain not severe Moderate pain, when provoked, settles immediately One or two provoking movements Eased with rest Symptoms present only with prolonged activity or sustained position at limit of range Sleep not disturbed, or Wakes but pain is eased with change of position, patient returns to sleep immediately	Subacute Chronic bouts require initial prolonged, vigorous activity Condition static or improving	Infrequent medication of mild analgesics as needed	No acute distress Patient looks well Patient moves easily Minimal functional loss	Minimal change in pain on movement Pain not severe Pain only at limit of range Pain builds or spreads only with sustained positions at the limit "Ache" during testing which settles immediately on cessation of movement or subsides quickly Soft tissue approximation on stretch with elastic, capsular end-feel	No evidence of neurologic deficit, or where present is most likely related to previous episodes

(Adapted from Grieve,[58] with permission.)

home exercise program, one solution would be to advise the patient to use a timer on the kitchen stove as a reminder to exercise. If the therapist instead asks questions so that the patient can arrive at the correct answer independently, the patient's mind is involved in the process of problem solving, and the solution is the patient's and will be better adhered to and remembered.

Communication Style

The communication style of the therapist is an essential element in promoting the patient's healing process. In order to get along with and make changes in the patient, the therapist must understand the patient's point of view as it relates to the problem. Then, from the patient's reality, the therapist is better able to assist the patient in the direction of health. A classic story involving Milton Erickson, the founder of modern hypnotherapy, illustrates this. Erickson went to work at a certain mental hospital, and within his first few weeks there he came across a patient who introduced himself as Jesus Christ. Erickson's response was, "Oh, you are a carpenter." He then told the man that he needed help with some carpentry and asked if he would help build some bookshelves in his new office. Erickson got the equipment, the man built some shelves, and from then on Erickson used carpentry as his way of developing that person. Eventually, the man left the hospital, went out into the community, and became a carpenter. He still believed he was Jesus Christ, so that aspect of his belief system was not changed, but he had become a functional member of the community as a carpenter.[53]

If one looked at only the negative aspects of this story, one would focus on the patient's delusion. This is not wrong, any more than looking at a half-full bottle of milk and saying that it is half empty is wrong. The facts can be viewed from many perspectives. In Erickson's example, if one is concerned with improving function rather than breaking the patient's delusional mode, one can do so by focusing the patient's thinking into a realistic function, in this case carpentry, that is consistent with his delusion. When we as therapists are confronted by patients who state that they are in pain and have certain functional limits, we should accept what they say as

truth. There may be symptom magnification, but practitioners should not allow that possibility to interfere with getting a real feeling of what the patient is experiencing. If therapists take what a patient says as the truth, because whatever we are told at that moment is true to the patient, we can get across to the patient that we believe him. Then the patient is more likely to regard us as allies in the healing process. We can then go on to use what we know about pain generators, pain behavior, and natural healing to move the patient in a direction of recovery.

Walking as Treatment

One of the most effective methods for treating injuries to the lumbar area is walking. Part of the therapist's job is to convince the patient that walking is the right thing to do. By showing the patient, through the use of visualization techniques, the segment that has been injured and what effect walking will have on it, the patient will get a graphic sense of the nature of the problem and the value of the treatment. This approach not only enlists patients in "becoming their own therapists," but also gives them a tool for visualization while walking. Briefly, have the patient place his hands on his own back and feel the contraction and relaxation of the muscles during walking, so the patient can visualize the pumping action of the muscles assisting in "lubricating" the injured area. This has the effect of enlisting the patient's positive energy in the healing process and contributes to a psychological advantage by helping the patient feel less powerless, while relieving negative emotions such as fear and anxiety.

In our sedentary culture, there is a high incidence of degenerative changes in the low lumbar segments in persons age 50 and over compared with people of age 20, even when they have not sustained an obvious injury to this area. In primitive cultures, where the people are physically active, the incidence of degeneration in the mobile segment from aging is less pronounced. In one study, 450 x-rays were taken of a group of 15- to 44-year-old members of the Bihl tribe in India and compared with x-rays from similar age groups in Sweden and the United States. The results indicated disk narrowing in 80% of a Swedish group of heavy laborers by age 55, 35 percent narrowing in a group of light workers in San Francisco, and only 9 percent in the Bihl tribe members at age 55. The incidence of disk narrowing was about 5 percent in all three series equally in the youngest age group studied.[54]

From this study one could conclude that the incidence of disk degeneration is not coincident with age, but has some correlation with such factors as activity, diet, and heredity. Therefore, one hypothesis would be that disk degeneration is not natural to the human body between the ages of 20 and 50, but rather a response to the stress placed on it. One might also hypothesize that maximizing nutrition of the mobile segment through positive activity would limit some of the aging changes that lead to low back disorders.

The job of the practitioner then becomes one of improving the nutrition of the mobile segment. This can be done through walking. In attempting to motivate patients to make behavioral changes, it can be helpful to use the following reasoning: State that walking is an effective treatment for lumbar injuries because it stimulates movement of cells, nutrients, and waste products directly from the blood supply of the vertebrae into the disk via imbibition and pumping action. Continue by telling patients that when they are sedentary, nutrition to the disk and other structures is impeded, but that if they walk 15 to 20 minutes regularly over a period of several months, circulation will be stimulated, facilitating recovery.

In addition to providing nutrition through the blood supply, synovial fluids function both as a lubricant and as a medium for nutrition of the cartilage of the zygapophyseal joints. Studies have demonstrated a rapid degeneration of the joint cartilage following immobility.[55] It has been hypothesized that this degenerative change is partly due to a decrease in nourishment of the cartilage, secondary to a decrease in synovial fluid movement.[36] Therefore, when muscle spasm and decreasing activity immobilize the joints of a mobile segment for longer than 48 hours, the cartilage can be expected to begin to undergo degenerative changes. The synovial fluids then begin to demonstrate chemical and physiologic changes, starting a process that is difficult and time-consuming to reverse. Walking produces repetitive movement of the joints, which mechanically increases the fluid lubrication and stimulates the secretion of normal synovial fluid by the synovial lining of the joint, aiding in regeneration and restoration of normal cartilage.[38,39]

In normal gait, the arms swing in alternation with the legs, imparting a cyclical motion to the spine. Spinal motions occurring in walking are flexion, lateral bending, and rotation, followed by extension, lateral bending, and rotation in the opposite direction. There are also small-magnitude strain deflection movements when the joints are subjected to the stress of weightbearing.[56] This strain deflection may stimulate the body to make the bone even stronger, since bone is living tissue and can adapt to stress, and careful training can increase its strength. Muscle contractions increase blood flow, and tiny electric voltages are generated within the bone that stimulate growth. However, a mild stress repeated thousands of times can cause the bone to develop minute fractures that can grow into full-scale fractures. These so-called stress fractures result from an attempt by the body to make the bone even stronger, but before new bone can be set in place, old bone must be removed by special demolition cells. Therefore, there is a moment in time when the bone is weaker than before and vulnerable to fracture. Hence, an important treatment principle— subjective though it may be—is derived from this theory. A brief period of rest will give the bone a chance to fill in, and then training can be resumed.[57] This conceptual framework is necessary in approaching a progressive walking program for back injuries.

The impact of walking is much broader than merely its effect on the mobile segment and muscles and nerves of the spinal column. It also:

1. Stimulates circulation of the blood, the cerebrospinal fluid, and the lymphatics.
2. Benefits cardiovascular and cardiopulmonary fitness and stimulates the endocrine system.
3. Reduces the viscosity of the nucleus of the disk, allowing for a better fluid exchange within the nucleus itself.
4. Assists mechanically in the exchange of fluid between the vertebrae and the nucleus by increasing and decreasing the pressure on portions of the disk. In other words, walking on the left leg

increases pressure on the left side of the disk and decreases pressure on the right side. When one then puts weight on the right leg, that pressure gradient is changed so that it is greater on the right side and less on the left. This reciprocal motion creates a pump-like action that increases pressure on one side of the disk and moves fluid into the vertebral body. Conversely, when the area is under decreased pressure, a sucking effect pulls fluid from the vertebra back into that area.

5. Stimulates the mechanoreceptors, facilitating the normal neurophysiologic status of the whole mobile segment.[30]
6. Improves coordination and strength of the muscles necessary to control the movement of the mobile segment. This is accomplished through the reciprocal contraction and relaxation of the muscles engaged in walking.
7. Impacts positively on the patient psychologically, maximizing the placebo effect.[47] It has been clinically observed that patients who have lost the ability to function subsequent to injury of the musculoskeletal system will heal more rapidly when their treatment plan consists of a repetitious activity with which they are already familiar. In contrast, if you ask the patient to learn a new motor skill such as the pelvic tilt, the patient not only must deal with the difficulties ensuing from the injury, but also must struggle with the stress involved in learning a new motor skill.
8. Allows patients to get away from the environment of the home, where they are frequently confronted with stressful emotional and mental conditions.
9. Moves the patient from the role of passive victim to one of active healer—a crucially important psychological shift in the promotion of wellness.

The amount of walking that is indicated depends on the stage of the pathology. One first must establish a base of activity that does not aggravate the underlying symptoms. For example, if what aggravates a patient's symptoms is sitting or standing more than half an hour, lifting more than 10 pounds from waist to shoulder level, lifting from the floor to the waist and from the shoulders to above the head, and walking more than 10 minutes, then this level of activity becomes the base. From this base, the patient slowly increases the amount of walking until an optimum level is reached, which should be maintained until the patient is well.

A moderate walking program is most effective at enhancing recovery. If the base level of the patient's walking activity is 10 minutes, the walking program then must be to walk four times a day for a 10-minute period, provided this does not increase the pain. Activity should be increased on alternate days, and as a general rule the patient should not increase the activity by more than 10 percent of the previous level. Slow increases in activity are preferable to sudden quick increases, and the body must be given less stress on alternate days. The stress of the activity on one day will cause the body to make adjustments that will weaken it on the next, but the body will then recover and be stronger because of this stress. Finally, the patient must walk frequently every day for a minimum of 15 to 20 minutes.

As the clinician assists the patient from the most acute stage of the injury through progressive improvement, the need for walking is critical at all levels except when strict bed rest is called for. At the acute stages, the patient may only walk for 2 minutes at a time, but the patient should walk as often as several times an hour. As the patient's condition improves, walking should increase to 5 minutes every hour, then 10 minutes every 2 hours, up to 15 minutes four times a day. The goal in walking is to get to where the patient can do a brisk half-hour to 40 minutes four times a day without discomfort. This amounts to anywhere from 6 to 8 miles a day. Once patients can walk that amount without aggravating symptoms, they need to stay at that level for anywhere from several weeks to a lifetime in order to maintain a healthy condition.

As the patient is recovering, the therapist can often relate the decrease in pain to the degree of healing that occurs. However, just because pain has been reduced to zero does not mean that there is 100 percent recovery. As the disk and other structures in the mobile segment heal, there is a point at which the patient will become asymptomatic. The therapist knows from clinical experience that this patient can be reinjured with excessive activity, even at this essentially asymptomatic stage.

By stressing the joint during examination, the therapist can determine its integrity. The structure can be considered recovered only when the segment is asymptomatic to all examination movements including end-range overpressure and combined movements. Further assessment of repetitive functional activity may be necessary to determine the endurance of the segment.

When teaching patients to become their own therapists, therapists must give them an understanding of the healing process so they can prevent themselves from being injured again. Patients may need to be taught to think in a common sense manner about injury and repair. These are not areas in which people are commonly instructed, and people frequently fear injury and do not understand the physiologic process of repair. To clarify the injury process and the normal repair process is to remove fear and give the patient more conscious control over what is going on. In a case of obvious injury to a mobile segment, even after reaching an asymptomatic level, the patient must continue to maximize disk nutrition. This process should continue for as long as is necessary for all the supportive structures in that segment to gain sufficient endurance to minimize the chance of reinjury.

CASE STUDY

The following case study was chosen because it illustrates many of the concepts presented in this chapter.

The patient, a 46-year-old male, 5 feet 10 inches tall and weighing 190 pounds, sustained a low back injury at age 19 when as a lifeguard he was carrying an accident victim from the water. He developed severe right sciatica with bladder paralysis and weakness of his right lower extremity. He was hospitalized for 3 weeks with total bladder paralysis, but recovered approximately 30 percent of function by use of massage, hot and cold compresses, and whirlpool. He was able to improve his condition an additional 25 percent by adhering for 5 months to a program that included swimming 5 hours a day and walking. For 20 years following that severe episode, he had minor incidents of low backache and occasional feelings of weakness in the leg. Otherwise he led an active life, which included expert skiing and playing racketball regularly.

Four years ago, while moving some heavy furniture from a warehouse to his office, he developed a severe recurrence of his right sciatica. His right foot began to drag, and he noted that the bladder weakness had returned. The symptoms gradually improved over the following year so that he could lie down and walk comfortably. But he had more problems walking uphill than on level ground, and prolonged sitting of more than 8 hours, such as was required on long plane flights, resulted in increasing pain.

At the time of the recurrence the patient had a CT scan which identified a calcified disk at the L5–S1 level, with possible foraminal stenosis on the right at the L4–L5 level. His neurologic examination revealed a decreased reflex in the right calf with 90 degrees of straight leg raise on the left and 80 degrees on the right. His standing posture was symmetrical with a slightly flattened lordosis. He had a limitation of full extension with a slight increase in low back pain. His flexion was 50 percent, and a left deviation accompanied the flexion. Lateral flexion left and right was within normal limits. Muscular strength tested as normal.

At that time, physical therapy treatment was initiated. It included end-range mobilization in rotation bilaterally and inversion gravity traction in flexion. This treatment resulted in a rapid resolution of his exacerbation, and within 1 month he had returned to his pre-exacerbation level of activity. He remained well until 9 months ago, when he sustained a further injury following the lifting of 150 pounds from waist level to overhead. He resorted to his home treatment program, which involved swimming a half-hour each morning and walking 2 miles a day, combined with inversion traction and repeated flexion in lying. He felt 40 percent relief following this program. However, for the next 4 months, despite cutting back on his activity level and avoiding lifting and sitting, he was unable to get back to a feeling of stability in his spine.

Physical therapy was then initiated involving gentle oscillatory transverse movements at the L4–L5 mobile segment. After these treatments the patient would feel significant relief of his pain, but he was unable to get sufficient relief to be able to resume his strengthening exercises without suffering exacerbation. He sought further medical advice and had another CT scan. The surgeon's opinion was that he had an unstable L5–S1 segment and a disk bulge at L4–L5. He recommended microsurgery at that disk and fusion of the L5–S1 motion segment. The patient was scheduled to have a myelogram to add further to this diagnostic and treatment decision, but before the scheduled myelogram, autotraction treatment was initiated. The autotraction treatment resulted in further improvement, and within six treatments he felt 70 percent recovered and was feeling better than he had since the exacerbation 9 months ago.

This patient's current functional level is such that he is walking 5 to 7 miles a day without pain. He stands and works 11 to 12 hours a day with minimal discomfort, avoids sitting except when driving, and stands for a maximum of 30 minutes at a time. Treatment progression will be to add spinal strengthening exercises to the autotraction program to teach protective body mechanics, allowing the patient to maintain an optimum neutral spinal posture for his condition at the same time as he performs stretching exercises of his lower extremity musculature.

Even before considering treatment, the therapist must first understand the patient as a human being. The therapist's sense of the patient in this case study was that he was a stoic and someone who had to be in control of his life. He was also someone who had to learn to limit himself so as not to exacerbate his condition.

To put this awareness to work, the therapist had to verify with the patient that he was in fact this type of person. This was accomplished by asking him if he considered himself a stoic who needed to be in control of his treatment in order to get better. When the patient agreed, the therapist added that he needed to learn to live within certain limits. The patient agreed here also. The important aspect of this question and affirmation process is that it enlists the patient's participation. It would be of little value for the therapist's assessment to be "right" if the patient did not agree. Since the patient has to make the changes, it is the patient's reality that matters, not the practitioner's.

It was then necessary for the therapist to understand what the patient was willing to live with. The patient wanted to be able to ski on the expert slopes, to play racketball, to lift weights, and to be relatively comfortable doing all of this. Therefore, in educating this patient, it was necessary for the therapist to emphasize to him that his injury was real, not emotional, and not something that would go away if he ignored it. At the same time, the therapist stated that the injury could be healed if the patient would do the right things in selectively stressing his low back to stimulate body repair to stabilize that injured mobile segment.

The next point the therapist emphasized was that as the patient increased his activity level and felt better, he could not ignore the fact that he still had a back problem. He therefore had to increase his activity level by no more than 10 percent at a time. If even that 10 percent was in fact too much, he would find that out by an increase in his symptoms, and he would then need to reduce his activity level. Through this trial and assessment process, the patient was able to monitor his level of discomfort and achieve the necessary stress to activate recovery without causing further injury to the mobile segment.

In this case, the surgeon's recommendation for surgery was based on hard signs such as CT scans and MRI findings which are not fully meaningful unless correlated clearly with the signs and symptoms. It can be a mistake to interpret those findings as completely explaining the patient's problem. Findings on CT scan and MRI explained the symptoms of instability the patient had in his spine and the pain he experienced, but they did not indicate that the only means of resolution of this problem was surgery.

The patient's case history indicated that the injury to the L5–S1 segment 25 years ago was a major injury. Yet the body was able to stabilize that injury through calcification of the disk. Thereafter the patient was able to conduct a very normal life, at least as normal as one could have expected had he had surgical intervention. In short, the physician from within did as good a job as one could have expected of any physician from without.

The patient's injury of 9 months ago might have stabilized in the same way as the prior injury did, or it might have reached a stage at which surgical stabilization was necessary. To make this decision entirely on the basis of the CT scan, MRI, myelography, and other standard tests would be to risk unnecessary surgery. Instead, all conservative approaches should be attempted first, including maximizing the positive psychological benefit of involving the patient in his own care and modifying any behavior that is detrimental to the resolution of the problem. Only if these approaches fail should one proceed with surgery.

The clinician must also be methodical in making decisions about what treatment to use. Three years earlier, mobilization at end range had resulted in rapid resolution of signs and symptoms and a return to optimum functioning that made that treatment the correct treatment at that time. More recently, the same approach to treatment did not result in the same rapid improvement. This then necessitated a change in approach, even though the aims were the same. Had the autotraction not been effective, another approach would have been used until all conservative approaches were exhausted, at which point surgical intervention to stabilize that mobile segment would have been a logical next step.

Throughout this patient's history, he consistently responded positively to movement, so long as it was performed repetitively and over an extended period of time in a way that did not increase the symptoms. For example, when he was initially injured he spent 5 months swimming in addition to his other activities. This could well have contributed to his initial recovery. The one thing the patient was able to do that 3 years ago would consistently relieve his symptoms was walk. The more he walked, the better he would feel, provided he did not go beyond his limits. As he got stronger and stronger, his limits became greater, until he was able to walk 5 to 6 miles a day.

The patient found that by getting up first thing in the morning and going for a 2- to 3-mile walk, he was far more comfortable during the day than if he got up and rushed off to work without walking. If he tried to do spinal stabilization exercises, play racketball, or ski before he could walk 5 to 6 miles a day, he would exacerbate his symptoms. Even when he could walk 5 to 6 miles a day, he needed to do that over an extended period of time before he became stable enough to be able to progress to the next stage of activity.

One approach to the treatment of the problem would be to categorize the patient as having a calcified disk, a disk bulge at L4–L5 with bladder paresis which indicates cauda equina involvement, a decreased gastrocnemius reflex, and weakness of the gastrocnemius muscle. Based on that list of signs, the treatment could be surgery, or pelvic traction and a corset.

Another approach is to make the same statements about the facts but to recognize that even given those same facts there are many different resolutions, many different ways to accomplish return to function. Also, the "history, signs, symptoms, and patient-focused" treatment approach recognizes the need to harness the power of patients to maximize their own progress and to let the signs and symptoms of the injury guide the treatment process.

This case study illustrates the following main principles:

1. The importance of the patient taking an active role in treatment
2. The need for the therapist to see the injury from the perspective of the patient
3. The need to activate the body's built-in healing methods through activities such as walking
4. The importance of the home treatment program being one of gradual and monitored increases in activity
5. The need for the patient to recognize and work within a necessary set of realistic limits
6. The need for the therapist to guide the treatment by the signs and symptoms, and by focusing on the patient rather than on a diagnostic label
7. The need to teach the patient to "become his own therapist"
8. The need to allow time for the body's natural healing process, the "physician from within," to work.

CONCLUSION

In physical therapy, patients often ask, "What's wrong with me?" Trying to explain what is wrong in terms of a diagnostic label often leads to more problems than it resolves. The essence of the medical model in Western medicine today is to examine a number of people with similar conditions and to study those conditions to try to come up with a general view as to etiology, pathology, and prognosis.

The diagnostic label is usually unclear to patients and gives them either a confused picture of the problem or one in which their knowledge of the negative aspects of the diagnosis dominates their awareness. We must give patients confidence so that they can assume an active role in freeing themselves from pain as they learn to be their own back doctors.

It is a natural human response to look at the worst case scenario in order to be prepared for the worst. The problem with this manner of thinking is that it can lead the patient to look only at the medical prognosis. But prognoses are based on statistical analyses of group means, not specific, individual patients. Therefore, patients who focus on the diagnostic label will be looking at a broad range of prognostic data that may or may not relate to them directly. This can lead the patient to self-program a negative outcome that may not be applicable. Patients create their own reality through their sets of expectations and beliefs. If a patient sees a negative outcome as reality, then that is often the reality the patient will experience.

Positive thinking maximizes the body's healing processes, whereas negative thinking is counterproductive.[11,47-49] Therefore, to focus a patient's thinking and understanding of the problem on specific factors that relate to his problem rather than the universe of people with that problem is to focus the patient in a constructive direction.

By clarifying the signs and symptoms that patients have, in a manner that is understandable, the therapist can assist patients in personalizing the problem as it relates to their own condition. Through this better understanding, patients will be better able to understand the problem and be in control of the condition rather than the victim of it.

There also is no clear relationship between the diagnostic label and the treatment. The therapist must attempt to clarify the diagnostic label for the patient by explaining it not as a pathology in the sense of a sickness or a disease, which is the common perception of pathology, but rather as a strain or sprain of a specific structure in the musculoskeletal system. When the diagnostic label does not specifically incriminate a structure, then the injury should be explained as occurring within a specific mobile segment. A further description of the movement characteristics can clarify the biomechanical nature of the disorder. One can describe that dysfunctioning mobile segment in terms of pain and pain patterns, or in terms of the pain's aggravation and easing with activity or rest.

A functional profile of a patient's disorder is far more meaningful to the patient than any diagnostic label. It is also more meaningful to those who have to deal with the problem, such as insurance carriers and employers. People will better understand a problem if they can live that problem in their own mind rather than try to understand a set of medical labels that have little relationship to their personal experience.

As clinicians, it is also important for us to remember that we cannot hasten the natural healing process. When we involve ourselves in treating the patient who has a problem that is resolvable by the patient's inner physician, we need to be very careful that we do not get in the way and interfere with the body's natural healing. Effective treatment is to minimize those factors that interfere with the natural healing process and simultaneously encourage that process through our art and science.

REFERENCES

1. Warwick R, Williams P (ed): Gray's Anatomy. 35th British Ed. WB Saunders, Philadelphia, 1973
2. McMinn RMH, Hutchins RT: Color Atlas of Human Anatomy. Year Book Medical Publishers, Chicago, 1977
3. Netter F: The CIBA Collection of Medical Illustrations. Vol. 1. Part 1. CIBA, West Caldwell, NJ, 1983
4. Bogduk N, Twomey L: Clinical Anatomy of the Lumbar Spine. Churchill Livingstone, Edinburgh, 1987
5. McNab I: Backache. Williams & Wilkins, Baltimore, 1977
6. Dixon ASJ: Diagnosis of low back pain — sorting the complainers. p. 77. In Jayson M (ed): The Lumbar Spine and Back Pain. Sector Publishing, London, 1976
7. Dvorak J, Dvorak V: Manual Medicine: Diagnostics. Thieme-Stratton, New York, 1984
8. Corrigan B, Maitland BD: Practical Orthopaedic Medicine. Butterworths, London, 1983

9. Yong-Hing K, Kirkaldy-Willis WH: The pathophysiology of degenerative disease of the lumbar spine. Orthop Clin North Am 14:491, 1983

10. Cyriax J: Textbook of orthopaedic medicine. 6th Ed. Vol. 1. Bailliere Tindall, London, 1975

11. Simonton O, Creighton J: Getting Well Again. Bantam, New York, 1980

12. Arey BL, Burrows W, Greenhill JP, Hewitt R (eds): Dorland's illustrated Medical Dictionary. 23rd Ed. WB Saunders, Philadelphia, 1959

13. Feinstein A: Clinical Judgement. Robert E. Krieger, Malabar, FL, 1967

14. Korr IM: The facilitated segment: a factor in injury to the body framework. p. 27. In Stark EH (ed): Clinical Review Series: Osteopathic Medicine. Publishing Sciences Group, Acton, 1975

15. Jull G, Janda V: Muscle and motor control in low back pain: assessment and management. p. 257. In Twomey L, Taylor J (eds): Physical Therapy of the Low Back. Churchill Livingstone, New York, 1987

16. Frank C, Akeson WH, Woo SL-Y, et al: Physiology and therapeutic value of passive joint motion. Clin Orthop 185:113, 1984

17. Macintosh J, Bogduk N: The anatomy and function of the lumbar back muscles and their fascia. p. 103. In Twomey L, Taylor J (eds): Physical Therapy of the Low Back. Churchill Livingstone, New York, 1987

18. McCall IW, Park WM, O'Brien JP: Induced pain referral from posterior lumbar elements in normal subjects. Spine 4:441, 1979

19. Mooney V, Robertson J: The facet syndrome. Clin Orthop 115:149, 1976

20. Wiberg G: Back pain in relation to the nerve supply of the intervertebral disc. Acta Orthop Scand 19:211, 1947

21. Hirsch C: An attempt to diagnose the level of a disc lesion clinically by disc puncture. Acta Orthop Scand 18:1132, 1949

22. Lindblom K: Technique and results in myelography and disc puncture. Acta Radiol 34:321, 1950

23. Perey O: Contrast medium examination of the intervertebral discs of the lower lumbar spine. Acta Orthop Scand 20:327, 1951

24. Collis JS, Gardner WJ: Lumbar discography—an analysis of 1,000 cases. J Neurosurg 19:452, 1962

25. Simmons EH, Segil CM: An evaluation of discography in the localization of symptomatic levels in discogenic disease of the spine. Clin Orthop 108:57, 1975

26. Wiley JJ, MacNab I, Wortzman G: Lumbar discography and its clinical applications. Can J Surg 11:280, 1968

27. Smyth MJ, Wright V: Sciatica and the intervertebral disc. An experimental study. J Bone Joint Surg 40A:1401, 1959

28. El Mahdi MA, Latif FYA, Janko M: The spinal nerve root innervation, and a new concept of the clinico-pathological interrelations in back pain and sciatica. Neurochirurgia 24:137, 1981

29. Boas RA: Post-surgical low back pain. p. 188. In Peck C, Wallace M (eds): Problems in Pain. Pergamon, Sydney, 1980

30. Wyke B: Neurological aspects of low back pain. p. 189. In Jayson M (ed): The Lumbar Spine and Back Pain. Sector Publishing, London, 1976.

31. Grieve GP: Common Vertebral Joint Problems. Churchill Livingstone, Edinburgh, 1981

32. Dommisse GF: The blood supply of the spinal cord. p. 37. In Grieve GP (ed): Modern Manual Therapy of the Vertebral Column. Churchill Livingstone, Edinburgh, 1986

33. Aki T, Toya S: Experimental study on the circulatory dynamics of the spinal cord by serial fluorescence and geography. Spine 9(3):262, 1984

34. Crock H, Goldwasser M: Anatomic studies of the circulation in the region of the vertebral end-plate in adult greyhound dogs. Spine 9(7):702, 1984

35. Hansen HJ: Comparative views of the pathology of disc degeneration in animals: Lab Invest 8:1242, 1959

36. Kahanovitz N: The effects of internal fixation on the articular cartilage of unfused canine facet joint cartilage. Spine 9:268, 1984

37. Wyke B: Neurological aspects of low back pain. In Jayson M (ed): The Lumbar Spine and Back Pain. Sector Publishing, London, 1976

38. Hunter L, Braunstein E, Bailey RW: Radiographic changes following anterior cervical fusion. Spine 5:399, 1980

39. Tredwell SJ, O'Brien JP: Apophyseal joint degeneration in the cervical spine following halo pelvic distraction. Spine 6:497, 1980

40. Evans P: The healing process at cellular level: a review. Physiotherapy 66:256, 1980

41. Maitland GD: Vertebral Manipulation. 5th Ed. Butterworths, London, 1986

42. Maitland GD: Examination and Recording Guide. 4th Ed. Lauderdale Press, Glen Osmond, South Australia, 1986

43. Magarey ME: Examination and assessment in spinal joint dysfunction. p. 481. In Grieve GP (ed): Modern Manual Therapy of the Vertebral Column. Churchill Livingstone, Edinburgh, 1986

44. Maitland GD: The Maitland concept: assessment, examination, and treatment by passive movements. p. 135. In Twomey LT, Taylor JR (eds): Physical Ther-

apy of the Low Back. Churchill Livingstone, New York, 1987

45. Berne E: Intuition and Ego States. Harper & Row, San Francisco, 1977

46. Grieve GP: Lumbar instability. p. 416. In Grieve GP (ed): Modern Manual Therapy of the Vertebral Column. Churchill Livingstone, Edinburgh, 1986

47. Borysenko J: Minding the Body, Mending the Mind. Addison-Wesley, Menlo Park, CA, 1987

48. Benson H, Proctor W: Beyond the Relaxation Repsonse. Berkley, New York, 1985

49. Pelletier K: Mind as Healer, Mind as Slayer. Dell Books, New York, 1977

50. Wiesel S, Tsourmas N, Feffer H, Citrin C, Patronas N: A study of computer-assisted tomography: The incidence of positive CAT scans in an asymptomatic group of patients. Spine 9:6, 1984

51. Gillstrom P: A Clinical and Objective Analysis of Autotraction as a Form for Therapy in Lumbago and Sciatica. Unpublished thesis, University of Stockholm, Sweden, 1985

52. Rumney I: The relevance of somatic dysfunction. Am Orthop Assoc 74:723, 1975

53. Haley J: Uncommon Therapy: The Psychiatric Technique of Milton Erickson. WW Norton, New York, 1973

54. Fahrni WH: Back Ache: Assessment and Treatment. Evergreen Press, Vancouver, 1978

55. Holm S, Nachemson A: Nutritional changes in the canine intervertebral disc after spinal fusion. Clin Orthop Rel Res 169:243, 1982

56. Farfan H: Mechanical Disorders of the Low Back. Lea & Febiger, Philadelphia, 1973

57. Padmore T: Limp in, jog out: Sports medicine up and running. Chronicle, p. 22. University of British Columbia, Spring, 1982

58. Grieve GP: Mobilization of the Spine. 4th Ed. Churchill Livingstone, Edinburgh, 1984

16

Surgical Treatment of the Lumbar Spine

DAVID ROUBEN

Medical and allied health professionals charged with the responsibility of evaluating, examining, and diagnosing spinal pain must be keenly attentive to the importance of appreciating each patient's problem as a unique and distinct entity. This is achieved by methodically analyzing the history presented by the patient, examining the physical idiosyncrasies of each patient, ordering and evaluating those clinically objective documentary tests that are available, making an assessment of the most plausible diagnosis, and deciding what can and should be done for the patients.

EVALUATING THE PATIENT

History

It is important for the treating physician or therapist eliciting the clinical history to appreciate that certain questions are of more significance in the evaluation of the back pain patient, and can easily direct them to a diagnosis.

Obviously, the sex and age of the patient are important. It is unlikely that a woman would have a disease such as ankylosing spondylitis, or that a 17-year-old would have symptoms of multiple myeloma, a disease most commonly seen in the elderly.

It is important to establish the nature of the complaint: How did it occur? Under what circumstances did it occur? When did it occur? How long have the symptoms been noticed? During what part of the day are the symptoms noticed? Do they occur at night or during the day? Are they only evident in the morning after the patient first awakens, or are they felt after the patient has been working all day? Are they related to a particular position or activity, or to the specific work that the patient does? Where is the pain located? Has the location changed over time? Does the patient perceive pain in one place and also sense it elsewhere in the body? Has there been any change in the perception of pain, its intensity, in location, or quality since the onset of any injury? Has it diminished or increased since the onset of any injury? How has the patient treated the condition until now, and have any of these treatments been effective?

A determination of any familial illnesses can be made through a family history and may prove enlightening.

Does the patient have any allergies? Are there any medical illnesses that the patient has had in the past or is presently being treated for that have any direct or indirect relation to the patient's symptomatology? What things seem to increase or decrease the pain, not only with respect to activity and exercise, but also with respect to the patient's environment at home, work, or play?

The differential diagnosis should be based on a complete and concise elicitation of the clinical history. The following case study illustrates this approach. The flowcharts in Figures 16-1 to 16-9 show the steps in evaluation that contribute to various diagnoses.

A 44-year-old white woman presented with pain in the right buttock and leg. Two years ago she

349

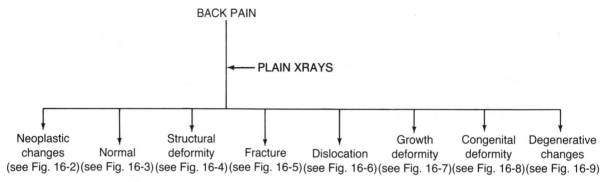

Fig. 16-1. Flowchart of differential diagnoses for back pain. The figure in parentheses beneath each diagnosis indicates the figure that continues the differential diagnosis for that cause.

was treated for a herniated disk. She underwent a chemonucleolysis procedure with chymopapain at the L4–L5 level, which until recently appeared to be completely successful. The patient is the mother of two, and appeared to be entering menopause because she had not had regular periods for some time.

While playing tennis with her daughters over the weekend, she noticed the onset of pain in her right buttock and leg. The pain was consistent and persistent. It was felt in her right buttock and down the posterolateral aspect of her right leg, distal to her knee, involving the posterior and lateral aspects of her calf and the lateral aspect of her foot, on both the dorsal and plantar aspects. Sexual relations with her husband were impossible because of the increased pain. The pain was accentuated by bending and by raising her leg in a straightened position.

The patient had tried bed rest and heat, but the heat did not diminish her pain. Lying on her back seemed to lessen the pain as long as she did not move quickly. The pain was accentuated when the patient would lay on her abdomen or on either side. She now had to walk in a crouched-over gait, because standing erect accentuated her pain. Sitting diminished her pain, but any fast motions accentuated it. She had not felt any pain in her middle or upper back.

The patient thought she felt the same type of pain that she had experienced when she had the herniated disk; however, it was now in the opposite leg. She had been healthy since her chymopapain injection. She was not allergic to any medications and was not taking anything other than Extra-Strength Tylenol, which did not diminish her pain significantly. She was able to sleep through the night, but when she got up in the morning she would feel the pain, and it was a persistent phenomenon throughout the day.

A review of her family history showed that both

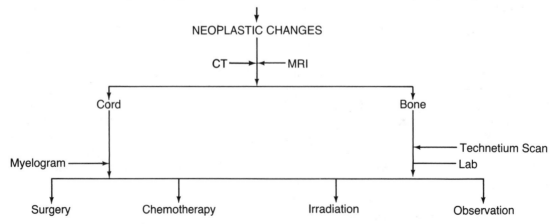

Fig. 16-2. Flowchart of evaluation and treatment of neoplastic changes.

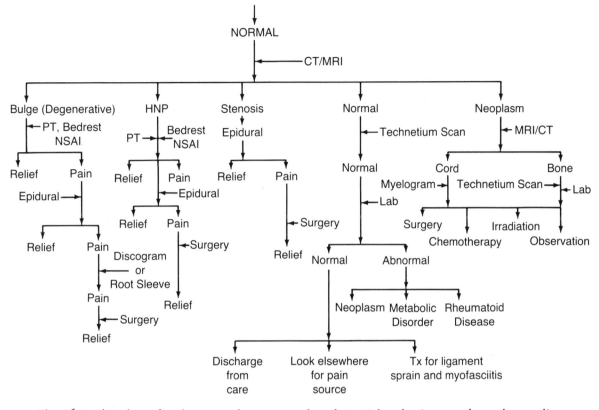

Fig. 16-3. Flowchart of evaluation and treatment when the initial evaluation reveals no abnormality.

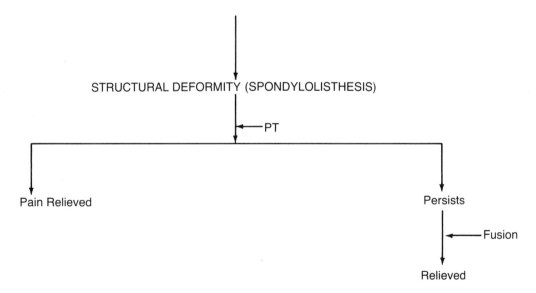

Fig. 16-4. Flowchart of evaluation and treatment of structural deformities.

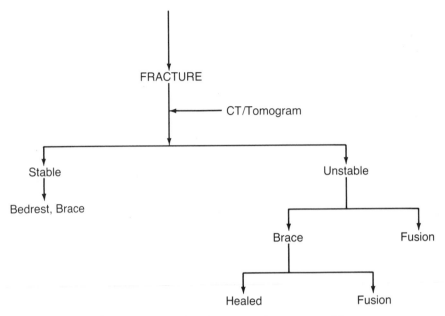

Fig. 16-5. Flowchart of evaluation and treatment of fractures.

her father and her mother were alive and healthy; however, the father suffered from hypertension and was taking medications for it.

The information presented in this case history answers the questions listed earlier in the chapter and gives us some direction for making a diagnosis. Read the list of questions again and find the answer to each question in the case study.

Physical Examination

The physical examination should be used as a means of verifying or excluding in possible diagnoses. It should be performed in such a way as to offer the greatest chance of proving or disproving any of the potential diagnoses. This is most efficiently done by performing physical examinations in the same sequence on each patient. For example,

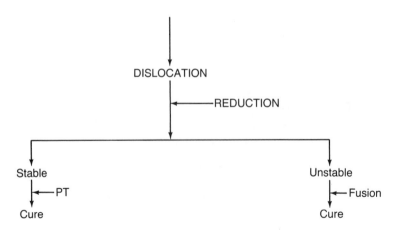

Fig. 16-6. Flowchart of evaluation and treatment of dislocations.

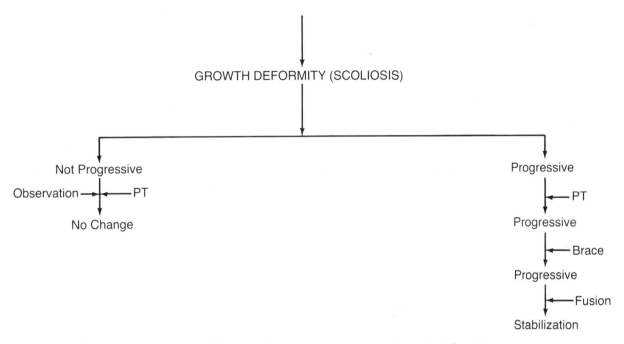

Fig. 16-7. Flowchart of evaluation and treatment of growth deformities.

clinicians start by examining the superior or cephalad aspect of the body, and continue in a caudad or inferior direction.

The physical examination should help uncover any pathologic findings that compromise the range of motion of the joints in the injured area. Is pain elicited during manipulation or motion of any of the joints? Are there weaknesses in any of the muscle groups in the area of the injury? Are there any objective findings that are associated with pain, such as muscular spasms, swelling, redness, or changes in skin temperature? Is there less awareness to light touch, temperature perception, and pressure? How does the patient ambulate, and how does the patient move when walking or getting in and out of a chair, or on and off a table?

Look for asymmetry when examining the body. What is the posture of the different parts of the torso

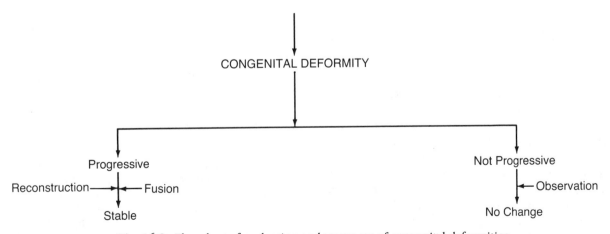

Fig. 16-8. Flowchart of evaluation and treatment of congenital deformities.

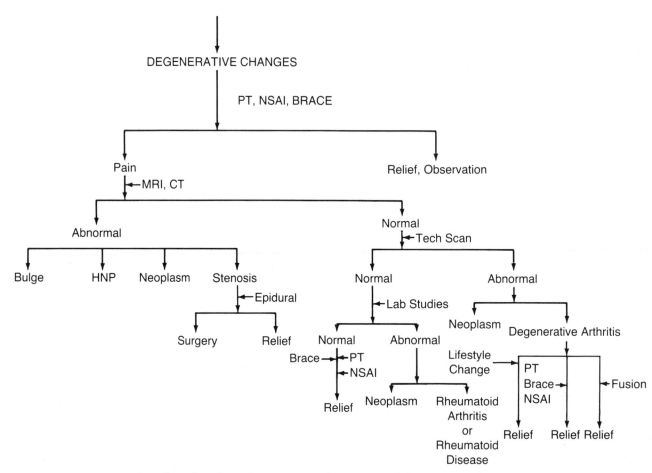

Fig. 16-9. Flowchart of evaluation and treatment of degenerative changes.

and of the extremities? Is there any evidence of dermatologic pathology, such as dimples, hairy patches, extra skin folds, or lesions, that help exclude or include possible diagnoses? Is there any evidence of atrophy, hypertrophy, or mass lesions over the involved parts of the body, or other parts of the body that may not be symptomatic, but may have some direct or indirect relationship to the problem?

It is important to correlate the subjective and objective abnormalities seen with respect to sensation and motor dysfunction with the motor and sen-

sory dermatome distributions illustrated in Figure 13-12 A.

Proper physical examination technique is illustrated in the continuation of the case study that follows.

The following findings were discovered upon physical examination. The patient stood in a semiflexed position, tending to obliterate some of the normal lumbar lordosis. When the patient ambulated she favored her right side with a slight limp, or at least the perception on visual examination was that there was discomfort during weightbearing. The pain was relieved when the patient sat or was supine with two pillows under her knees. She had a positive straight leg raising sign in her right leg. She had normal patellar tendon reflexes, and somewhat diminished but bilaterally symmetrical achilles tendon reflexes. There was no gross evidence of motor weakness to ankle, foot, knee, or hip function. However, there was a marked straight leg raising sign at 60 degrees, with discomfort in the buttocks and posterior thigh, and enhancement of discomfort with the knee extended and forceful dorsiflexion of the ankle. There was no contralateral discomfort with straight leg raising on the left side. Stressing the sacroiliac joint by placing the foot on top of the contralateral knee and then forcing the leg into external rotation did not elicit typical discomfort. There was discomfort on flexion at the waist as compared to extension, and no enhanced discomfort was felt on rotation or lateral bending at the waist.

Upon completion of the history and physical examination, a careful discussion of your findings with the patient is indicated. By this time you have collectively assessed the information from the history as well as the confirmatory findings retrieved from the physical examination. You should now be able to direct your attention toward confirmation of your presumed differential diagnosis.

Laboratory Tests

Ancillary laboratory and radiographic tests are often used to confirm a diagnosis. The tests most often used in the evaluation of patients with back pain include, complete blood count, erythrocyte sedimentation rate, SHA 18, human leukocyte antibody (HLAB) 27, rheumatoid antigen, antinuclear antibody (ANA), serum protein electrophoresis, urinalysis with urine culture and sensitivity, assessment of blood bacterial contamination (i.e., blood cultures); technetium bone scan, gallium scan, indium scan, magnetic resonance imaging (MRI), computed tomography (CT), myelography, discogram, facet blocks, root sleeve injections, and thermography.[1]

After the history and physical examination have been used to narrow the diagnosis, appropriate tests are ordered to prove or disprove the clinician's

theories. A basic understanding of what each test is and what information it can provide is important. See Figures 16-2 to 16-9 for an idea of which tests are indicated for different findings.

An evaluation for traumatic injury to the spine would certainly include an assessment of the urine as well as plain radiography, CT, MRI, and possibly myelography, and a technetium scan. Patients being assessed to differentiate between mechanical pain for either degenerative arthropathy or discogenic pain would certainly benefit from MRI and CT scans and possibly myelography. These are followed by discography, root sleeve injections, and facet injections where clinically indicated.[1-6] The next part of the case study describes the laboratory tests that were performed on the case study patient.

A CT scan and MRI of the lumbosacral spine were performed. Other than findings supporting the history of previous chemical dissolution of the L4–L5 disk, there was no evidence to support any persistent mechanical entrapment or pressure upon any of the neurologic structures within the spine. A technetium scan was also ordered to rule out any neoplastic phenomenon as the source of the pain; this too was normal. A sedimentation rate was ordered to determine the possibility of an inflammatory process due to neoplasm, infection, or rheumatism; the sedimentation rate proved normal.

These results created a most perplexing dilemma. The patient presented with a history consistent with neurologic compression upon a specific root, causing pain to the dermatome of the S1 root to the right lower extremity. The physical examination was consistent with some type of inflammatory process involving the S1 root to the right lower extremity. Nevertheless, all the usual modalities of diagnostic confirmation gave normal results. Re-examination of the patient revealed no new information.

The patient was admitted to the hospital for bed rest and myelography. The myelogram was normal. However, the patient's symptoms persisted in spite of 10 days' bed rest in the hospital. During her hospitalization a root sleeve injection was performed to the right S1 root. Xylocaine block of the S1 root relieved her pain for approximately 2 hours.

The root sleeve injection proved that there was some pathology irritating the S1 root. The patient had to have had some irritative focus upon the S1 root distal to the transverse process of the spinal column. Since the patient was a woman, and the lumbar and sacral roots exit into the leg close to the posterior aspect of the pelvic wall, this prompted an investigation of the anatomic structures within the pelvis.

The patient was referred to a gynecological surgeon, and a careful bimanual examination was performed, which reproduced her pain to the right lower extremity. A pelvic soft tissue CT scan delineated a 5 × 6 cm mass emanating from the right ovary, adherent to the posterior aspect of the pelvic wall. The patient underwent excision of the lesion; postoperatively her pain totally resolved and she returned to a normal, active life-style.

TREATMENT

The initial treatment for any patient with acute back pain has always been a course of bed rest. It has been shown that mechanical stresses on the spine are most reduced in a supine position. It has also been shown that in most cases of traumatically induced back pain, bed rest alone is enough to relieve the patient's symptoms within 10 days to 6 weeks.[1,6,7] Bed rest is therefore the initial treatment of choice to be followed by a carefully supervised return to normal function under the direction of a licensed physical therapist.

The physical therapist should educate the patient through basic back therapy techniques, and offer the patient technical treatments designed to diminish and alleviate the pain. Techniques such as massage, heat, iontophoresis, phonophoresis, ultrasound, traction, and soft tissue desensitization and mobilization are used. The physical therapist should be aware of all these techniques and their appropriate indications.

Once the patient has perceived a significant reduction in discomfort, careful progressive muscular strengthening through exercises to the back and abdomen are indicated as a direct means of lessening the chance of recurrent back pain syndrome.

Injections

Epidural cortisone injections are used primarily as a means of diminishing the inflammation around a specific root and/or disk and the neurostructures near the area. This technique can offer significant long-standing relief.[1]

Corticosteroid facet injections are used to diminish inflammation around the anatomic facet joint. They should be performed by either a spinal surgeon or a neuroradiologist with a fluoroscope to ensure the appropriate anatomic deposition of the medicine. This technique has been successful in offering significant long-term relief to patients with chronic inflammations secondary to arthritic arthropathy to the lumbar spine. Epidural morphine sulfate injections, although used in a number of centers around the country, do not seem to offer any greater adjunctive relief of pain than a simple epidural injection.

Orthotics

Lumbosacral bracing of many types is utilized to diminish motion at the lumbar and sacral spine, and in so doing diminish the patient's perceived pain. This, however, is done at the cost of diminished muscular strength. Lumbosacral cushions to use when sitting, whether in a chair or car seat, also seem to hold the appropriate posture for at least the lower back, and in so doing diminish the recurrence of discomfort to patients with long-standing back pain.[2,3]

Many clinicians advocate the use of shoe lifts, on the theory that loading and unloading of the lumbosacral spine and pelvis by changing the height of the shoe, as well as changing the normal carrying angle of the pelvis, can diminish the pain and reduce its recurrence rate in patients with discogenic or facet arthropathy inflammation.

Surgical Intervention

If conservative modalities of treatment fail, surgical intervention may be indicated. For patients with proven discogenic pain, in which the disk acts as a mechanical compressive force upon the neurologic structures, formal laminotomy and diskectomy are certainly indicated (Fig. 16-10). When bony hypertrophy of the neural foramina progresses to a point where impingement upon the nerve root is noted, bony decompression through foraminotomy is indicated. When both soft tissue and bony compres-

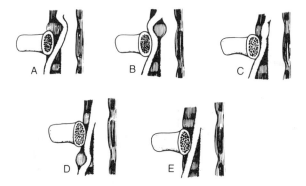

Fig. 16-10. Disk herniation may occur in one of several positions. Always identify the nerve root before incising the presumed herniation. (From Yong-Hing,[10] with permission.)

sive forces are appreciated, as in a patient with spinal stenosis, formal and often extensive bony and soft tissue débridement and decompression can and should be performed.[1] In many cases of spinal stenosis, especially in older patients, serial epidural steroid injections have been found to be most efficacious and should be tried before resorting to operative decompression (Fig. 16-11). If, as a result of bony decompression, both facet joints at a specific level or multiple facet joints involving multiple levels are disrupted, the spine may be considered unstable. If this phenomenon is not appreciated, the patient may experience intolerable pain postoperatively. The surgeon should recognize this situation preoperatively and plan on stabilizing the patient by means of standard techniques of bony fusion.[1-3,7-9]

When a patient suffers from intolerable pain related to joint arthropathy and inflammation from the disk, and it can be proven that the disk is not compressing upon the neurologic structures, and if epidural injection and facet joint injection and other modalities of conservative treatment fail, then bony fusion at the inflamed levels is certainly indicated. Whether the surgeon used internal fixation or not is a controversial subject, and has yet to be settled in the literature.

A number of surgical modalities of treatment have been publicized over the last few years, especially the technique of chemical dissolution of the nucleus of the disk through the injection of chymopa-

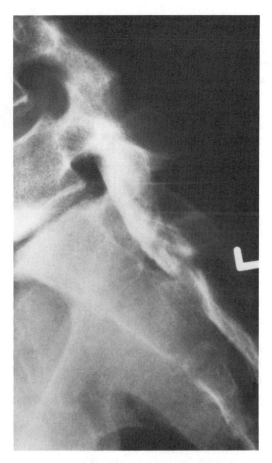

Fig. 16-11. Technique of selective third lumbar spinal nerve and first sacral nerve block. The sacrum has been cut away in a sagittal plane through its anterior and posterior foramina. (From Yong-Hing,[10] with permission.)

pain. When this procedure was first approved in the United States in 1983, it was publicized as the panacea for all forms of disk disease. It certainly has not proved to be that in any case. The procedure has been shown to be successful when performed on one disk that is laterally displaced and not extruded and separated from the confines of the annulus itself. Where multiple disks were injected, and when there was diffuse bulging of the nuclear and annular material, many of these cases failed and showed persistent pain and disability. Chymopapain injections also have been criticized because of recurrence of pain in patients who initially were considered cured, but who demonstrated collapse of the

Fig. 16-12. Disk removal. Avoid damaging the nerve by inserting the pituitary forceps with its jaws closed. Avoid damaging the great vessels by referring to the depth mark scored on the forceps. (From Yong-Hing,[10] with permission.)

intervertebral heights and compression of the neurostructures by a bulging annulus and/or bony stenosis.

Microdiskectomy, which has gained a lot of attention in the neurosurgical literature, as well as in the lay literature, may have its place, but it has not yet shown consistently good results to justify its routine use with any degree of success[1] (Fig. 16-12).

The most recent publicized technique for eliminating the pathologic compressive phenomenon seen in disk herniation has been the removal of nuclear disk material by insertion of a small suction cannula into the center of the disk under fluroscopic control. Although under limited use, outpatient percutaneous diskectomy may prove to be an excellent adjunct to disk disease treatment. It is a safe procedure and, when used for the proper indications, offers good results.[1]

The careful assessment, evaluation, and confirmation of a back pain patient's problems is a complex exercise for any clinician no matter how experienced. Adherence to the basics of taking a good history, making a careful physical examination, ordering the proper confirmatory tests, and formulating a logical diagnosis will afford clinician and patient a reasonably good chance of making the proper treatment decision.

REFERENCES

1. American College of Orthopaedic Surgeons. Orthopaedic Knowledge Update I. p. 237. American College of Orthopaedic Surgeons, Chicago, 1984
2. American College of Orthopaedic Surgeons. Orthopaedic Knowledge Update II. pp. 159, 303. American College of Orthopaedic Surgeons, Chicago, 1987
3. Rockwood CA, Green DP: Fractures in Adults. p. 1036. JP Lippincott, Philadelphia, 1984
4. Hoppenfield S, de Boer P: Surgical Exposures in Orthopaedics. p.281. JB Lippincott, Philadelphia, 1984
5. Crenshaw AH: Campbell's Operative Orthopaedics. 7th Ed. Vol. IV. pp. 3091, 3143, 3255. CV Mosby, St. Louis, 1987
6. White AH, Rothman RH, Rey CD (eds): Lumbar Spine Surgery: Techniques and Complications. CV Mosby, St. Louis, 1987
7. MacNab N: Back Ache. Williams & Wilkins, Baltimore, 1977
8. Feffern HL. Complications of invasive diagnostic procedures of the spine. Lesson 36. Orthopaedic Surgery Update Series. Case Western Reserve University, Cleveland, 1982
9. Eismont FJ: Lumbosacral spine. Maine Orthop Rev 151, 1985
10. Yong-Hing K: Surgical techniques. p. 315. In Kirkaldy-Willis WH (ed): Managing Low Back Pain. 2nd Ed. Churchill Livingstone, New York, 1988

17

Manual Therapy Techniques for the Thoracolumbar Spine

ROBERT W. SYDENHAM

Spinal mobilization and manipulation are arts that have been practiced since ancient times. Early recordings of such treatments were made by Hippocrates, Galen, Paré, Pott, Paget, and many others.[1,2] The literature indicates that primitive forms of manipulation were used by the ancient Greeks and Romans, by the Japanese, by South American civilizations, and in India, Egypt, China, and Europe.[1-4] In 1876 the renowned British surgeon Sir James Paget (1814–1899) published his famous lecture, "Cases that Bonesetters Cure," in the *British Medical Journal.* However, orthodox medicine at that time found the rationale behind bonesetting untenable, despite support from patients.[5] Today these services are provided by osteopaths, chiropractors, allopathic physicians, physical therapists, and various others.

Osteopathy owes its origin and development to Andrew Taylor Still (1828–1917), who founded the American School of Osteopathy in 1892 at Kirksville, Missouri.[5] The practice of chiropractic had its origin with Daniel David Palmer, who after reading some of Still's works founded the first chiropractic school in Davenport, Iowa, in 1897.[5] Although only a few allopathic physicians use mobilization or manipulative techniques, some have been paramount in the development and integration of mobilization and manipulation techniques that are in use today. James Mennell, his son John, and James Cyriax have contributed immensely by their individual efforts and their publications, with which most therapists are familiar.[6,7]

Therapists today are able to credit their own colleagues, such as Grieve, Maitland, Paris, Kaltenborn, and McKenzie, for the significant change over the last 20 years in the manner in which manual therapy is practiced by physical therapists.[5,8-11] The increasing interest in the interrelationship between the biomechanical effects of mobilization and manipulation and the neurophysiologic mechanisms that come into play has resulted in investigations into the efficiency of mobilization and manipulation in an effort to determine their mechanisms of action.

A significant step in this direction was initiated by the National Institutes of Health. The National Institute of Neurological and Communicative Disorders and Stroke held a conference, which resulted in the publication edited by Goldstein in 1975 on "The Research Status of Spinal Manipulative Therapy."[12] Of special interest is the work by Sato and Perl in that publication.[13,14] This conference was followed by another in Italy in 1978 at which Granit and Pompeiano presented additional research applicable to manual therapy.[15] Freeman and Wyke in 1967 coined the expression "articular neurology."[16] Additional research by Wyke and Polacek, further supported by Wyke's publication, "The Neurology of Low Back Pain," with its exhaustive bibliography, further explained the neurophysiologic ramifications of manual therapy.[17-22] Research by Polacek and Halata also contributed to our understanding of articular neurology.[23,24]

Another meeting of the clinical and scientific

359

worlds took place in Melbourne, Australia, in 1979, at a conference sponsored by the Lincoln Institute of Health Sciences on "Manipulative Therapy in the Management of Musculo-Skeletal Disorders."[25] This conference was significant in that it brought together clinicians, researchers, and scientists from many different schools of thought, from all over the world.

Until recently manipulation and mobilization have been considered empirical treatment procedures. However, researchers have put forth theories to explain why mobilization and manipulation play an important part in treating somatic dysfunction. Unfortunately, the saving of lives and the accurate diagnosis of a broad spectrum of medical conditions have a prior claim on the time and effort of the medical profession. The time spent in medical school studying the assessment and treatment of musculoskeletal disorders is not in proportion to the number of patients who attend a medical, or especially a physical therapy practice. However, there is an increased awareness in the undergraduate programs that manual therapy is a vital part of our skills, and many postgraduate courses are available, with specialization in many areas in preparation or in place. The more time spent in raising the level of expertise in the diagnosis and treatment of musculoskeletal disorders, the better off our patients will be.[25]

TERMINOLOGY

Mobilization

Mobilization has been described by Grieve as the attempt at restoration of full, painless joint function by rhythmic, repetitive, passive movements within the patient's tolerance and within the voluntary and accessory range, and graded according to examination findings. The patient is at all times able to stop the movement if he or she so wishes. Mobilization may affect the whole vertebral region or may be localized to a single segment.[8] The term thus applies to a wide variety of techniques.

Kaltenborn advocates various mobilization techniques such as translating or gliding movements, and angular or rolling movements, in addition to different degrees of traction, all of which form part of some very exacting, specific techniques.[26]

Maitland's approach to mobilization is heavily based on assessment of range of motion, pain, stiffness, and spasm, with alterations in signs and symptoms used as indicators for modification of further treatment.[9,27] Maitland's techniques are quite gentle, are easily controlled by the patient, and vary in intensity from grades I to IV.

Mennell's approach to mobilization is based on the restoration of joint play or accessory joint movements, with techniques aimed at restoration of joint dysfunction, followed by exercises to maintain the newly restored range.[7,28]

Although not known for his mobilization techniques per se, James Cyriax developed a detailed and comprehensive examination involving contractile and noncontractile tissue, normal and abnormal end-feels of joint movement, and classification of joint restrictions into capsular and noncapsular patterns.[6]

Articulation

Articulation is an osteopathic term that refers to the same type of movement as occurs in mobilization; however, the effects are intended to be localized to a single spinal segment, in an attempt to improve the restricted range of a single movement of that segment.[8] It is the osteopathic belief that these articulatory techniques gradually stretch contracted muscles, ligaments, or joint capsules, in addition to restoring the normal movements of which the joint is capable. Articulatory techniques also attempt to ensure that the movements that normally are not under voluntary control of the joint are also free. In addition to the mechanical aspects of articulatory techniques, reference is made to the nutritional and circulatory factors that influence the joint. Articulatory techniques are frequently used in preparation for specific manipulations, as there may be less reactive tissue response and the benefit may be more lasting.[29]

Articulation differs from simple passive movement in that the operator should be constantly sensing the feedback from the tissue under his hand and measuring the intensity of pressure or stretch that the operator feels is necessary, according to what he or she is feeling. Articulation is often combined with a small "bounce" at the end of the range of motion to test tissue reactivity.[30] Localized mobilizations or articulations are often distinguished by the use of direct contact through soft tissues with the bony apophyses of a single vertebral body.[27]

Manipulation

Manipulation is often described as an accurately localized, single, quick, and decisive movement of small amplitude following careful positioning of the patient. It is not necessarily energetic and is completed before the patient can stop it. Manipulation may have a regional or a more localized affect, depending on the technique of the therapist and the positioning of the patient.[8]

Manipulation has also been defined as a passive manual maneuver during which the three-joint complex is suddenly carried beyond its normal physiologic range of movement, without exceeding the boundaries of anatomic integrity. The usual characteristic is a brief, sudden, and carefully administered "impulsion" given at the end of the normal passive range of movement. Usually it is accompanied by a cracking noise.[31,32]

Many forms of manipulation involve variations of leverage, thrust, and momentum. The effectiveness of one group of techniques over another is probably due more to the skill of the clinician than to the superiority of a particular procedural technique.

Manipulation has also been referred to as spinal manipulative therapy (SMT)[12] and high velocity thrust (HVT).[33]

Soft Tissue Techniques

Soft tissue techniques involve stretching of connective and/or muscle tissue in an abnormal state that generally crosses joints, for example, spasm, weakness, wasting, tightness, and ultimately some degree of fibrosis, all of which prohibit normal painless joint range of motion.[8] Stretching techniques, both specific and general, have proven to be most effective and are illustrated and described in great detail by Olaf Evjenth and Jern Hamberg.[34] Their most common use, however, is to prepare the tissue for and reduce the stress of articulatory techniques. A few such techniques are illustrated in Figures 17-1 through 17-10.

Nonspecific Soft Tissue Techniques for the Lumbar Spine

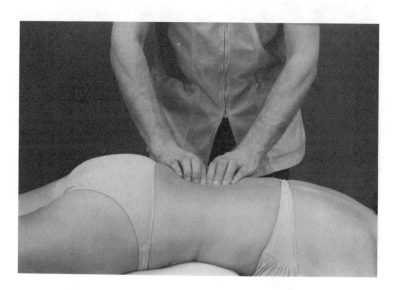

Fig. 17-1. The patient is prone, with the lumbar spine in a neutral position. The therapist, with fingertips in a row lateral to the spinous process, uses a pulling motion to stretch the erector spinae muscle mass at right angles to the spine.

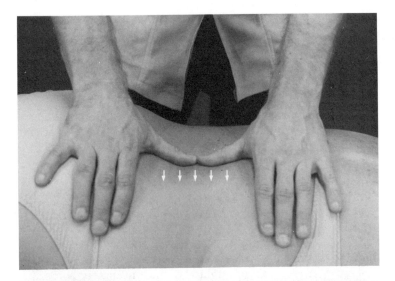

Fig. 17-2. This technique uses the same principles as in Fig. 17-1. The therapist's thumbs push the opposite erector spinae laterally, at right angles to the spinous processes. A scooping motion of the thumb assists with the lateral movement of the muscle.

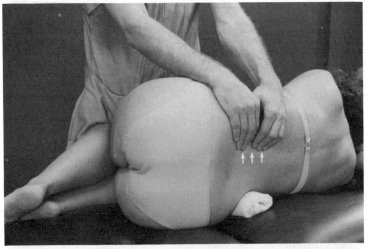

Fig. 17-3. The therapist flexes the patient's knees and, with his thighs, pushes against the patient's knees causing the lumbar spine to flex. With the erector spinae in some degree of stretch, the therapist pulls the erector spinae mass in a transverse direction. Altering pressure on the knees varies the tension on the erector spinae muscle.

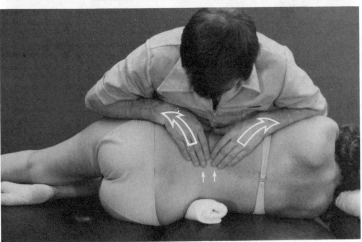

Fig. 17-4. The therapist applies outward pressure with both forearms, causing the lumbar spine to arch and stretching the quadratus lumborum and erector spinae muscles. Arching is assisted by a roll under the patient's lumbar spine and flexing the patient's bottom hip, and by the therapist pulling up with the fingers on the erector spinae mass.

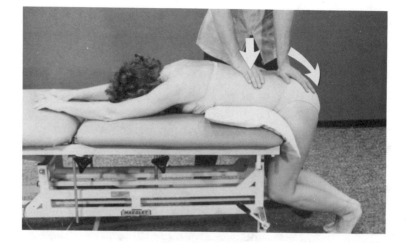

Fig. 17-5. While increasing the flexion of the lumbar spine in the prone position, the therapist stabilizes the T12–L1 segment and presses against the patient's sacrum. Further stretch may be achieved by the therapist pushing downward along the patient's thighs.

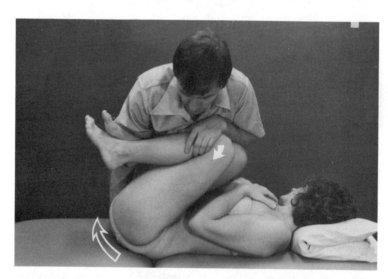

Fig. 17-6. The therapist stretches the lumbar extensors by pressing on the patient's knees while simultaneously lifting the patient's sacrum. Further stretch may be achieved by pushing downward along the patient's thighs.

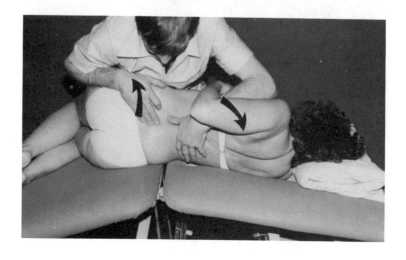

Fig. 17-7. Technique to increase extension, left rotation, and right sidebending. A cushion under the waist may be used to produce right sidebending if the bed does not elevate in the middle. As the patient exhales, the therapist pushes the left shoulder and thorax posteriorly and cranially while pulling the left ilium forward and caudally.

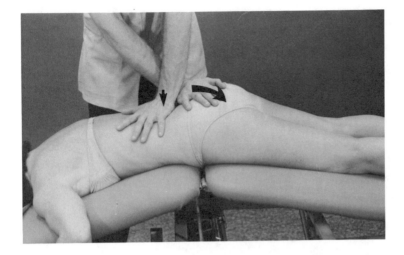

Fig. 17-8. Technique to increase the flexion of L5 on S1. The middle of the couch is elevated. A roll may be placed under the abdomen. As the patient exhales, the therapist pushes the sacrum caudally and ventrally. This technique may be used for all the lumbar segments. The therapist's hypothenar eminence stabilizes the proximal lumbar segment.

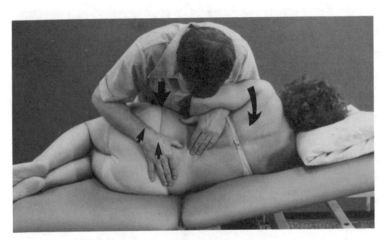

Fig. 17-9. Technique to increase flexion and left rotation and sidebending at L2–L3. The pelvis may be stabilized with a belt. As the patient exhales, the therapist pushes the patient's left shoulder and thorax backward. The head of the bed is progressively elevated to sidebend the lumbar spine to the left. Rotation may be enhanced by pulling the right arm and shoulder forward. The pelvis is stabilized between the therapist's chest and forearm and by the therapist's hand over the sacrum. The patient's upper leg may be extended, and a roll may be put under the lower lumbar spine.

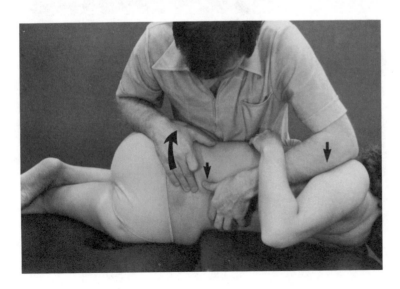

Fig. 17-10. Technique to increase flexion and left rotation and sidebending of L5 on S1. The upper lumbar spine is flexed and right sidebent, causing right rotation, thus locking the upper lumbar segments. If the midsection of the bed will not lift, use a roll. As the patient exhales, the therapist pulls the pelvis forward and cranially.

Traction

Traction is a combination of distraction and gliding movements between two joints or surfaces. Various types of traction can be applied to the lumbar spine. Often, for the therapist's benefit, a mechanical apparatus is used to achieve the effects of traction. Continuous traction is generally applied for several hours at a time with minimal weight and is not considered very effective in causing mechanical separation of the vertebrae.[35] Sustained traction involves shorter periods of constant pull, varying in time up to one-half hour.[35] A variation is intermittent mechanical traction, in which the pressure is applied and released in a rhythmic fashion. Efficiency is increased with the use of a traction table, the caudal half of which is on rollers, thus reducing friction. Manual traction can be used as a treatment technique or in determining the patient's tolerance to traction or to find the most comfortable position in which to apply a traction force (see Figs. 17-11 through 17-13).

An alternative method of applying manual traction is by vertical adjustive traction[29] (see Fig. 17-14).

Three-dimensional traction allows the patient's position to be precisely adjusted by means of pillows, foam wedges, sand bags, or, if available, a three-dimensional mobilization table (see Fig. 17-15). Autotraction uses a two-segment traction table that can be individually angled and rotated according to the patient's response as treatment progresses.

Gravity lumbar traction is applied in a variety of ways. In one technique the patient is tilted up on a circular or elevating bed into an approximately vertical position, while at the same time being suspended by a vest around the chest. In this position, the free weight of the legs and hips exerts a traction force on the lumbar spine equal to approximately 40 percent of body weight.[36,37]

Probably the most prevalent type of gravity traction uses inversion boots worn in conjunction with a gravity guider.[38] A variation of this technique uses another apparatus in which the patient bends forward at the waist and is able to hang inverted while being supported on the anterior thighs with the hips and knees flexed approximately 90 degrees. However, the patients who would benefit the most from this type of treatment are usually in too much pain even to get on the machine.

Traction Techniques for the Lumbar Spine

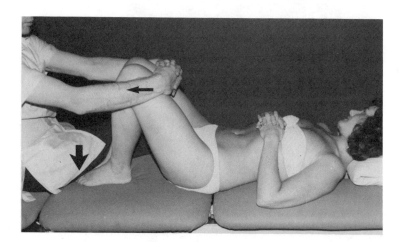

Fig. 17-11. A surprisingly effective manual traction may be applied in crook lying through the patient's hips when the therapist leans back. The therapist's thighs fix the patient's feet. The angle of pull may be guided by the patient's response.

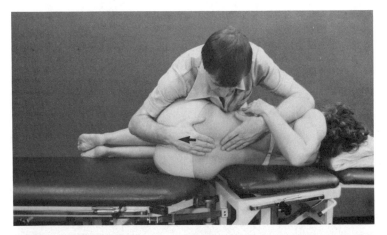

Fig. 17-12. Specific distraction in lumbar flexion is facilitated by the use of a mobilization bed to sidebend, and the use of accessories to assist with distraction. The patient's pelvis is stabilized by the therapist's shoulder, chest, forearm, and hand.

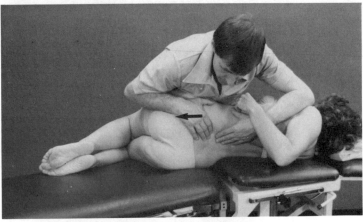

Fig. 17-13. Specific distraction in lumbar extension. The patient's pelvis may also be stabilized with a belt. Sidebending of the lumbar spine may be prevented by a pillow if the bed does not lift.

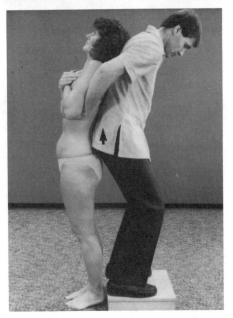

Fig. 17-14. The patient is lifted up with relative ease if patient and therapist are of the same height. A small platform may be used to position the therapist's sacral base at the desired level of the patient's lumbar spine. Straightening of the therapist's knees and forward flexion lift the patient off the floor. Traction is exerted by the therapist coming up onto the balls of the feet, then rapidly dropping onto the heels. Various degrees of sidebending or rotation may be used. The patient should be able to extend the lumbar spine, or else the technique may cause discomfort.

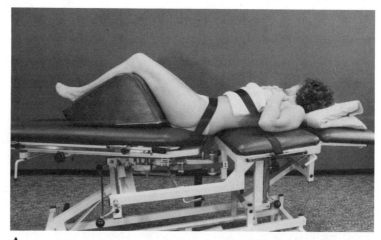

A

Fig. 17-15. Various degrees of rotation and sidebending may be incorporated to accommodate discomfort. Traction may be applied by the therapist or the patient with the use of appropriate accessories.

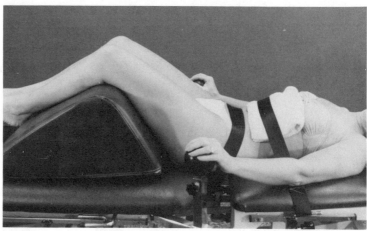

B

Strain and Counterstrain

Strain and counterstrain techniques involve putting the joint into the position of greatest comfort, thus relieving pain by reduction and arrest of the continuing inappropriate proprioceptor activity. The tender point is shut off by markedly shortening the muscle that contains a malfunctioning muscle spindle by applying mild strain to its antagonist[39] (see Figs. 17-16, 17-17).

Strain in this context refers to overstretching of muscles, tendons, ligaments, or fascia, along with the associated altered neuromuscular reflex. Treatment is directed at the neuromuscular reflexes rather than tissue stretching. Generally the position in which there is spontaneous release of tissue tension assumes the disorder as being unilateral and moves to the position of greatest ease of the abnormally tense side. The position of the patient in the treatment position often mimics the position in which the original strain was experienced. Selected anterior and posterior lumbar dysfunction techniques are illustrated in Figures 17-18 through 17-22.

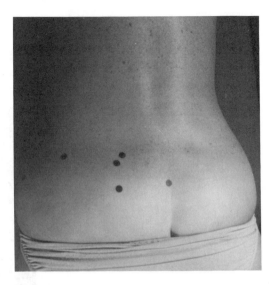

Fig. 17-17. Tender points for posterior lumbar dysfunctions.

Counterstrain Techniques for Lumbar Spine

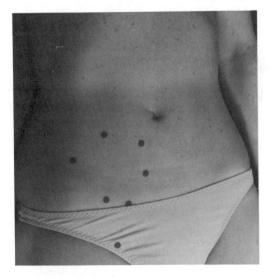

Fig. 17-16. Tender points for anterior lower thoracic and lumbar dysfunctions.

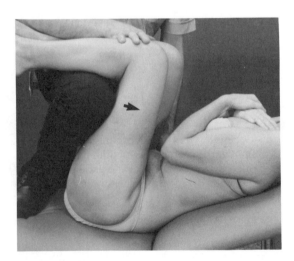

Fig. 17-18. Treatment for a forward bending dysfunction of L1. Assist flexion of the thoracolumbar junction by lifting the end of the bed. Further flexion is produced by the therapist's knees against the back of the patient's thigh, with slight rotation of the patient's knee toward the side of tenderness. The position is one of marked flexion, rotation away, and sidebending toward. The position is held and the tender spot monitored for 90 seconds.

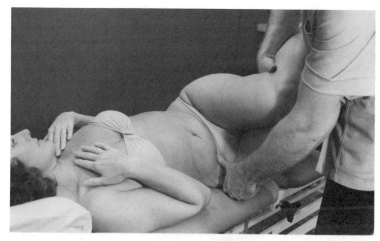

Fig. 17-19. Treatment for abdominal L2 dysfunction. The hips are flexed and the pelvis rotated to the right, and the patient's feet are lifted to the left to sidebend the lumbar spine. Adductor strain can be reduced by slightly lifting behind the upper knee.

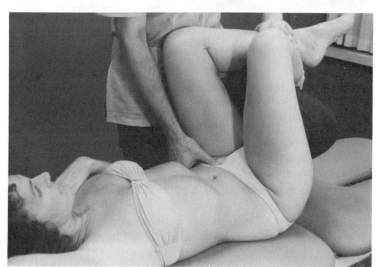

Fig. 17-20. Treatment for iliacus dysfunction. A tender point is located in the iliac fossa. The hips are flexed, the ankles crossed, and the thighs externally rotated.

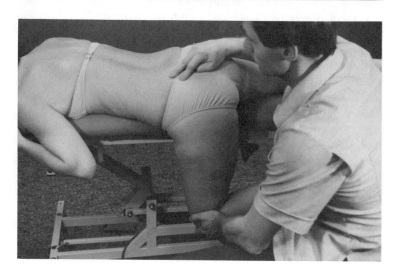

Fig. 17-21. Treatment for L5 dysfunction. Approximately 20 degrees of pelvic rotation plus adduction of the thigh reduces the tender spot under the index finger. The third finger marks the posterior superior iliac spine.

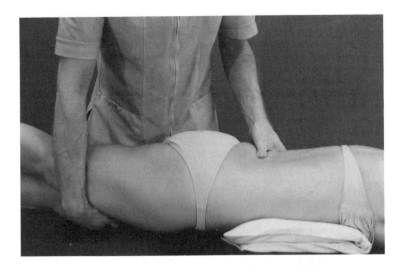

Fig. 17-22. Treatment for L3, L4, and L5 dysfunctions. Adduction of the thigh is necessary at all levels. More rotation is needed for L3, whereas L5 requires more extension.

Functional Techniques

Functional technique is a method of treating joints in which the direction of movement of the joint is that of least resistance and greatest comfort. The technique thus reduces exaggerated spindle responses from facilitated segments of spinal muscles and restores normal joint mobility. The end position is that in which the tensions of tissues around the joint are equal; this position is known as "dynamic neutral." [40] This technique is similar to that of strain and counterstrain in that the position of spontaneous release is the same, and direction of movement is toward immediate ease and comfort. However, functional technique differs in that the dynamic neutral concept seeks a balance of tissue tension fairly near the anatomic neutral position (see Fig. 17-23). This reduction in tissue tension is obtained when the spinal segment is put through various physiologic motions that relax or reduce tissue tension. The process of finding the easy physiological motion, following it until decreased tissue tension starts, and rechecking may go through one or two directions until a state of equilibrium is found in which tissue texture indicates relaxation or ease of movement. Neurophysiologically, Korr postulated that the segmental resistance to motion may be due to high discharge of the gamma fibers, causing sustained contraction of the intrafusal fibers, which

Functional Techniques for the Lumbar Spine

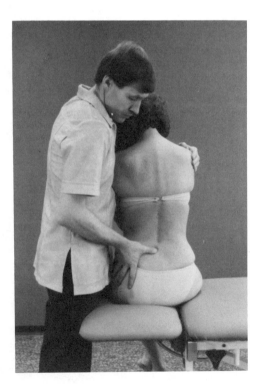

Fig. 17-23. Starting position for a functional technique for lumbar dysfunction. The therapist palpates changes in tissue tension with the right thumb.

keep the annulospiral endings firing continuously. This maintains, in the muscle, a high resistance to stretching, and perhaps this is the tension or the bind that is encountered as a segment is moved in a specific direction.[41] The functional technique concept is one of positioning the joint such that the facilitated muscle spindle is shortened, thus reducing its apparent discharge from the primary annulospiral ending. The central nervous system subsequently decreases the gamma motor neuron discharge.[42] The patient's palpable muscular tension provides information to the practitioner as to what movement is required.[41] In functional techniques all the possible parameters of movement and direction are utilized, and the movements that cause and result in the greatest ease are summed and combined to maximize the relaxation of a particular segmental level[30] (see Fig. 17-24).

Muscle Energy

The muscle energy technique developed by Fred Mitchell, Sr., involves active, distinct, controlled muscle contraction in a precisely controlled position, in a specific direction, against a distinct counterforce.[43] The aim of muscle energy techniques is to restore the normal neurophysiology of the segment. The guiding principle is that the joint is taken up to the sense of a barrier in the three separate cardinal planes. The therapist resists the isometric contractions of the patient and prevents any actual movement from taking place. Only minimal amounts of pressure are necessary, as it is the neurophysiologic effect that is of primary importance in the reduction of abnormal tissue tension in the segment. The position is held momentarily, and after a few seconds the tension relaxes and the therapist then moves the joint further toward the barrier, which should be found to have moved. When the new barrier has been located, the therapist asks the patient to again perform an isometric contraction while the therapist resists any movement. This is repeated three to four times while the therapist monitors any increase in range of motion and alteration of tissue tension.[44] Selected techniques are illustrated below.

Muscle Energy Techniques for the Lumbar Spine

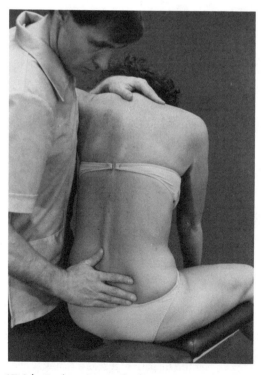

Fig. 17-24. End position of a functional treatment technique. The point of greatest tissue relaxation determines the movement and position of the patient.

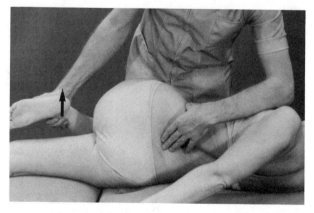

Fig. 17-25. Technique for correcting an L5 that is flexed, rotated right, and sidebent right (FRSR). The aim of treatment is to extend, rotate, and sidebend left (ERSL). The patient resists lifting up of the left ankle. The patient may look over the left shoulder to reduce stress on the upper thoracic spine.

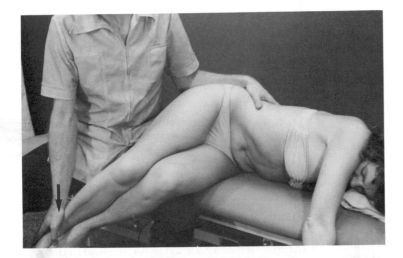

Fig. 17-26. Technique for correcting an L5 that is extended, rotated right, and sidebent right (ERSR). The aim of treatment is to flex, rotate, and sidebend left (FRSL). The patient resists pushing down of both feet. The therapist protects the patient's left thigh from the edge of the bed by supporting it with his or her own left thigh.

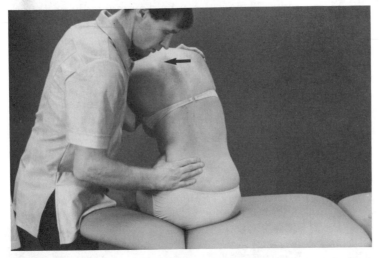

Fig. 17-27. Technique for correcting an L4 that is ERSR in a sitting position. The therapist flexes and rotates the patient to the segment involved; the patient resists sidebending further to the left. The aim of treatment is FRSL of L4.

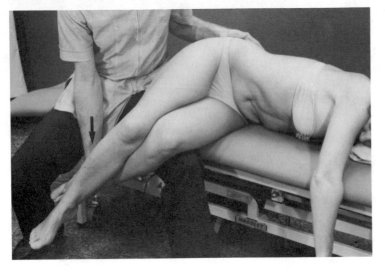

Fig. 17-28. Technique for correcting a forward left sacral torsion (L/L). This is an often-forgotten technique to restore full function of the L5–S1 segment. The aim of treatment is to restore symmetry and motion to the sacrum by reciprocally inhibiting the right piriformis by contracting the left. The patient resists pushing down with the left leg, but allows the right to fall in the relaxation phase, or to be gently stretched.

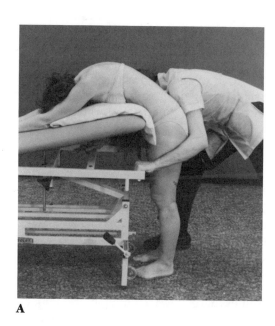

A

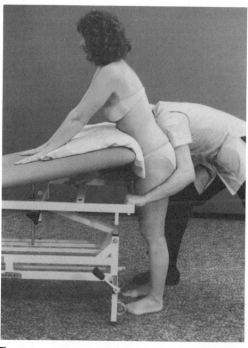

B

Fig. 17-29. An acute sacral torsion is often termed a bilateral flexed L5. The patient presents with a significantly kyphotic lumbar spine. Correction is by stabilizing the patient's sacrum against the end of the bed (**A**) and having the patient walk his hands up the bed (**B**) until an upright position of the lumbar spine is achieved (**C**). Two or three attempts may be required. Caution is warranted, as the symptoms are similar to those of an acute lumbar disk prolapse. Clinical examination should differentiate.

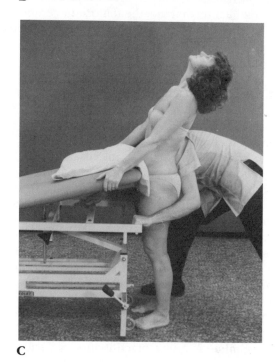

C

Cranial Techniques

Cranial osteopathy, originally developed by William Sutherland in the early 1900s, embraces the concept that there is mobility between the cranial bones. The rhythmic movement of 6 to 12 cycles per minute is very small, but is a measurable 10 to 25 microns.[45] Sutherland suggested that distortions in the movement pattern of the cranium, the sacrum, and the dural membrane system can be responsible for signs and symptoms locally and elsewhere.[46] The guiding principles of craniosacral therapy can be listed under five headings:

1. The existence of inherent mobility of the central nervous system (i.e., the brain and spinal cord)
2. Production, resorption, and pulsatility of the cerebrospinal fluid (CSF)
3. The existence of reciprocal tension membranes, namely, the dura, which forms the periosteum of the cranial vault, attaching to the foramen magnum, C2–C3, and the sacrum (S2); the vertical membranes, the falx cerebri and cerebelli; and a horizontal membrane, the tentorium cerebelli.
4. The mobility of the cranial bones around articular axes
5. Mobility of the sacrum between the ilia.

To those not familiar with this concept, these principles may seem rather unusual. However, they are palpable phenomena, and documented evidence supports their existence.

The craniosacral rhythmic impulses can be felt throughout the body but are strongest when contact is with the cranial bones, which are the vehicle through which cranial techniques are classically performed. A whole series of holds designed to influence different aspects of the above-listed points have been worked out.[47] These techniques utilize fine palpation skills and the specific direction of minute forces to alter osseous or membrane restrictions.[48] They can produce quite specific and sometimes dramatic results in a number of cases, and they form a very useful addition to the categories of reflex techniques. Adept practitioners can successfully treat many seemingly remote symptoms, such as headaches due to a lumbar sacral lesion or restriction, as well as local symptoms originating from a craniosacral dysfunction.[30]

INDICATIONS FOR TREATMENT

Following the history taking and the usual review of medical information such as medication and radiographic reports, a decision must be made as to what approach or direction should be taken with respect to treatment. In some situations, such as joint hypomobility due to sprains or surgery in which some form of splinting or casting is involved, the choice and direction of treatment may seem fairly obvious.

Neurophysiologic Indications

In some situations, however, no specific pathology can be identified. Often the term *syndrome* is used, implying a certain diagnostic vagueness, and frequently characterized by numerous approaches to treatment.[49] It is well known that it is extremely difficult, if not impossible, to make a precise diagnosis in many cases of low back pain.[50-54]

Empirical observations of the nonradicular pain syndromes have been gaining more importance through the experimental neurophysiologic work of Korr, Simons, and Wyke.[17,19,55-57] Different authors, with their own language and terminology reflecting their own opinion or school of thought, often describe the same somatic phenomenon, for example, Brugger,[58,59] Feinstein et al.,[60] Hohermuth,[61] Jones,[39] Mitchell et al.,[44] Hoover,[40] Sutter,[62] Sutter and Frohlich,[63] and Waller[64] (Table 17-1). The result of this diversity of terminology and theories is that these valuable clinical observations have found limited diagnostic utilization in the mainstream of medicine.[65-68] However, these ob-

Table 17-1. Common Nonradicular Spondylogenic Reflex Syndromes

Syndrome	References
Referred pain	Kellgren,[70,71] Sinclair et al.,[72] Hockaday and Whitty[73]
Myofascial trigger points	Melzack,[74,75] Reynolds,[76] Rubin,[77] Simons,[56,57] Travell and Rinzler,[78] Travell[79,80]
Pseudoradicular	Brugger[58,59,81,82]
Tender points	Mitchell et al.,[44] Jones,[39] Hoover,[40] Lewit[83]
Spondylogenic reflexes	Sutter,[62] Maigne,[69] Caviezel,[84,85] Sell,[86] Jones[39]

(Data from Dvorak et al.[68])

servations together indicate that the reflex is mediated through the reflexogenic pathways of the central nervous system, and is the reproducible, causative factor linking the skeletal segmental dysfunction and the soft tissue changes. These have been described by Maigne as "dérangements intervertebrales mineurs." [69] Causes of the segmental dysfunction with its consequential soft tissue changes include trauma, muscle imbalance, uncoordinated or sudden movement, chronic strain, and degenerative joint changes.[87]

However, not all syndromes with respect to low back pain need be so controversial. Experience plus awareness of the literature facilitates the therapist's choice of approach in managing somatic dysfunction. Often the neurophysiologic approach seemingly may be less appropriate in light of a more direct or mechanical means of treatment.

Mechanical Indications

McKenzie described "three syndromes that have characteristics, definition, causes of development, clinic presentation, and specific treatment procedures." [11] He proposed that uncomplicated mechanical spinal pain is caused by mechanical deformation of soft tissues containing nociceptive receptors.

Postural Syndrome

Patients are usually under the age of 30, have sedentary occupations, and often do not exercise regularly. Pain is never produced by movement, and is never referred or constant. There is no loss of range of motion and no pathology, and there are no signs on examination. The pain is due to the mechanical deformation or prolonged stretching of normal spinal tissue, probably ligamentous, causing stimulation of the nociceptors.

Dysfunction Syndrome

The patient is usually over 30 (unless trauma is the cause), generally exhibits poor posture, and frequently lacks exercise. Pain is always felt at the end-range of motion, never during motion, and unless there is an adherent nerve root, pain is never referred. Loss of range of motion — loss of extension is the most frequent — is generally due to long-standing poor posture causing adaptive shortening or contracture of fibrous tissue, which forms an inextensible scar. Pain results immediately from the stretching of the inextensible but unidentifiable shortened tissue, causing deformation of the nociceptors. Selected techniques to increase extension of the lumbar spine are illustrated below.

Techniques to Increase Extension of the Lumbar Spine

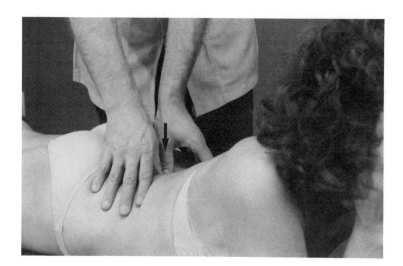

Fig. 17-30. Specific posteroanterior central pressure to increase extension.

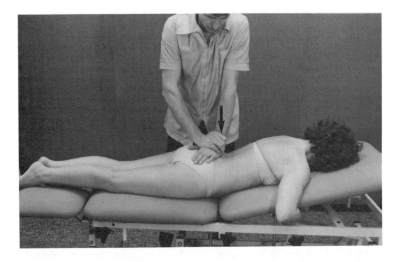

Fig. 17-31. Specific extension mobilization with the pisiform. As mobility increases, the end of the bed may be elevated further.

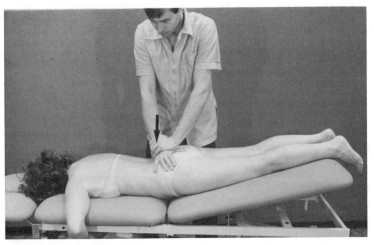

Fig. 17-32. Specific extension mobilization with the pisiform as a contact. The caudal end of the bed is elevated as much as mobility allows.

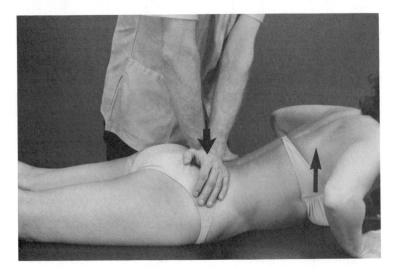

Fig. 17-33. Specific stabilization over the transverse processes as the patient attempts extension.

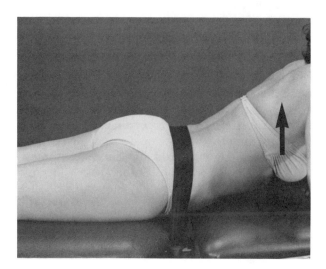

Fig. 17-34. Specific stabilization using a belt as the patient attempts extension.

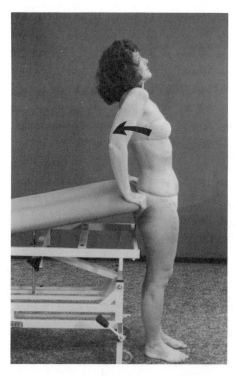

Fig. 17-35. Nonspecific extension over the end of the bed. Be sure that the patient's knees do not flex.

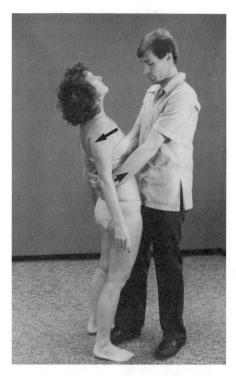

Fig. 17-36. Specific stabilization of the lumbar segment by the therapist's hypothenar eminences. Extension may be assisted by pulling forward with the hands as the patient leans back. The patient's pelvis is stabilized by the therapist's thigh.

Derangement Syndrome

Patients are usually 30 to 50 years of age, have poor sitting posture, and often experience an acute onset of pain for no apparent reason. Symptoms may be painful and localized, or be referred in the form of pain, paresthesia, or numbness. The symptoms usually are directly affected by certain movements and postures; therefore a discogenic origin must be considered. Although the pain may fluctuate in intensity, it is usually fairly constant because of the anatomic disturbance within the intervertebral disk complex. Selected techniques that are frequently successful in the clinic are illustrated below.

Techniques to Correct Lumbar Derangements

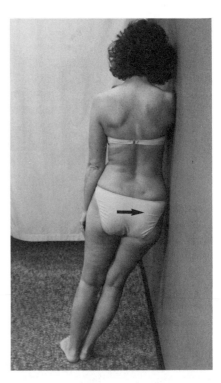

Fig. 17-38. Self-correction of a right lumbar shift. Alternatively, the patient may stand in a doorway and let the pelvis sag to the right.

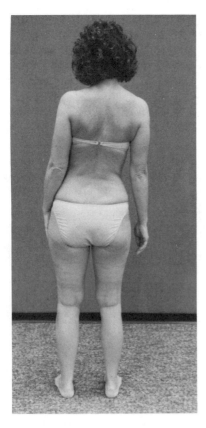

Fig. 17-37. Typical presentation in which the lumbar spine is slightly shifted to the right.

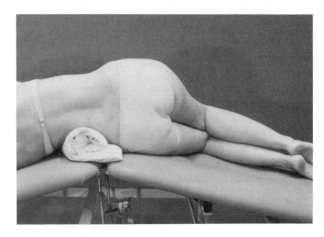

Fig. 17-39. Positional traction in side-lying to correct a right lumbar shift to the left.

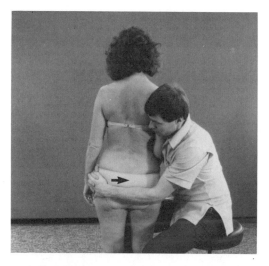

Fig. 17-40. The therapist assists in correction of a right-deviated spine. The therapist stabilizes with the shoulder while pulling on the patient's pelvis. A slow constant pull is most beneficial. A slight overcorrection may be needed.

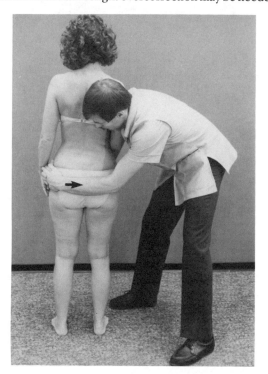

Fig. 17-41. The therapist assists in correction of a right-deviated lumbar spine. This technique is not recommended because it involves poor body mechanics by the therapist, and frequently the stabilization provided by the therapist's shoulder is too high.

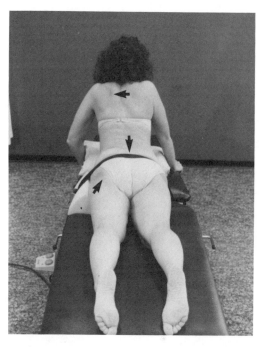

Fig. 17-42. Correction of a right-deviated lumbar spine in the prone position. The technique is assisted by belt stabilization, a foam wedge under the hip opposite the deviation, and extending to the left when pressing up. If a three-dimensional mobilization bed is used instead, it may be adjusted accordingly.

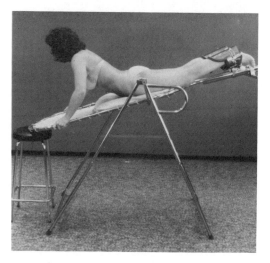

Fig. 17-43. Extension exercises with the assistance of progressive inversion for reducing persistent pain.

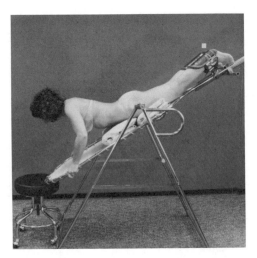

Fig. 17-44. Same technique as in Fig. 17-43 but with more inversion. If the pain is to one side, extension exercises accommodating for unilateral pain may be helpful.

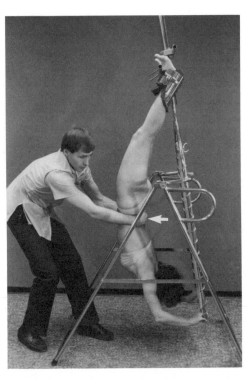

Fig. 17-46. The therapist assists with extension of the lumbar spine, with persisting central pain.

Mobilization

A joint is usually suitable for treatment if the symptoms are aggravated by certain movements or postures and relieved by rest or other movements or positions.[88] The patient may not always present with true articulatory signs; however, the symptoms generally will respond to mobilization techniques.

It must be kept in mind that visceral pathology may cause spinal pain, but this pain is not typically aggravated by spinal movement. Manual therapy techniques are either contraindicated or of no value.

The degree of intensity of mobilization depends upon the examination findings and has an almost direct relationship to the number of factors assessed. Observation of the patient and the history will indicate the necessity of a gentle approach. Such findings as indicated by Grieve[88] are:

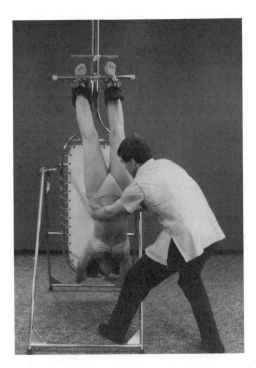

Fig. 17-45. The therapist assists with extension and correction for a right-deviated lumbar spine with persisting referred pain to the left.

Much joint irritability
Severe pain accompanying all movements

Severe pain in certain postures
Severe limb pain
Interruption of sleep
Protective spasm
Long-standing severe pain
Distal pain produced by coughing and sneezing.

The examination reveals the following:

Facial distortion due to increased pain on
    movement
Distal limb pain on spinal movement
An increase of pain or paresthesia after testing
An increase of spasm
Distal pain or paresthesia with gentle pressure
Presence of a neurologic deficit
Increase of pain after minimal examination.

Obviously, more vigorous mobilization may commence on reassessment when there is reduced or minimal spasm, pain, paresthesia, or distal symptoms as a result of previous examination and treatments. The indications and steps for progression of treatment have been meticulously set out by Grieve.[88] The importance of a thorough and efficient examination can not be overemphasized.

Manipulation

Manipulation is a natural progression from a grade IV mobilization if the maximum improvement in signs and symptoms has not been achieved. Manipulation is of benefit if there are no articular signs but only hypomobility of the segment, and if minimal pain does not appear until near the end of the range of motion.

The clinical difficulty in the selection of patients for manipulation is partly due to a lack of clear understanding of pathogenesis and of objective examination techniques, as well as differing intentions with regard to manipulation. There appear to be five different philosophies regarding the effects of manipulation, and thus five differing purposes. These consist of (1) the mobilizing or oscillating techniques, affecting soft tissue; (2) osteopathy, concerned with restoration of joint motion; (3) chiropractic, concerned with putting a vertebra that is "out" back in place; (4) laymen and bonesetters, who seek to cause a "click" in the joint when it is manipulated; and (5) Cyriax techniques, affecting the disk or a loose fragment of the disk. Although each school of thought has its degrees of success, a thorough examination with an understanding of anatomy will result in greater consistency of success than the blind following of a particular doctrine. Regardless of ideology, clinically certain conditions seem to benefit from the application of manipulative techniques.[89]

Uncomplicated Low Back Pain

Patients who develop uncomplicated low back pain of recent onset in the absence of radicular signs were found to be more responsive to manipulation than to a placebo treatment.[90] In a further study by Bergquist-Ullman and Larsson, they were found to respond most favorably if their onset of symptoms was less than 9 days before treatment.[91] Potter also noted that patients with acute low back pain had the highest rate of improvement (93 percent) following manipulation.[92]

Complicated Acute Low Back Pain

Patients with acute onset of low back pain complicated by leg pain or neurologic symptoms appeared to respond very well to spinal manipulation.[93,94] Both Potter and Edwards found that over 75 percent of patients with pain radiating into the buttock or down into the leg recovered or improved considerably following spinal manipulation.[92,95] Buerger, in a blind clinical trial, has shown that a painful limited straight leg raise was shown to improve following manipulation.[96] Many practitioners, however, become very cautious when frank neurologic deficit or signs are present.[93,97] Research has indicated that patients with neurologic signs that have been subjected to spinal manipulation have not experienced rewarding results.[92,98]

Uncomplicated Chronic Low Back Pain

By definition, patients with uncomplicated chronic low back pain are not recovering spontaneously. Potter showed that although improvement in this group was less than in the group of uncomplicated low back pain patients, 71 percent showed improvement of their symptoms.[92] A similar study by Riches indicates that improvement occurs in as many as 86 percent.[99] The results of another study by Kirkaldy-Willis and Cassidy showed considerable variation depending upon the pathogenic diagnosis. However, 65 percent of patients showed some degree of improvement.[100]

Complicated Chronic Low Back Pain

Manipulation of patients with complicated chronic low back pain yielded results similar to those in patients with complicated acute pain in that likelihood of success of treatment decreased considerably when neurologic signs were present.[92] It was noted, however, that previous back surgery did not appear to play a significant role in the outcome of treatment and was not considered a contraindication to manipulation.

Disk Degeneration and Herniation

The causative effect of spinal manipulation on intervertebral disk dysfunction is very controversial. Such authors as Cyriax, as well as Matthews and Yates, claim that manipulation seems to have some beneficial effect on the intervertebral disk.[97,101] Chrisman and associates, as well as Kirkaldy-Willis and Cassidy, were unable to achieve favorable results in those patients that demonstrated lumbar disk protrusion.[98,100] In light of this controversy, manipulation is often used on those patients diagnosed as having degenerative disk without frank herniation or neurologic deficits.[29,97,102]

Facet Syndrome

Many practitioners believe that the primary effect of manipulation is on a fixated or blocked facet joint.[7,103,104] However, it appears that the basis for this belief is merely that there is an increase in mobility of the spine following manipulation.

Sacroiliac Syndromes

If the diagnosis is one of sacroiliac syndrome, manipulation appears to be a very effective choice of treatment.[99,100] Many practitioners place a great deal of emphasis on the ability to analyze sacroiliac motion, or lack thereof, and choose an appropriate manipulative technique according to their findings.[105-107] Kirkaldy-Willis and Cassidy and Riches claim that over 90 percent of patients with this diagnosis show improvement following manipulation.[99,100]

Spondylolisthesis

Kirkaldy-Willis and Cassidy et al. found that they were able to improve back pain in 85 percent of cases.[100,108] However, they made it quite clear that spinal manipulation did not influence the spondylolisthesis itself but rather that spondylolisthesis was an incidental finding. In the study by Cassidy et al. great care was taken to ensure that manipulative forces were minimized at the level of instability but rather were aimed at the sacroiliac joints or the facet joints at a higher level.

Spinal Stenosis

Kirkaldy-Willis and Cassidy and Potter reported that a significant number of patients with lateral or central spinal stenosis experienced some improvement following manipulation.[100,109] Very few of these patients ever became symptom free, which is not surprising, and often relief was only temporary.[110]

Whatever the diagnosis or etiology, the objective remains the same: restoration of full, painless joint motion. Faulty mechanics prevent normal function, leading in turn to compensatory mechanisms. A functional diagnosis based on mechanical faults is more pertinent than a static positional evaluation.[111] When the body's adaptive potential both locally and regionally is exhausted, dysfunction ensues. Goldthwait et al. were among the first to recognize a link between faulty mechanics and disease.[112]

PRINCIPLES AND RULES OF MOBILIZATION AND MANIPULATION

Regardless of the profession, nationality, or school of thought, all rational treatment must have a reasoned basis. The following list summarizes the principles and rules of procedures offered by such notable clinicians as Grieve, Maitland, Cyriax, Stoddard, and others.[8,9,26,97,113] The order of presentation is not an indication of relative significance.

Remember contraindications and conditions requiring extra care.

Do no harm to the patient — or to yourself.

A thorough and structured examination is fundamental.

Make as accurate a diagnosis as possible, based on a solid knowledge of anatomy.

All pain arises from a lesion.

For treatment to be effective, it must reach the lesion.

Constantly reassess to determine the effect of the techniques being used.

Progress is governed by the response to previous treatment.

Discontinue techniques that are not productive.

Use the minimum of force consistent with achieving the objective.

If possible, use the patient's own weight to do the work.

Get the patient to relax; reduce the patient's anxiety and fear.

Timing is essential in the application of technique so that the effects of its various components will be cumulative.

Do not force through a protective muscle spasm.

A slight alteration of joint position or angle of thrust often allows a technique to be much more effective.

In general, manipulate only if the expected degree of improvement is not being achieved with mobilization.

Warn patients of the potential for posttreatment soreness.

Do not overtreat; stop when symptoms abate.

Aim for restoration of normal, painless mobility.

PREVENTION OF COMPLICATIONS

The main factors to consider with respect to prevention of complications are diagnostic assessment and procedural cautions that reduce the risk of complications from manipulation.

Assessment

The diagnostic assessment includes a patient history, physical examination, and radiologic examination.

History

The history is probably the most underrated portion of the examination. The significance and necessary detail of a case history have been discussed previously by Mennell,[7] Stoddard,[114] Maigne,[94] Matthews,[115] and many others.

Physical Examination

The importance of a complete physical examination is recognized when conditions such as abdominal aneurysms, occlusive vascular disease, hypertension, elevated temperature, prostatic enlargement, and abnormal lymph nodes are found.[116]

Radiologic Examination

Radiographs should always be obtained to rule out contraindications (e.g., underlying overt disease). The absence of either a thorough clinical examination or a radiologic examination is an overriding contraindication for manipulation.[116]

Procedures

The most common and important accident to prevent in the lumbar spine is the rupture of the intervertebral disk with resultant cauda equina syndrome, characterized by paralysis, weakness, pain, reflex changes, and bowel and bladder disturbances.[116–118] Reports indicate that an uncomplicated herniated disk can be reduced by manipulation, possibly as a result of centripetal force.[97,101,119] Manipulation can, however, aggravate the symptoms when serious disk lesions are present.

The following screening tests, described in detail by Kleynhans and Terrett,[116] reduce the risk of disk rupture from lumbar spine manipulation:

Straight leg raise (Laseque/buckling sign)

Well leg raise (Laseque contralateral/crossed Laseque)

Deyerle's sciatic tension test (bowstring test)

Prone knee flexion test

Dejerine's triad (coughing, sneezing, Valsalva's test)

PRECAUTIONS

Although the following are not absolute contraindications, prudence and care must be observed in their presence.[119]

Mobilization

Mobilization procedures should be undertaken with caution in the presence of any of the following:

Neurologic signs—avoid procedures that reduce the intervertebral foramen on the painful side

Rheumatoid arthritis—mobilization may be performed if there is no acute inflammation and bone consistency is kept in mind

Osteoporosis—approximately 40 percent of bone structure is lost before osteoporosis becomes radiologically evident

Spondylolithesis—when treating adjacent levels, avoid stressing the level of instability

Previous malignant disease—if possible, rule out the presence of metastasis

Hypermobility

Pregnancy.

Manipulation

Some of the more common restricted indications for manipulation appear in Table 17-2.[116]

CAUSES OF COMPLICATIONS

Complications resulting from manipulations may be related to either the practitioner or the patient.

Practitioner-Related Complications

Practitioner-related complications may result from diagnostic errors. Medical practitioners often do not have the diagnostic skills necessary to prescribe manipulations.[139] An exacting knowledge of tissue structure and of the conditions that cause signs and symptoms is necessary.[140] It must be remembered that referral by a physician does not necessarily mean that manipulation should be performed. The final decision as to the indications, contraindications, technique, and execution of manipulation rests with the practitioner, and cannot be made by referral.[122] A radiologic examination is a necessary part of the patient assessment; diagnostic errors may result if it is omitted.[141]

Another possible cause of complications is practitioner lack of skill. A practitioner with excellent diagnostic ability but with inadequate training and inferior skills in mechanical diagnosis is just as great a threat to the safe practice of manipulation as are those unqualified manipulators who lack diagnostic expertise.[82,142-144] The literature lists many cases of death or damage in which lack of skill and experience were replaced by brute force.[123,142,145,146]

The application of manipulation without any formal training is probably one of the greatest problems in manipulation. Reading a textbook or attending a weekend course does not make one a skilled practitioner of manipulation. Like any other skilled procedure, the results and complications depend on the ability of the clinician. Absence of manipulative skills on the practitioner's part should be a contraindication to manipulation.[89]

A third cause of practitioner-related complications is lack of interprofessional consultation. One situation in which this is especially important is the patient on anticoagulant therapy, because of the increased risk of hemorrhage.[147] Heparin, because of its anticoagulant and lipid-clearing characteristics, is widely used for the treatment of coronary artery disease, myocardial infarction, and venous thrombosis; in conjunction with vascular surgery; and as a prophylaxis against thromboembolism in pregnancy. Heparin-associated osteoporosis with resulting weakness, fracture, and pain is a well-documented entity.[148]

Patient-Related Complications

Other causes of complications stem from the patients themselves. Examples of patients in whom treatment is prone to complications include:

1. Patients with psychological intolerance of pain or discomfort[94,114,149]
2. Patients in whom minimal stress causes a disproportionate vasoconstrictive response (this reaction can be enhanced in emotionally unstable individuals)[150]

Table 17-2. Relative Contraindications to Manipulation

Condition	References
Articular derangements	
Ankylosing spondylitis after acute stage	Bollier,[120] Rinsky et al.,[121] Sandoz and Lorenz,[122] Stoddard[114]
Articular deformity	Cyriax[97]
Basilar impression	Kaiser[123]
Congenital anomalies	Grillo,[124] Janse,[125] Maigne,[94] Sandoz,[126] Valentini,[127] Yochum[128]
Hypertrophic spondyloarthritis	
Osteoarthritis	Sandoz and Lorenz[122]
Osteochondrosis with defective "holding apparatus"	Stoddard[114]
Bone weakening and modifying disease	
Hemangioma	Siehl[129]
Paget's disease	Sandoz and Lorenz,[122] Nwuga,[5] Lindner[130]
Scheuermann's disease	Beyeler,[131] Hauberg,[132] Janse,[125] Maigne,[94] Nwuga[5]
Spondylolisthesis, spondylolysis	Hauberg,[132] Sandoz and Lorenz[122]
Disc lesion	
Posterolateral and posteromedial disk protrusions	
Degenerative disease	Jaquet,[133] Odom,[134] Stoddard[114]
Neurological dysfunction	
Myelopathy	Cyriax,[97] Stoddard[114]
Dysfunction of nonvertebral origin	Nwuga,[5] Stoddard[114]
Pyramidal tract involvement	Cyriax[97]
Radicular pain from disk lesion	Gutmann,[135] Stoddard[114]
Viscerosomatic reflex pain	Gutmann,[135] Nwuga,[5] Stoddard[114]
Unclassified	
Abdominal hernia	Sandoz and Lorenz[122]
Asthma	Beyeler,[131] Sandoz[136]
Basilar ischemia	Bourdillon,[137] Cyriax,[97] Nwuga[5]
Dysmenorrhea	Sandoz[136]
Epicondylitis	Droz[138]
Postspinal operations	Nwuga[5]
Peptic ulcer	Janse[125]
Pregnancy	Cyriax,[97] Nwuga,[5] Sandoz and Lorenz[122]
Scoliosis	Stoddard[114]
Lumbar Spine	
Accessory sacroiliac joints	
Baastrup's disease	Maigne,[94] Grillo[124]
Cleft vertebra in sagittal plane	Grillo[124]
Facet tropism	Grillo,[124] Janse[125]
Knife clasp syndrome	
Nuclear impression	Grillo[124]
Pseudosacralization	Grillo,[124] Janse[125]
Sacralization, lumbarization	Grillo,[124] Janse[125]
Spina bifida occulta	Janse[125]
Spondylolisthesis	Janse[125]

3. Patients with an excessive pain response due to ethnic background or to certain conditions that preclude manipulation[94,149,151]

4. Patients in whom uncomplicated sciatica becomes a unilateral radiculopathy with distal paralysis of limbs, sensory loss in the sacral distribution, and sphincter paralysis — these patients do not respond to manipulation and should be considered a surgical emergency[152]

5. Patients who develop a psychological dependence on manipulation — this is not uncommon, and the therapist must decide on the importance of the inevitable physical signs that any spine may produce, as treatments are doomed to failure if the patient is allowed to orient his or her neurosis around the spine

6. Patients who have recently undergone treatments with another practitioner — enough time

must be allowed for latent symptoms to develop or reactions to settle down

7. Patients in whom, on examination, the signs and symptoms do not match—experienced practitioners often encounter situations in which there is no direct or obvious contraindication, but the practitioner develops an intuition that manipulation should not be attempted

8. Patients involved in litigation.

CONTRAINDICATIONS
Mobilization

Grieve[119] has suggested the following contraindications to mobilization:

1. Malignancy involving the vertebral column
2. Cauda equina lesions producing disturbances of bladder and/or bowel function
3. Signs and symptoms of:
   a. Spinal cord involvement
   b. Involvement of more than one spinal nerve root on one side, or two adjacent roots in one lower limb only
4. Rheumatoid collagen necrosis of vertebral ligaments—the cervical spine is especially vulnerable
5. Active inflammatory and infective arthritis
6. Bone disease of the spine.

Manipulation

Besides the contraindications listed in Table 17-3, Grieve[88] also listed the following:

1. Evidence of involvement of more than two adjacent nerve roots in the lumbar spine
2. Lower limb neurologic symptoms due to cervical or thoracic joint dysfunction
3. Undiagnosed pain
4. Protective joint spasm
5. Segments adjacent to the level being manipulated that are too irritable or hypermobile to allow stress to be applied for positioning prior to or during manipulation
6. Inability of the patient to relax
7. Rubbery end-feel of the joint.

Inversion Therapy

The use of inversion therapy or gravity traction is not without risks. Certain conditions or situations must be addressed and may restrict or preclude the use of inversion therapy in conjunction with manual techniques. Elevation of blood pressure, especially ophthalmic arterial pressure, increases the risk of subconjunctival and retinal hemorrhage.[155] Patients with a history of hypertension, cardiovascular disease, or stroke are at especially high risk.[155-158] Other pertinent factors include cardiac arrhythmias, heart murmurs, diabetes, thyroid problems, hiatal hernia, migraine headaches, glaucoma, asthma, sinusitis, recent surgery, and artificial joints.[159]

The same principles and rules apply as for other manual procedures. A gradual increase in the degree of inversion as well as its duration will allow the patient to become familiar with and accommodate to the unusual feeling and the physiologic changes, thus reducing certain risks. Further study is required on the influence of gravitational stress on cardiovascular regulation during inversion therapy.[160]

MOBILIZATION AND MANIPULATION TECHNIQUES

Manual therapy is both a diagnostic and a treatment approach to somatic disorders. The choice of a treatment technique not only depends upon the proper analysis of spinal mechanics, which involves exacting palpatory skills, but also must be suited to the patient's age, physical type, and general state of health, as well as the therapist's size, strength, weight, and manual dexterity.

It is impossible to illustrate every technique or even all the variations of a single basic technique. Many of the procedures selected are classic ones and are used by many disciplines. The variations of these techniques can be easily and successfully applied in the clinical situation.

There is an increasing awareness of the neurophysiologic component in addition to the mechanical effect of manual therapy. This awareness is reflected in Table 17-1, and by the recognition on the

Table 17-3. Contraindications for Manipulation

Condition	References
Articular derangements	
Arthritides	
Acute arthritis of any type	Hauberg,[132] Janse,[125] Maigne,[94] Maitland,[9] Stoddard,[114] Yochum,[128] Haldeman,[89] Grieve[88]
Rheumatoid arthritis	Bourdillon,[137] Janse,[125] Maigne,[94] Stoddard,[114] Yochum,[128] Grieve,[88] Haldeman[89]
Acute ankylosing spondylitis	Bollier,[120] Droz,[138] Hauberg,[132] Janse,[125] Nwuga,[5] Stoddard,[114] Haldeman,[89] Grieve[88]
Hypermobility	Gutmann,[135] Kaltenborn,[26] Maitland,[9] Stoddard,[114] Grieve,[88] Haldeman[89]
Bone weakening and destructive disease	
Calvé's disease	Lindner[130]
Fracture	Gutmann,[152] Heilig,[153] Maigne,[94] Nwuga,[5] Rinsky et al.,[121] Siehl,[129] Stoddard,[114] Haldeman[89]
Malignancy (primary or secondary)	Bourdillon,[137] Gutmann,[135] Maigne,[94] Maitland,[9] Nwuga,[5] Timbrell-Fisher,[154] Stoddard,[114] Grieve,[88] Haldeman[89]
Osteomalacia	Lindner[130]
Osteoporosis	Bollier,[120] Bourdillon,[137] Maigne,[94] Nwuga,[5] Siehl,[129] Stoddard,[114] Grieve,[88] Haldeman[89]
Osteomyelitis	Hauberg,[132] Nwuga,[5] Sandoz and Lorenz,[122] Stoddard[114]
Tuberculosis (Pott's disease)	Bourdillon,[137] Hauberg,[132] Maigne,[94] Siehl,[129] Stoddard,[114] Timbrell-Fisher[154]
Disk lesions	
Prolapse with serious neurologic changes (including cauda equina syndrome)	Bourdillon,[137] Cyriax,[97] Hooper,[118] Jaquet,[133] Jennett,[152] Nwuga,[5] Odom,[134] Stoddard,[114] Haldeman,[89] Grieve[88]
Neurologic dysfunction	
Micturition with sacral root involvement	Cyriax,[97] Stoddard,[114] Haldeman,[89] Grieve[88]
Painful movement in all directions	Maigne[94]
Unclassified	
Infectious disease	Maigne,[94] Nwuga[5]
Patient intolerance	Maigne,[94] Lescure[148]

(Modified from Haldeman.[161])

part of many clinicians of these seemingly unorthodox treatment approaches.

The use of arrows in the following illustrations gives a general indication of direction. Keep in mind individual anatomic variations, and the fact that most joint motion occurs in a curvilinear plane.

Mobilization Techniques

Flexion

Fig. 17-47. One of the basic positions for applying lumbar flexion. The patient's knees rest on the therapist's abdomen, and the therapist's left hand guides the knees into flexion, as the therapist sidebends or sways at the hips. The fingers of the therapist's right hand palpate the interspaces for movement.

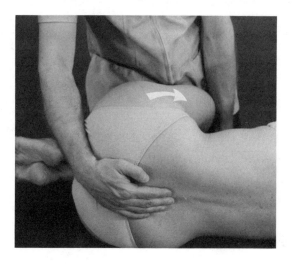

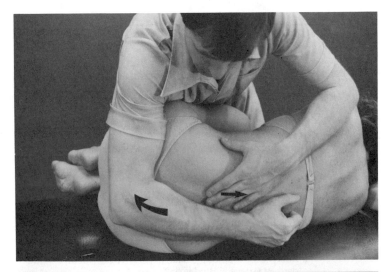

Fig. 17-48. Very strong flexion is applied by a combination of full hip flexion and a strong pull with the therapist's right forearm against a firm pull by the therapist's left hand on a spinous process. Strain on the therapist's back is reduced by leaning on the patient's left hip, which assists in stabilization. The therapist must adopt a wide stance.

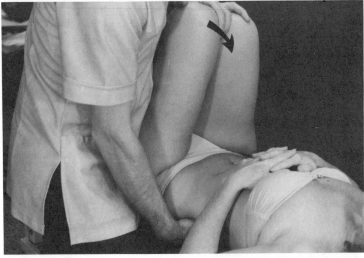

Fig. 17-49. Suitable techniques for light subjects. The therapist flexes the patient's hips with the left hand. The therapist's right hand may palpate the intraspinous process or stabilize the spinous process.

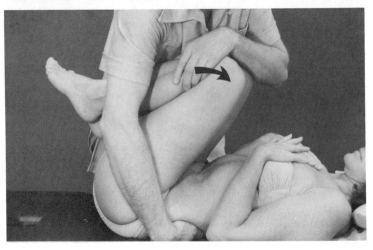

Fig. 17-50. Fairly forceful flexion may be applied by the therapist leaning on the patient's knees. The therapist guides with the left hand, and palpates or stabilizes with the right.

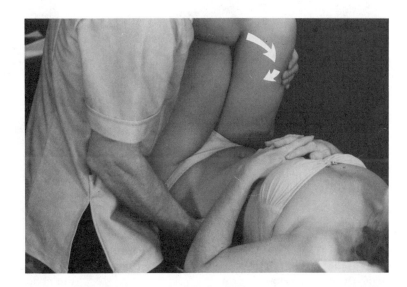

Fig. 17-51. Crossing the patient's knees induces slight sidebending; the therapist's left hand adds flexion. The right hand palpates or stabilizes the spinous process.

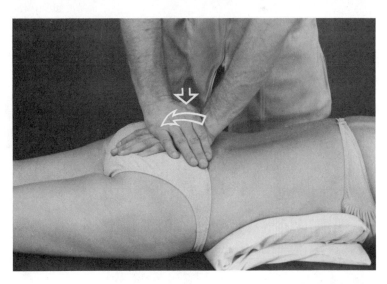

Fig. 17-52. The therapist applies firm ventral pressure over the sacrum, then applies a rocking motion caudally, to flex the lumbosacral joint. A pillow under the patient's abdomen is recommended.

Extension

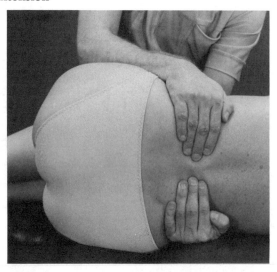

Fig. 17-53. The patient's knees are pushed toward the pelvis as the therapist pulls ventrally on the lumbar segment, causing extension.

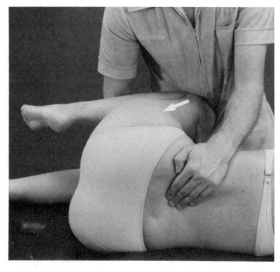

Fig. 17-55. The therapist flexes the patient's left hip to about a right angle and supports the patient's knee with the abdomen and right forearm. The therapist pushes along the patient's thigh, pushing the left side of the pelvis back, and causing extension and left rotation of the lumbar vertebrae. Stabilization can be provided by placing the thumb against the side of the spinous process, or the fingers may palpate for mobility.

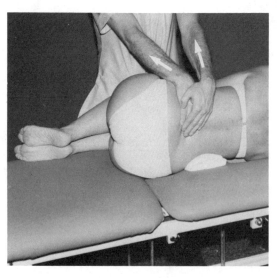

Fig. 17-54. An alternate method for extending the lumbar spine. This method is not as forceful or as localized as that shown in Fig. 17-53.

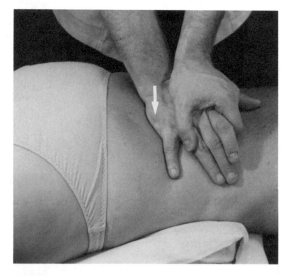

Fig. 17-56. Specific extension over the spinous process with the pisiform bone of one hand, reinforced by the other hand. The therapist's arms are straight. Note the quality and quantity of movement of each lumbar segment.

Selected Sidebending Techniques

Sidebending

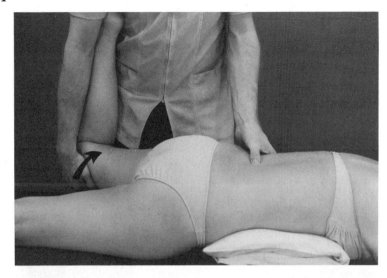

Fig. 17-57. Specific technique to assess or increase left sidebending of the lumbar segment with the patient prone. The therapist's thumb palpates the lateral aspect of the interspinous space. Lumbar spine extension may be increased without the use of a pillow. The therapist steadies the patient's leg and knee with a firm grip while abducting the patient's hip beyond its physiologic barrier.

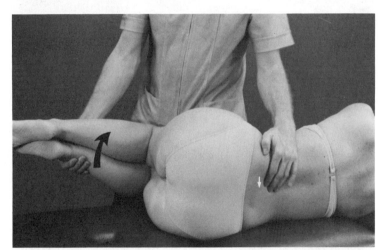

Fig. 17-58. Specific technique to assess or increase left sidebending in side-lying. The patient's knees are supported in the therapist's abdomen or groin. The therapist palpates the lateral aspect of the interspinous space while lifting up on the patient's leg above the ankle.

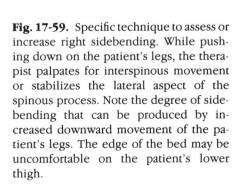

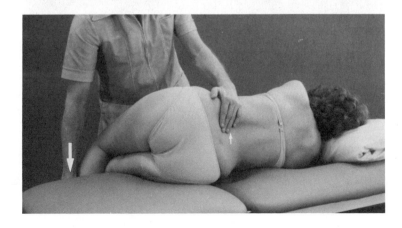

Fig. 17-59. Specific technique to assess or increase right sidebending. While pushing down on the patient's legs, the therapist palpates for interspinous movement or stabilizes the lateral aspect of the spinous process. Note the degree of sidebending that can be produced by increased downward movement of the patient's legs. The edge of the bed may be uncomfortable on the patient's lower thigh.

Lateral Shifting

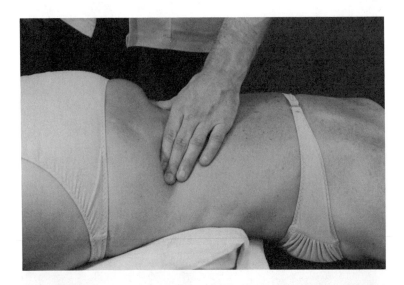

Fig. 17-60. Basic hand position used to apply side-to-side rocking of a lumbar segment. The thumb and index finger are over the transverse process of the vertebrae.

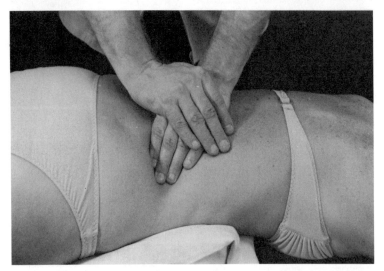

Fig. 17-61. With support from the other hand, the therapist rocks the lumbar segment from side to side. Pressure is applied to attempt a lateral shift motion rather than sidebending.

Selected Rotation Techniques

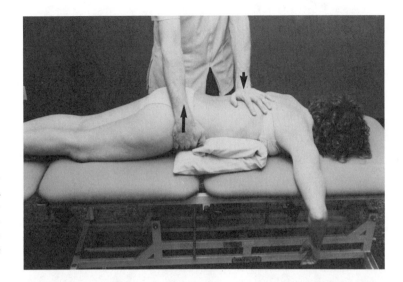

Fig. 17-62. Nonspecific technique to increase left rotation of the lumbar spine. A pillow may be used to reduce lumbar extension. The therapist fixes the thoracolumbar junction and lifts with a comfortable but firm grip of the ilium over the anterior superior iliac spine.

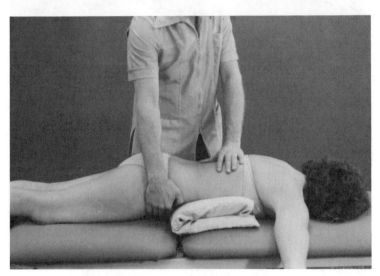

Fig. 17-63. Specific technique to increase or assess left rotation of a lumbar segment. The therapist stabilizes the cranial vertebrae by pressure against the lateral aspect of the spinous process, and lifts with a comfortable grip over the anterior superior iliac spine.

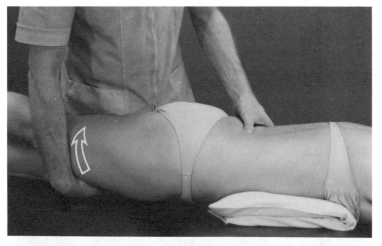

Fig. 17-64. Minimal effort is required to lift the patient's crossed right thigh with the right forearm, causing rotation of the pelvis to the right. The therapist's right hand grasps the patient's anterior left thigh. The patient's thighs are stabilized at the edge of the bed by the therapist's right thigh.

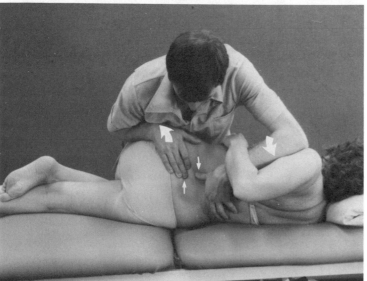

Fig. 17-65. Probably the most common basic position for treating a rotation restriction of the lumbar spine. The patient's left knee is flexed until movement is palpated at a specific lumbar level. The patient's right shoulder is then pulled forward, and the left shoulder is rotated backward to lock the thoracolumbar spine at the desired level. This is further assisted by pressure of the left thumb on the lateral aspect of the cranial spinous process. Gapping of the left apophyseal joint is accomplished by (1) simultaneous opposing thrusts of the therapist's left and right forearms; (2) the therapist pulling forward with the right hand; and (3) the therapist lifting upward with the index or middle finger of the right hand on the underside of the caudal spinous process.

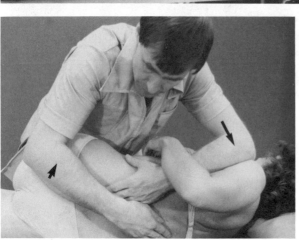

Fig. 17-66. A variation of a nonspecific basic position in which the therapist uses the inner aspect of the forearm against the posterior ilium, allowing for more extension. The therapist palpates with the fingers of the left hand and stabilizes the patient's left shoulder with the left forearm.

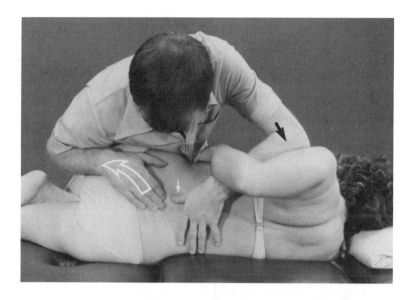

Fig. 17-67. A variation of a specific position in which the patient's left shoulder, is stabilized as well as the cranial lumbar segment, by the therapist's left thumb. The fingers of the therapist's right hand pull up on the underside of the spinous process. The patient's left knee lies over the edge of the table, with the left foot hooked comfortably behind the right knee. If the edge of the midsection of the bed does not lift up, a cushion may be placed under the patient's side. Additional distraction may be applied by the therapist's right hand and forearm.

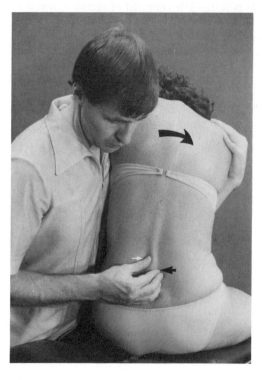

Fig. 17-68. The therapist's left arm is placed under the patient's folded arms, and the therapist reaches across the patient's chest while firmly holding the right shoulder. The patient leans forward as the therapist rotates the patient to the left. The therapist assists the rotation with the right thumb pushing on the lateral aspect of the spinous process, while stabilizing the caudal spinous process with the second finger, reinforced by the third. Alternatively, the therapist may resist rotation of the caudal spinous process by stabilizing with the thumb instead of the fingers.

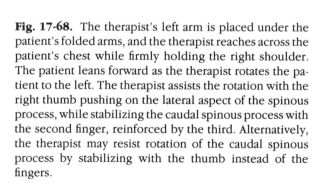

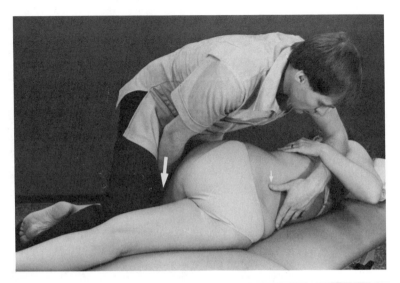

Fig. 17-69. Specific technique to gap the left lumbosacral facet joint. With the patient lying close to the edge of the bed, the left knee is flexed and allowed to hang over the edge of the bed. If the patient cannot comfortably keep the left foot behind the right knee, the therapist can place his or her own flexed right knee on the bed, allowing the patient's left ankle to rest on the posterior aspect of the therapist's right leg. The therapist places thumb and index finger on each side of the patient's left knee, the popliteal space covered by the web of the hand. The therapist's right forearm is along the posterior aspect of the patient's left thigh. Leaning well forward, the therapist thrusts through the popliteal space. Stabilization of L5 is by the therapist's left forearm and thumb, which is on the lateral aspect of the spinous process of L5. As there is a wide range of angles for the lumbosacral facets, the degree of left hip flexion will vary to accommodate the saggital or more coronal joint plane.

ACKNOWLEDGMENT

I would like to express my thanks to Jennie Turner for her expert photographic assistance.

REFERENCES

1. Lomax E: Manipulative therapy: a historical perspective from ancient times to the modern era. In Goldstein M (ed): The Research Status of Spinal Manipulative Therapy. NINCDS Monograph No. 15. DHEW Publication No. (NIH) 76-998. National Institute of Neurological and Communicative Disorders and Stroke, Bethesda MD, 1975

2. Schiotz EH: Manipulation treatment of the spinal column from the medical-historical viewpoint. Tidsskr Nor Laegeforen 78:359, 372 (NIH library translation, 1958)

3. Gibbons RW: Chiropractic in America. The historical conflicts of cultism and science. Presented at the 10th Annual History Forum of Duquesne University, Pittsburgh, 1976

4. Schaefer RD: Chiropractic Health Care. 2nd Ed. Foundation for Chiropractic Education and Research, Des Moines, IA, 1976

5. Nwuga V: Manipulation of the Spine. Williams & Wilkins, Baltimore, 1976

6. Cyriax J: Textbook of Orthopaedic Medicine. 6th Ed. Vol. 1. Bailliere Tindall, London, 1975

7. Mennell JM: Back pain—Diagnosis and Treatment

Using Manipulative Techniques. Little, Brown, Boston, 1960

8. Grieve GP: Common Vertebral Joint Problems. p. 376. Churchill Livingstone, Edinburgh, 1981

9. Maitland GD: Vertebral Manipulation. 4th Ed. Butterworth, London, 1977

10. Paris SV: The spinal lesion. Pegasus, Christchurch, New Zealand, 1965

11. McKenzie RA: The lumbar spine. Mechanical Diagnosis and Therapy. Spinal Publications, Waikanoe NZ, 1981

12. Goldstein M: The Research Status of Spinal Manipulative Therapy. NINCDS Monograph No. 15. PHEW Publication No. (NIH) 76-998. National Institute of Neurologic and Communicative Disorders and Stroke, Bethesda MD, 1975

13. Sato A: The somato-sympathetic reflexes: their physiological and clinical significance. p. 163. In Goldstein M (ed): The Research Status of Spinal Manipulative Therapy. National Institute of Neurological and Communicative Disorders and Stroke, NINCDS Monograph No. 15. DHEW Publication No. (NIH) 76-998. Bethesda MD, 1975

14. Perl E: Pain, spinal and peripheral nerve factors. In Goldstein M (ed): The Research Status of Spinal Manipulative Therapy. NINCDS Monograph No. 15. DHEW Publication No. (NIH) 76-998. National Institute of Neurological and Communicative Disorders and Stroke, Bethesda MD, 1975

15. Granit R, Pompeiano O: Reflex control of posture and movement. Prog Brain Res 50:1, 1979

16. Freeman MAR, Wyke BD: The innervation of the knee joint. An anatomical and histological study in the cat. J Anat 101:505, 1967

17. Wyke BD: The neurological basis of thoracic spinal pain. Rheumatol Phys Med 10:356, 1967

18. Wyke BD: Neurological mechanisms in the experience of pain. Acupuncture Electrother Res 4:27, 1979

19. Wyke BD: Neurology of the cervical spinal joints. Physiotherapy 65:72, 1979

20. Wyke BD: Perspectives in physiotherapy. Physiotherapy 32:261, 1980

21. Wyke BD, Polacek P: Structural and functional characteristics of the joint receptor apparatus. Acta Chir Orthop Traumatol Cech 40:489, 1973

22. Jayson MIV: The Lumbar Spine and Back Pain. 2nd Ed. Pitman, London, 1980

23. Polacek P: Receptors of the joints: their structure, variability and classification. Acta Fac Med Univ Brunensis 23:1, 1966

24. Halata Z: The ultrastructure of the sensory nerve endings in the articular capsule of the knee joint of the domestic cat (Ruffini corpuscles and Pacinian corpuscles). J Anat 124:717, 1977

25. Maitland GDL: Foreword. In Glasgow EF, Twomey LT, Scull ER, Kleynhans AM (eds): Aspects of Manipulative Therapy. 2nd Ed. Churchill Livingstone, Melbourne, 1985

26. Kaltenborn FM: Mobilization of the Extremity Joints. Olaf Norlis Bokhandel, Oslo, 1980

27. Maitland GD: Peripheral Manipulation. 2nd Ed. Butterworth, London, 1977

28. Mennell JM: Joint Pain—Diagnosis and Treatment Using Manipulative Techniques. Little, Brown, Boston, 1964

29. Stoddard A: Manual of Osteopathic Technique. Hutchinson of London, London, 1974

30. Hartman LD: Handbook of Osteopathic Technique. N.M.K. Publishers, Herts, England 1983.

31. Sandoz R: Some physical mechanisms and effects of spinal adjustments. Ann Swiss Chiropract Assoc 6:91, 1976

32. Sandoz R: Some reflex phenomena associated with spinal derangements and adjustments. Ann Swiss Chiropract Assoc 7:45, 1981

33. Gainsbury JH: High velocity thrust and pathophysiology of segmental dysfunction. In Glasgow EF, Twomey LT, Scull ER, Kleynhans AM (eds): Aspects of Manipulative Therapy. 2nd Ed. Churchill Livingstone, Melbourne, 1985

34. Evjenth O, Hamberg J: Muscle Stretching in Manual Therapy—A Clinical Manual—The Spinal Column and the TM Joint. Vol. 2. Alfta Rehab, Alfta, Sweden, 1984

35. Judovich B: Lumbar traction therapy. JAMA 159:549, 1955

36. Burton C: Low Back Pain. 2nd Ed. Philadelphia, JB Lippincott, 1980

37. Burton D, Nida G: The Sister Kenny Institute Gravity Lumbar Reduction Therapy Program. Publication No. 731. Sister Kenny Institute, Minneapolis, 1982

38. Martin RM: The Gravity Guiding System. Essential Publishing, San Marino CA, 1981

39. Jones LH: Strain and Counterstrain. American Academy of Osteopathy, Colorado Springs CO, 1981

40. Hoover HV: Functional Technic. In: 1958 Yearbook. Academy of Applied Osteopathy, Carmel CA, 1958

41. Korr I: Muscle spindle and the lesioned segment. p. 45. In: Proceedings of the International Federation of Orthopaedic Manipulative Therapists, Vail CO, 1977

42. Lee D: Principles and practices of muscle energy and functional techniques. p. 640. In Grieve GP (ed): Modern Manual Therapy of the Vertebral Column. Churchill Livingstone, New York, 1986

43. Goodridge JP: Muscle energy techniques: definition, explanation, methods of procedure. Osteopath Assoc 81:249, 1981

44. Mitchell FL, Moran PS, Pruzzo NA: An Evaluation and Treatment Manual of Osteopathic Muscle Energy Procedures. Mitchell, Moran and Pruzzo, Valley Park MO, 1979

45. Upledger JE, Vredevoogd JD: Craniosacral Therapy. Eastland Press, Chicago, 1983

46. Magoun HI: Osteopathy in the Cranial Field. 3rd Ed., Sutherland Cronial Teaching Foundation, Meridian, Idaho, 1976

47. Gehin A: Atlas of Manipulative Techniques for the Cranium and Face. Eastland Press, Seattle, 1985

48. Brookes D: Lectures on Cranial Osteopathy. A Manual for Practitioners and Students. Thorsons Publishers, Wellingborough, England, 1981

49. Anderson JAD: Problems of classification of low back pain. Rheum Rehabil 16:34, 1977

50. Cailliet R: Low Back Pain Syndrome. 3rd Ed. FA Davis, Philadelphia, 1983

51. Jayson MIV: Preface. In Jayson MIV (ed): The Lumbar Spine and Back Pain. 2nd Ed. Pitman Medical, Tunbridge Wells, England, 1980

52. Nachemson A: A critical look at conservative treatment for low back pain. In Jayson MIV (ed): The Lumbar Spine and Back Pain. 2nd Ed. Pitman Medical, Tunbridge Wells, England, 1980

53. Yates DAH: Treatment of back pain. In Jayson MIV (ed): The Lumbar Spine and Back Pain. 2nd Ed. Pitman Medical, Tunbridge Wells, England, 1980

54. Dixon AS: Diagnosis of low back pain—sorting the complainers. In Jayson MIV (ed): The Lumbar Spine and Back Pain. 2nd Ed. Pitman Medical, Tunbridge Wells, 1980

55. Korr IM: Proprioceptors and somatic dysfunction. J Am Osteopath Assoc 74:638, 1975

56. Simons DG: Electrogenic nature of palpable bands and local twitch response associated with myofascial trigger points. In Bonica JJ, Albe-Fessard D (eds): Advances in Pain Research and Therapy. Vol I. Raven Press, New York, 1976

57. Simons DG: Muscle pain syndromes. Am Phys Med 54:289, 1975; 55:15, 1976

58. Brugger A: Pseudoradikuläre Syndrome. Acta Rheumatol 19:1, 1962

59. Brugger A: Die Erkrankungen des Bewegungsapparatus und seines Nervensystems. Fisher, Stuttgart, 1977

60. Feinstein F, Langton JNK, Jameson RM, Schitter F: Experiments on pain referred from deep somatic tissues. J Bone Joint Surg 36A:981, 1954

61. Hohermuth HJ: Spondylogene Kniebeschwerden. Vortrag anlablich der 4. Deutsch-schweizerischen Forbildungstagung für Angiologie und Rheumatologie, Rheinfelden, Switzerland, May 1981

62. Sutter M: Wesen, Klinik und Bedeutung spondylogener Reflexsyndrome. Schweiz Rundsch Med Prax 64:42, 1975

63. Sutter M, Frohlich R: Spondylogene Zusammenhänge im Bereich der oberen Thorax-Apparatus. Report of the Annual Meeting of the Swiss Society for Manual Medicine, 1981

64. Waller U: Pathogenese des spondylogenen Reflexsyndroms. Scweiz Rundsch Med Prax 64:42, 1975

65. Dvorak J: Manuelle Medizin in USA in 1981. Manuelle Med 20:1, 1982

66. Gibson RW: The evolution of chiropractic. In Haldeman S: Modern Developments in the Principles and Practice of Chiropractic. Appleton-Century-Crofts, New York, 1980

67. Wardwell WI: The present and future role of the chiropractor. In Haldeman S: Modern Developments in the Principles and Practice of Chiropractic. Appleton-Century-Crofts, New York, 1980

68. Dvorak J, Dvorak V: Manual Medicine Diagnostics. Georg Thieme Verlag, Stuttgart, 1984

69. Maigne R: Wirbelsäulenbedingte Schmerzen. Hippokrates, Stuttgart, 1970

70. Kellgren HL: Observation of referred pain arising from muscles. Clin Sci 3:175, 1938

71. Kellgren HJ: On the distribution of pain arising from deep somatic structures with charts of segmental pain areas. Clin Sci 4:35, 1939

72. Sinclair DC, Feindel WH, Weddell G, Falconer MA: The intervertebral ligaments as a source of segmental pain. J Bone Joint Surg 30B:515, 1948

73. Hockaday JM, Whitty CWM: Patterns of referred pain in normal subject. Brain 90:481, 1967

74. Melzack R: Phantom body pain in paraplegics: evidence for central "pattern generating mechanisms" for pain. Pain 4:195, 1978

75. Melzack R: Myofascial trigger points: relation to acupuncture and mechanisms of pain. Arch Phys Med 62:114, 1981

76. Reynolds MD: Myofascial trigger point syndromes in the practice of rheumatology. Arch Phys Med 62:111, 1981

77. Rubin D: Myofascial trigger point syndromes: an approach to management. Arch Phys Med 62:107, 1981

78. Travell J, Rinzler SH: The myofascial genesis of pain. Postgrad Med 2:425, 1952

79. Travell J: Myofascial trigger points: clinical view. In Bonica JJ, Albe-Fessard DG (eds): Advances in Pain

Research and Therapy. Vol. 1. Raven Press, New York

80. Travell J: Identification of myofascial trigger point syndromes: a case of atypical facial neuralgia. Arch Phys Med 62:100, 1981

81. Brugger A: Uber die tendonomyse. Dtsch Med Wochenschr 83:1048, 1958

82. Brugger A: Pseudoradikuläre Syndrome des Stommes. Huber, Bern, 1965

83. Lewit K: Muskelfazilitations und Inhibitionstechniken in der manuellen Medizin. Manuelle Med 10:12, 1981

84. Caviezel H: Beitrag zur Kenntnis der Rippenläsionen. Manuelle Med 5:110, 1974

85. Caviezel H: Klinisch Diagnostik der Funktionsstörung an den Kopfgelenken. Schweiz Rundsch Med Prax 65:1037, 1976

86. Sell K: Spezielle manuelle Segment-Technik als Mittel zur Abklärung spondylogener Zusammenhangsfragen. Manuelle Med 7:99, 1969

87. Northup GWL: Osteopathic Medicine: An American Reformation. American Osteopathic Association, Chicago, 1966

88. Grieve GP: Mobilization of the Spine. 3rd Ed. Churchill Livingstone, Edinburgh, 1979

89. Haldeman S: Spinal Manipulative Therapy in the Management of Low Back Pain. In Finneson BE (ed): Low Back Pain. 2nd Ed. JB Lippincott, Philadelphia, 1981

90. Glover JR, Morr JG, Khosia T: Back pain: a randomized clinical trial of rotational manipulation of the trunk. Br J Ind Med 31:59, 1974

91. Bergquist-Ullman M, Larsson U: Acute low back pain in industry. Acta Orthop Scand (suppl.) 170:1, 1977

92. Potter GE: A study of 744 cases of neck and back pain treated with spinal manipulation. J Can Chiropract Assoc 21(4):154, 1977

93. Fisk JW: A Practical Guide to Management of the Painful neck and Back. Charles C Thomas, Springfield IL, 1977

94. Maigne R: Orthopaedic Medicine. A New Approach to Vertebral Manipulations (translated by WT Liberson). Charles C Thomas, Springfield IL, 1972

95. Edwards BC: Low back pain and pain resulting from lumbar spine conditions: a comparison of treatment results. Aust J Physiother 15(3):104, 1969

96. Buerger AA: A clinical trial of rotational manipulation. Pain Abstracts 1:248. Second World Congress on Pain. International Association for the Study of Pain, Montreal, Canada, 1978

97. Cyriax J: Textbook of Orthopaedic Medicine. 8th Ed. Vol. 2. Bailliere-Tindall, London, 1971

98. Chrisman OD, Mittnacht A, Snook GA: A study of the results following rotatory manipulation in the lumbar intervertebral disc syndrome. J Bone Joint Surg 46A:517, 1964

99. Riches EW: End results of manipulation of the back. Lancet, p. 957, May 3, 1930

100. Kirkaldy-Willis WH, Cassidy JO: Effects of manipulation on chronic low back pain. Presented at a conference on Manipulative Medicine in the Management of Low Back Pain. Sponsored by the University of Southern California and the North American Academy of Manipulative Medicine, Los Angeles, October 1978.

101. Matthews JA, Yates DAH: Reduction of lumbar disc prolapse by manipulation. Br Med J 20:696, 1969

102. White AA, Panjabi MM: Clinical Biomechanics of the Spine. JB Lippincott, Philadelphia, 1979

103. Gillet H, Liekens M: Belgian Chiropractic Research Notes. 10th Ed. Belgium Chiroproct. Association, Brussels, 1973

104. Lewit D: Manuelle Medizin. Im Rahmen der Medizinischen Rehabilitation. 2nd Ed. Johann Ambrosius, Leipzig, 1977

105. Gitelman R: A chiropractic approach to biomechanical disorders of the lumbar spine and pelvis. In Haldeman S (ed): Modern Developments in the Principles and Practice of Chiropractic. Appleton-Century-Crofts, New York, 1980

106. Gonstead CS: Gonstead Chiropractic Science and Art. Sci-Chi Publications, 1968

107. Logan VF, Murray FM (eds): Textbook of Logan Basic Methods. LBM, St. Louis, 1950

108. Cassidy JD, Potter GE, Kirkaldy-Willis WH: Manipulative management of back pain in patients with spondylolisthesis. J Can Chiropract Assoc 22(1):15, 1978

109. Potter GE: Chiropractors (letter). Can Med Assoc J 121:705, 1979

110. Henderson DJ: Intermittent claudication with special reference to its neurogenic form as a diagnostic and management challenge. J Can Chiropract Assoc 23(1):9, 1979

111. Bowles CH: Functional Orientation for Technique. In: 1957 Year Book. Academy of Applied Osteopathy, Carmel CA, 1957

112. Goldthwait JE, Brown LT, Swain LT, Kuhns JG: Essentials of Body Mechanics in Health and Disease. p. 1. JB Lippincott, Philadelphia, 1945

113. Fryette HH: Principles of Osteopathic Technique. Academy of Applied Osteopathy, Carmel CA, 1954

114. Stoddard A: Manual of Osteopathic Practice. Hutchinson of London, London, 1969

115. Matthews JA: The Scope of manipulation in the management of rheumatic disease. Practitioner 208:107, 1972

116. Kleynhans AM, Terrett AG: The prevention of complications from spinal manipulative therapy. In Glasgow EF, Twomey LT, Scull ER, Kelynhans AM (eds): Aspects of Manipulative Therapy. 2nd Ed. Churchill Livingstone, Edinburgh, 1985

117. DePalma AF, Rothman RH: The Intervertebral Disc. WB Saunders, Philadelphia, 1970

118. Hooper J: Low back pain and manipulation paraparesis after treatment of low back pain by physical methods. Med J Aust 1:549, 1973

119. Grieve GP: Common Vertebral Joint Problems. p. 460. Churchill Livingstone, Edinburgh, 1981

120. Bollier W: Inflammatory infections and neoplastic disease of the lumbar spine. Ann Swiss Chiropract Assoc 1960

121. Rinsky LA, Reynolds GG, Jameson RM, Hamilton RD: Cervical spine cord injury after chiropractic adjustment. Paraplegia 13:233, 1976

122. Sandoz R, Lorenz E: Presentation of an original lumbar technic. Ann Swiss Chiropract Assoc 1:43, 1960

123. Kaiser G: Orthopedics and traumatology (translated from the German). Beitr Orthop 20:581, 1973

124. Grillo G: Anomalies of the lumbar spine. Ann Swiss Chiropract Assoc 1:56, 1960

125. Janse J: Principles and practice of chiropractic: an anthology. In R Hildebrandt (ed): National College of Chiropractic, Lombard IL, 1976

126. Sandoz R: Newer trends in the pathogenesis of spinal disorders. Ann Swiss Chiropract Assoc 5, 1971

127. Valentini E: The occipito-cervical region. Ann Swiss Chiropract Assoc 4:225, 1969

128. Yochum TR: Radiology of the Arthritides (lecture notes). International College of Chiropractic, Melbourne, 1978

129. Siehl D: Manipulation of the spine under anaesthesia. In: 1967 Yearbook. Academy of Applied Osteopathy, Carmel CA, 1967

130. Lindner H: A synopsis of the dystrophies of the lumbar spine. Ann Swiss Chiropract Assoc 1:143, 1960

131. Beyeler W: Scheuermann's disease and its chiropractic management. Ann Swiss Chiropract Assoc 1:170, 1960

132. Hauberg GV: Contraindications of the Manual Therapy of the Spine (translated from the German). p. 231. Hippokrates, Stuttgart, 1967

133. Jaquet P: Clinical chiropractic—a study of cases. Chrounauer, Geneva, 1978

134. Odom GL: Neck ache and back ache. In: Proceedings of the NINCDS Conference on Neck Ache and Back Ache. Charles C Thomas, Springfield IL, 1970

135. Gutmann G: Chirotherapie, Grundlagen, Indikationen, Genenindikationen and objektivier Barkeit. Med. Welf. Bd. 1978

136. Sandoz R: About some problems pertaining to the choice of indications for chiropractic therapy. Ann Swiss Chiropract Assoc 3:201, 1965

137. Bourdillon JF: Spinal Manipulation. W Heinemann, London, 1973

138. Droz JM: Indications and contraindications of vertebral manipulations. Ann Swiss Chiropract Assoc 5:81, 1971

139. Wolff H.D. Remarks on the present situation and further development of manual medicine with special regard to chirotherapy. Presented to the Deutsche Gesellschaft für Manuelle Medizin, February 1972

140. Smart M: Manipulation. Arch Phys Med p. 730, December 1946

141. Robertson AHM: Manipulation in cervical syndromes. Practitioner 200:396, 1968

142. Bollier W: Chiropractic and medicine—editorial. Ann Swiss Chiropract Assoc 1960

143. Lewit K: Complications following chiropractic manipulations. Deutsch Medizinische Wochenshrift 97:784, 1972

144. Livingston M: Spinal manipulation causing injury. Br Columbia Med J 14:78, 1971

145. Oger J: 1966 The dangers and accidents of vertebral manipulations (translated from the French). Rev Rhum 33:493, 1966

146. Kuhlendahl H, Hansell V: Nil nocere. Shaden bei Wirbelsäulenreposition (translated from the German). Med Wochenschr 100:1738, 1958

147. Dabbert O, Freeman DG, Weis W: Spinal meingeal hematoma, warfarin therapy and chiropractic adjustment. JAMA 214:11, 1970

148. Lescure R: Incidents, accidents, contreindications des manipulations de la colonne vertebrae. (translated from the French). Med Hyg 12:456, 1954

149. Ladermann JP: Accidents of spinal manipulations. Ann Swiss Chiropract Assoc 7:161, 1981

150. Janse J: Unpublished lecture notes. National College of Chiropractic, Lombard IL, 1961

151. Peters RE: Heparin Therapy—Contraindications to Manipulation. Charter House Publishing, Wagga Wagga, Australia, 1983

152. Jennett WB: A study of 25 cases of compression of the cauda equina by prolapsed IVD. J Neurol Neurosurg Psychiatry, 8:19, 1956

153. Heilig D: Whiplash—mechanics of injury, management of cervical and dorsal involvement. In: 1965 Yearbook. Academy of Applied Osteopathy, Carmel CA, 1965

154. Timbrell-Fisher AG: Treatment by Manipulation. HK Lewis, London, 1948

155. Klatz RM, Goldman RM, Pinchuk BG, Nelson KE, Tarr RS: The effects of gravity inversion on hypertensive subjects. Phys Sports Med 13(11):85, 1985

156. Goldman RM, Tarr RS, Pinchuk BG, et al: The effects of oscillating inversion on systemic blood pressure, pulse, intraocular pressure and central retinal arterial pressure. Phys Sports Med 13(3):93, 1985

157. Klatz RM, Goldman RM, Pinchuk BG, Nelson KE, Tarr RS: The effects of gravity inversion procedures on systemic blood pressure and central retinal arterial pressure. J Am Osteopath Assoc 82:853, 1983

158. Lemarr JD, Golding LA, Crehan KD: Cardiorespiratory responses to inversion. Phys Sports Med 11(11):51, 1983

159. Cooperman J, Scheid D: Guidelines for the use of inversion therapy. Clinical Management, Vol. 4, No. 1, pp. 6-9, 1984. In Physical Therapy published by American Physical Therapy Association, Alexandria Virginia

160. Zito M: Effects of two gravity inversion methods on heart rate, systolic brachial pressure, and ophthalmic artery pressure. Phys Ther 68:20, 1988

161. Haldeman S (ed): Modern Developments in the Principles and Practice of Chiropractic. Appleton-Century-Crofts, New York, 1980

18

Evaluation and Treatment of Dysfunction in the Lumbar-Pelvic-Hip Complex

ALLYN L. WOERMAN

This chapter emphasizes the interrelatedness of the main components of the lumbar-pelvic-hip complex, especially the pelvis. The lumbar spine is discussed in Chapters 15, 16, and 17, so in this chapter only those aspects that are directly involved with pelvic and/or hip function are discussed. By establishing the relationship among these three functional components of the kinetic chain, the clinician can better evaluate the patient and formulate more effective treatment programs.

Many texts offer detailed anatomic and kinesiologic descriptions of the lumbar spine, hip, and pelvis as well as a plethora of evaluative and treatment techniques for these areas. This chapter will give the reader sufficient information to be able to render accurate assessment and treatment for the syndromes described. For simplicity's sake, and for continuity, most illustrations and anatomic descriptions are taken or adapted from Kapandji.[1] The reader must keep in mind the possible effects and influences of other components of the kinetic chain such as the foot, the ankle, and the knee in order to

complete the picture of dysfunction. The assessment and treatment techniques described are primarily osteopathic in nature and utilize the so-called muscle energy techniques popularized by Fred Mitchell, Sr.

FUNCTIONAL ANATOMY AND MECHANICS OF THE HIP

Osteology of the Hip

The hip joint is formed by the articulation of the head of the femur with the acetabulum of the pelvis. This joint is a classic example of a ball-and-socket joint and has three degrees of freedom of motion.[1]

The head of the femur is ellipsoid in shape, forming roughly two-thirds of a sphere approximately 4 to 5 cm in diameter. It is covered with hyaline cartilage, which is thicker centrally and thinner at the periphery. Two basic functional adaptations have been identified in the structure of the femoral head (Fig. 18-1). In the first (type I), the femoral head is greater than two-thirds of a sphere with maximal angles. Its shaft is slender and the associated pelvis is small and high slung. This adaptation is suited for speed and movement. The type II adaptation has a femoral head that is nearly a full hemisphere and minimal angles. Its shaft is thick and its associated

The opinions expressed herein are solely those of the author and are not to be construed as reflecting official doctrine of the U.S. Army Medical Department.

403

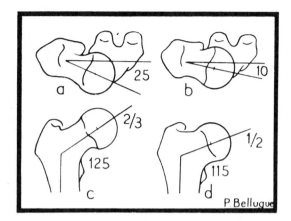

Fig. 18-1. Functional adaptations of the femoral head and neck. Type I **(A, C)** has a head equal to two-thirds of a sphere and maximal angles; type II **(B, D)** has a head greater than half a hemisphere and minimal angles. The angle of inclination is shown in **C, D** and the angle of declination is shown in **A, B**. (From Kapandji,[1] with permission.)

pelvis is broad. This adaptation is for power and strength.

The femoral neck projects laterally from the head and fans out. This projection is usually between 120 and 125 degrees in adults and is known as the angle of inclination (Fig. 18-1). In infants, this head-to-neck angle can be as much as 150 degrees. The decrease in this angle from infancy to adulthood is the result of compression and bending forces acting on the head during weightbearing. From a mechanical standpoint, this head-neck relationship may be likened to a gibbet and strut. The gibbet is an overhang. Vertical forces exerted on it are transmitted to the shaft by means of a horizontal lever. Shear forces are produced near the junction of the horizontal and vertical beams, and so a strut must be interposed to counteract the shear. The struts in the hip are the trabecular systems.

There are two main trabecular systems and one accessory system in the femoral head and neck, and these systems correspond to the lines of force (Fig. 18-2). The medial system begins in the cortical layer of the lateral femoral shaft and ends on the inferior aspect of the cortical layer of the femoral head (arcuate bundle of Gallois). The lateral system arises from the internal aspect of the shaft and the inferior part of the neck and ends in the superior cortical

bone of the head (supporting bundle). The accessory system has two bundles, which arise in the trochanter and fan out from there. The intersection of these systems forms a structure similar to gothic arches with keystones, one of the strongest architectural forms known. One gothic arch is formed by the intersection of the trochanteric bundle of the accessory system and the lateral set of the main system. Its inner pillar is less dense and weakens with age. The other gothic arch is formed by the intersection of the

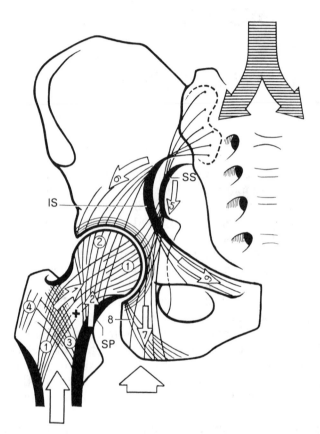

Fig. 18-2. Trabecular systems of the hip and pelvis. Main system: (1) arcuate and (2) supporting bundles. Accessory system: (3) and (4). The intersection of (1) and (3) and (1) and (2) forms the main gothic arches of the hip. A third arch, of less importance, is formed by the intersection of (3) and (4). Sacroacetabular trabeculae (5) and (6) take stress away from the sacroiliac joint. Set (5) converges with set (1) from the femur, while set (6) converges with set (2). Sacroischial trabeculae (7) and (8) intersect to bear the body weight in sitting. (Adapted from Kapandji,[1] with permission.)

medial and lateral systems and forms very dense bone (nucleus of the head). It rests on extremely strong cortical bone at the inferior spur of the neck known as the vault of Adams. Between these two arches is a zone of weakness; this weakness increases with age and is the site of basal neck fractures.

The femoral head and neck project anteriorly in relation to the femoral condyles. The angle formed is known as the angle of declination (Fig. 18-1) and is usually 23 to 26 degrees in the adult. If this angle is significantly increased, the condition known as anteversion (toe-in) occurs. If the angle is significantly decreased, the condition known as retroversion (toe-out) occurs.

A 5 to 7 degree angle exists in the shaft of the femur with respect to the vertical plane, thus causing an anteroposterior bend. This bend produces

strength to withstand ground reaction forces.

The acetabulum or socket portion of the hip joint is formed by the junction of the ilium, ischium, and pubic bones of the pelvis (Fig. 18-3A). It is ellipsoidal and not quite hemispheric. Its orientation is directed laterally, inferiorly, and anteriorly 30 to 40 degrees with the horizontal. A fibrocartilaginous ring called the labrum inserts into the acetabular rim. The labrum is triangular in shape and serves to deepen the acetabulum. It bridges the acetabular notch along with the transverse acetabular ligament (Fig. 18-3B). Within the acetabulum is a horseshoe-shaped hyaline cartilage lining, which is thicker and broader at the roof and thinner and narrower at the floor. No cartilage exists in the central fossa. Instead, a fat pad covers the floor since there is no compression or contact by the head there.

The ligamentum teres, comprised of three bun-

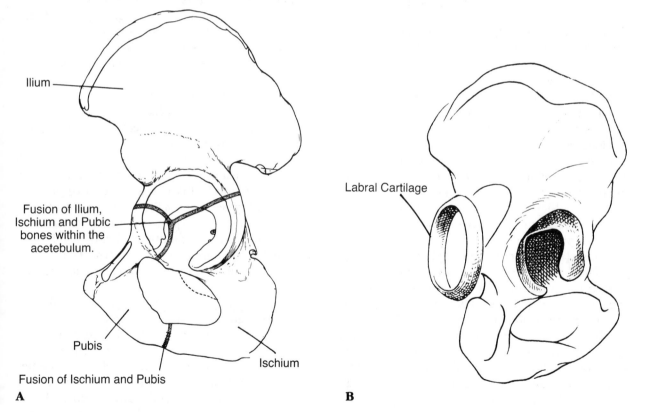

A

Ilium

Fusion of Ilium, Ischium and Pubic bones within the acetebulum.

Pubis

Ischium

Fusion of Ischium and Pubis

B

Labral Cartilage

Fig. 18-3. The innominate, acetabulum, and labrum. **(A)** Left innominate, lateral view. Note the junction of the ischium, ilium, and pubic bones in the fossa of the acetabulum (adapted from Warwick and Williams,[3] with permission); **(B)** acetabulum and three-sided circular labral cartilage (adapted from Kapandji,[1] with permission).

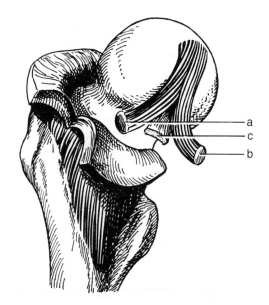

Fig. 18-4. Ligamentum teres. The ligamentum teres consists of three bundles: (a) posterior ischial bundle; (b) anterior pubic bundle; (c) intermediate bundle. (Adapted from Kapandji,[1] with permission.)

dles, is a flattened fibrous band 3 to 3.5 cm long that arises from the acetabular notch and inserts into the fovea capitis. It lies in the floor of the acetabulum and has minimal if any mechanical function in the hip joint, as it only comes under tension in adduction. Its main function is to protect the delicate posterior branch of the obturator artery, which supplies the head of the femur (Fig. 18-4).

The osteology of the pelvis is described in greater detail in the discussion of the sacroiliac joints. For now the pelvis can be described as a closed ring comprised of the two innominate bones, which are conjoined anteriorly by the pubic symphysis and posteriorly by the interposed sacrum and the resulting two sacroiliac joints. The pelvis functions to transmit vertical forces from the vertebral column to the hips via the sacroiliac joints and to transmit ground reaction forces from the legs and hips to the vertebral column, also via the sacroiliac joints. These force transmissions and dissipations are accomplished through two trabecular systems, the sacroacetabular system and the sacroischial system. The sacroacetabular system resists the forces of compression and traction through the kinetic chain, whereas the sacroischial system resists the forces of compression applied to the pelvis. The sacroischial system especially bears the trunk weight when the individual is seated (Fig. 18-2).

Arthrology of the Hip

Maximal joint congruence of the hip is achieved only in 90 degrees flexion, slight abduction, and slight external rotation.[1] In the erect posture, the femoral head is not completely covered by the acetabulum but is exposed superiorly and anteriorly. It is only in the "all-fours" position that the two joint surfaces come into true physiologic congruence.

The capsule of the hip is comprised of four sets of fibers: longitudinal, oblique, arcuate, and circular (Fig. 18-5). The circular fibers form the zona orbicularis around the neck of the femur and divide the joint cavity into two spaces, medial and lateral. The medial capsule inserts into the acetabular rim and the transverse ligament and is intimate with the rectus femoris tendon. The lateral capsule inserts into the base of the femoral neck along the trochanteric line and posteriorly just above the groove and into the trochanteric fossa. The frenulum (pectinofoveal fold of Amantini) is the longest part of the inferior capsule and unpleats itself, especially in abduction, thereby lengthening the capsule and increasing range of motion.

The closed-packed position of the hip is at 0 to 15 degrees extension, 30 degrees abduction, and slight internal rotation.[2] This is the position of greatest joint stability because of the combination of ligamentous tightness and joint congruity. The capsular pattern of restriction of motion is limitation of internal rotation and abduction *more than* flexion and extension *more than* external rotation and adduction.

The anterior ligaments of the hip form a Z-shaped pattern and are analogous to the glenohumeral ligaments of the shoulder (Fig. 18-6). The iliofemoral ligament (the Y-shaped ligament of Bigelow) is made up of two bands: the iliotrochanteric (superior) band and the inferior band. The superior band is the stronger of the two and is 8 to 10 mm thick; it is strengthened by the iliotendinotrochanteric ligament. The inferior band inserts into the lower trochanteric line. The other anterior ligament, the pubofemoral, blends medially with the pectineus

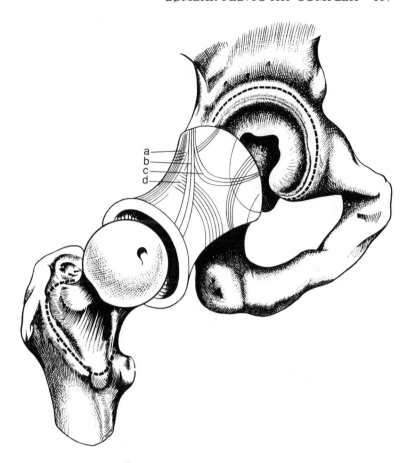

Fig. 18-5. Hip capsule fibers. The directions in which the fibers of the hip capsule are oriented resist stresses placed on the hip: (a) longitudinal; (b) oblique; (c) arcuate; (d) circular. (Adapted from Kapandji,[1] with permission.)

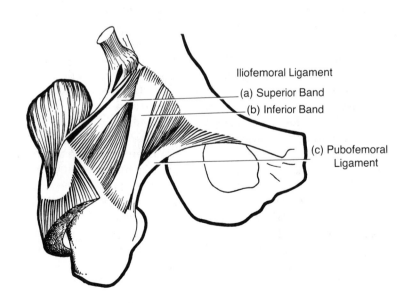

Fig. 18-6. Anterior capsular ligaments of the hip. Capsular ligaments are thickenings of the capsule to reinforce it. The iliofemoral ligament has two bands: (a) superior and (b) inferior. The pubofemoral ligament (c) blends with the pectineus muscle. (Adapted from Kapandji,[1] with permission.)

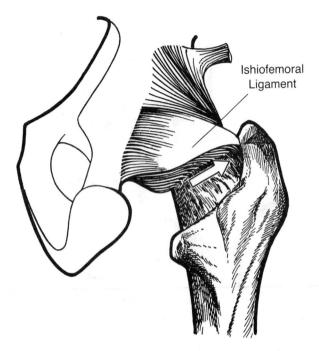

Ishiofemoral
Ligament

Fig. 18-7. Posterior capsular ligament of the hip. The ischiofemoral ligament is coiled in the same direction as the anterior capsular ligaments. (Adapted from Kapandji,[1] with permission.)

muscle and attaches anteriorly into the trochanteric fossa. Between the arms of the Z the capsule is thinner. The iliofemoral bursa lies over this area beneath the iliopsoas tendon.

The posterior ligament of the hip, the ischiofemoral ligament (Fig. 18-7), arises from the posterior acetabular rim and the labrum and attaches into the trochanteric fossa and tendon of the obturator externus muscle. Both the anterior and posterior ligaments are coiled in the same direction around the hip as a result of bipedal stance. In the erect posture, all ligaments are under modest tension. In extension, all ligaments tighten, especially the inferior band of the iliofemoral ligament, which checks posterior tilting of the pelvis. In flexion, all ligaments relax. In external rotation, all anterior ligaments tighten and the posterior relaxes. Just the reverse occurs with internal rotation. With adduction, the iliotrochanteric band tightens, the pubofemoral ligament slackens, and the ischiofemoral ligament relaxes. In abduction, the pubofemoral ligament tightens, the iliotrochanteric band slackens, and the ischiofemoral band tightens.

Neurovascular Supply of the Hip

The nerve supply of the hip joint is derived from the L3 somite with basic spinal cord connections from L2, L3, and L4.[3] The nerve supply is derived directly from the femoral nerve through its muscular branches the obturator, the accessory obturator, the nerve to the quadratus femoris, and the superior gluteal nerve.

The arterial supply is derived from the obturator artery, the medial and lateral circumflex femoral arteries, and the superior and inferior gluteal arteries. The venous supply comes from the femoral vein and the medial and lateral circumflex femoral veins.

Lymphatic drainage is accomplished primarily by the deep inguinal lymphatic chain, especially the upper and middle nodes in the femoral canal and the lateral part of the femoral ring and the extrailiac lymph nodes.

Myology of the Hip

Posterior Musculature

Gluteus Maximus

The gluteus maximus is innervated by the inferior gluteal nerve, L5, S1, and S2.[1,3-5] This muscle is primarily an extensor of the hip and assists in pelvic stability at heel-strike during the gait cycle. It is a phasic muscle and tends to weaken with dysfunction.

Gluteus Medius

The gluteus medius is innervated by the superior gluteal nerve, L5–S1. It is primarily an abductor, but its anterior fibers can flex and internally rotate the hip while the posterior fibers externally rotate. It is the main lateral stabilizer of the pelvis. Its fibers run parallel to the femoral shaft. It is not a very strong muscle until the femur is abducted 30 degrees or more, bringing its fibers more perpendicular to the shaft. It is a phasic muscle and tends to weaken with dysfunction, producing the Trendelenburg gait pattern.

Gluteus Minimus

The gluteus minimus lies deep to the medius and is likewise innervated by the superior gluteal nerve, L5–S1. It functions as a medial-lateral stabilizer of the hip. It is a phasic muscle and tends to weaken with dysfunction.

Piriformis

The piriformis muscle arises on the anterior surface of the sacrum (S2–S4), the sacroiliac capsule, and the ilium, and its tendon passes through the greater sciatic foramen to the greater trochanter of the femur. It is a two-joint muscle, acting on both the sacrum and the femur. External rotation of the femur, especially when the hip is flexed, is its primary action, although it may also extend and abduct. When acting on the sacrum, it will produce torsion of the sacrum to the opposite side. The piriformis derives its innervation from the L5–S2 nerve roots. The nerves of the sciatic plexus and the inferior gluteal vessels run intimately together. In 90 percent of individuals these nerves and vessels pass under the piriformis. In 10 percent of the population, the nerves and vessels pierce the body of the muscle, passing through it. Dysfunction can compress the sciatic nerve against the foramen. The piriformis is a postural muscle and tends to tighten with dysfunction, producing external rotation of the femur and a restriction of internal rotation. Dysfunction of the piriformis can thus cause problems with both the sacroiliac joint and the hip.

Superior and Inferior Gemelli, Obturator Externus and Internus, Quadratus Femoris

All these muscles are external rotators of the hip and function best when the hip is in extension. They run close to the capsule and help reinforce it. They are postural muscles and tend to tighten with dysfunction. The obturator externus is innervated by the posterior obturator nerve, L3–L4, and the obturator internus is innervated by the nerve to the obturator internus, L5–S1. All the others are innervated by nerve roots L5 and S1.

Hamstrings

The hamstrings are two-joint muscles acting at both the knee and the hip. They are most effective in extension of the hip when the knee is extended. They are postural muscles and tend to tighten with dysfunction. Bilateral tightness or contracture produces a posterior pelvic tilt. The semitendinosus is innervated by the tibial division of the sciatic nerve, L5–S2, as is the semimembranosus. The biceps femoris has its long head innervated by the tibial division of the sciatic nerve, L5–S2, whereas the short head is innervated by the peroneal division.

Medial Musculature

The medial muscles as a group arise from the pubis and insert on the posterior and posteromedial aspect of the femur. They are postural muscles and tend to tighten with dysfunction. Tightness unilaterally produces a lateral pelvic tilt high to the involved side, giving the appearance of a long leg.

Adductors

The adductor longus is innervated by the anterior obturator nerve, L2–L4; the adductor magnus is innervated by the obturator nerve and the tibial division of the sciatic nerve, L2–L4; the adductor brevis is innervated by the obturator nerve, L2–L4.

Pectineus

The pectineus muscle, along with the iliopsoas and the adductor longus, forms the floor of the femoral triangle. It is innervated by the accessory obturator nerve, L2–L3, and the femoral nerve, L2–L3.

Gracilis

The gracilis is the only two-joint adductor and is innervated by the obturator nerve, L2–L3.

Anterior Musculature

Iliopsoas

The iliopsoas is formed as the iliacus from the iliac fossa unites with the psoas major, which arises from the transverse processes of L1 through L5, inserting by a common tendon into the lesser trochanter of the femur. The iliopsoas is a two-joint muscle: When the spine is stable, it flexes the hip (and adducts and externally rotates it to some degree); when the femur is stable, it extends the lumbosacral spine. Unilateral contraction sidebends the spine to the same side and rotates the spine to the opposite side. It is a primary stabilizer of the hip in erect posture. Being a postural muscle, it tightens with dysfunction, producing hip flexion and increased lumbar lordosis. The iliopsoas is innervated by the femoral nerve, L2–L3, and the lumbar nerves, L1–L3.

Rectus Femoris

The rectus femoris has two heads: The straight head arises from the anterior superior iliac spine (ASIS); the reflected head arises from the margins of the hip joint capsule. It inserts into the common quadriceps tendon and into the tibial tubercle. It is a hip flexor when the knee is extended and tends to tighten with dysfunction. It is innervated by the femoral nerve, L2–L4.

Sartorius

The sartorius obliquely crosses the thigh from the ASIS to the superomedial tibia. It flexes, abducts, and externally rotates the hip. It forms the lateral border of the femoral triangle (the superior border is the inguinal ligament, and the medial border is the adductor longus). It tightens with dysfunction and is innervated by the femoral nerve, L2–L3.

Lateral Musculature

Tensor Fasciae Latae

The tensor fasciae latae arises from the iliac crest, the ASIS, and the fascia and inserts into the iliotibial band along with the superior fibers of the gluteus maximus to form the "deltoid" of the hip. It is primarily an abductor, but it can also flex and internally rotate the hip. It has a very long lever arm, as the iliotibial band crosses the knee. It tightens with dysfunction. Unilateral tightness produces a lateral pelvic tilt low to that side. Bilateral tightness produces an anterior pelvic tilt. The tensor fasciae latae is innervated by the superior gluteal nerve, L4–L5.

Entrapment Syndromes of the Hip and Pelvis

Several peripheral nerve entrapment syndromes that can occur in and around the hip and pelvis[6] are briefly mentioned here not only to alert the clinician to the possibility of neurogenic pain in this region, but to emphasize their anatomic considerations as well.

Femoral Nerve

The femoral nerve, L2–L4, descends through the psoas and travels on top of the iliacus. It exits the pelvis behind the inguinal ligament. It lies close to the femoral head, from which it is separated only by a small amount of muscle and capsule. Trauma or hematoma here may cause entrapment, producing pain and muscle weakness in the iliopsoas, sartorius, pectineus, and quadriceps muscles. The major complaint is pain that starts below the inguinal ligament and can encompass the anteromedial surface of the thigh and the medial surface of the leg down to the medial surface of the foot. Local tenderness in the groin is almost always present. Muscle stretch reflexes of the knee will be diminished.

Sciatic Nerve

The sciatic nerve, L4–S2, usually passes deep to the piriformis muscle. If the nerve pierces the piriformis, it is usually the lateral division that does so. The lateral division forms the peroneal trunk. It is postulated by some that the basis for the piriformis syndrome is a hip flexion posture with a compensatory lordosis, which tightens the sciatic nerve against the notch. A true neuropathy will result in a flail leg and foot, but neuropathy secondary to direct external trauma at the sciatic notch is rare. The sciatic nerve innervates the hamstrings, the adductor magnus, and all the muscles of the leg and foot. It provides sensory innervation to the posterolateral leg and the plantar and dorsal aspects of the foot (see section on the piriformis under "Myology of the Hip").

Obturator Nerve

The two most common causes of obturator nerve (L2–L4) entrapment are obturator hernia and osteitis pubis. Both conditions entrap the nerve in the obturator foramen. Obturator nerve entrapment is characterized by groin pain to the inner thigh, increasing during Valsalva maneuver and not relieved with rest. True neuropathy will cause pain and weakness in its distribution. The obturator nerve provides motor innervation to the adductors, the gracilis, the obturator externus, and occasionally the pectineus. Its pain reference is the medial thigh from the groin. Motion of the hip in a neuropathy will cause pain. Patients may exhibit a waddling gait pattern due to pain and adductor weakness and in an attempt to restrict hip motion.

Ilioinguinal Nerve

The ilioinguinal nerve, (L1–L2), is vulnerable to entrapment in the region of the ASIS. This nerve follows the pattern of an intercostal nerve and arrives in the region of the ASIS. Here it turns medially and traverses the abdominal muscles in a stepwise fashion, piercing the transversus abdominis and internal oblique to reach the spermatic cord under the external oblique muscle. Entrapment of this nerve will cause pain into the groin, with some radiation to the proximal inner surface of the thigh. It is aggravated by increasing tension in the abdominal wall upon standing erect and by hip motion, especially extension. There is a high incidence of lower back difficulties associated with this condition. Pressure over a point medial to the ASIS will cause pain to radiate into the area of innervation.

Lateral Femoral Cutaneous Nerve

The lateral femoral cutaneous nerve, L2–L3, is vulnerable to entrapment in the region of the ASIS where the nerve passes through the lateral end of the inguinal ligament. This condition is known as meralgia paresthetica. It is characterized by a burning pain in the anterior and lateral portions of the thigh. Pressure over the ASIS should aggravate the pain. The mechanism of onset may be traumatic, but very often the condition is without known cause. Pelvic tilt or a short leg resulting in postural alterations may be associated with this condition.

FUNCTIONAL ANATOMY AND MECHANICS OF THE PELVIS

The pelvis is considered to be a closed ring comprised of three functional pieces: the two pelvic halves (innominates) and the sacrum. The two innominates are conjoined anteriorly by the pubic symphysis and posteriorly by the interposed sacrum and the resulting two sacroiliac joints. The pelvis functions to attach the spine and the lower limbs, transmitting vertical forces between them as part of the kinetic chain, and also to protect the viscera. Many practitioners are mistakenly taught that the articulations of the pelvis (the pubic symphysis and the sacroiliac joints) have no functional movements except in childbirth, and therefore do not contribute to complaints of pain or dysfunction except in rare instances such as disease and trauma. However, the pelvic joints do indeed move[3] and are probably involved directly or indirectly in the greater percentage of mechanical low back problems.[7,8]

Osteology of the Pelvis

Innominate Bones

The innominate bones (left and right pelvic halves) are each formed by the fusion of the ilium, ischium, and pubic bones. This fusion is complete, with no movement between them whatsoever. Their common junction is in the acetabulum. As there is no functional movement between the bones of the innominates, each half is a functional unit by itself (Fig. 18-3A).

The left and right innominate bones are joined anteriorly in the midline by the pubic symphysis (Fig. 18-8). This articulation is bound together by the superior pubic ligament and inferiorly by thick arcuate fibers. Between the two halves is a fibrocartilaginous disk. A cavity (nonsynovial) may often be found in the disk, especially in women, and may extend the length of the disk. The pubic symphysis receives muscle attachments from the external oblique abdominal and the rectus abdominis muscles.

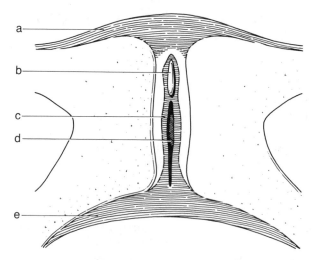

Fig. 18-8. Pubic symphysis. (a) Superior pubic ligament; (b) hyaline cartilage; (c) fibrocartilaginous disk; (d) nonsynovial cavity; (e) inferior pubic ligament. (Adapted from Kapandji,[1] with permission.)

Sacrum

The iliac portions of the posterior innominate bones are joined together through the sacrum. The articulations here form the sacroiliac joints. The sacrum is formed by the fusion of the five sacral vertebrae and sits as a wedge between the innominates. The base of the sacrum (S1) forms the lumbosacral junction with the fifth lumbar vertebra. Its anterior projecting edge is known as the sacral promontory. The sacral apex (S5) articulates with the coccyx. The sacrum is curved ventrally, increasing the capacity of the true pelvis for visceral contents and childbearing. Posteriorly, the sacrum encases the spinal canal and the end of the cauda equina.

The sacroiliac joints are synovial articulations. Some classify the sacroiliac joint as a syndesmosis because of its synovial nature,[3] whereas others consider it to be a synchondrosis because of its fibrous articulation.[9] In the adult, the joint has an auricular shape and is characterized by irregularities (elevations and depressions) in the joint surfaces. These irregularities fit reciprocally with one another, lending to the strength of the joint, but also tend to restrict its movements. The sacral surface is fibrocartilaginous whereas the iliac surface is of hyaline cartilage.

Sacroiliac Ligaments

The ligaments surrounding the sacroiliac joint are the strongest in the body and serve as attachments and origins for some of the strongest muscles in the body.[10] The strength of these ligaments has led some authorities to the belief that the sacroiliac joint is relatively immobile and consequently rarely the source of pain or pathology,[11,12] or that the sacrum moves only as a unit with the innominates.[13] However, the fact that the sacroiliac joints do move has been convincingly proven as experimental methods have improved. For example, Frigerio, Stowe, and Howe,[14] using stereoradiography and computer vector analysis demonstrated movement of up to 26 mm between the sacrum and the innominates in vivo. Others[15,16] have documented similar findings. Turek[17] stated that the sacroiliac joints have motion of 3 to 5 degrees until late middle age. For simplicity, the sacroiliac ligaments are presented here in two groups: intrinsic and extrinsic.

Intrinsic Ligaments

The anterior sacroiliac (capsular) ligament is a thickening of the capsule and is relatively weak compared to its other supporting structures. It is considered by some[3] to be continuous with the iliopsoas and occasionally the piriformis, having origins from each muscle. It surrounds the joint surfaces completely and is continuous with the periosteum caudally, where it is about 1 mm thick, becoming better developed at the level of the arcuate line (Fig. 18-9). The interosseous ligaments are massive and form the chief bond between the two joint surfaces. The deep cranial and caudal bands blend with a more superficial sheet which also has cranial and caudal portions, which form the short posterior sacroiliac ligaments (Fig. 18-10). The dorsal ligaments overlie the interosseous ligaments. Their lower fibers may form a separate fasciculus known as the long posterior sacroiliac ligament. This ligament blends with the sacrotuberous ligament and the thoracolumbar fascia. Because of the directions of fiber arrangements of the anterior and posterior sacroiliac ligaments, some authors tend to group them into caudal and cranial groups, indicating their functional capacities.[1,18]

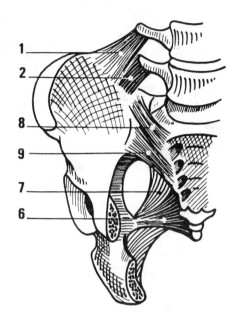

Fig. 18-9. Anterior sacral joint capsule and ligaments. (1) and (2) are the iliolumbar ligaments; (8) and (9) are anterior sacroiliac ligaments consisting of a superior and an inferior band; (6) sacrospinous ligament; (7) sacrotuberous ligament. (From Kapandji,[1] with permission.)

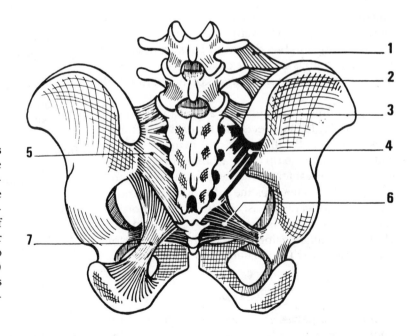

Fig. 18-10. Posterior view of the pelvis showing the ligamentous support of the sacroiliac joint. (1) and (2) are the iliolumbar ligaments; (3) intermediate plane ligament from the iliac crest to the transverse process of S1; (4) posterior fibers of the interosseous ligaments; (5) anterior plane of the sacroiliac ligaments (deep fibers of the interosseous ligaments; (6) sacrospinous ligament; (7) sacrotuberous ligament. (From Kapandji,[1] with permission.)

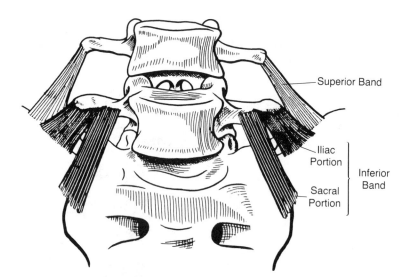

Fig. 18-11. Iliolumbar ligaments. (From Kapandji,[1] with permission.)

Extrinsic Ligaments

The sacrotuberous and sacrospinous ligaments bind the sacrum to the ischium. The lower fibers of the sacrotuberous ligament blend with the gluteus maximus and the biceps femoris. This ligament functions to resist the upward tilting of the lower sacrum under the downward thrust of the weight of the trunk imparted to the sacral base from above. The sacrospinous ligament connects the spine of the ischium to the lateral margins of the sacrum and coccyx.

The iliolumbar ligaments have two bands: a superior band, which connects the tip of the L4 transverse process to the iliac crest, and an inferior band, which connects the tip of the L5 transverse process to the iliac crest anteromedially to the superior band (Fig. 18-11). Sometimes the inferior band can display two distinct divisions: one strictly iliac portion and one portion that is strictly sacral. The influence of the iliolumbar ligaments on lumbosacral motion is discussed later (see "Lumbopelvic Rhythm").

Pelvic Types

Four types of pelves are described in *Gray's Anatomy*[3]: anthropoid, android, gynaecoid, and platypelloid. The differences mainly depend on the sex of the individual. These pelvic types differ in the dimensions of the superior and inferior apertures, the greater sciatic notch, and the subpubic arches. There are also proportional differences between the fore and hind pelves as well as the anterior and posterior transverse diameters of the inlets.

Sexual differences between male and female pelves have to do with function. Although the primary function in both pelves is locomotion, the major difference is in the female role in childbirth. The male pelvis is more heavily built, and the general architecture, being more angular in orientation, is more for power and strength. The female pelvis is broader and deeper, with its iliac wings more vertically set but shallower than in the male pelvis.

The pelvis functions to transmit vertical forces from the vertebral column to the hips via the sacroiliac joints or to transmit ground reaction forces from the legs and hips to the vertebral column via the sacroiliac joints. These force transmissions and dissipations are accomplished through two trabecular systems previously mentioned, the sacroacetabular system and the sacroischial system (see "Osteology of the Hip").

Innervation

The innervation of the sacroiliac joint is not always symmetrical.[3] The joint is most consistently found to be innervated by segments S1 and S2 dorsally and segments L3 to S2 ventrally. Participation of the obturator nerve in the innervation of the sacroiliac joint is not confirmed.[10]

Muscular Influences

Solonen[10] noted that the sacroiliac joint is normally in a state of stable equilibrium and that much force is required to disturb this equilibrium. He further pointed out that the strongest muscles in the body surround the sacroiliac joint but that none have the primary function of moving it. Thus, he concluded, there are no voluntary movements of the sacroiliac joint, and what movements do occur are produced by other movements of the body, especially weight changes and postural influences. Such movements are referred to by some as joint play motions[19,20] or accessory joint motions.[3]

Some authorities[9,21-24] believe that the following muscle or muscle groups can indirectly impart force upon the sacroiliac joint either through their primary actions or by their reverse actions, depending on the points of fixation: the iliopsoas, rectus femoris, hip abductors and adductors, sartorius, external rotators and piriformis, gluteus maximus, hamstrings, abdominals, quadratus lumborum, and multifidus. Rather than give a detailed synopsis of each muscle by its morphology, each muscle or group will be presented according to its action.

Iliopsoas

With the femur and pelvis fixed, the iliopsoas produces powerful ipsilateral flexion of the lumbar spine with rotation contralaterally. It flexes the lumbar spine relative to the pelvis, increasing lordosis. If the lumbar spine and pelvis are fixed, the iliopsoas produces flexion of the hip as well as some lateral rotation of the hip and may have some adduction function. Some fibers, especially from the iliacus, blend with the anterior sacroiliac ligament and joint capsule. Bilateral contraction of the iliopsoas produces an anterior force on the pelvis, causing anterior motion of the innominate as well as an anterior force on the sacrum because of its attachment on the sacral ala. Unilateral contraction may cause an anterior force ipsilaterally, resulting in anterior rotation of the innominate, and may produce anterior movement of the sacrum on that side. Si-

multaneously, it may produce a torsion of the sacrum to the opposite side.

Rectus Femoris

The rectus femoris can simultaneously flex the hip and extend the knee. If the pelvis is fixed, it will flex the thigh on the pelvis. If the thigh is fixed, it will flex the pelvis on the thigh. If the thigh and the lumbar spine are both fixed, with the pelvis free to move, the rectus femoris has the potential to cause anterior rotation of the innominate.

Sartorius

The sartorius can simultaneously flex the knee and the hip. It assists with hip abduction and external rotation. It may exert an anterior influence on the innominate when the knee is fixed in some flexion and the hip is extended.

Hip Abductors

The hip abductors indirectly influence the sacroiliac joints through the pubic symphysis (see the sections on "Myology of the Hip," "Evaluation," and "Treatment").

Tensor Fasciae Latae

See the section on "Myology of the Hip."

Gluteus Maximus

The gluteus maximus extends a flexed thigh and prevents the forward momentum of the trunk from causing flexion of the hip during the gait cycle. It is inactive in standing, but powerfully rotates the pelvis backward in the raising of the trunk from a forward bent position. It can be a strong lateral rotator of the thigh and abductor as it exerts influence on the iliotibial tract. Bilateral contraction may assist in trunk extension if the femur is fixed. Bilateral contraction produces posterior movement of the innominates through the sacrotuberous and posterior sacroiliac ligaments. Unilateral contraction produces a posterior force on the innominate ipsilaterally, causing posterior rotation on that side.

Hip Adductors

The hip adductors exert indirect action on the sacroiliac joints through the pubis (see sections on "Evaluation" and "Treatment"). Tightness or weakness of the adductors may influence hip position, which in turn influences the sacroiliac joints.

Hamstrings

The hamstrings as a group are the primary knee flexors, but they can extend the hip when the hip is flexed and the knee is in extension (see "Myology of the Hip"). They work to convert the posterior ligaments, especially the sacrotuberous ligament, into dynamic movers. Tightness or weakness of the hamstrings can cause either an anterior or a posterior rotation of the pelvis on the hip (see "Lumbopelvic Rhythm").

External Rotators and Piriformis

Bilateral contraction of the piriformis will produce an anterior force on the sacrum and cause it to flex forward. Unilateral contraction may produce an anterior force on the side of contraction, causing rotation to occur to the opposite side. Tightness or spasm of the piriformis may have significant influence on the sacroiliac joint (see sections on "Myology of the Hip," "Gait and Body Position," "Sacral Torsions," "Evaluation," and "Treatment").

Quadratus Lumborum

The quadratus lumborum fixes the twelfth rib and can be an accessory muscle of inspiration. Bilateral contraction results in stabilization of the lumbar spine, preventing deviation from the midline. Unilateral contraction produces ipsilateral sidebending when the pelvis is fixed. Some elevation and rotation anteriorly occur with unilateral contraction. Bilateral contraction may produce an anterior flexion of the sacrum through its attachments onto the base and ala. A unilateral contraction may produce an ipsilateral sacral flexion, with rotation to the side opposite the contraction.

Multifidus

Along with the rotatores (transversospinalis group), the multifidus is primarily a postural muscle and stabilizes the lumbar spinal joints. A bilateral contraction extends the vertebral column from the prone or the forward bent position and, conversely, performs in controlled forward bending (eccentric contraction). In the lumbar spine during rotation, the contralateral group is more active. A bilateral contraction may produce a posterior force on the pelvis through its attachments with the erector spinae, the posterior superior iliac spine (PSIS), and the posterior sacroiliac ligaments. A unilateral contraction may produce a posterior rotation of the vertebrae on that side.

Abdominals

The importance of the abdominals in relation to the lumbar spine and the pelvis is in lifting. By exerting pressure internally (Valsalva), the abdominals significantly reduce axial compressive forces. The abdominals resist the shear forces produced by the multifidus and the psoas on the lumbar facets.[25] A bilateral contraction, especially of the rectus abdominis, produces a posterior rotation of the pelvis when the vertebral column and the sternum are fixed. Lack of abdominal tone will result in an increased lumbar lordosis and increased sacral flexion position.

Anatomic Considerations for Sacroiliac Dysfunction

According to Cyriax,[12] sacroiliac joint problems are more common in females than in males. The following anatomic factors may explain why the occurrence of sacroiliac dysfunctions in the general population is six times greater in females than in males (see "Functional Anatomy and Mechanics of the Pelvis").

1. The lateral dimension of the pelvic foramen is greater in females than in males
2. The bone density of the male pelvis is greater
3. The sacroiliac joint surfaces are smaller in females
4. The sacroiliac joint surfaces are flatter in females
5. The sacroiliac joints are located farther from the hips in females than in males

6. The iliac crests are set farther apart in the female pelvis than in the male pelvis
7. The vertical dimension of the pelvis is greater in the male pelvis
8. The more rectangular the shape of the sacrum, the more stable it is within the innominates
9. The more vertical the orientation of the sacrum within the innominates, the flatter or less lordotic is the lumbar spine—this increases compressive forces upon the lumbar spine
10. The more horizontal the orientation of the sacrum within the innominates, the greater will be the lumbar lordosis—this increases the shear forces across the lumbosacral angle
11. Three types of sacral articular surfaces have been classified according to shape:
    a. Average or normal auricular surface
    b. Smooth and convex anteroposteriorly (this is the type of articular surface in which the rare inflare and outflare dysfunctional lesions of the innominates occur)
    c. Extremely irregular and concave auricular surfaces (these are very stable and usually uniform bilaterally but occasionally may be asymmetrical in shape).

Orientation Planes of the Pelvis

To understand the relationships of the structure and movements of the sacrum, lumbar spine, and lower extremities to one another, one must understand and be able to relate the reference planes of the pelvis to the cardinal planes of the body. Knowing these planes, one is then able to describe the direction and degree of motion of any given pelvic landmark in relation to any other specified landmark.

The cardinal planes of the body are (1) the transverse plane, which bisects the body through the center of gravity into upper and lower halves; (2) the sagittal plane, which bisects the body in the midline through the center of gravity into right and left halves; and (3) the frontal plane which bisects the body through the shoulders anteroposteriorly into ventral and dorsal halves.

The orientation planes of the pelvis are (1) the pelvic frontal plane, which is parallel to the frontal plane, running through the anterior edge of the symphysis pubis to the ASIS; (2) the pelvic trans-

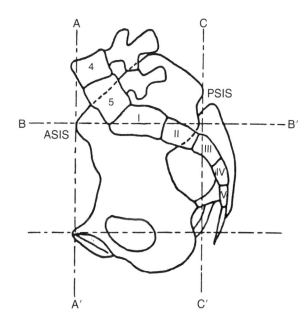

Fig. 18-12. Orientation planes of the pelvis. A–A', pelvic frontal plane; B–B', pelvic transverse plane; C–C', pelvic dorsal plane. (Adapted from Mitchell.[26])

verse plane, which is parallel to the transverse plane and runs through the ASIS to the PSIS; (3) the pelvic dorsal plane, which is parallel to the pelvic frontal plane and runs through the PSIS. These reference planes are shown in Figure 18-12.

Principal Pelvic Axes of Motion

The movements of the pelvic joints can be somewhat confusing if one does not understand the axes about which these movements occur. It is important to realize that these movements are conjoined and do not occur as pure movements in pure planes (Fig. 18-13).

Pubis

The pubis has its axis in the frontal plane, which allows anteroposterior rotation of one innominate against the other. Movement in any other plane at this joint is pathologic. Its greatest functional movements occur in the gait cycle (see "Gait and Body Position").

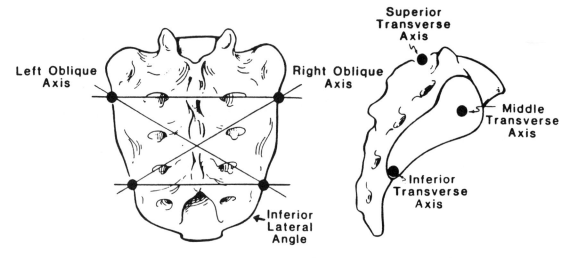

Fig. 18-13. Principle axes of sacral motion. (From Saunders,[27] with permission.)

Sacroiliac Joint

The sacroiliac joint can be considered as two joints: the iliosacral and the sacroiliac. The term *iliosacral* implies the innominates moving on the sacrum. Conversely, the term *sacroiliac* implies the sacrum moving within the innominates. Functionally, and from a treatment standpoint, these designations hold true, since they are based on the recruitment of motion and transmission of forces from the spine or lower members through the pelvis even though it is one and the same joint.

Iliosacral motion occurs primarily in the sagittal plane about the inferior transverse axis (anterior and posterior rotation of the innominates; see "Gait and Body Position"). Iliosacral motion is conjoined with rotation at the pubis and through the sacrum at the contralateral oblique axis.

Sacroiliac motions occur about multiple axes, two transverse and two oblique. The principal axis of regular sacroiliac movement (nutation/counternutation) is the middle transverse axis. However, because iliosacral motion is conjoined with the pubis, the sacrum must make adaptive movements about the two oblique axes alternately (see sections on "Gait and Body Position" and "Sacral Torsions"). The superior transverse axis is often referred to as the respiratory axis. This axis is actually a fulcrum formed by the attachments of the posterior sacroiliac ligaments and the thoracodorsal fascia. As one inhales, the sacrum extends (counternutates), and as one exhales, the sacrum flexes (nutates).

Functional Integration of Related Areas

The transmission of vertical forces from the spine to the lower members, and of ground reaction forces from the lower limbs to the spine, (Fig. 18-14) occurs through trabecular lines (see "Osteology of the Hip"). The manner in which these forces are transmitted and dispersed (i.e., from the top down versus from the bottom up) helps explain why certain dysfunctional lesions of the pelvis occur regularly with certain actions or activities as will be discussed later.

Lumbopelvic Rhythm

The concept of normal functional integration among the lumbar spine, pelvis, and hip joints is basic to the understanding of dysfunction in this region. In the total forward bending of the spine, there is synchronous movement in a rhythmic rotation of the lumbar spine to that of pelvic rotation about the hips.[13,27]

As one bends forward, the lumbar lordosis reverses itself from concave to flat to convex. At the same time, there is a proportionate amount of pelvic

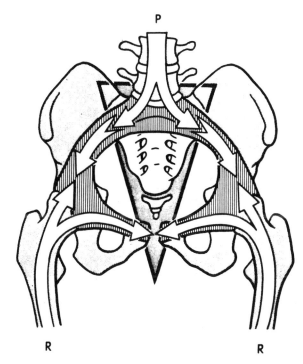

Fig. 18-14. Transmission of ground reaction forces and vertical compression forces from the upper body through the sacroiliac joints and pubic rami. (From Kapandji,[1] with permission.)

rotation about the hips. The amount of movement between lumbar levels will vary, with the most movement occurring at L5–S1 and lesser amounts at successively higher levels. Nonetheless, the rhythm between levels should be smooth and precise, rendering a balance between lumbar reversal and pelvic rotation (Fig. 18-15). Obviously, the ability of a person to bend forward will be influenced by this rhythmic balance or lack of it. Many factors can influence this rhythm, such as facet restriction, degenerative joint disease, or tight hamstring muscles. Thus, in order to achieve full forward bending, the lumbar spine must fully reverse itself, and the pelvis must rotate to its fullest extent. During these movements, the sacrum is also moving within the ilia. Initially, the sacrum nutates (flexes), but as motion in the lumbar spine is recruited and the hamstrings begin to tether the pelvis in its rotation around the hips, the sacrum begins to counternutate (extend) within the ilia.

At the same time as these movements are occur-

ring in the sagittal plane, there is a backward translation of the pelvis and the hips in the horizontal plane. This represents a shift in the pelvic fulcrum so that the center of gravity is maintained over the feet. If this did not occur, the person would fall forward.

As the person returns to the standing position, just the reverse process should occur in an equally smooth manner. It is a fallacy to think that just because a person can bend forward and touch his toes he has full range of motion of the lumbosacral spine. Such an individual may very well have loose hamstrings, which never engage the pelvis to tether it. Thus, the lumbar spine is allowed to remain relatively concave or flat, and the sacrum in relative nutation. Conversely, the hamstrings may be tight and can markedly restrict pelvic rotation about the hips. Should this person try to force flexion of the trunk as in lifting, a strain may occur in the lumbosacral area. The point is made to encourage the clinician to assess closely the integration of motion between the lumbar spine and pelvic components.

Sacroiliac movement in forward bending occurs first at the middle transverse axis. As one approaches the middle of forward bending, a small amount of sacral extension occurs. This is followed by the base moving slightly anterior and the apex to the middle transverse axis. In forced forward bending, the movement shifts more to the superior transverse axis, and the base of the sacrum moves posteriorly and superiorly and the apex anteriorly.

The iliolumbar ligaments directly influence the integration of movement between the lumbar and pelvic components of the complex. The superior and inferior bands are selectively stretched during various movements and serve to greatly limit motion and stabilize the lumbosacral junction. In side-bending, the iliolumbar ligaments become taut contralaterally and relax ipsilaterally. They allow only 8 degrees of movement of L4 relative to the sacrum.[1] In flexion, the inferior band is relaxed and the superior band tightens. In extension, the inferior band tightens and the superior band relaxes.

To reiterate, certain motions in the pelvic complex must be differentiated from each other. Although the joint is called the sacroiliac joint, and that motion occurring at this joint can rightly be called sacroiliac motion, the term must be narrowed

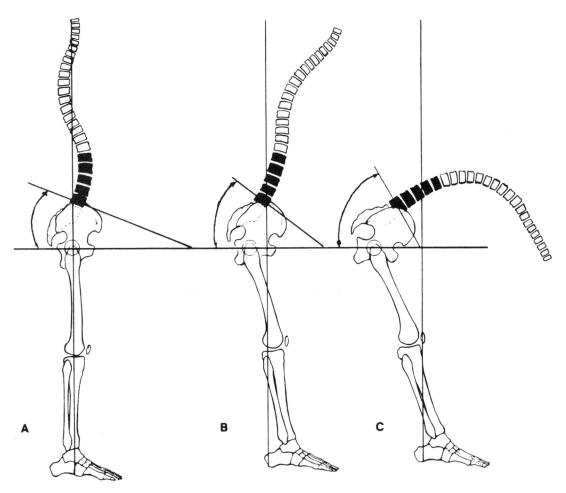

Fig. 18-15. Lumbopelvic rhythm. **(A)** Normal standing posture with lumbar concavity; body weight superimposed directly over the hip joints; normal pelvic inclination with respect to horizontal. **(B)** Flattening of the lumbar spine; the pelvis begins to rotate anteriorly around the hips; hips and pelvis more posteriorly in the horizontal plane. **(C)** Reversal of the lumbar spine into lumbar convexity; the pelvis rotates anteriorly to the fullest extent; hips and pelvis are posteriorly displaced in the horizontal plane. (From Saunders,[27] with permission.)

somewhat. In certain contexts, *sacroiliac motion* will be viewed as motion of the sacrum within the two innominates. Motion of the innominates on a fixed sacrum will be termed *iliosacral motion*. These two categories of movement comprise sacroiliac motion in the broader sense (see "Principal Pelvic Axes of Motion").

MECHANICS OF DYSFUNCTION

The following descriptions fit a model for sacroiliac dysfunction as taught by osteopathic practitioners.[9,21-23] It must be remembered that very few if any motions in the human body occur in a single plane about a single axis. So it is in the sacroiliac joint. The models described give concepts of motion about the principal axes and form a basis for examination and a rationale for treatment. The seven most common dysfunctions will be presented in some detail. The other less common ones will be briefly mentioned (see "Signs of Sacroiliac Problems").

Innominate Rotations

There are two principal rotatory dysfunctions of the innominates: anterior (forward) and posterior (backward). The axis through which these rotations occur is the transverse axis through the pubic symphysis in the horizontal plane. To visualize this, form an open ring with your hands between the tips of the long fingers. The space between the thumbs represents where the sacrum would be placed to complete the ring. The pubic symphysis is represented by the touching of the fingertips. Rotating one hand up or down in relation to the other represents the motion of one innominate in relation to the other (Fig. 18-16). Dysfunctional innominates are thus described as either anterior or posterior according to the side of involvement (e.g., left posterior, right anterior). By far the most common of these dysfunctional rotations is the left posterior innominate, and the next most common is the right anterior innominate.[21] Some practitioners believe that left anterior and right posterior dysfunctions almost never occur,[21] whereas others believe that

their incidence is related to the type of population being treated and the types of stresses sustained in working situations (military, mining, business, industrial, etc.; Stratton SA: personal communication).[28]

Posterior innominate dysfunctions occur most frequently in the following situations: (1) repeated unilateral standing; (2) a fall onto an ischial tuberosity; (3) a vertical thrust onto an extended leg; (4) lifting in a forward bent position with the knees locked; (5) intercourse positions in females (hyperflexion and abduction of the hips). Anterior innominates occur most frequently in the following situations: (1) golf or baseball swing; (2) horizontal thrust of the knee (dashboard injury); (3) any forceful movement on a diagonal (ventral PNF) pattern.

Sacral Torsions

Sacral torsions are perhaps the hardest dysfunctions to conceptualize. They occur as fixations on either of the oblique axes, usually during the gait cycle, and are held in this dysfunctional position by the piriformis (see "Gait and Body Position"). Torsions might be thought of as half the sacrum flexing and the other half extending on one of the two oblique axes.[29] Torsions do not occur purely on the oblique axes but have a sidebending component as well as a flexion component. To visualize the concept of sacral torsion, take a matchbook cover to represent the

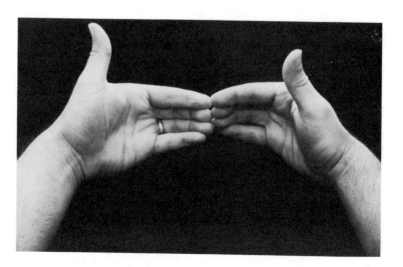

Fig. 18-16. Innominate rotations.

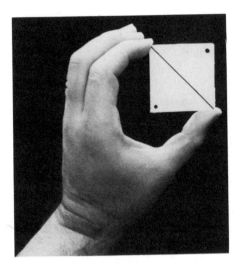

Fig. 18-17. Left oblique axis.

sacrum in three-dimensional space. Holding the top left corner and the bottom right corner between the thumb and long finger (the diagonal between them representing the left oblique axis (LOA); (Fig. 18-17), push forward on the top right corner and allow the "sacrum" to rotate between the fingers; the effect approximates that of a sacral torsion to the left on the left oblique axis (Fig. 18-18). It must be remembered that all anatomic referencing is from the standard anatomic model, and what is considered to be forward or backward must be in relation to this position. Clinically, however, patients with back problems are viewed from the posterior aspect, and sometimes confusion arises as to what is

forward and backward with regard to sacral torsions. Thus, in the model described, the sacrum is labeled according to the *direction* of motion and the *axis* on which the motion occurred: left forward torsion *on* the left oblique axis, or a left-on-left forward torsion (L on L).

By simply changing the finger holds on the matchbook to the opposite diagonal corners and pushing forward on the top left corner (Fig. 18-19), one now approximates a right forward torsion on the right oblique, axis of a right-on-right forward torsion (R on R). (Note: Forward torsions are *only* left-on-left or right-on-right.)

Backward torsions positionally in space appear to be identical to forward torsions. They are, however, quite different. To visualize this concept, take the matchbook and, while holding it on the left oblique axis (top left and bottom right corners), pull the top right corner backward (Fig. 18-20). This approximates a right backward torsion on the left oblique axis, or a right-on-left backward torsion (R on L). Grasping the opposite diagonal corners (top right and bottom left) and pulling the top left corner backward approximates a left backward torsion on the right oblique axis (L on R). (Note: Backward torsions are *only* left-on-right or right-on-left.).

Unilateral Sacral Flexions

Sacral flexion lesions might be thought of as failure of one side of the sacrum to extend (counternutate) from the flexed (nutated) position.[28] In this situa-

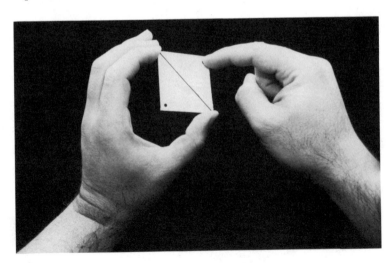

Fig. 18-18. Left-on-left forward sacral torsion.

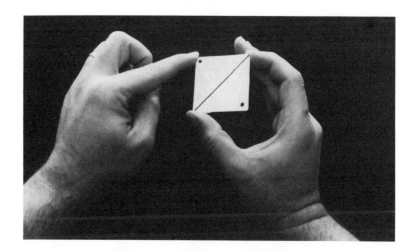

Fig. 18-19. Right-on-right forward sacral torsion.

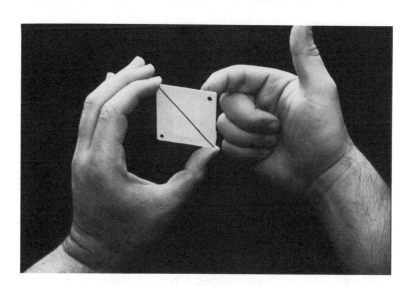

Fig. 18-20. Right-on-left backward sacral torsion.

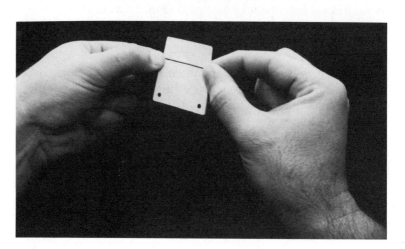

Fig. 18-21. Unilateral sacral flexion lesion.

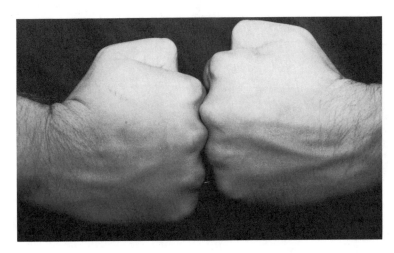

Fig. 18-22. Pubic shear lesion.

tion, the sacrum has flexed on the middle transverse axis. As the dysfunction occurs, the sacrum is forced down the long arm of the joint, where it becomes restricted. Thus, there is a large sidebending component in this dysfunction as well as a flexion component. Because of this restriction, the sacrum is unable to extend on that side. Sacral flexion lesions tend to be traumatic in nature and usually do not occur as the result of everyday stresses and strains.

Again using the matchbook cover, holding the cover about one-third the way down on each side simulates the middle transverse axis. Turning the cover forward between the fingertips simulates nutation. Now, by turning forward with one hand and turning backward with the other, adding also a little bending to the side that is turning backward, the sacral flexion lesion is approximated (Fig. 18-21).

Pubic Shear Lesions

Pubic shears are, as the name implies, a sliding of one joint surface in relation to the other in either a superior or an inferior direction. To visualize this dysfunction, place the knuckles of your two fists together and slide one fist superiorly one knuckle width (Fig. 18-22).

Pubic shears are probably the most commonly overlooked pelvic dysfunction. However, their recognition and proper treatment are mandatory for success in treating pelvic dysfunctions. Pubic shears very frequently occur with innominate rotations and upslips and are often the cause of groin pain as a presenting symptom (see "Evaluation").

Superior Innominate Shear (Upslip)

Innominate shears, either superior or inferior, were once usually thought of as rather rare. However, Greenman[30] has indicated that their occurrence is much more common than previously thought. As the name suggests, an innominate shear is a sliding of one entire innominate superiorly (upslip) or inferiorly (downslip) in relation to the other. These shears are usually traumatic in nature and result from a fall onto an ischial tuberosity or as an unexpected vertical thrust onto an extended leg.

Etiology of Sacroiliac Joint Dysfunction

Sacroiliac joint dysfunctions are fairly characteristic of one another in that certain disease processes or mechanical factors may manifest themselves in localized sacroiliac pain. Diseases such as ankylosing spondylitis, Paget's disease, or tuberculosis all may give rise to sacroiliac pain as an initial complaint.[14,31] In the general population, acute strains with joint involvement are actually rare. This may not be true in certain populations such as athletes and the military.[32] Far more common in terms of mechanical dysfunction are structural and muscular imbalances and joint hypermobilities which give rise to sacroiliac complaints.

Signs of Sacroiliac Problems

The types of pain that can occur with sacroiliac dysfunction are variable.[7-9,21,23,33] The pain may be sharp or dull, aching or tingling, and so on. The pain is most often unilateral and local to the joint (sulcus) itself, but it may refer down the leg (usually posterolaterally and not below the knee) because of innervation from the L2 through S2 segments. There are no associated neurologic symptoms with sacroiliac dysfunction. A straight leg raise test may be positive but only for pain, and usually in the higher arc above 60 degrees. The pain is usually worse with walking and stair climbing, and the patient usually limps (with a Trendelenburg or similar gait pattern). Pain intensity usually does not increase with prolonged sitting; however, when the condition is acute, the patient may sit shifted onto one ischium. The patient often maintains lumbar lordosis in forward bending, recruiting motion around the acetabuli (see "Lumbopelvic Rhythm"), and may also complain of some lumbar pain. The clinician may note ipsilateral tension over the erector spinae muscles and may see a slight swelling over the dorsal aspect of the sacrum. Pain may often arise from the nonblocked side (i.e., the dysfunctional side may be nonpainful but is causing the opposite side to become hypermobile and painful). Finally, sacroiliac pain is more common in females in the general population (see "Anatomic Considerations for Sacroiliac Dysfunction").

Gait and Body Position

A patient with sacroiliac joint dysfunction will often complain of pain during walking or stair climbing. An understanding of the relative positions and movements of the sacrum, innominates, and other body parts will help account for the pain produced during locomotion. The following is a synthesis of an article by Mitchell on this topic.[9,21,26] The cycle of movement of the pelvis in walking is described in sequence as though the patient were starting to walk by advancing the right foot first:

1. Trunk rotation in the thoracic region occurs to the left, accompanied by left sidebending of the lumbar spine, forming a convexity to the right.

2. The body of the sacrum begins a torsional movement to the left, locking the lumbosacral junction and shifting the body weight to the left sacroiliac. This locking mechanism establishes movement of the sacrum on the left oblique axis. As the sacrum can now turn torsionally to the left, the sacral base must also move down on the right to conform to the lumbar convexity that has formed on the right.

3. As the right leg accelerates forward through action of the quadriceps, tension accumulates at the junction of the left oblique axis and the inferior transverse axis and eventually locks. As the body weight swings forward, slight anterior movement is increased by the backward thrust of the restraining left leg as the right heel strikes the ground.

4. Tension in the right hamstrings begins with heel-strike. As the body weight moves forward and upward toward the right crest of femoral support, there is a slight posterior movement of the right innominate on the inferior transverse axis. This movement is also increased by the forward thrust of the propelling leg action. This ilial rotational movement is also influenced, directed, and stabilized by the torsional movement of the pubic symphysis on its transverse axis. Also at heel-strike, the right piriformis contracts to fixate the left oblique axis at the inferior lateral angle, thus allowing for a left forward torsion of the sacrum on the left oblique axis (left-on-left forward torsion). From the standpoint of total pelvic movement, one might consider the transverse pubic symphyseal axis as the postural axis of rotation for the entire pelvis.

5. As the right heel strikes the ground, trunk rotation and accommodation begin to reverse themselves. At midstance, as the left foot passes the right and the body weight passes over the crest of femoral support, the accumulating forces move to the right. At this point, the sacrum changes its axis to the right oblique axis, which then allows the left sacral base to move forward and torsionally to the right. The cycle of movements is then repeated in identical fashion on the left.

Vertebral Motion

Frequently, in attempting to describe the motion of a vertebral segment, terms become confused. Sometimes terms describing motion are inappropriately interchanged with terms that describe posi-

Table 18-1. Standard Vertebral Motion Terminology

Term	Definition
Flexion	Forward bending of the trunk in the sagittal plane about a transverse axis
Extension	Backward bending of the trunk in the sagittal plane about a transverse axis
Sidebending	Movement (left or right) in the coronal plane about an anteroposterior axis
Rotation	Movement (left or right) in the transverse plane about a vertical axis

tion. This section defines the terms for both vertebral segment motion and vertebral segment positioning. These must be clearly differentiated to ensure accurate communication.

A vertebral motion segment consists of two adjacent vertebrae, specifically, the inferior half of the superior vertebra and the superior half of the inferior vertebra, which includes the posterior intervertebral facet joints and the intervertebral disk anteriorly.[1] Vertebral motion occurs in a plane around an axis and is named for the superior segment moving on the inferior segment. Table 18-1 defines the standard motion terms with regard to anatomic planes and axes.

Early in this century, Fryette described the coupling of the various spinal motions with one another.[34] His observations have, with certain clarifications, remained substantially valid over the years. These "laws" of spinal motion are summarized in Table 18-2 and Figures 18-23 and 18-24.

The range of vertebral motion may be considered as either active or passive. Active vertebral motion is the result of the patient's voluntary activity. It involves multiple segmental activity and is frequently compound in nature. Passive vertebral motion is the

Table 18-2. Laws of Physiologic Spinal Motion (Fryette's Laws)

I.	If the vertebral segments are in the neutral (or easy normal) position without locking of the facets, rotation and sidebending are in opposite directions (type I motion) (see Fig. 18-23)
II.	If the vertebral segments are in full flexion or extension with the facets locked or engaged, rotation and sidebending are to the same side (type II motion) (see Fig. 18-24)
III.	If motion is introduced into a vertebral segment in any plane, motion in all other planes is reduced.

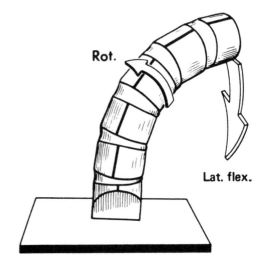

Fig. 18-23. First law of physiologic spinal motion: Sidebending and rotation are in opposite directions when the spine is in a neutral posture. (From Kapandji,[1] with permission.)

result of clinician activity or an external force. It may involve one or multiple segments and may be simple or compound in nature. Vertebral segment dysfunction may be compensatory as a result of long-standing postural imbalance, inequality of muscle tone, or single-segment dysfunction above or below. It may also be traumatic in nature.

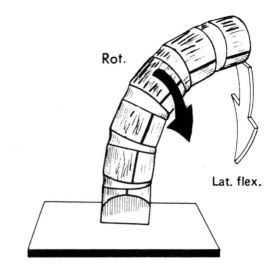

Fig. 18-24. Second law of physiologic spinal motion: Sidebending and rotation are in the same direction when the spine is in flexion or extension. (Adapted from Kapandji,[1] with permission.)

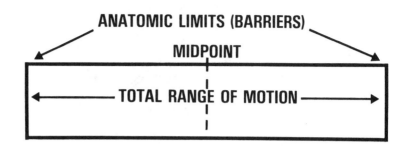

Fig. 18-25. Total range of motion for any joint. (Adapted from Kimberly,[23] with permission.)

Quality of Vertebral Motion

The ease with which a patient moves through a range of motion is as significant as the total range of motion itself. With careful palpation, the clinician can assess subtle aberrations in the freedom of motion within a segment or group of segments that appear to have a normal range of motion. Thus, the clinician must be able to evaluate quality as well as quantity of motion for diagnostic as well as therapeutic considerations. Segments with restricted range of motion (usually symmetrical) may have normal degrees of freedom or ease. Hypermobility is increased range and freedom (laxity) of joint motion. Hypermobile segments are frequently symptomatic, and thrust mobilizations are generally contraindicated. Hypermobile joints are most frequently the result of compensatory change due to restricted motion (above or below the joint) or are traumatic in origin.[21]

Barrier Concept of Vertebral Motion Restriction

Not every object moving in space has six degrees of freedom of motion; however, the vertebral segment does.[27] A normal functional range of motion exists in or across the three planes of motion for each segment. If, for whatever reason, motion becomes restricted in one plane, motion in the other two planes is also reduced (Fryette's third law). This may be perceived as a restriction in overall movement during an analysis of spinal movement.

Somatic dysfunction has been described as impaired or altered function of related components of the somatic (body framework) system. Somatic dysfunction is characterized by impaired mobility, which may or may not occur with positional alteration.[9,21,22,35] Figure 18-25 illustrates the total range of motion for any given joint. It is bounded at its extremes by its anatomic limits (barriers). A barrier is an obstruction or a restriction to movement. Anatomic barriers include the bone contours and/or soft tissues, especially the ligaments, that serve as the final limit to motion in an articulation beyond which tissue damage will occur. Physiologic barriers are the soft tissue tension accumulations that limit the voluntary motion of an articulation. Further motion toward the anatomic barrier can be induced passively.

Figure 18-26 illustrates the divisions of active and

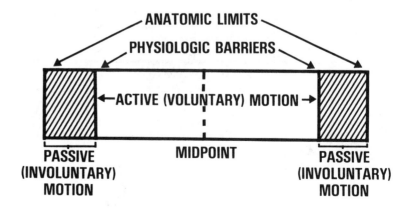

Fig. 18-26. Active and passive divisions in somatic dysfunction. (Adapted from Kimberly,[23] with permission.)

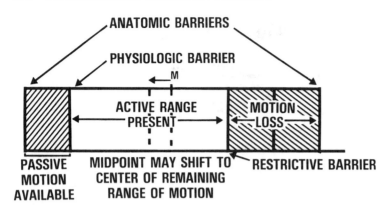

Fig. 18-27. Minor motion loss in somatic dysfunction. (Adapted from Kimberly,[23] with permission.)

passive motion within the total range of motion of a given joint. Active motion is movement of an articulation by the individual between the physiologic barriers. Passive motion is movement induced in an articulation by the clinician. It includes the range of active motion as well as the movement between the physiologic and anatomic barriers permitted by soft tissue resiliency that the individual cannot initiate voluntarily. Soft tissue tension accumulates as the joint is passively moved from its active range through physiologic barriers toward anatomic barriers. Thus, when the clinician tests a joint for end-feel or joint play, it is these barriers that are being tested and compared.

In somatic dysfunction, minor motion loss sometimes occurs, implying that a restrictive barrier has formed somewhere within the normal active range of motion, thus limiting the ability of the joint to complete its full, pain-free range of motion. A minor motion loss is one in which the barrier does not cross the midpoint of the joint's normal range of motion. This concept is illustrated in Figure 18-27.

A major motion loss occurs when the motion barrier crosses the normal midpoint of the active range of motion of the joint. This is illustrated in Figure 18-28. Motion loss, whether major or minor, is maintained until something occurs to change the barrier. Various factors influence these restrictions, such as taut joint capsules, shortened ligaments and fascias, muscles shortened due to spasm or fibrosis, or a shift in the gamma gain mechanism.[36] Long-standing lesions lead to changes in the adjacent tissues (adnexae), especially in circulatory (edema with dilation or vasoconstriction), neural (pain, tenderness, hyperesthesia, itching), and myofascial components (muscle contraction, fibrosis). These can lead to changes in segmentally related tissues, especially circulatory (usually vasoconstriction) and neural (altered efferent or afferent flow).

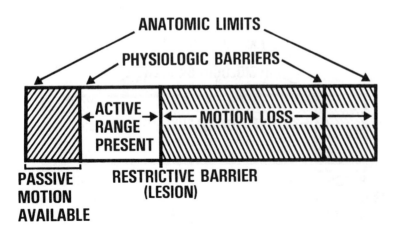

Fig. 18-28. Major motion loss in somatic dysfunction. (Adapted from Kimberly,[23] with permission.)

Nomenclature for Vertebral Segment Dysfunction

Asymmetry in position and restriction in motion of the vertebral segment(s) (superior segment on inferior segment) must be differentiated.[21,37] Table 18-3 illustrates this point. The example given is of the L3 vertebra, which has been found to be in a flexed, left rotated, and left sidebent position. The motion restriction of this segment (what it cannot do) is just the opposite of the dysfunctional position: The segment cannot extend, right rotate, or right sidebend. Note that the major differences between the terms describing position and motion is in the suffixes used. The positional terms use the past participle, whereas the motion terms are in the present tense (Table 18-4).

The intervertebral facet joints function primarily to guide motion of the spinal segment. Table 18-5 depicts facet function in relation to trunk motion. Factors that restrict vertebral motion may be interpreted as interfering with the ability of the facets to open or close.

The clinician must be able to accurately assess mechanical problems of the spine by differentiating between the positions that the vertebral segments assume or fail to assume during active motion.[9,21,23] The following examples typify why this concept is important. To the casual observer, the two schematics in Figure 18-29 of a right sidebent vertebral segment may look the same. In reality, they represent two different lesions and must be treated differently if the clinician hopes to be successful in caring for this patient.

In Figure 18-29A, the left facet will not close (extend). Thus, when the patient is asked to perform backward bending, the right transverse process becomes more prominent. The reason is that, as motion is recruited through the segment from top to bottom, the right facet, which is already in a rela-

Table 18-3. Differentiation Between Vertebral Motion Position and Restriction

Motion Segment	Position	Motion Restriction
L3 on L4	Flexed	Extension
	Left rotated	Right rotation
	Left sidebent	Right sidebending

Table 18-4. Suffixes for Vertebral Segment Positioning and Corresponding Motion Restriction

Position	Motion
Flex*ed*	Extens*ion*
Extend*ed*	Flex*ion*
Right rotat*ed*	Left rotat*ion*
Left side*bent*	Right sidebend*ing*

tively closed (extended) position, is carried along into more extension as a part of the whole spinal movement. In forward bending, both transverse processes become more equal. This occurs because as motion is recruited, the right facet opens from its relatively extended position to become equal with the left facet in its blocked (flexed) position. Knowing this, the clinician can now make a *positional diagnosis* of this dysfunctional vertebral segment in three-dimensional space: The segment is *Flexed, right Sidebent,* and *right Rotated* (FRS right). Therefore, the *motion restriction* of the segment (what it cannot do) is just the opposite of the positional diagnosis: *Extension, left Sidebending,* and *left Rotation.* The clinician will thus select a technique that will facilitate motion in the directions of the restriction (see "Treatment").

In Figure 18-29B the right facet will not open (flex). Thus, when the patient is asked to forward bend, the right transverse process becomes more prominent. This occurs because as motion is recruited from the top down through the spinal segment, the right facet (which is in a relatively extended position) is carried along by the overall spinal movement in this extended position. There is no restriction to the left facet, which is already in a relatively opened position. Thus, the right transverse process becomes more prominent. When the

Table 18-5. Control of Vertebral Motion by Facet Function

Trunk Motion	Facet Function
Forward bending (flexion)	Facets open
Backward bending (extension)	Facets close
Sidebending right	Right facet closes, left facet opens
Sidebending left	Left facet closes, right facet opens

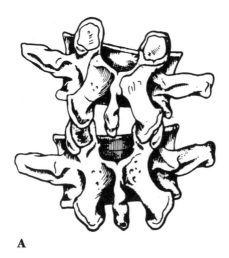 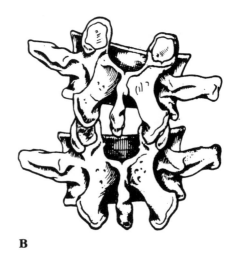

A　　　　　　　　　　　　　　　　**B**

Fig. 18-29. Lumbar facet restrictions. **(A)** The left facet will not *close* (extend); **(B)** the right facet will not *open* (flex). (Adapted from Kapandji,[1] and Greenman,[37] with permission.)

patient is asked to backward bend, both transverse processes become more equal, because the left

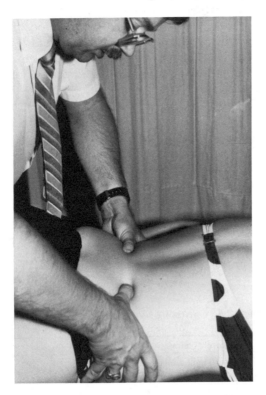

Fig. 18-30. Palpation of transverse processes through fascial planes.

facet is able to close, bringing its transverse process into line with the right one. Knowing this, the clinician can now state the *positional diagnosis* of the affected segment: *Extended, right Sidebent,* and *right Rotated* (ERS right). The motion restriction of the segment is *Flexion, left Sidebending,* and *left Rotation.* A treatment technique appropriate to the motion restriction is then selected (see "Treatment").

The reader should now be able to appreciate that, in the neutral position, the two lesions described would appear to be the same. However, through the use of positional diagnosis and assessment of motion restriction, they are found to be quite different. Thus, they must be treated by different techniques.

The value of using the transverse processes through a flexion-extension arc of spinal motion is that it clearly distinguishes normal vertebral motion from dysfunctional motion. Use of the transverse processes gives the clinician the ability to discern structural from functional asymmetry and has been shown to be a consistently accurate method among examiners and with the same examiner over time.[9,21,23]

Palpation of the transverse processes is done through the fascial planes of the paravertebral muscles (erector spinae) (Fig. 18-30). Indirect contact is made with the tips of the transverse processes with the clinician's thumbs. Even pressure is applied so as to appreciate the relative anteroposterior position of the left transverse process to the right one (see sections on "Evaluation" and "Treatment").

Adaptation

The lumbar spine must make certain adaptations to the position of the sacrum.[9,21,23,29] It has already been noted that L5 and S1 are coupled through the iliolumbar ligaments and that the sacrum nutates and counternutates in response to lumbar flexion and extension (lumbopelvic rhythm). It has also been noted that certain spinal movements are coupled together consistently and have been defined as Fryette's laws (type I = neutral and type II = nonneutral). *Neutral mechanics* refers to the situation where the vertebral weightbearing is on the vertebral bodies, and the introduction of sidebending results in the vertebral bodies twisting out from under the load (in the opposite direction of the sidebending). *Nonneutral mechanics* of the spine refers to the situation where there has been sufficient sagittal plane motion that the vertebral arches (facets), either through stretch or compression, influence motion so that the introduction of sidebending results in a vertebral body twisting into the intended concavity, thus permitting sidebending to occur. Neutral mechanics are usually grouped (three to five segments), and nonneutral mechanics are usually single segment.

It may be easier to think of the sacrum as behaving like a sixth lumbar vertebra when considering the functional integration of total spinal motion. Normally, if the sacrum should sidebend left, L5 would sidebend right. In neutral (type I) spinal mechanics, if the L5 segment is sidebent right, rotation to the left is coupled to it. Thus, if the sacrum is left-sidebent and the L5 vertebra is found to be left rotated, one can presume, according to type I mechanics, that the spine has made a normal adaptation to the dysfunctional sacral position (Fig. 18-31). When attempting to assess the presence of neutral adaptations in the lumbar spine, the clinician should start at the bottom and work up to the first segment with dysfunction. Then everything relates to the last segment that was found to be normal.

Normal neutral adaptive lumbar spinal behavior occurs over three to five segments and produces a minimal flexion or extension restriction to overall spinal movement. The principal restriction to motion is sidebending. The sacrum should *always* face the concavity of the lumbar spinal curve if the lumbar spine is normally adaptive. This is the usual situation in forward sacral torsion lesions.

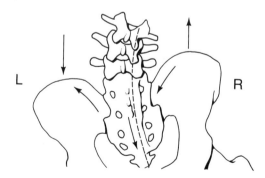

Fig. 18-31. Posterior view of the lumbar spine and pelvis showing a left-on-left forward sacral Torsion lesion. The lumbar vertebrae are normally adapting into right sidebending and left rotation following type I mechanics. (Adapted from Pratt,[29] with permission.)

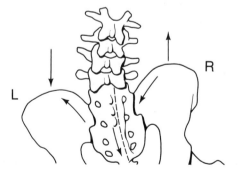

Fig. 18-32. Posterior view of the lumbar spine and pelvis showing a left-on-left forward sacral torsion lesion. The fourth and fifth lumbar vertebrae are nonadapting into right rotation and right sidebending following type II mechanics. (Adapted from Pratt,[29] with permission.)

Nonneutral or type II restrictions are coupled with sidebending and rotation to the same side. Here the facets influence the motion to a greater extent, and the flexion or extension component is part of the restriction. In the L4 and L5 segments, the iliolumbar ligaments greatly influence these mechanics if flexion or extension is great enough to produce tension in them. A nonneutral restriction will restrict the segment above and below it. Thus, if the sacrum is left sidebent and it is found that the L5 vertebra is right rotated and right sidebent, one can presume, according to type II mechanics, that the lumbar spine has not made a normal adaptation to the sacral dysfunction (Fig. 18-32). Nonadaptive lumbar responses to sacral positioning are highly significant in patients who do not get better or have chronic recurrences. These responses must be treated before the underlying sacral lesion. Nonadaptive lumbar responses are very common in backward sacral torsion lesions.

EVALUATION
Development of the Tactile Sense

The clinician specializing in musculoskeletal disorders must hone his or her palpatory skills to a fine degree. Through palpation, the clinician should be able to (1) detect a tissue texture abnormality; (2) detect asymmetry of position of comparable body parts visually and tactilely; (3) detect differences in the quality as well as the range of joint movement; (4) sense position in space, both the patient's and his or her own; and (5) detect changes in the palpatory findings from one examination to the next.

Development of palpatory skills involves three components within the neurophysiologic makeup of the clinician: reception of information through the fingertips and eyes, transmission of this information to the brain, and interpretation of the information.

The sensitivity or tactile discriminatory power of the fingertips is extremely fine. A good exercise for practicing palpatory skills is to take a 25-cent piece, close one's eyes, and then try to palpate George Washington's nose on the coin.[20] Another exercise is to pluck a single hair from one's head and, without

looking, place it on a hard surface under a piece of paper, and then locate the hair and trace its length with the fingertip.[28]

The clinician's palpatory examination should begin with light touching over the area under observation. This allows a sort of scanning examination of the area and will reveal the presence of any large abnormalities in the superficial or deep layers of tissue. The clinician can then identify the structures or planes as the compression increases. The clinician may use shear movements across the tissues to determine the various structures, planes, or extent or size of a lesion. The palpatory examination takes concentration, and errors in reception result from too much pressure and too much movement of the palpating fingertips.

Layer Palpation

Somatic dysfunction is the impaired or altered function of related components of the somatic (body framework) system: skeletal, arthrodial, and myofascial structures and related vascular, lymphatic, and neural elements.[21,23] The discussion in this section is based on work by Philip Greenman.[39]

The goal of palpatory diagnosis is to identify and define areas of somatic dysfunction. Once such an area is defined, the goal of manual therapy is to improve function in that area, that is, to improve the mobility of tissues (bone, joint, muscle, ligament, fascia, fluid) and to restore normal physiologic motion, if and as much as possible.

Table 18-6. Diagnostic Criteria for the Palpatory Examination ("PART")

P	Pain
A	Asymmetry of related parts of the musculoskeletal system either structurally or functionally (e.g., shoulder height by observation, height or iliac crest by palpation, contour and function of thoracic area
R	Range-of-motion abnormality of a joint, several joints, or a region of the musculoskeletal system by either hypomobility (restriction) or hypermobility. This is ascertained by observation and palpation utilizing both active and passive patient cooperation.
T	Tissue texture abnormality of the soft tissues of the musculoskeletal system (skin, muscle, or ligament). These are ascertained by observation and palpation.

The diagnostic criteria for the palpatory examination may be easily remembered through the simple mnemonic "PART" (Table 18-6).

Differentiation of Structural and Functional Asymmetry

Structural asymmetry is the rule, not the exception, particularly in the lower lumbar and sacral spine. If the relative position of comparable anatomic parts (right and left transverse processes, right and left inferior lateral angles of the sacrum, etc.) is observed to remain constant throughout the full flexion-extension range of motion, then the perceived positional asymmetry is due to *structural variation* of the anatomic part. If, however, the relative position of the comparable anatomic parts changes within the full flexion-extension range of motion, then the perceived asymmetry is due to *functional alteration* of the anatomic parts.

Key Landmarks for Pelvic Girdle Evaluation

The clinician must be able to accurately and consistently palpate the following anatomic landmarks and be able to relate their relative positions to the pelvic and cardinal planes of motion already discussed. Only then will the clinician be able to assess dysfunction and be able to test, retest, and evaluate the effects of treatment.

Iliac Crest

The iliac crests are compared with the patient in the standing and prone positions. Soft tissue must be moved out of the way by pushing it superiorly and medially above the crests. The crests are evaluated for their superoinferior relationship (Fig. 18-33).

Anterior Superior Iliac Spine

The clinician must be able to locate the anterior-medial aspect of the inferior slope of the ASIS with the patient standing and in the supine position and assess their relative positions (superoinferior and/or mediolateral; Fig. 18-34).

Pubic Tubercles

With the patient supine, the anterior aspects of the pubic tubercles are palpated for their relative anteroposterior position. Then the superior aspects of the tubercles are examined by pushing the soft tissue out of the way cephalically in order to assess their relative cephalocaudal position (Fig. 18-35).

Posterior Superior Iliac Spine

The PSIS is a most important landmark and must be assessed in the standing, seated, and prone positions by locating the inferior slope of the posterior aspect of the prominence. Its relative position must be assessed as superoinferior and/or mediolateral (Fig. 18-36).

Inferior Lateral Angle

Another very important landmark, the inferior lat-

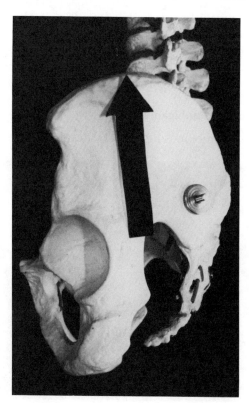

Fig. 18-33. Skeletal model, iliac crests.

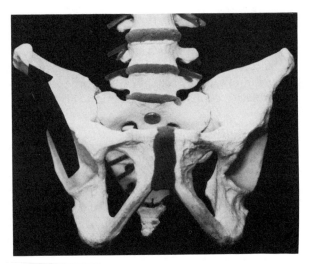

Fig. 18-34. Skeletal model, anterior superior iliac spine.

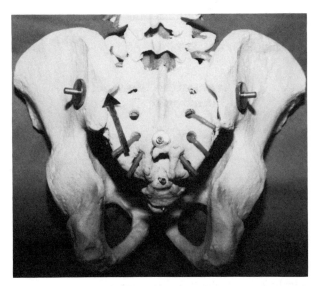

Fig. 18-36. Skeletal model, posterior inferior iliac spine.

eral angle (ILA), is found by palpating laterally approximately 1 to 1½ inches from the sacral cornua. Its posterior aspects must be assessed for their anteroposterior relationship, and its inferior aspects must be assessed for their superoinferior relationship (Fig. 18-37).

Sacrotuberous Ligament

The sacrotuberous ligament is located between the

ILA and the ischial tuberosity and needs to be compared for equality of tension and tenderness (Fig. 18-38).

Ischial Tuberosity

The ischial tuberosities are palpated at their inferior aspects in the prone position and are assessed for

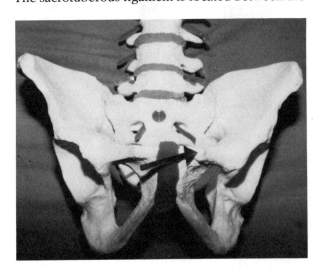

Fig. 18-35. Skeletal model, pubic tubercles.

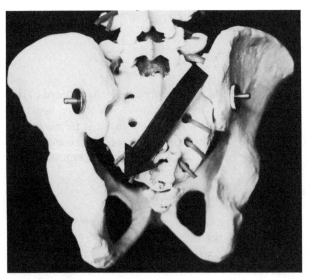

Fig. 18-37. Skeletal model, inferior lateral angle of the sacrum.

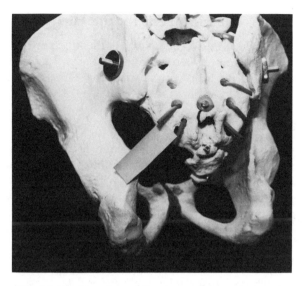

Fig. 18-38. Location of the sacrotuberous ligament.

their relative superoinferior position (Fig. 18-39).

Medial Malleolus

The inferior slopes of the medial malleoli must be located in both the supine and the prone position. They are then compared for their relative superoinferior positions (see Fig. 18-40).

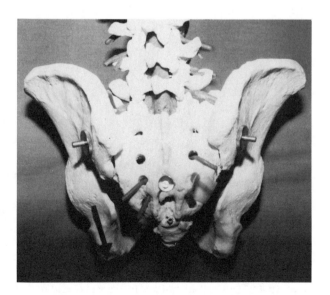

Fig. 18-39. Skeletal model, ischial tuberosity.

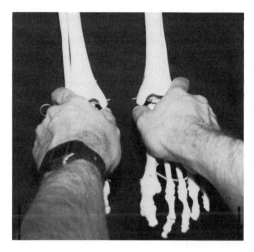

Fig. 18-40. Skeletal model, medial malleolus.

Lower Quarter Screening Examination

The patient positions used in the examination of pelvic girdle dysfunction are standing, seated, supine, and prone. To avoid unnecessary movement of the patient from one position to the other, which wastes time and may exacerbate the patient's condition, as many relevant tests should be done in one patient position as possible. The lower quarter screening examination is included here for completeness in that aspects of it might be needed in a pelvic dysfunction examination for the purpose of ruling out certain diagnoses. The advantage of this examination sequence is that the clinician can rapidly evaluate many areas and functions and be assured of not missing any major dysfunction (see appropriate chapters for related tests and their meanings).

The areas included in the examination are the thoracic spine (T6–T12), the lumbar spine, the sacroiliac joint, the pubic symphysis, the hip, the knee, the ankle, and the foot.

The examination begins with an inspection of the patient's posture, with attention to the following:

1. Feet
2. Knees
3. Pelvis
4. Thoracolumbar spine

Next the following functional tests are performed:

1. Standing position:
   a. Active range of motion in the lumbar spine, all planes
   b. Active clearing test for peripheral joints (full squat)
   c. Toe walking (S1, S2)
   d. Heel walking (L4, L5)
2. Sitting position:
   a. Active and passive rotation of the thoracolumbar spine
   b. Knee jerk (L3, L4)
3. Supine position:
   a. Straight leg raising; (the Kernig, Lesague, and bowstring tests may also be included)
   b. Long sitting test for the sacroiliac joint (the patient must have a normal straight leg raising test)
   c. Range of motion of the hip, all planes (check for sign of the buttock[12])
   d. Resisted hip flexion (L1, L2); test for range of motion and pain
   e. Resisted knee extension (L3, L4); test for range of motion and pain
   f. Resisted ankle dorsiflexion (L4); test for range of motion and pain
   g. Resisted eversion of the foot (L5, S1); test for range of motion and pain
   h. Knee clearing tests (full extension, varus and valgus stress)
4. Prone position:
   a. Femoral nerve stretch
   b. Ankle jerk (SI)
   c. Resisted knee flexion (SI); test for range of motion and pain
   d. Observation of gluteal mass
   e. Prone knee flexion to 90 degrees (SI)
   f. Spring testing (thoracolumbar spine and sacrum)
   g. Ankle clearing tests.

Remember that the screening examination only indicates the area in which the lesion lies. Do a detailed examination of the area if a problem is detected. Do not persist in the examination if it is apparent that the condition is being exacerbated.

Clearing Tests for the Hip

Should the clinician need to clear the hip in order to differentiate between hip and lumbar or sacroiliac problems, the following special procedures are recommended for this purpose.

Log Roll

The log roll is a joint play movement for internal and external rotation of the hip in extension. The clinician simply rolls the thigh under his or her hands to get an end-feel of the joint in internal and external rotation. By watching the excursion of the feet, the clinician can estimate range of motion (Fig. 18-41).

Thomas Test

The Thomas test detects tightness of the long and short flexor muscles of the hip. While lying with one leg freely hanging over the edge of an examination table, the patient flexes the opposite hip toward the chest to a point where the lumbar spine flattens against the table. The freely hanging leg is then observed for its position in space. The knee should be flexed to 70 to 90 degrees, and the hip should be in 0 degrees extension. If the knee is flexed sufficiently but the hip is found to be in flexion, this indicates tightness of the iliopsoas group. If the hip is in 0 degrees extension but the knee lacks suffi-

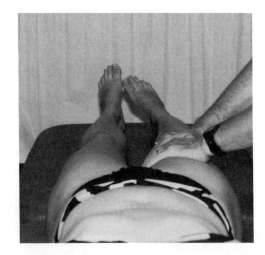

Fig. 18-41. Log roll technique for capsular end-feel of the hip joint.

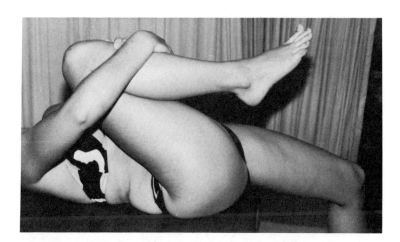

Fig. 18-42. Thomas test for assessing tightness of the long and short hip flexor muscles.

cient flexion, this indicates tightness of the rectus femoris (Fig. 18-42).

Scour Test

The scour test is done to "feel" the acetabular rim. The clinician literally scours the femoral head around the acetabular rim from the point of maximal flexion, adduction, and internal rotation to the point of maximal extension, abduction, and external rotation, with axial compression being applied to the hip through the knee. The clinician thus "palpates"

for joint crepitation and for "bumps" in the smoothness of the range of motion that may indicate degenerative joint disease (Fig. 18-43).

FABERE Test

See "Objective Examination of the Sacroiliac Joint."

Piriformis Tightness

See "Objective Examination of the Sacroiliac Joint."

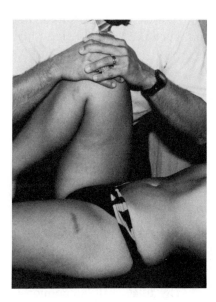

Fig. 18-43. Scour test for the hip joint.

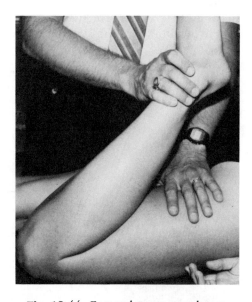

Fig. 18-44. Femoral nerve stretch test.

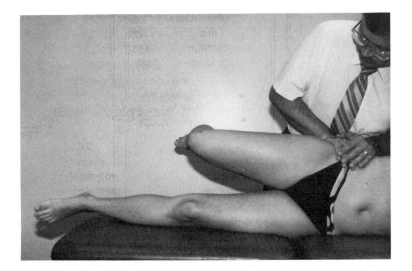

Fig. 18-45. Ober test for tightness of the lateral hip musculature.

Femoral Nerve Stretch

With the patient in the prone position, the clinician passively flexes the knee in an attempt to bring the patient's heel to the buttock (Fig. 18-44). If the femoral nerve is entrapped, this movement should produce neurologic pain in the femoral nerve distribution of the anterior thigh. This test may also be used to test rectus femoris tightness. Normal muscle length should allow an individual to touch his heel to his buttock. If tightness exists, the clinician will observe the pelvis rising on that side as the hip flexes in response to the passive knee flexion. (See "Entrapment Syndromes of the Hip and Pelvis.")

Ober Test

The Ober test is used to determine the presence of tight hip abductor muscles, especially the gluteus medius and the tensor fasciae latae. The patient lies on his side, facing away from the clinician. The clinician asks the patient to raise (abduct) his leg toward the ceiling with the knee flexed to 90 degrees. This relaxes the iliotibial tract and fascia lata. Using his or her own body weight to stabilize the pelvis above the level of the hip joint, the clinician instructs the patient to lower his leg. Normal muscle length should allow the patient's thigh to cross the midline and touch the downside leg (Fig. 18-45).

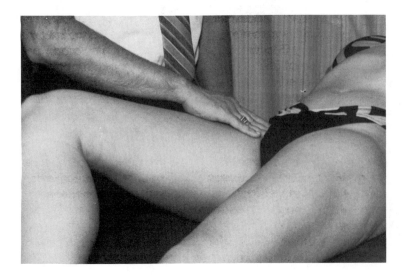

Fig. 18-46. FABERE position and area of palpation for the femoral triangle.

Femoral Triangle Palpation

Palpation of the structures of the femoral triangle is important in distinguishing soft tissue problems in and around the hip. The borders of the femoral triangle are the inguinal ligament superiorly, the sartorius laterally, and the adductor longus medially. The floor of the femoral triangle is formed by portions of the adductor longus, the pectineus, and the iliopsoas muscles. Within the borders of the triangle may be found the femoral artery, the psoas bursa, and the hip joint. The inguinal ligament runs between the ASIS and the pubic tubercles and should be palpated for tenderness and tightness. The FABERE position is best for the examination of the femoral triangle (Fig. 18-46).

Common Hip Syndromes

Sacroiliac and pubic dysfunctions can give rise to pain, which is felt in the groin area. The clinician evaluating a patient with complaints in this area must be able to differentiate between complaints of hip origin and those of pelvic origin. The following discussion gives some of the signs and symptoms of several common hip problems that must be considered in any evaluation of this region.[17,31,40]

Degenerative Joint Disease (Osteoarthrosis)

Degenerative joint disease is the most common disease process affecting the hip. The degenerative tissue changes that occur with symptomatic degenerative joint disease are usually reactions to increased stress to the joint over time. Some predisposing factors include congenital hip dysplasia, osteochondrosis, slipped capital femoral epiphysis, leg length disparity, a tight hip capsule, and shock loading.

The patient is usually middle-aged or older, with an insidious onset of groin or trochanteric pain, which becomes more noticeable after use of the joint (walking, running, etc.). Typically, the pain is felt first in the groin and later in the L2 and L3 distributions (anterior thigh and knee). Later it progresses to the lateral and posterior regions. The pain rarely extends below the knee. The usual complaints include morning stiffness and stiffness when arising from the sitting position, with pain by day's

end. This progresses to a constant ache at night and loss of functional abilities such as tying one's shoes and climbing stairs.

The clinician should assess range of motion of the hip, paying attention to loss of the motions of abduction and external rotation. The clinician should use the log roll test, the scour test, the Thomas test and the FABERE test as well as palpate the femoral triangle.

When early or even moderately advanced signs of degenerative joint disease of the hip are found, the clinician may elect to use capsular stretch techniques and long axis distraction techniques for pain control and improvement in function (see Chapter 24).

Iliopectineus Bursitis

The iliopectineal bursa lies anterior to the hip joint between the capsule and the iliopsoas tendon. Inflammation is fairly common and can be confused with degenerative joint disease of the hip and vice versa. The bursa can communicate with the hip.

The pain from an iliopectineal bursitis is insidious. It is felt in the groin with some radiation into the L2 and L3 distributions. The clinician should check for a restriction in the capsular pattern of motion to rule out joint effusion or capsular involvement.

Pulsed ultrasound directed into the bursa may be beneficial in the treatment of iliopectineal bursitis, coupled with the use of nonsteroidal anti-inflammatory agents.

Trochanteric Bursitis

The onset of trochanteric bursitis is usually insidious. Occasionally there is an acute history where the patient heard a "snap" in the posterolateral region of the hip (e.g., when getting into a car). The pain is in the lateral hip. There may be some radiation into the L5 distribution along the lateral thigh to the knee and lower leg. Occasionally it may radiate proximally to the lumbar region and mimic an L5 spinal lesion. A tight tensor fasciae latae tendon may also produce a "snap" over the trochanter and result in a friction syndrome in this area.

The pain of a trochanteric bursitis is a deep aching sclerotogenous pain rather than the sharp dermatomal L5 pain of nerve root involvement. Stair climbing and side-lying, both of which compress the bursa, will be painful. The patient may stand in a lateral pelvic shift away from the side of involvement, which also increases valgus stress at the knee.

The clinician tests the bursa by fully flexing the patient's hip passively and then moving it into adduction and internal rotation. This maneuver compresses the stretched bursa under the gluteus maximus. The clinician may also palpate the bursa, but it is located behind the trochanter rather than directly on top of it.

Ultrasound and the use of a hydrocortisone-based coupling agent (phonophoresis), iontophoresis, ice massage, and nonsteroidal anti-inflammatory agents may prove helpful in the treatment of trochanteric bursitis. If a tensor fasciae latae friction syndrome is suspected, stretching exercises may be indicated for it and the iliotibial tract.

Subjective Examination

Evaluation of the lumbopelvic unit begins with the subjective examination. A careful, detailed history is essential to proper diagnosis and management of these problems. The following outline by Maitland[41] gives a concise historical picture and tends to focus the clinician's attention toward particular trouble spots.

Location of Pain

Use of a body chart is helpful. Note the length (proximal to distal), width (medial to lateral), depth (superficial to deep), type (burning, aching, etc.), and intensity (sharp, dull, etc.) of the pain. Also note any areas of paresthesia or anesthesia.

Present History (Fig. 18-47A)

Behavior of Symptoms (Fig. 18-47B)

Previous History

The clinician should get a detailed account to the best of the patient's recollection of the first episode of similar lower back pain. Many times this is a vivid memory, and the patient will have no trouble in relating the episode. The clinician gathers information about subsequent episodes of the same problem as to frequency of occurrence, the ease of the cause, what the patient did to lessen the pain, recovery time, and any previous treatments, whether successful or not.

Effect of Rest

The clinician then obtains answers to the following questions:

1. How does rest affect the pain? (Pain of musculoskeletal origin usually gets better with rest.)
2. Does the pain ever awaken the patient during the night? (Night pain that awakens an individual from a sound sleep may suggest neoplastic activity.)
3. What is the pain like in the morning? (Does the patient awaken painfree and then experience worsening of symptoms as the day goes on, or does he awaken with the same pain, which remains at a constant level throughout the day?)
4. Is there any stiffness? (The clinician should suspect rheumatologic or degenerative processes.)

Particular Questions for the Pelvic Joints

1. Have you experienced a sudden sharp jolt to the leg, for example, after unexpectedly stepping off a curb? (This is a very common mechanism for innominate rotations and shears.)
2. Have you recently experienced a fall directly onto your buttocks? (This is a very common mechanism for innominate rotations, shears, and sacral flexion lesions.)
3. What is the effect on the pain of sitting, standing, walking, or maintaining a sustained posture? (If pain, especially radicular pain, increases with sitting, then a discogenic etiology is more suspect; if pain increases with standing, then the sacroiliac joint may be implicated, especially if the patient habitually stands unilaterally a great deal; if the pain increases with walking, then the sacroiliac joint is very much implicated, and sacral torsion is especially likely.)
4. Have you recently experienced a sudden trunk flexion with rotation? (This is a common mechanism for sacroiliac strain.)

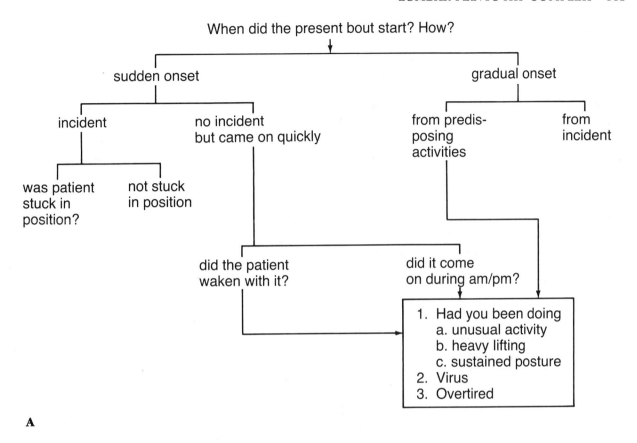

A

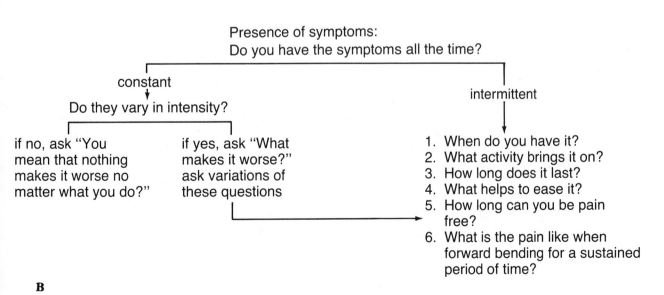

B

Fig. 18-47. (A) Flowchart of patient's present history; **(B)** flowchart for determining presence of symptoms.

Special Questions for Contraindications

1. How is your general health? (This is a very important question, especially if the clinician should find a history of carcinoma, chronic disease, or general malaise that speaks of nonmusculoskeletal origin.)
2. Have you had a recent unexplained weight loss? (Recent unexplained weight loss implicates neoplastic activity.)
3. Are you currently taking any medications? (It is helpful to know what a patient may be taking and for what reasons.)
4. Have you had any recent radiographs of your spine? (In cases of trauma, radiographs are always mandatory. In chronic cases of back pain, radiographs should probably be no more than 1 year old.)

Objective Examination

As with any musculoskeletal complaint, the examination begins as the patient walks into the office. The clinician should observe how the patient walks, moves, sits, and so on, especially if the patient does not know that he is being observed.

The following outline for planning the objective examination is based on the work of Maitland.[41]

The Cause of Pain

1. Name as the *possible* source of *any part* of the patient's pain every joint and muscle that must be examined:
   a. Joints that lie under the painful area
   b. Joints that refer pain into the area
   c. Muscles that lie under the painful area
2. Are you going to do a neurologic examination?
3. List the joints above and below that must be cleared.

Influence of Pain on the Examination

1. Is the pain severe?
2. Does the subjective examination suggest an easily irritable disorder?
3. Are the symptoms local or referred? Which is the dominant factor?

4. Give an example of:
   a. An activity that causes increased pain
   b. The severity of the pain so caused
   c. Duration before the pain subsides
5. Does the nature of the pain indicate caution?
   a. Pathology (osteoporosis, rheumatoid arthritis, etc.)
   b. Episodes easily caused
   c. Imminent nerve root compression.

Kind of Examination Indicated

1. Do you think you will need to be gentle or moderately vigorous with your examination of movements?
2. Do you expect a comparable sign to be easy or hard to find?
3. Do you think you will be treating pain, resistance, or weakness?

The Cause of the Cause of the Pain (Other Factors)

1. What associated factors must be examined as reasons for the present symptoms that might cause recurrence? (Posture, muscle imbalance, muscle power, obesity, stiffness, hypermobility, instability, deformity in a proximal or distal joint, etc.)
2. In planning the treatment (after the examination), what patient education measures would you use to prevent or lessen recurrences?

Objective Examination of the Sacroiliac Joint

Evaluation of the lumbopelvic-hip complex by the osteopathic system of positional diagnosis uses a commonsense approach in the correlation of comparable signs. This means that a given dysfunctional lesion will reflect a fairly consistent pattern of findings, which when viewed together yield a diagnosis of the affected segment in three-dimensional space and in relation to adjoining segments. The clinician simply collects the raw data using his or her palpatory and observational skills, formulates a diagnosis, and then applies a specific technique to the affected segment based on that diagnosis. It should be kept in mind that each test viewed by itself does not make a diagnosis. Only when all data are gathered and correlated can the clinician make the diagnosis. The following outline of clinical testing procedures and their meanings is categorized according to patient position and follows a sequence that will minimize patient position changes.

Standing Position

Posture

Make sure that the feet are hip width apart and that the knees are fully extended. Assessment needs to be made from the anterior, posterior, and lateral aspects (Fig. 18-48) for the general postural conditions of the patient (e.g., scoliosis, kyphosis, lordosis, protracted shoulders, forward head, slope of waist, distances of arms from sides).

Gait

Observe the patient's gait pattern. Frequently, sacroiliac lesions may produce a Trendelenburg gait or a gluteus maximus gait, or they may sidebend the trunk away from the affected side. The patient may walk with difficulty or may limp.

Alignment and Symmetry

Observations of alignment and symmetry begin with the general postural assessment, but now the following are checked.

Iliac Crest Height   Iliac crest height is best observed by using the radial borders of the index fingers and the web spaces of the hands to push the soft tissue up and medially out of the way, and then pushing down on each crest with equal pressure.

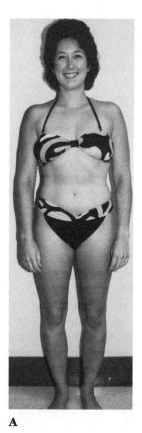 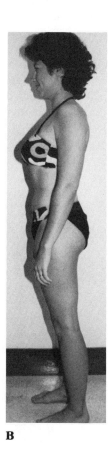 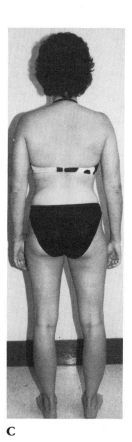

A   B   C

Fig. 18-48. Postural assessment. **(A)** Anterior aspect; **(B)** lateral aspect; **(C)** posterior aspect.

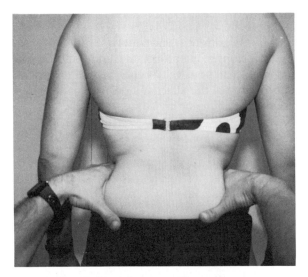

Fig. 18-49. Palpation of iliac crests.

The clinician's eyes must be level with his or her hands to assess whether one side is more caudad or cephalad in relation to the other (Fig. 18-49). This

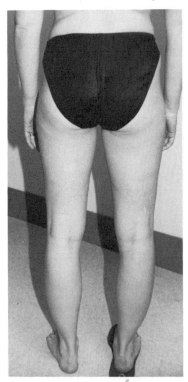

Fig. 18-50. Use of lift blocks to induce symmetry of muscle tone and balance the pelvis for landmark palpation and motion testing.

method has been found to be quite accurate and precise in the detection of leg length discrepancies.[42] If an asymmetry is found, a lift of appropriate dimension should be placed under the short side before any of the other motion tests in the standing position are executed (Fig. 18-50). This is done to achieve symmetry of muscle tone and balance the pelvis in space before testing motion. Placing a lift under the foot does not imply that a determination has been made as to whether the asymmetry is due to a structural or functional leg length discrepancy.

Posterior Superior Iliac Spine In the standing position, localization of the PSIS is very important (see "Key Landmarks for Pelvic Girde Evaluation"). An assessment needs to be made as to the relative superoinferior and mediolateral relationships in positions. This may be done with the ulnar borders of the thumbs or the tips of the index fingers, hooking them under the inferior aspect to the posterior spine. Again, the clinician must be at eye level with the PSISs in order to make an accurate assessment (Fig. 18-51). If the patient has an iliosacral dysfunction (anterior or posterior innominate), the iliac crests and the PSIS positions will be unlevel but in opposite directions.

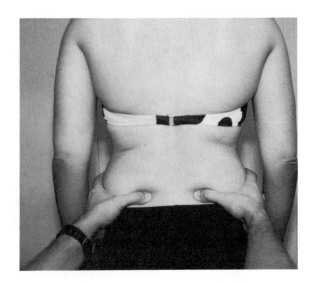

Fig. 18-51. Palpation of the PSIS.

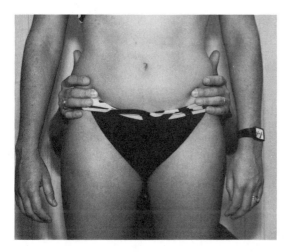

Fig. 18-52. Palpation of the ASIS from behind the patient in the standing position.

Anterior Superior Iliac Spine Position As with the PSIS, the relative position of the ASISs must be assessed as to their superoinferior and mediolateral relationships. This may be accomplished from behind the patient with the clinician's arms extended (Fig. 18-52) or from the front by visual inspection and thumb palpation (Fig. 18-53).

Trochanteric Levels Trochanteric levels are palpated by the same method as for the iliac crests, with

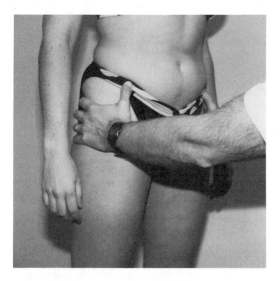

Fig. 18-53. Palpation of the ASIS from in front of the patient in the standing position.

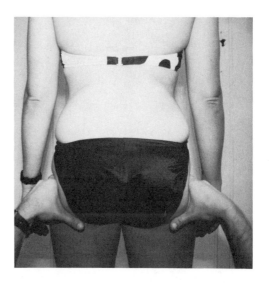

Fig. 18-54. Palpation of the greater trochanters.

the radial borders of the index fingers and the web spaces resting on the tops of the greater trochanters (Fig. 18-54). Levelness here and unlevelness at the iliacs would indicate pelvic dysfunction producing an apparent leg length discrepancy. Unlevelness here would indicate a structural leg length discrepancy below the level of the femoral neck.

Standing Flexion Test (Forward Bending of the Trunk)

The standing flexion test of iliosacral motion is accomplished by localization of the PSISs, noting their relative position. The patient is asked to bend forward as if to touch the toes. The head and neck should be flexed, and the arms should hang loose from the shoulders. As the patient bends forward, the examiner should note the cranial movement of the PSISs (Fig. 18-55). The side that moves first or the farthest cranially is the blocked side. The standing flexion test may be thought of as iliosacral motion recruited from the top down.

Gillet's Test (Sacral Fixation Test)

Gillet's test is also a test of iliosacral motion, but recruitment here is from the bottom up. The PSISs are again localized. The patient is asked to stand first on one leg and then on the other while pulling the

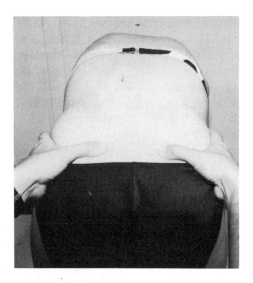

Fig. 18-55. Palpation of PSIS movement during the standing flexion test.

opposite knee up toward the chest (Fig. 18-56). The PSIS on the unblocked side will move farther inferiorly. The blocked side will move very little. An alternate method of assessment uses the S2 spinous process as a fixed reference point for the relative PSIS movement as the patient alternately pulls the knees toward the chest (Fig. 18-57). Hip flexion must reach at least 90 degrees.[7,43,44]

Active Lumbar Movements

Since lumbar lesions often occur along with iliosacral and sacroiliac dysfunctions, restrictions of lumbar movement must be assessed as well. Often when a sacroiliac dysfunction exists, sidebending of the lumbar spine toward the affected side will cause an exacerbation of pain (Fig. 18-58). Pain on backward bending may be indicative of a lumbar lesion as well (Fig. 18-59).

Sitting Position

The sitting position fixes the innominates to the chair or table and eliminates the influence of the hamstrings on the pelvis. This allows for sacroiliac movement within the innominates when testing motion. Additionally, active trunk rotation can best be tested since hip and pelvic motions are stabilized. The clinician should also note the posture of the patient in this position; the patient with sacroiliac dysfunction often tends to sit on the unaffected buttock. The sitting position also facilitates the neu-

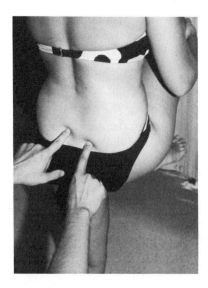

Fig. 18-56. Palpation of PSIS movement during the sacral fixation (Gillet's) test. Here the examiner compares the inferior movement of one PSIS to the other as the patient alternates stance and hip being flexed.

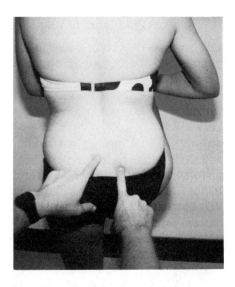

Fig. 18-57. Palpation of PSIS movement during the sacral fixation (Gillet's) test. Here the examiner compares PSIS movement to the relatively fixed reference point of the S2 spinous process.

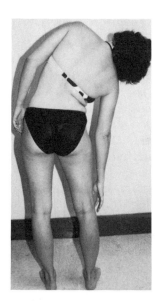

Fig. 18-58. Active sidebending of the lumbar spine in the standing (neutral) position. The patient is asked to lean to the side as if to touch the knee until the opposite foot begins to come up off the floor.

rologic examination, which consists of testing muscle strength, sensation, and muscle stretch reflexes (see chapters on the thoracolumbar spine).

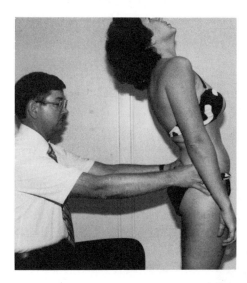

Fig. 18-59. Active backward bending of the lumbar spine in the standing position. The patient's pelvis is stabilized by the examiner, who observes segmental deviations in the midline.

Neurologic Examination

The examiner tests the following:

1. Muscle stretch reflexes (deep tendon reflexes)
2. Sensation
3. Resistive muscle tests.

Sitting Flexion Test (Forward Bending of the Trunk)

The clinician must again be at eye level after having localized the PSISs. The patient is asked to cross the arms across the chest and pass the elbows between the knees as if to touch the floor. The patient's feet should be in contact with the floor, or be resting on a stool if seated on the edge of an examination table (Fig. 18-60). The involved PSIS will move first or farther cranially (i.e., the blocked joint moves solidly as one, while the sacrum on the unblocked side is free to move through its small range of motion with the lumbar spine). If a blockage is detected in this test, and it is more positive (greater) than the restriction noted in the standing flexion test, then the test is indicative of a sacral dysfunction. If the two PSISs move symmetrically, then an innominate dysfunction is present (if a positive standing flexion or Gillet's test was noted). If the standing flexion test and the sitting flexion test are both equally positive, then a soft tissue lesion is suspected.

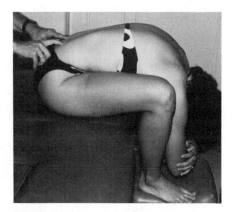

Fig. 18-60. Palpation of PSIS movement during the sitting flexion test.

Supine Position

Straight Leg Raising

The straight leg raising test is one of the most common clinical tests used in the evaluation of low back pain. It is perhaps one of the most commonly misinterpreted clinical tests as well.[45] The test applies stress to the sacroiliac joint in the higher ranges of the arc and can indicate the presence of a unilateral torsional dysfunction of the joint. It could also be indicative of a coexisting lumbar problem. The following guidelines are helpful in interpreting the results of the straight leg raising test:

0 to 30 degrees: hip pathology or severely inflamed nerve root
30 to 50 degrees: sciatic nerve involvement
50 to 70 degrees: probable hamstring involvement
70 to 90 degrees: sacroiliac joint is stressed.

The patient is supine on the examining table. The clinician lifts one of the patient's legs by supporting the heel while palpating the opposite ASIS (Fig. 18-61). The leg is raised until the clinician can appreciate motion of the pelvis occurring under the fingertips of the palpating hand. This determines the hamstring length in the leg being raised.[4] The other side is then similarly tested.

Leg Lengthening and Shortening Test

The leg lengthening and shortening test assesses the ability of the sacroiliac joints to move in response to external forces that passively rotate the innominates. The relative levelness of the medial malleoli is assessed following the symmetrization maneuver described in Figure 18-62 (Wilson-Barstow maneuver).[9] One leg is then passively flexed on the abdomen and then abducted and externally rotated and then extended (Fig. 18-63). The malleoli are then compared again for their relative levelness. The leg so moved should appear longer. The same leg is then flexed on the abdomen, adducted, internally rotated, and then extended (Fig. 18-64). The malleoli are again compared. This time, the leg should appear to have shortened. Failure of the leg to either lengthen or shorten may indicate pelvic dysfunction. The opposite leg is similarly tested.

Long Sitting Test

The long sitting test indicates an abnormal mechanical relationship of the innominates moving on the sacrum (iliosacral motion) and helps determine the presence of either an anterior innominate or a posterior innominate by a change in the relative length of the legs during the test. The malleoli are assessed

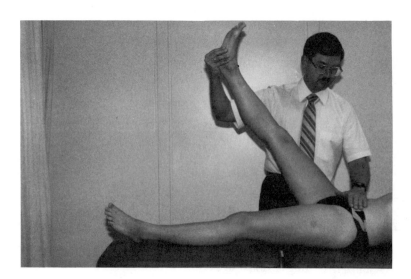

Fig. 18-61. Performance of the straight leg raising test.

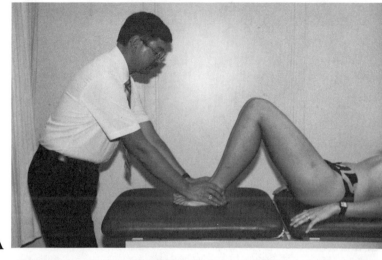

A

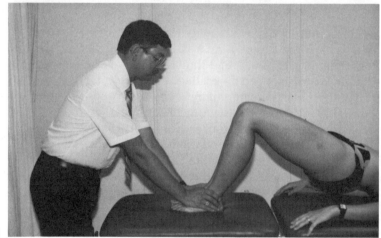

B

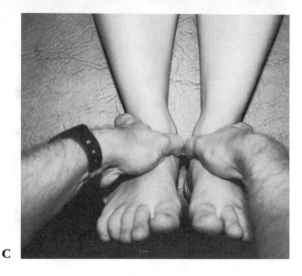

C

Fig. 18-62. Wilson-Barstow maneuver for leg length symmetry.[9] **(A)** The examiner stands at the patient's feet and palpates the medial malleoli using the ulnar borders of the thumbs at the most distal prominence of the tibia. The patient is asked to bend the knees. **(B)** The patient is then asked to lift the pelvis from the examining table. **(C)** The patient returns the pelvis to the table, and the examiner *passively* extends the patient's legs toward himself and compares the positions of the malleoli to one another using the borders of the thumbs.

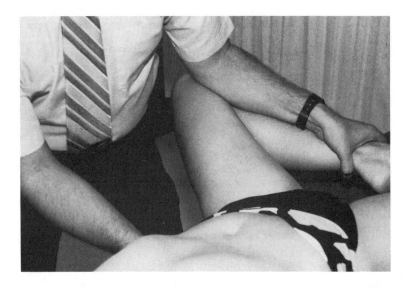

Fig. 18-63. Lengthening maneuver for sacroiliac mobility.

as to levelness as depicted in Figure 18-62. The patient is then asked to perform a sit-up, keeping the legs straight (Fig. 18-65). The clinician observes the change, if any, between the malleoli. The presence of a posterior innominate will make the leg in question (side of the positive standing flexion test) appear to be getting longer from a position of relative shortness (short to long or equal to long). This phenomenon occurs because, in the posterior innominate, the posterior rotation of the innominate moves the acetabulum in a superior direction and carries the leg along with it. Thus, the leg appears short-

ened. Just the opposite occurs in the anterior innominate. When the long sitting test is performed, the leg in question will appear to move from long to short or from equal to short.[46] These mechanisms are shown in Figure 18-66.

Pelvic Rocking

The pelvic rocking test involves simply getting an end-feel for the relative ease or resistance to passive overpressure for each innominate. The clinician places his or her hands on the ASISs and gently

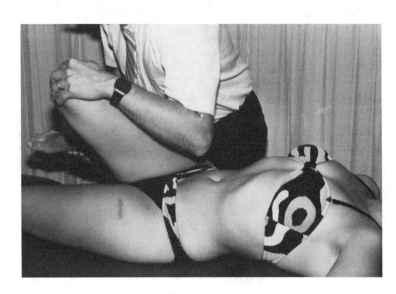

Fig. 18-64. Shortening maneuver for sacroiliac mobility.

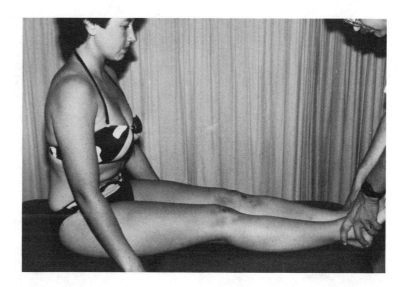

Fig. 18-65. Comparison of medial malleoli in the long sitting test.

springs the innominates alternately several times to assess the end-feel to this motion (Fig. 18-67). A harder end-feel indicates a probable restriction of movement on that side.

Compression-Distraction Tests

Compression-distraction tests are used to ascertain the presence of joint irritability, hypermobility, or serious disease such as ankylosing spondylitis, Paget's disease, or infection. The clinician may leave his or her hands on the ASISs as in the pelvic rocking test or may cross them to opposite ASISs (Fig. 18-68). The clinician then applies pressure down upon them to take up any slack and gives a sudden, sharp spring to the ASISs. This action compresses the sacroiliac joints posteriorly and gaps the joints anteriorly. The clinician then moves his or her hands to the lateral iliac wings and repeats the same maneuver (Fig. 18-69). In doing so, the clinician compresses the anterior and distracts the posterior sacroiliac joints. Pain as a result of either of these maneuvers is considered to be a positive sign.

FABERE (Patrick's) Test

The FABERE test is useful in differentiating between hip and sacroiliac pain. The hip is *F*lexed, *AB*ducted, and *E*xternally *R*otated, with the lateral malleolus being allowed to rest upon the opposite

thigh above the knee. The opposite ASIS is stabilized, and pressure is applied to the other externally rotated leg at the knee (Fig. 18-70). Pain caused in the groin or anterior thigh is more indicative of hip pathology. Pain in the sacroiliac joint is indicative of sacroiliac involvement.

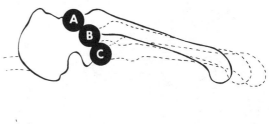

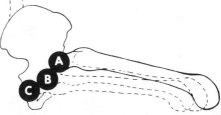

Fig. 18-66. Mechanism of the long sitting test in the posterior and anterior innominate dysfunctions. **(A)** In the supine position, posterior rotation of the ilium on the sacrum would appear to shorten the leg *(A)*, and anterior rotation to lengthen it *(C)*. **(B)** In the sitting position, the reverse occurs: Posterior rotation appears to lengthen the leg *(A)*, and anterior rotation appears to shorten it *(C)*. (From Saunders,[27] with permission.)

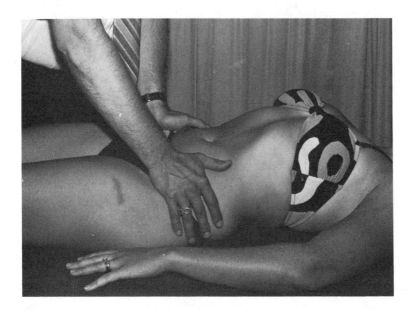

Fig. 18-67. Pelvic rocking technique.

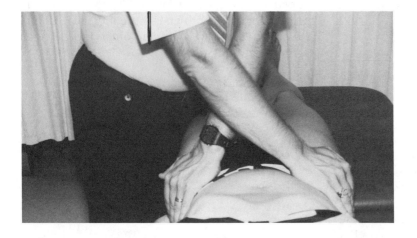

Fig. 18-68. Compression-distraction test using the crossed hands method.

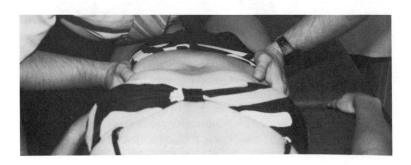

Fig. 18-69. Compression-distraction test from the lateral aspect.

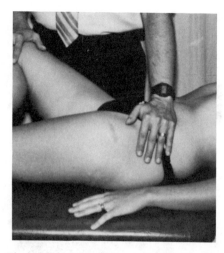

Fig. 18-70. Patrick's test (FABERE test).

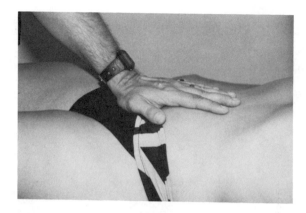

Fig. 18-72. Locating of the pubic tubercles by sliding the heel of the hand down the abdomen to make contact with the pubic bone.

Piriformis Tightness

Tightness of the piriformis muscles is easily checked by flexing the hip and knee to 90 degrees and then passively rotating the hip into internal rotation through the lower leg (Fig. 18-71). Relative end-feel and range of motion can be assessed.

Pubic Tubercles

The pubic tubercles are assessed for their relative superior-inferior and anteroposterior relationships. If unlevelness is detected, the positive side is correlated to the side of the positive standing flexion and/or Gillet's test. To avoid embarrassment and unnecessary probing in this region, it is recommended that the clinician slide the heel of his hand down the abdomen until contact is made with the pubic bone (Fig. 18-72). The tubercles may then be easily located with the fingertips (Fig. 18-73). In

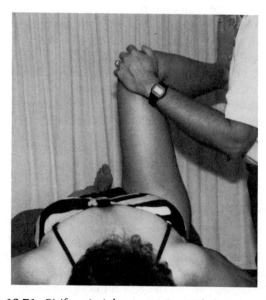

Fig. 18-71. Piriformis tightness testing with the patient in the supine position.

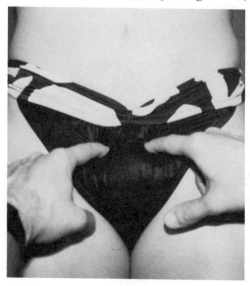

Fig. 18-73. Palpation of the pubic tubercles with the fingertips.

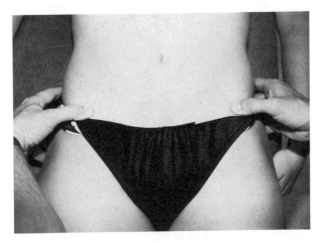

Fig. 18-74. Palpation of the ASISs to determine superinferior and mediolateral relationships.

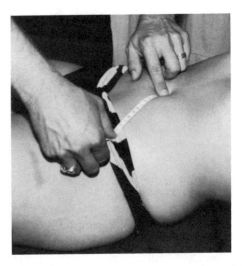

Fig. 18-76. Use of a tape measure between the umbilicus and the ASIS to determine the possibility of iliac inflare or outflare dysfunction.

most men and some women, because of the strength of the abdominal muscles, it is sometimes helpful to ask the patient to flex the knees a little to relax the muscles. Palpation is further facilitated by asking the patient to take a breath; upon exhalation the clinician slides his or her fingers over the top and presses down upon the tubercles (see "Key Landmarks for Pelvic Girdle Evaluation").

Anterior Superior Iliac Spine

Positioning of the ASISs must be assessed for any change from the standing position. The superoinferior and mediolateral relationships are assessed by the clinician placing his or her thumbs under the lip of the ASIS and sighting in their plane from a position perpendicular to the midline (Fig. 18-74). To determine the anteroposterior relationship of the ASISs, the clinician places the fingertips on the tips of the ASISs and sights along the plane of the abdomen (Fig. 18-75). The umbilicus also becomes a reference point for the mediolateral positioning. A tape measure may be used from the umbilicus to the inside border of the ASIS to determine the presence of an iliac inflare or outflare (Fig. 18-76).

Prone Position

Palpation

Depth of the Sacral Sulci (Medial PSIS) The depths of the sacral sulci are best determined if the clinician uses the tips of the long fingers while curling his or her fingers around the posterior aspects of the iliac crests (Fig. 18-77). The clinician assesses not only the relative depth of each sulcus but the quality of the ligaments under the fingertips as well, for tightness and swelling. If one side is found to be

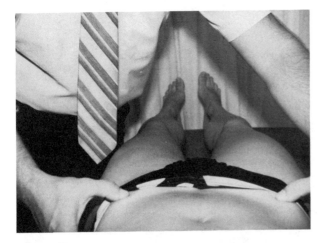

Fig. 18-75. Palpation of the ASISs to determine their anteroposterior relationship.

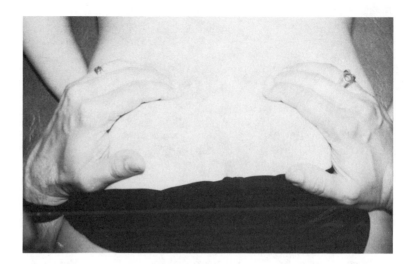

Fig. 18-77. Palpation of depth of the sacral sulci.

deeper than the other, this could indicate the presence of a possible sacral torsion or an innominate rotation.

Inferior Lateral Angles The ILAs are compared as to their relative caudad/cephalad and anteroposterior positions (Fig. 18-78). If one side is found to be more caudad and/or posterior, then a sacral lesion exists. If the ILAs are level and a deep sacral sulcus has been appreciated, then the lesion is in one of the innominates.(See "Key Landmarks for Pelvic Girdle Examination.")

Symmetry of the Sacrotuberous and Sacrospinous Ligaments These ligaments must be palpated through the gluteal mass (Fig. 18-79). The clinician must assess changes in tension and springiness from one side to the other. If such changes are noted, they are due to positional changes of the ilium.

Tenderness of the Sacral Sulcus If a sacroiliac problem exists, tenderness in the sulcus is well localized. This can be elicited during the test for sacral sulcus depth.

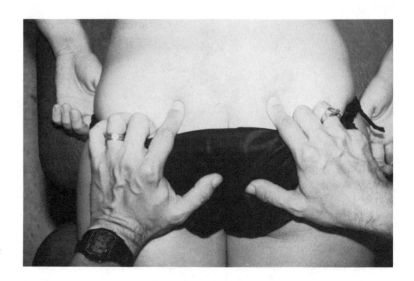

Fig. 18-78. Palpation of the ILAs of the sacrum.

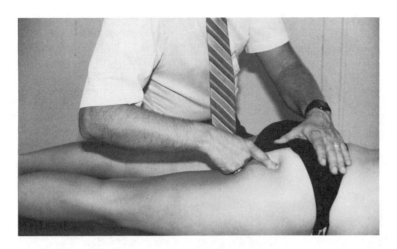

Fig. 18-79. Palpation of symmetry in the sacrotuberous and sacrospinous ligaments. This is very difficult because of their depth within the gluteal mass.

Piriformis Tightness The piriformis was tested in the supine position while on stretch. It is now tested while not on stretch by having the patient flex the knees to 90 degrees and internally rotate the hips by allowing the legs to move laterally (Fig. 18-80).

Ischial Tuberosities The clinician checks for the relative anteroposterior and cephalad/caudad relationships of the ischial tuberosities by using the thumbs to push soft tissue out of the way (Fig. 18-81). A change in the anteroposterior relationship may indicate an innominate rotation, whereas a change in the cephalad/caudad relationship may indicate an ilium upslip or downslip (see "Key Landmarks for Pelvic Girdle Evaluation").

Rotation of L4 and L5 Testing for rotation of L4 and L5 is done according to the method described in the section on the lumbar spine in this chapter (see Nomenclature for Vertebral Segment Dysfunction, ERS, and FRS Lesions). Rotation of these segments may indicate a compensated or noncompensated lumbar curve in response to a sacroiliac dysfunction.

Sphinx Test (Press-up or Backward Bending)

The patient is asked to come up from the prone position onto his elbows and rest his chin in his hands (Fig. 18-82). The clinician then palpates the following structures.

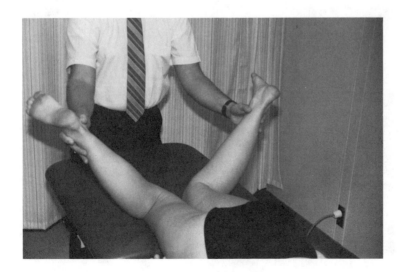

Fig. 18-80. Bilateral test of piriformis tightness with the patient in the prone position.

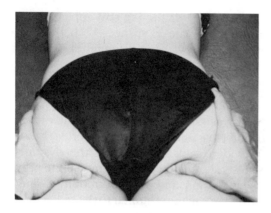

Fig. 18-81. Palpation of the ischial tuberosities.

Sacral Sulci The clinician now determines if there has been a change in the relative depth of the sacral sulci from that noted in the neutral prone position. If a sacroiliac dysfunction exists, the side that is blocked will remain shallow, and the side that is free to move will go deeper (remember that in backward bending of the lumbar spine there is relative nutation of the sacrum; see Fig. 18-77).

Inferior Lateral Angles The clinician now determines if there has been a change in the position of

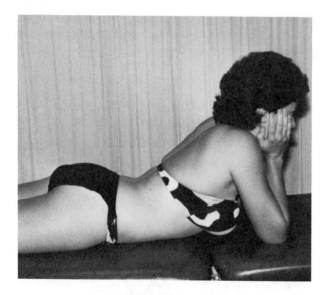

Fig. 18-82. Sphinx position.

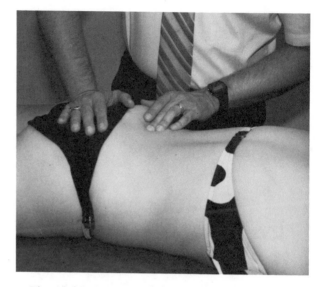

Fig. 18-83. Passive mobility testing of the sacrum.

the ILAs. If the ILA opposite to the deep sacral sulcus became more posterior by movement into the sphinx position, this indicates the presence of a forward sacral torsion. If the angle became more inferior on the same side as the deep sacral sulcus, it indicates the presence of a unilateral sacral flexion (Fig. 18-78).

Mobility Test

To test the passive mobility of the sacrum within the innominates, the clinician palpates the sacral sulci while applying negative posteroanterior pressure on the sacrum (Fig. 18-83). Hypermobility or hypomobility is assessed by the relative amount of movement that occurs between the PSIS and the dorsal aspect of the sacrum.

Spring Test

The standard spring test is applied to the lumbar spine to rule out the possibility of a lumbar lesion (Fig. 18-84).

Prone Knee Flexion to 90 Degrees

The clinician stands at the foot of the examination table and holds the patient's feet in a symmetrical position with thumbs placed transversely across the

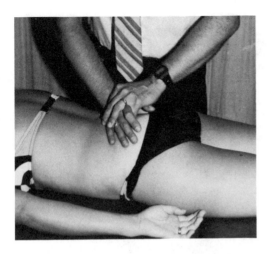

Fig. 18-84. Lumbar spring test.

soles of the feet just forward of the heel pad. Sighting through the plane of the heel with eyes perpendicular to the malleoli (Fig. 18-85), the clinician assesses the relative length of the legs in the prone position (the short side may not be the same as in the supine or standing position). If one leg appears shorter, it is the positive side. The knees are then simultaneously flexed to 90 degrees (Fig. 18-86). Care must be taken to maintain the feet in the neutral position and to bring the feet up in the midline. Deviation to either side will cause a false impres-

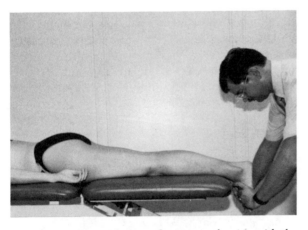

Fig. 18-85. The prone knee flexion test begins with the examiner bringing the patient's feet into a neutral position and checking for a leg length difference at the level of the malleoli.

sion (Fig. 18-87). If the leg still appears short, an anterior innominate is suspected. If the leg that seemed short now appears longer, a posterior innominate should be suspected.

Sacral Provocation Tests

Sacral provocation tests should be done only when applicable, that is, when the above series of tests has not provided a clear picture of the dysfunction. These tests should not be performed if the previous tests have demonstrated a hypermobility. They are performed in a manner similar to the sacral mobility test (Fig. 18-83). In chronic sacroiliac pain, provocation should increase symptoms as a result of adaptive shortening of the soft tissues having taken place.

1. Anteroposterior pressure on the sacrum at its base (this encourages sacral flexion)
2. Anteroposterior pressure on the sacrum at its apex (this encourages sacral extension)
3. Anteroposterior pressure on each side of the sacrum just medial to the PSISs (this encourages motion about the vertical axis)
4. Cephalad pressure on the sacrum applied near the apex (note pain or movement abnormalities)
5. Cephalad pressure on the sacrum applied near the base (note pain or movement abnormalities)
6. If a sulcus is found to be deep, pressure is applied on the opposite ILA to see if the sulcus comes up (this encourages torsional movement about an oblique axis).

Physical Findings and Diagnosis of Pelvic Girdle Dysfunctions

The following positive physical findings characterize the seven most common pelvic girdle dysfunctions.

Posterior Innominate

Posterior innominate is a unilateral iliosacral dysfunction. It is by far the most common pelvic dysfunction, whether iliosacral or sacroiliac. The following findings are those for a left posterior innominate:

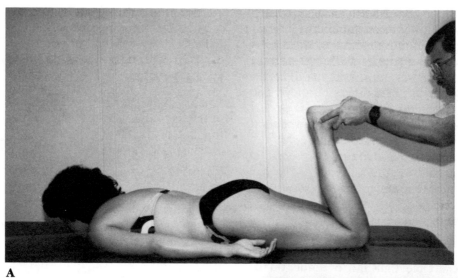

A

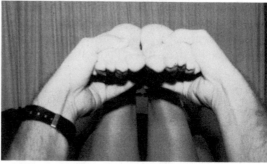

B

Fig. 18-86. The prone knee flexion test is completed as the examiner passively flexes the patient's knees to 90 degrees and sights through the plane of the heel pads to see whether a change in position has occurred.

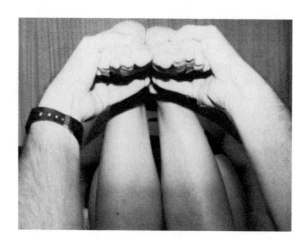

Fig. 18-87. False positive prone knee flexion test due to the examiner allowing the legs to move away from the midline, thus shortening one leg in relation to the other.

1. Iliac crests: high on the left
2. PSIS: low and posterior on the left
3. ASIS: high and anterior on the left
4. Standing flexion test: the left PSIS moves first or farthest superiorly
5. Gillet's test: the left PSIS moves inferiorly and laterally less than the right
6. Long sitting test: the left malleolus moves short to long
7. Sitting flexion test: negative (unless a sacral lesion coexists)
8. Pubic symphysis: negative (may be superior if also involved)
9. Hip: may lie in some external rotation
10. Sulci: deep on the left
11. ILA: usually no change in position
12. Tensor fasciae latae: tight and/or tender on the right
13. Other findings: sacroiliac ligament may be tense; decreased lumbar lordosis; pain usually well defined in the sulcus and/or unilateral buttock pain

Anterior Innominate

Anterior innominate is also a unilateral iliosacral dysfunction and is essentially the reverse of the posterior innominate. The following findings are those for a right anterior innominate:

1. Iliac crests: low on the right
2. PSIS: high and anterior on the right
3. ASIS: low and posterior on the right
4. Standing flexion test: the right PSIS moves first and/or farther superiorly
5. Gillet's test: the right PSIS moves less inferiorly and laterally compared to the left
6. Sitting flexion test: usually negative (unless a sacral lesion coexists)
7. Long sitting test: the right medial malleolus moves long to short
8. Pubic symphysis: usually no change
9. Hip: the right leg may lie in some internal rotation
10. Sulci: shallow on the right
11. ILA: usually no change in position
12. Tensor fasciae latae: may be tender on the left
13. Other findings: possibly increased lumbar lor-

dosis; possible complaint of cervical and/or lumbar symptoms

Sacral Torsion (Left-on-Left Forward Torsion)

The left-on-left forward torsion is the most common of the sacroiliac lesions. The primary axis of dysfunction is the left oblique axis. The findings listed will be just the opposite for the less common right-on-right torsion:

1. Iliac crests: usually no change
2. PSIS: may be posteriorly situated in relation to the sacral dorsal plane on the right
3. ASIS: negative
4. Standing flexion test: may be negative
5. Gillet's test: may be negative
6. Sitting flexion test: the blocked side moves first
7. Prone knee flexion test: the left malleolus is short
8. Pubic symphysis: no change
9. Hip: the left hip lies in external rotation in the supine position
10. Sulci: deep on the right, shallow on the left
11. ILA: posterior and inferior in the pelvic dorsal plane on the left
12. Piriformis and tensor fasciae latae: both are tender on the right
13. Other: usually a history of a pelvic twist injury.

Sacral Torsion (Right-on-Left Backward Torsion)

Backward sacral torsion also occurs most often on the left oblique axis. The findings listed will be opposite for the much less common left-on-right backward torsion:

1. Iliac crests: usually no change
2. PSIS: posterior on the right in relation to the orientation planes but anterior to the sacral base
3. ASIS: may be carried posterior and superior on the right or anterior and inferior on the left in the supine position
4. Standing flexion test: may be negative
5. Sitting flexion test: the blocked side moves first
6. Prone knee flexion: the medial malleolus is short on the left

7. Pubic symphysis: no change
8. Hip: the right leg may lie in slight external rotation
9. Sulci: shallow on the right, deep on the left
10. ILA: superior and anterior on the left in the pelvic dorsal plane
11. Piriformis: tender and tight on the right
12. Other: 90 percent of all sacroiliac torsions occur on the left oblique axis.

Unilateral Sacral Flexion

Unilateral sacral flexion occurs primarily around the middle transverse axis of the sacroiliac joint. It might be thought of as failure of one side of the sacrum to counternutate from a fully nutated position. When this occurs, a sidebending component takes place, driving the sacrum down the long arm of the joint. Findings for a right unilateral sacral flexion are the following:

1. Iliac crests: usually no change
2. PSIS: posterior in relation to the sacral base on the right but may not be in relation to the orientation planes
3. ASIS: carried posterior and superior on the right
4. Standing flexion test: the blocked side probably moves first
5. Sitting flexion test: the blocked side probably moves first
6. Prone knee flexion test: long on the right
7. Pubic symphysis: no change
8. Hip: no change
9. Sulci: deep on the right
10. ILA: inferior and posterior on the right (the positional relationship of the left side is unchanged)
11. Tensor fasciae latae: the left tensor is tight and tender

Superior Pubis

Dysfunctions of the pubic symphysis are probably the most commonly overlooked lesions of the pelvis. The lesions that usually occur at this joint are shear lesions, either in a superior or an inferior direction. Anterior and posterior shears are rare and, if present, are usually the result of trauma. Findings for a left superior pubis are the following:

1. Iliac crests: may be high on the left
2. PSIS: posterior in relation to the pelvic dorsal plane and anterior to the sacral base in the prone position
3. ASIS: superior on the left; may be slightly posterior
4. Standing flexion test: the blocked side will move first; the side that is blocked (in this case the left) will indicate the type of pubic lesion (superior or inferior)
5. Sitting flexion test: probably negative
6. Long sitting test: may be equal or shorter on the left before becoming longer
7. Pubic symphysis: the left pubic tubercle will be superior and tender
8. Hip: no change
9. Sulci: shallow on the left
10. ILA: no change
11. Other: almost all of these lesions occur simultaneously with the posterior innominate.

Superior or Inferior Innominate Shear (Upslip/Downslip)

Usually considered uncommon, vertical shear lesions of an entire innominate have been shown to occur more frequently than originally thought.[30] Signs of a left superior shear are the following (signs for an inferior shear are just the opposite):

1. Iliac crest: high on the left
2. PSIS: high on the left
3. ASIS: high on the left
4. Standing flexion test: positive on the left
5. Gillet's test: positive on the left
6. Long sitting test: positive on the left, short to long
7. Pubic symphysis: high on the left
8. Hip: no change
9. Sulci: the left sulcus may be shallow
10. ILA: no change
11. Piriformis: no change
12. Other: high left ischial tuberosity

The following pelvic dysfunctions are quite rare. Their combined occurrence may represent fewer than 5 to 10 percent of all pelvic dysfunctions. For the sake of completeness, their findings are included.

Iliac Inflare

Use of a tape measure may be helpful in assessing inflare. Measure the relative distances between the ASISs and the umbilicus. An unequal measurement coupled with the findings below may indicate an iliac inflare (on the right):

1. Iliac crests: no change
2. PSIS: the right moves away from the sagittal plane
3. ASIS: the right moves medially toward the sagittal plane
4. Standing flexion test: the blocked right side may move first if coupled with an anterior innominate
5. Gillet's test: may be positive if an anterior innominate exists
6. Long sitting test: no changes
7. Pubic symphysis: no change
8. Hip: may lie in some internal rotation on the right
9. Sulci: right sulcus widens
10. ILA: no change
11. Piriformis and tensor fasciae latae: no changes
12. Other: iliac inflare is a rare finding by itself; it can be the result of muscle imbalance; it occurs only with a convex sacral articulation; it is best examined supine.

Iliac Outflare

Iliac outflare is essentially the opposite of an iliac inflare. If a tape measure is used, a longer measurement (ASIS to umbilicus) coupled with the following findings may indicate the presence of an iliac outflare (on the right):

1. Iliac crests: no change
2. PSIS: the right moves toward the sagittal plane
3. ASIS: the right moves laterally away from the sagittal plane
4. Standing flexion test: the blocked right side may move first when coupled with a posterior innominate
5. Gillet's test: may be positive if a posterior innominate also exists
6. Long sitting test: no change unless there is anterior or posterior innominate involvement

7. Pubic symphysis: no change
8. Hip: the right leg may lie in some external rotation
9. Sulci: the right sulcus is narrowed
10. ILA: no change
11. Piriformis and tensor fasciae latae: no change
12. Other: iliac outflare is a rare finding by itself; it can be the result of muscle imbalance; it occurs only with a convex sacral articulation and is best examined supine.

Unilateral Sacral Extension

Unilateral sacral extension is essentially the opposite of unilateral sacral flexion. It might be thought of as the failure of one side of the sacrum to nutate (flex) from the fully counternutated position. (extended) The following findings are those for a right unilateral sacral extension lesion:

1. Iliac crests: usually no change
2. PSIS: anterior in relation to the sacral base on the right
3. ASIS: carried anterior and inferior on the right
4. Standing flexion test: the blocked side may move first
5. Sitting flexion test: the blocked side may move first
6. Prone knee flexion test: short on the right
7. Pubic symphysis: no change
8. Hip: no change
9. Sulci: shallow on the right
10. ILA: superior and anterior on right
11. Piriformis and tensor fasciae latae: no change
12. Other: this lesion is very rare.

Bilateral Sacral Flexion

Bilateral sacral flexion may be thought of as failure of the sacrum to return from a fully nutated position. The findings are as follows:

1. Iliac crests: no change
2. PSIS: equal bilaterally but approximated
3. ASIS: no change
4. Standing and sitting flexion tests: probably no difference
5. Long sitting and prone knee flexion tests: no change

6. Pubic symphysis: no change
7. Hip: no change
8. Sulci: deep bilaterally
9. ILA: posterior and inferior bilaterally
10. Tensor Fasciae Latae: possible tenderness and tightness bilaterally
11. Other: the sacrotuberous and sacrospinous ligaments are under tension and are painful bilaterally.

Bilateral Sacral Extension

Bilateral sacral extension is the opposite of bilateral sacral flexion and may be thought of as the failure of the sacrum to return from the fully counternutated position. The findings are as follows:

1. Iliac crests: no change
2. PSIS: equal in relation to each other bilaterally; both are anterior in relation to the sacral base
3. ASIS: no change
4. Standing and sitting flexion tests: probably no difference
5. Pubic symphysis: no change
6. Hip: no change
7. Sulci: shallow bilaterally
8. ILA: anterior and superior bilaterally
9. Tensor fasciae latae: possible tenderness and tightness bilaterally
10. Other: the individual is usually slouched and has a reversed or kyphotic lumbar curve and often cannot straighten up

TREATMENT

Because of the conjoining of the various lumbar, pelvic, and hip components into an interrelated unit, the clinician should treat dysfunctions in a certain order when multiple lesions exist:

1. Pubic
2. Nonadapting lumbar compensations
3. Sacral lesions
4. Innominate lesions.

This treatment order takes advantage of the axes of motion, so that unlocking a restriction in one area facilitates the unlocking of a restriction in another. For example, a very common combination of lumbopelvic dysfunctions consists of left superior pubic shear, left-on-left forward sacral torsion, and left posterior innominate. The lumbar spine is usually adaptive in response to these dysfunctions and does not need correction.

Muscle Energy Techniques

A muscle energy technique (MET) is any manipulative treatment procedure that uses a voluntary contraction of the patient's muscles against a distinctly controlled counterforce from a precise position and in a specific direction. MET is considered to be an active technique, as opposed to a passive technique in which the clinician does the work, and it requires direct positioning (where the motion restriction barrier is engaged but not stressed). MET may be used to lengthen shortened muscles, strengthen weakened muscles, reduce localized edema, and mobilize restricted joints.[9,21-23] The focus of this section will be on the utilization of MET in mobilization of joint restrictions.

Types of Muscle Contraction

MET may employ various forms of muscle contraction for the purposes outlined above. The contractions are usually isotonic and isometric, but may also be isokinetic and isolytic.[21]

An *isotonic* muscular contraction is one in which the proximal and distal attachments approximate (i.e., a shortening or concentric contraction). An isotonic contraction may also occur when the proximal and distal attachments separate (i.e., a lengthening or eccentric contraction). An example is raising and lowering a weight.

An *isometric* muscular contraction is one exerted against an unyielding resistance in which the proximal and distal attachments neither separate nor approximate (i.e., no joint motion is produced).

An *isolytic* contraction is a contraction of modulated intensity against a force of greater intensity in the opposite direction, so that the joint motion produced is opposite that of the muscular contraction. Examples are certain PNF techniques.

An *isokinetic* contraction is one against a resistance in which speed is the controlled variable. Specialized equipment is usually required to produce this type of exercise contraction, but it may be performed manually as well.

Techniques[9,21,23,28,47]

Anterior Innominate

Pelvic examination: ASIS is low, PSIS is high
Positive standing flexion test
Positive long sitting test: long to short (on side of the positive standing flexion test)
Positive prone knee flexion test: short to short
Check hip musculature for symmetry

Muscular correction of this positional fault utilizes muscles that can rotate the innominate in a posterior direction. In this case, the major mover is the gluteus maximus. The technique is as follows:

1. The patient is supine with the opposite leg hanging free from the edge of the treatment table, supported at approximately the level of the ischium.
2. The hip and knee are flexed on the involved side

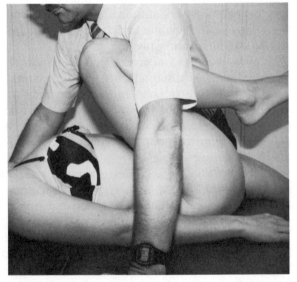

Fig. 18-88. Muscle energy technique for anterior innominate.

until the freely hanging leg begins to come up.
3. The clinician may then stabilize the flexed knee with his or her shoulder or instruct the patient to hold the knee in that fixed position with his own hands (Fig. 18-88).
4. The patient is then instructed to push his knee (on the involved side) against his own hands (or the clinician's shoulder) with a submaximal sustained contraction (isometric) for about 7 to 10 seconds, all the while breathing in a smooth, relaxed manner. Note that the hip is not allowed to move into extension at any time, only flexion.
5. As soon as the contraction ends, the slack is taken up by further flexing the hip and knee toward the chest until the new barrier is reached. This occurs as the opposite, freely hanging leg begins to rise further. The contraction is repeated and then relaxed and the slack taken up. The procedure is repeated three or four times or until all slack is taken up.
6. The patient is now re-examined for any change, usually by the long sitting test or the standing flexion test. The treatment is repeated if necessary.

This treatment may be given to the patient to do as a home program two to three times per day for the next several days. It should be noted that this technique is a powerful rotator of the innominate and can be easily overdone unless specific guidelines are given.

Posterior Innominate

Pelvic examination: ASIS is high, PSIS is low
Positive standing flexion test
Positive long sitting test: short to long (on side of the positive standing flexion test)
Positive prone knee flexion test: short to long
Check hip musculature for symmetry

Muscular correction of this positional fault utilizes muscles that can rotate the innominate in an anterior direction. In this case, the rectus femoris is the major mover:

1. The patient is supine with the involved leg hang-

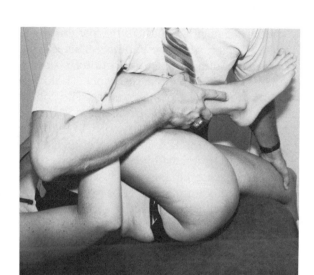

Fig. 18-89. Muscle energy technique for posterior innominate.

ing free over the edge of the treatment table as described previously. The hip is extended and the knee is flexed.

2. The opposite hip and knee are flexed in a similar manner as previously described until the freely hanging leg begins to come up. The patient is instructed to hold the flexed knee and hip in that position with his hands. The clinician may assist this effort with a hand, arm, or shoulder.

3. The clinician places the other hand on the anterior supracondylar area of the freely hanging knee and gently pushes down to take up the slack (Fig. 18-89).

4. The patient is then instructed to push the freely hanging leg up against the clinician's hand with a submaximal force, holding it constant for 7 to 10 seconds while breathing in a relaxed, smooth manner. It is important for the clinician to give unyielding resistance to the contraction.

5. As the patient relaxes the contraction, the slack is taken up by the clinician by pushing down on the freely hanging leg and assisting the patient in pulling the flexed hip and knee up somewhat to the new barrier. The contraction is then again executed in the new position. This procedure is repeated three or four times.

6. The patient is now re-examined for any changes produced by these efforts, usually by the long

sitting test. Treatment is repeated if necessary.

The patient can be instructed in a modification of this technique for home use simply by telling him to hang the uninvolved leg from the edge of his bed or other raised surface and flex the opposite hip and knee to the chest. The patient should then hold that position for 2 to 3 minutes and perform slow, relaxed breathing. The purpose of the breathing techniques used for both the anterior and the posterior innominate procedures is to take advantage of rotatory motion of the innominate around the superior transverse (respiratory) axis of the sacroiliac joints.

Forward Sacral Torsion (Left-on-Left or Right-on-Right)

Forward sacral torsion is diagnosed by:

A deeper sacral sulcus on the *opposite* side
A more posterior and inferior ILA on the *same* side
Positive sitting flexion test usually on the *opposite* side (but may vary)
Positive prone knee flexion test short on the *same* side
Sphinx test: sulci become equal or less asymmetrical

Muscular correction of forward sacral torsion utilizes muscles that will cause the sacrum to move backward on an oblique axis. This technique employs reciprocal inhibition of one piriformis by the opposite internal hip rotators (unlocks the axis) while the other piriformis moves the sacrum from the faulty position.

1. The patient lies on the side that corresponds to the axis of involvement. In other words, a patient with a left-on-left torsion would lie on the left side.

2. The clinician stands at the side of the table, facing the patient.

3. The patient should be as close to the edge of the table as possible. The downside arm should rest behind the trunk (the hand may be used to stabilize the patient by having him grip the edge of the treatment table behind him). The topside arm hangs over the edge of the table closest to the

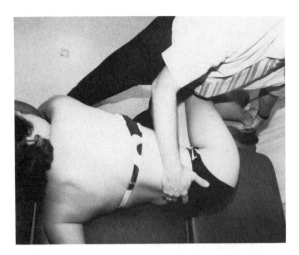

Fig. 18-90. Muscle energy technique for left-on-left forward sacral torsion dysfunction.

clinician as the trunk of the patient is rotated forward and the chest approximates the table.

4. The clinician's cephalad hand palpates the lumbosacral junction while the caudad hand flexes the patient's knees and hips to approximately 70 to 90 degrees or until the clinician can appreciate motion occurring at the lumbosacral junction. This is best achieved by grasping both legs together at the ankles and moving the hips passively into flexion. The patient's knees should be resting in the hollow of the clinician's hip as he translates his body laterally toward the patient's head, thus flexing the patient's hips and lumbar spine up to the lumbosacral junction (Fig. 18-90).

5. The clinician now moves his or her hand from the lumbosacral junction and places it on the patient's shoulder near the edge of the treatment table. The patient is instructed to "take a deep breath," and as he exhales to "reach toward the floor." As the patient does this, the clinician assists by pressing downward on the patient's shoulder to help take up the slack. This is repeated two or three times.

6. The clinician now returns that hand to the lumbosacral junction and, using the hand holding the ankles, lowers the ankles toward the floor until resistance is met and/or motion is felt at the lumbosacral junction (Fig. 18-91).

7. The clinician now instructs the patient to "lift both ankles toward the ceiling." This is a submaximal contraction, and the clinician must be sure to give unyielding resistance (hold-relax contraction) to the patient's effort. The contraction is held for 7 to 10 seconds and is then relaxed.

8. As the contraction is relaxed, the clinician takes up the slack by translating his or her body cephalad (to increase flexion) and lowers the ankles toward the floor until resistance is met or motion felt at the lumbosacral junction (to increase side-bending), and the patient reaches toward the floor with the hanging arm (to increase rotation).

9. Steps 7 and 8 are repeated two or three times, and then the patient is retested to check for any changes in sacral position. The treatment is repeated if necessary.

In some instances, the edge of the treatment table is uncomfortable to the patient's downside thigh during performance of the contractions in step 7. The clinician must sometimes support the patient's knees with his or her own thigh or may sit on the

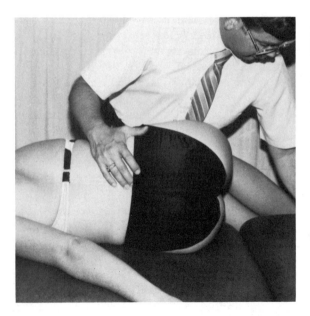

Fig. 18-91. Muscle energy technique for left-on-left forward sacral torsion dysfunction.

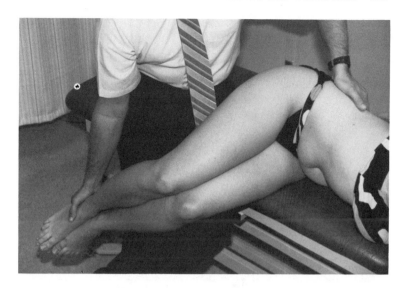

Fig. 18-92. Alternate method of muscle energy technique for left-on-left forward sacral torsion dysfunction.

treatment table and perform the technique from that position (Fig. 18-92).

Backward Sacral Torsion (Left-on-Right or Right-on-Left)

Backward sacral torsion is diagnosed by:

A deeper sacral sulcus on the *opposite* side
A more posterior and inferior ILA on the *same* side
Positive sitting flexion test on the *same* side
Positive prone knee flexion test on the *opposite* side
Sphinx test: sacral sulci become *more* asymmetrical.

Muscular correction of backward sacral torsion utilizes muscles that will cause the sacrum to move forward on an oblique axis. The technique described uses the gluteus medius and the gluteus maximus for this purpose:

1. The patient lies on the side corresponding to the axis of involvement. This means that a patient with a left-on-right torsion would lie on his right side.
2. The patient lies as close to the edge of the table as possible, and the clinician stands at that edge facing the patient.
3. The patient's trunk is now rotated so that the

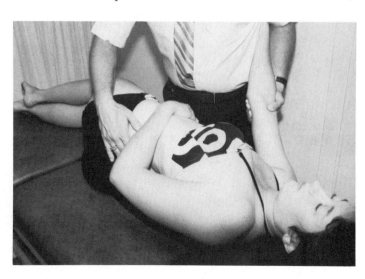

Fig. 18-93. Muscle energy technique for left-on-right backward sacral torsion dysfunction.

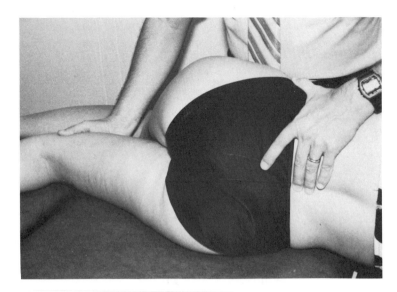

Fig. 18-94. Muscle energy technique for left-on-right backward sacral torsion dysfunction.

back approximates the table surface. This is accomplished by the clinician grasping the patient's downside arm (usually above the elbow) and pulling it out from under the patient (Fig. 18-93). The clinician now flexes the patient's topmost leg somewhat at the hip and knee. The downside leg is allowed to remain straight for the moment.

4. The clinician now palpates the patient's lumbosacral junction with the cephalad hand. With the other hand, the clinician reaches behind the patient's topside flexed knee and passively extends the patient's bottom hip by pushing the leg posteriorly. The clinician does this until motion is perceived occurring at the lumbosacral junction (Fig. 18-94).

5. The clinician now repositions his or her hands so that the caudal hand now palpates the lumbosacral junction and the cephalad hand is moved to the patient's shoulder.

6. The clinician now uses the forearm of his or her caudad arm to stabilize the pelvis and instructs the patient to "take a deep breath." As the patient exhales, the clinician presses downward

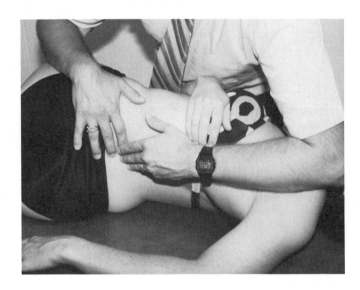

Fig. 18-95. Muscle energy technique for left-on-right backward sacral torsion dysfunction.

on the shoulder, causing greater trunk rotation, and further approximating the trunk to the table surface (Fig. 18-95). This maneuver is repeated two or three times to take up all the slack. The clinician must be careful not to allow the pelvis to move and change its alignment.

7. Maintaining trunk rotation and pelvic alignment, the clinician instructs the patient to "straighten the topside knee and allow the leg to hang freely" from the table. Being careful not to change pelvic alignment, the clinician slides the caudad hand down the thigh to the lateral supracondylar area of the patient's knee.

8. The patient is then instructed to "lift the knee toward the ceiling" while the clinician provides unyielding resistance to the effort. The contraction is held for 7 to 10 seconds and is then relaxed (Fig. 18-96).

9. Slack is taken up by the clinician moving the downside leg back a little (to increase extension), rotating the trunk a little (to increase rotation), and pushing down on the hanging leg until resistance is met (to increase sidebending).

10. Steps 8 and 9 are repeated two or three times, and the patient is then retested to check for positional changes of the sacrum. Treatment is repeated if necessary.

Unilateral Sacral Flexion

Unilateral sacral flexion is diagnosed by:

A deep sacral sulcus on the *same* side
An inferior and posterior ILA on the *same* side
Positive prone knee flexion test *short* on the *opposite* side
Positive sitting flexion test on the *same* side
Sphinx Test: no change.

Muscular correction of this sacral positional fault takes advantage of the normal nutation-counternutation movement of the sacrum during respiration. By accentuating the breathing pattern and applying direct pressure to the sacrum, it can be made to move up the long arm of the joint axis to its normal resting position:

1. The patient is prone.

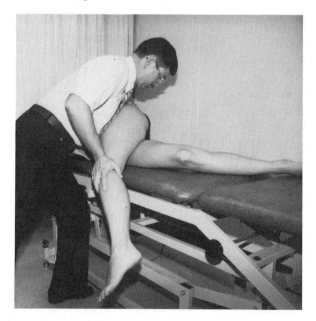

Fig. 18-96. Muscle energy technique for left-on-right backward sacral torsion dysfunction.

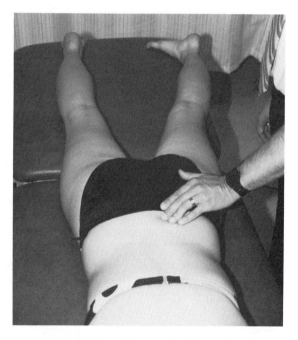

Fig. 18-97. Palpation of the sacral sulcus and positioning of the hip for application of muscle energy technique for a unilateral sacral flexion dysfunction.

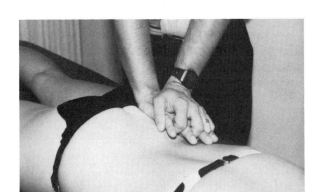

Fig. 18-98. Muscle energy technique for unilateral sacral flexion dysfunction.

2. The clinician stands on the *same* side as the lesion.
3. The clinician palpates the sacral sulcus on the side of the lesion with a finger and abducts the patient's hip on the involved side approximately 15 degrees and then internally rotates that same hip. This hip position is maintained throughout the procedure (Fig. 18-97).
4. Using a straight arm force, the clinician places a constant downward pressure on the ILA on the side of the lesion with the heel of the hand in the direction of the navel (Fig. 18-98).
5. The clinician instructs the patient to take in his breath in "small sips" (as through a soda straw) until he can hold no more air, then hold his breath with lungs maximally filled.
6. After several seconds, the clinician instructs the patient to release his air while the clinician maintains the constant downward pressure on the ILA.
7. Steps 5 and 6 are repeated three or four times, and then the patient is retested for positional changes of the sacrum. Treatment is repeated if necessary.

For a home self-treatment program, the patient may be instructed to sit in a chair with his legs abducted. He then takes a deep breath, holds it, and flexes his trunk between his spread knees, passing his elbows between the knees (Fig. 18-99). After several seconds, he releases his air and straightens his trunk. This procedure is repeated several times two or three times per day.

Superior Pubic Shear

Superior pubic shear is diagnosed by:

Positive standing flexion test on one side
Pubic tubercle *superior* on the same side as the positive standing flexion test
Tense and/or tender inguinal ligament on the same side

Muscular correction of this very common pelvic dysfunction utilizes the combined forces of the rectus femoris and the hip adductor group to effect the mobilization:

1. The patient is supine with the leg on the involved side freely hanging from the edge of the table (ischial contact).
2. The clinician stands on the same side as the lesion.
3. The lower portion of the freely hanging leg is passively extended at the knee and is held in this

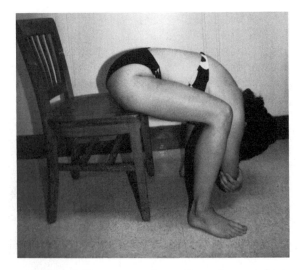

Fig. 18-99. Self-treatment for unilateral sacral flexion dysfunction.

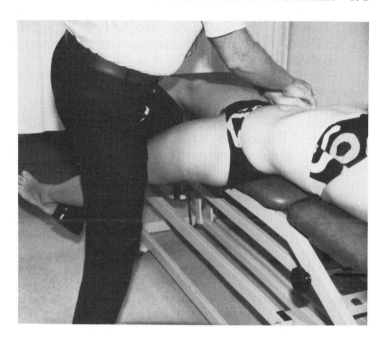

Fig. 18-100. Support of the lower leg by the clinician's leg in positioning the patient for application of muscle energy technique for a superior pubic shear dysfunction.

position, supported between the legs of the clinician (Fig. 18-100).

4. The clinician then reaches across the patient and places one hand on the ASIS opposite the side of involvement to stabilize it.

5. With the other hand, the clinician gently presses down on the supracondylar area of the freely

hanging leg of the patient and takes up the available slack at the hip. The clinician does this maintaining the position of the knee in passive extension between his or her own legs (Fig. 18-101).

6. The patient is then instructed to "squeeze your thigh against the table and push your leg up

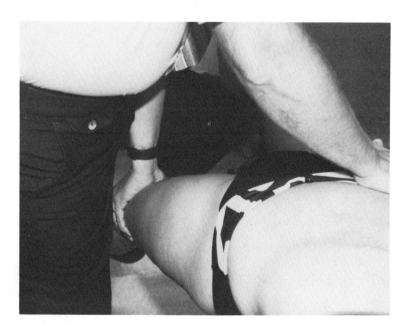

Fig. 18-101. Taking up of slack in the pelvic ligaments and the hip while supporting the patient's freely hanging lower leg prior to application of muscle energy technique for a superior pubic shear dysfunction.

against my hand.'' The clinician offers unyielding resistance to the upward contraction, and the table offers unyielding resistance to adduction. The knee must be maintained in passive extension as the patient tries to raise the leg. Note: The forces generated are to be submaximal — probably 10 pounds is sufficient to accomplish the task. The contraction is held for 7 to 10 seconds, and the patient is then instructed to relax.

7. As the patient relaxes, the slack is taken up into hip extension. Stabilization of the opposite ASIS is important during this step. When the new barrier to motion is reached, step 6 is repeated (usually steps 5 and 6 are repeated a total of three or four times).
8. Retest. Repeat the treatment if needed.

Inferior Pubic Shear

Inferior pubic shear is diagnosed by:

Positive standing flexion test on one side
Pubic tubercle *inferior* on *same* side as the positive standing flexion test
Possible tense and/or tender inguinal ligament on the same side

Muscular correction of this pelvic dysfunction is similar to the technique for the anterior innominate and uses the action of the gluteus maximus in combination with some direct pressure onto the ischium from the clinician. This allows the pubis to slide superiorly from the dysfunctional inferior position:

1. The patient is supine on the treatment table.
2. The clinician stands on the side of the patient *opposite* the side of involvement.
3. The patient is now instructed to flex the hip and knee completely on the involved side.
4. The clinician now reaches across the patient and grasps the edge of the treatment table on the opposite side. The clinician allows the patient's flexed knee on the involved side to rest against the axilla of his or her shoulder (Fig. 18-102).
5. The clinician now makes a fist and brings it to bear against the ischial tuberosity, taking up all available slack, and then relaxes (Fig. 18-103).
6. The patient is then instructed to "attempt to straighten your leg" on the involved side as the clinician resists this motion. This effort by the patient should only be in the range of 5 to 10 pounds of force and should be exerted for 7 to 10 seconds. He is then instructed to relax.
7. Step 5 is now repeated to take up the slack created by the muscular effort of step 6. Step 6 is then repeated. This sequence of steps 5 and 6 is repeated a total of three or four times each.

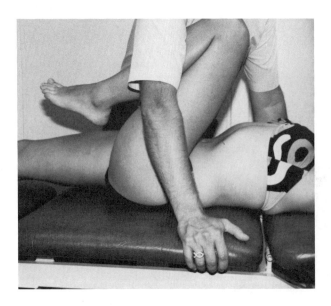

Fig. 18-102. Positioning for application of muscle energy technique for an inferior pubic shear dysfunction.

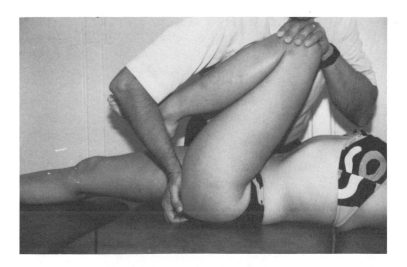

Fig. 18-103. Taking up available slack before and between applications of muscle energy technique for an inferior pubic shear dysfunction.

8. The patient is now retested and treatment repeated if necessary.

Combined Treatment for Superior and Inferior Pubic Subluxations

This technique is a powerful mover of the pubic symphysis. It first employs the hip abductors to "gap" the joint and then the hip adductors to "reset" the joint in its normal position.

1. The patient is supine with his knees flexed and together. He should be positioned toward the end of the treatment table so that his toes are near the end of the table.
2. The clinician stands at the end of the table facing the patient.
3. The clinician places his or her hands on either side of the patient's knees and instructs the patient to "push your legs apart" (abduct the knees) (Fig. 18-104). This is done with maximal force, and the clinician resists this effort by pushing against the lateral aspects of the patient's knees. This isometric contraction is held for 7 to 10 seconds. The patient is then instructed to relax.
4. The patient is then instructed to allow his legs to "fall apart" (abduct the knees). The clinician guides this action so that the feet are held together and the legs abduct 30 to 45 degrees. Step

3 is now repeated in this new position, with the patient giving a *maximal* contraction into abduction while the clinician resists this effort (Fig. 18-105).
5. As soon as the patient has ceased his contraction, the clinician quickly places his or her forearm between the patient's knees (the clinician's hand and elbow make contact with the medial aspects of the patient's knees), and the patient is instructed to "squeeze your knees together against

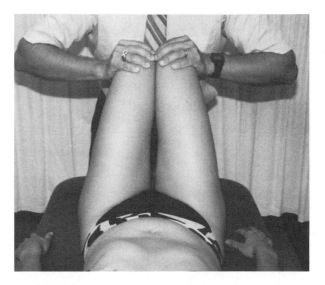

Fig. 18-104. Muscle energy technique for combined pubic shear dysfunction: first step.

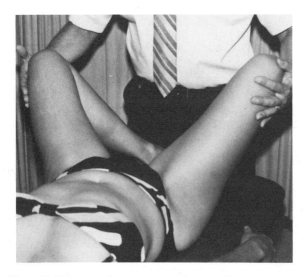

Fig. 18-105. Muscle energy technique for combined pubic shear dysfunction: second step.

my arm" (adduct the knees). This is also done with a maximal contraction (Fig. 18-106).
6. The contraction is held for a few seconds and then relaxed. It may need to be repeated once or twice more before repositioning the patient on the table to retest. Treatment may be repeated if necessary.

Many times an audible "pop" is heard during this treatment. This represents a separation of the pubic symphysis and allows them to reset themselves. This technique can be used separately or in combination with the specific pubic subluxation techniques previously described.

Superior Iliac Subluxation (Upslip)

Superior iliac subluxation is diagnosed by:

Superior iliac crest
Superior ASIS on same side
Superior PSIS on same side
Superior pubic tubercle on same side
Superior ischial tuberosity on same side

This technique is a direct action thrust technique but applies principles of "closed-packed" versus "loose-packed" joint mechanics to effect the mobilization.

1. The patient is prone, and the clinician stands at the foot of the treatment table on the side of the lesion.
2. The clinician grasps the patient's distal lower leg above the ankle and raises the entire leg into approximately 30 degrees of hip and lumbar extension, and abduction of 30 degrees, and then internally rotates the leg. This approximates the closed-packed position of the hip as much as possible.
3. The clinician then instructs the patient to grasp the top table edge with his hands. The clinician then proceeds to take up the slack by distracting the leg along its long axis until tightness is perceived along the kinetic chain (Fig. 18-107).
4. The clinician now applies a quick caudal jerk on the leg.
5. The patient is then retested and treatment is repeated if necessary.

By employing the closed-packed position of the hip, the effect of the distraction is applied to the innominate instead of the hip. Mobilization of the hip is done supine in the loose-packed position.

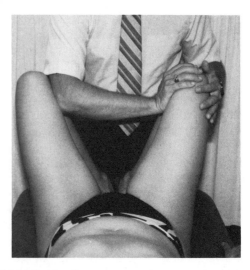

Fig. 18-106. Muscle energy technique for combined pubic shear dysfunction: last step.

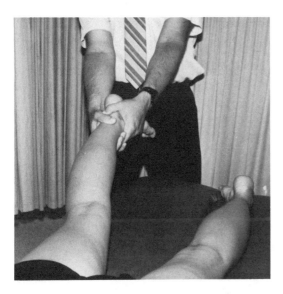

Fig. 18-107. Long axis distraction technique for correction of superior iliac shear (upslip).

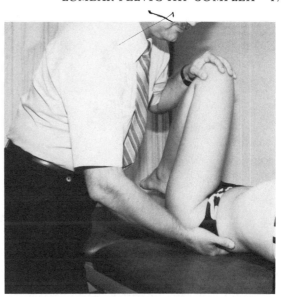

Fig. 18-108. Palpation of the sacral sulcus and PSIS in positioning the patient for application of muscle energy technique for correction of an iliac inflare dysfunction.

Iliac Inflare

Iliac inflare is diagnosed by:

Positive standing flexion test on the *same* side
Wide sacral sulcus on the *same* side
ASIS closer to the midline on the *same* side
PSIS farther from the midline on the *same* side

Muscular correction of this positional fault primarily utilizes the hip adductors, but from extreme positions in order to generate an effect on the pelvis:

1. The patient is supine on the treatment table.
2. The clinician stands on the same side as the lesion. With the cephalad hand, the clinician reaches under the patient and palpates the sacral sulcus and the PSIS (Fig. 18-108).
3. With the other hand, the clinician now grasps the patient's knee on the involved side and flexes the hip until motion is perceived at the sacral sulcus by the palpating hand. At this point, the clinician then abducts the hip, moving it to its limit. This position must be maintained (Fig. 18-109).
4. The clinician now moves the palpating hand to the opposite ASIS to stabilize the pelvis, then

shifts the other hand from the patient's knee to the medial aspect of the patient's ankle, grasping it. The clinician then produces external rotation of the hip by moving the foot medially to its limit,

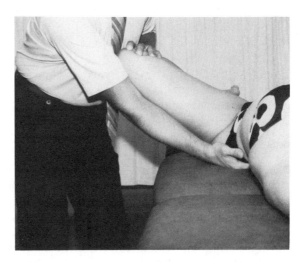

Fig. 18-109. Positioning of the patient's hip into flexion and abduction while palpating the sacral sulcus in preparation for application of muscle energy technique for an iliac inflare dysfunction.

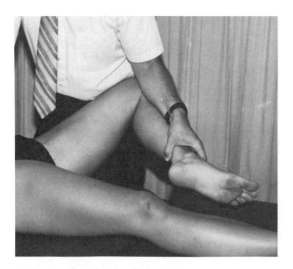

Fig. 18-110. External rotation of the patient's hip in the flexed and abducted position prior to application of muscle energy technique for an iliac inflare dysfunction.

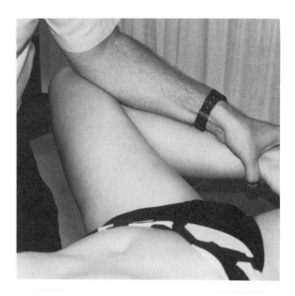

Fig. 18-111. Application of muscle energy technique for an iliac inflare dysfunction. The patient is instructed to adduct the thigh against the clinician's elbow from this position of flexion, abduction, and external rotation.

while maintaining the flexed-abducted position achieved in step 3 (Fig. 18-110).

5. While holding the patient's ankle, the clinician places his or her elbow against the medial aspect of the patient's knee and then instructs the patient to adduct his leg against the unyielding resistance of the clinician (Fig. 18-111). Note that both the clinician's hands are busy: One continues to support the opposite ASIS while the other maintains the flexed, abducted, and externally rotated position of the hip on the involved side.

6. The patient maintains the isometric contraction for 5 to 7 seconds and is then told to relax. During the relaxation, slack is taken up into gaining additional abduction and external rotation of the hip.

7. Steps 5 and 6 are repeated three or four times. At the conclusion of the last contraction and relaxation, the clinician straightens the hip and knee to their extended, neutral resting position, while maintaining the abducted and externally rotated position through the hand and elbow on the involved side and stabilizing the pelvis on the opposite ASIS (Fig. 18-112).

8. The patient is retested and treatment is reapplied if necessary.

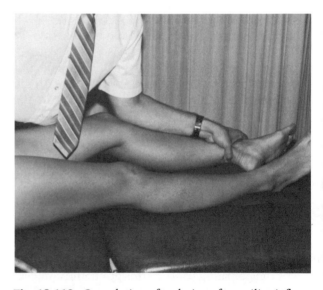

Fig. 18-112. Completion of technique for an iliac inflare dysfunction. The clinician extends the patient's hip and knee from the flexed, abducted, and externally rotated position.

Iliac Outflare

Iliac outflare is diagnosed by:

Positive standing flexion test on the *same* side
Sacral sulcus narrowed on the *same* side
The ASIS is moved away from the midline on the *same* side
The PSIS is moved toward the midline on the *same* side

This technique is a combination of direct traction by the clinician coupled with the muscular effort generated primarily by the hip abductors.

1. The patient is supine on the treatment table with the clinician standing on the same side as the lesion.
2. The clinician slips his or her cephalad hand under the patient until the fingertips come to rest in the sacral sulcus on that side. The clinician then exerts lateral traction on the PSIS, pulling toward himself (Fig. 18-113).
3. With the other hand, the clinician grasps the patient's knee on that side and produces hip and knee flexion to 90 degrees.
4. The clinician now leans his or her shoulder against the lateral aspect of the patient's knee, causing adduction of the hip. While supporting the foot to maintain hip and knee flexion, the hip is moved into its limit of adduction.
5. The clinician now produces internal rotation of the hip by moving the foot laterally to its limit (the clinician's shoulder is the fulcrum). This position must be maintained (Fig. 18-114).
6. While maintaining the position obtained with the caudad hand and shoulder, and the other hand applying lateral traction to the PSIS, the clinician instructs the patient to push his hip against the resistance.
7. The contraction is held for 5 to 7 seconds before the patient is instructed to relax. During the re-

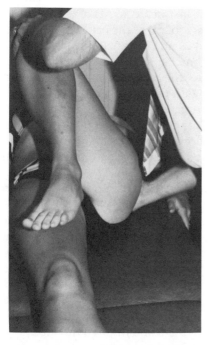

Fig. 18-113. Palpation and application of lateral traction on the sacral sulcus and PSIS prior to application of muscle energy technique for an iliac outflare dysfunction.

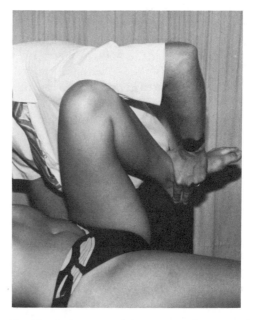

Fig. 18-114. Positioning of the patient's hip into adduction and internal rotation with the clinician's shoulder as the fulcrum. Application of muscle energy technique for an iliac outflare dysfunction is performed from this position.

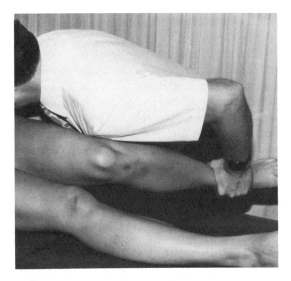

Fig. 18-115. Completion of technique for an iliac out-flare dysfunction. The clinician extends the patient's hip and knee from the flexed, adducted, and internally rotated position.

laxation, slack is taken up into additional adduction and internal rotation.

8. Steps 6 and 7 are repeated two or three times. At the conclusion of the final contraction, the clinician returns the leg to its neutral resting position, while maintaining the adducted and internally rotated position of the hip with the caudad hand and shoulder, and lateral traction on the PSIS with the cephalad hand (Fig. 18-115).

9. The patient is then retested and treatment reapplied if necessary.

Treatment Techniques for Lumbar Lesions

A description of the multiplicity of techniques that might be devised for the treatment of lumbar ERS and FRS lesions, as described previously in Figure 18-29, is beyond the scope of this chapter. The two techniques that are the most simple and probably the most used are included as a starting point for the reader.

FRS Right: Lateral Recumbent Technique

Positional diagnosis: FRS right
Motion restriction: Extension, left sidebending, left rotation

1. The patient is side-lying on the treatment table on the side of the more posterior transverse process (in this case, the right). The clinician stands facing the patient.

2. The patient's head is supported by a pillow, and the lower leg is straight. The upper leg is in some flexion of the knee and hip.

3. With the left hand, the clinician palpates the interspinous space of the involved segment. With the right hand, the clinician reaches behind the flexed upper knee to the thigh of the lower leg and passively extends the patient's lower hip until motion is felt at the interspinous space (Fig. 18-116).

4. The clinician now repositions the hands so that the right hand is palpating the interspinous space and the left hand introduces trunk rotation by grasping the patient's upper arm and pulling it toward him. Thus, the patient's upper shoulder approximates the table surface. This is continued until the clinician perceives motion arriving at the interspinous space (Fig. 18-117).

5. The patient is instructed to grasp the edge of the table behind him with the upper hand. The patient is instructed to "take a deep breath and then let it out." As the patient does so, the clinician takes up any remaining slack.

6. The clinician now repositions the hands and palpates the interspinous space with the left hand. With the right hand, the clinician grasps the patient's uppermost leg at the ankle.

7. Using the crook of the hip as the pivot point and the elbow as the fulcrum, the clinician lifts the patient's leg upward and introduces sidebending into the segment. The clinician then slowly extends the hip of the upper leg until extension is felt at the segment (Fig. 18-118).

8. At this point, the patient is instructed to "pull your ankle down toward the floor" and hold the contraction for 5 to 10 seconds and then relax.

9. The clinician then relocalizes movement to the segment by taking up the slack created by rotating the patient's trunk further, sidebending the trunk by lifting the ankle a little higher and extending the trunk through the hip.

10. Steps 8 and 9 are repeated three or four times before retesting the patient. Treatment is repeated if necessary.

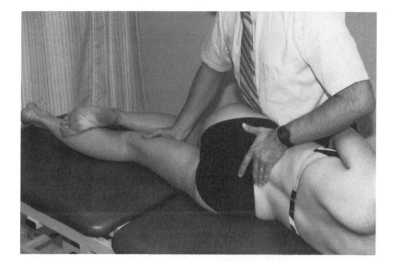

Fig. 18-116. Positioning for application of muscle energy technique for a right flexed, rotated, and sidebent (FRS right) lumbar facet restriction.

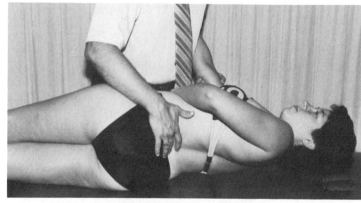

Fig. 18-117. Positioning and taking up of slack for application of muscle energy technique for a right flexed, rotated, and sidebent (FRS right) lumbar facet restriction.

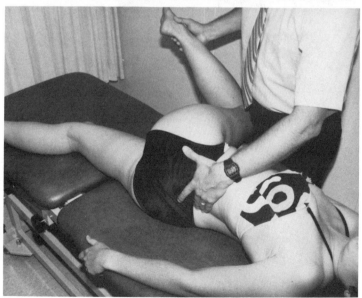

Fig. 18-118. Positioning and application of muscle energy technique for a right flexed, rotated, and sidebent (FRS right) lumbar facet restriction.

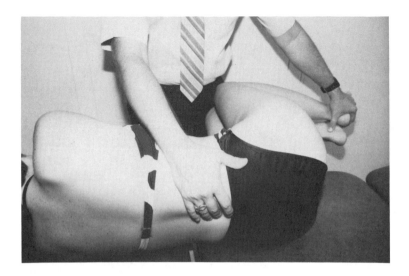

Fig. 18-119. Positioning for application of muscle energy technique for a right extended, rotated, and sidebent (ERS right) lumbar facet restriction.

ERS Right: Lateral Recumbent Technique

Positional diagnosis: ERS right
Motion restriction: Flexion, left rotation, left sidebending

1. The patient is side-lying on the treatment table with the affected side up (the side of the most prominent transverse process). In this case, the patient will be lying on his left side.
2. The clinician stands facing the patient. The clinician palpates with the left hand the interspinous space at the level below the one to be treated,
while flexing the patient's hips with the other hand until he can appreciate motion being introduced into the segment being palpated (Fig. 18-119).
3. While supporting the patient's knees against the crook of his or her own hip or body, the clinician lowers the patient's legs toward the floor until sidebending (left) can be perceived being introduced into the segment.
4. The patient is then instructed to "reach toward the floor with your uppermost arm." This introduces left rotation into the segment. Note: At times this step can be omitted since rotation may

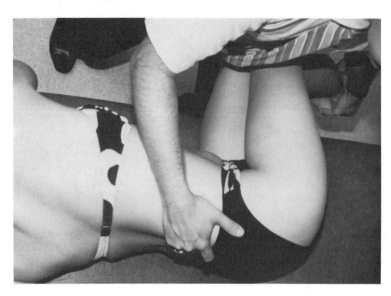

Fig. 18-120. Positioning and application of muscle energy technique for a right extended, rotated, and sidebent (ERS right) lumbar facet restriction.

be localized simultaneously with sidebending.

5. The clinician instructs the patient to "lift both ankles toward the ceiling." The clinician offers unyielding resistance to the patient's effort (right sidebending) for 5 to 10 seconds before the patient is told to relax. The force required is approximately 5 to 10 pounds (Fig. 18-120).

6. The clinician takes up the slack created by increasing the sidebending, flexion, and rotational components until motion is relocalized to the segment.

7. Steps 5 and 6 are repeated three or four times before the patient is retested. Treatment is repeated if necessary.

Manipulation

The focus of the treatment techniques presented in this chapter has been on the "patient-active" muscle energy techniques. A variety of high-velocity thrust mobilizations for the sacroiliac joints exist. They primarily produce rotatory forces on the innominates and are thus more appropriate for the iliosacral lesions. One particularly effective thrust technique is included for completeness:

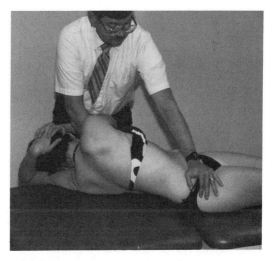

Fig. 18-122. Positioning for sacroiliac joint manipulation and application of thrust to the ASIS.

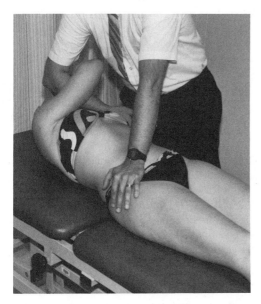

Fig. 18-121. Positioning for sacroiliac joint manipulation.

1. The patient is supine with hands locked behind the head (fingers interlaced).

2. The clinician stands opposite the affected side and makes hand contact on the patient's ASIS (on the affected side) with the caudad hand.

3. With the cephalad hand, the clinician reaches through the crook of the patient's elbow (on the affected side) from behind and allows the dorsum of his hand to contact the patient's chest (Fig. 18-121).

4. Using the dorsum of the hand as a fulcrum against the patient's chest, the clinician rolls the patient's torso toward him. The clinician instructs the patient to "relax, hang on to your head, and allow me to turn you."

5. The clinician takes up the slack through the pelvis using a stiff arm with the direction of force applied down and away.

6. The clinician instructs the patient to "take in a deep breath and let it out." As the patient does so, the clinician takes up the remainder of the slack through the torso and pelvis and gives a quick thrust to the pelvis through the ASIS (Fig. 18-122).

ACKNOWLEDGMENTS

The author thanks Linda, Scott, and Sean for their understanding, patience and encouragement along the way to completion of this work. Special thanks to Steve Stratton for his inspiration to excel and for his advice, and to Barbara Springer for modeling.

REFERENCES

1. Kapandji IA: The Physiology of the Joints. 2nd Ed. Vol. III. The Trunk and the Vertebral Column. p 53. Churchill Livingstone, Edinburgh, 1974

2. Kaltenbourn FM: Mobilization of Extremity Joints: Examination and Basic Treatment Techniques. 3rd Ed. p 154. Olaf Norlis Bokhandel, Oslo, 1980

3. Warwick R, Williams P (eds): Gray's Anatomy. 35th British Ed. p 242–244, 344–358, 442–450, 559–570. WB Saunders, Philadelphia, 1973

4. Kendall FP, Kendall-McCreary E: Muscles, Function and Testing. 3rd Ed. p 148. Williams & Wilkins, Baltimore, 1983

5. Janda V: Muscle Function Testing. p 157. Butterworths, London, 1983

6. Kopell HP, Thompson WAL: Peripheral Entrapment Neuropathies. p 59. Robert E Krieger, Huntington NY, 1976

7. Kirkaldy-Willis WH: Managing Low Back Pain. p 92. Churchill Livingstone, New York, 1983

8. Stoddard A: Manual of Osteopathic Technique. pp 81–85, 211–228. Hutchinson, London, 1978

9. Mitchell FL Jr, Moran PS, Pruzzo NA: An Evaluation and Treatment Manual of Osteopathic Muscle Energy Procedures. Mitchell, Moran and Pruzzo Associates, Valley Park MO, 1979

10. Solonen KA: The sacroiliac joint in the light of anatomical, roentogenological and clinical studies. Acta Orthop Scand, suppl. 27, 1–115, 1957

11. Hoppenfeld S: Physical Examination of the Spine and Extremities. p 144. Appleton-Century-Crofts, New York, 1976

12. Cyriax J: Textbook of Orthopaedic Medicine. 7th Ed. Vol 1. Diagnosis of Soft Tissue Lesions. p 572. Bailliere-Tindall, London, 1978

13. Cailliet R: Low Back Pain Syndrome. 2nd Ed. FA Davis, Philadelphia, 1982, pp 10, 23–26.

14. Frigerio NA, Stowe RR, Howe JW: Movement of the sacroiliac joint. Clin Orthop Rel Res 100:370, 1974

15. Colachis SC, Werden C, Bechtol C, Strohm B: Movement of the sacroiliac joints in the adult male. A preliminary report. Arch Phys Med Rehab 44:490, 1963

16. Egund N, Olsson TH, Schmid H, Selvik G: Movements in the sacroiliac joints demonstrated with roentgen stereophotogrammetry. Acta Radiol (Stockholm) 19:833, 1978

17. Turek SL: Orthopaedics: Principles and Their Applications. 4th Ed. pp 431, 736, 1663–1665. JB Lippincott, Philadelphia, 1984

18. Weisl H: Movements of the sacro-iliac joint. Acta Anat 23:80, 1955

19. Mennell JM: Back Pain. Little, Brown, Boston, 1960

20. Paris SV: Course Notes: The Spine. Institute of Graduate Health Sciences, Atlanta, 1979

21. Course Notes: Tutorial on Level I Muscle Energy Techniques. Michigan State University College of Osteopathic Medicine, East Lansing, MI, 1986

22. Goodridge JP: Muscle energy technique: definition, explanation, methods of procedure. J Am Osteopath Assoc 82(4):249, 1981

23. Kimberly PE (ed): Somatic Dysfunction: Principles of Manipulative Treatment and Procedures. Kirksville College of Osteopathic Medicine, Kirksville MO, 1980

24. Nyberg R: The lumbar and pelvic musculature. Unpublished manuscript, 1978

25. Farfan H: Muscular mechanism of the lumbar spine and the position of power and efficiency. Orthop Clin North Am 6(1): 135, 1975

26. Mitchell FL Sr: Structural pelvic function. AAO Yearbook II: 178, 1965.

27. Saunders HD: Evaluation, Treatment and Prevention of Musculoskeletal Disorders. p 77. 2nd Ed. H Duane Saunders, Minneapolis, 1985

28. Stratton SA: Course Notes: Muscle Energy Techniques. U.S. Army-Baylor University Program in Physical Therapy, Fort Sam Houston TX 1983–1984

29. Pratt WA: The lumbopelvic torsion syndrome. J Am Osteopath Assoc 51(7):335, 1952

30. Greenman PE: Innominate shear dysfunction in the sacroiliac syndrome. Manual Med 2:114, 1986

31. DiAmbrosia RD: Musculoskeletal Disorders. pp 258–260, 271, 273. JB Lippincott, Philadelphia, 1977

32. Nitz PA, Woerman AL: Acute sacroiliac joint strain in young adult males as evidenced by bone scan. Preliminary research. 1988

33. Grieve GP: Common Vertebral Joint Problems. pp 29–31, 39, 307–310. Churchill Livingstone, New York, 1981

34. Fryette HH: Principles of Osteopathic Technique. p

113. American Academy of Osteopathy, Carmel CA, 1954

35. Greenman PE: The manipulative prescription. Mich Osteopath J, December 1982

36. Korr I: Proprioceptors and somatic dysfunction. J Am Osteopath Assoc 74:638, 1975

37. Greenman PE: Restricted vertebral motion. Mich Osteopath J, March 1983, p 31

38. Clemente CD: Anatomy: A Regional Atlas of the Human Body. #376. Lea & Febiger, Philadelphia, 1975

39. Greenman PE: Motion sense. Mich Osteopath J, January 1983, p 39

40. Kessler RM, Hertlig D: Management of Common Musculoskeletal Disorders. p 379. Harper & Row, Philadelphia, 1983

41. Maitland GD: Vertebral Manipulation. Butterworths, London, 1977

42. Woerman AL, Binder-MacLeod S: Leg length discrepancy assessment: accuracy and precision in five clinical methods of evaluation. J Orthop Sports Phys Ther 5:230, 1984

43. Kirkaldy-Willis WH, Hill RJ: A more precise diagnosis for low-back pain. Spine 4(2):102, March–April 1979

44. Liekens M, Gillets H: Belgian Chiropractic Research Notes. 10th Ed. Brussels, 1973

45. Mooney V, Robertson J: The facet syndrome. Clin Orthop Rel Res 115:149, March/April 1976

46. Bemis T, Daniel M: Validation of the long sit test on subjects with iliosacral dysfunction. J Orthop Sports Phys Ther 8(7):336, 1987

47. Grieve GP: Mobilization of the Spine. 4th Ed. p 188. Churchill Livingstone, New York, 1984

SELECTED READINGS

Beal MC: The sacroiliac problem: review of anatomy, mechanics and diagnosis. J Am Osteopath Assoc 81(10):667, 1982

Bourdillon JF: Spinal Manipulation. 3rd Ed. Appleton-Century-Crofts, New York, 1982

Bowen V, Cassidy JD: Macroscopic and microscopic anatomy of the sacroiliac joint from embryonic life until the eighth decade. Spine 6(6):620, 1981

Erhard R, Bowling R: The recognition and management of the pelvic component of low back and sciatic pain. Bull Orthop Sect Am Phys Ther Assoc 2(3):4, Winter 1977

Grieve GP: The sacroiliac joint. Physiotherapy 62(12):384, 1976

Johnston WL: Hip shift: testing a basic postural dysfunction. J Am Osteopath Assoc 63:923, 1964

Retzlaff EW, Berry AH, Haight AS, et al: The piriformis muscle syndrome. J Am Osteopath Assoc 73:799, 1974

Stoddard A: Conditions of the sacro-iliac joint and their treatment. Physiotherapy 44(4):97, 1958

Sutton SE: Postural imbalance: Examination, and treatment using flexion tests. J Am Osteopath Assoc 77:456, 1978

Walheim G, Olerud S, Ribbe T: Mobility of the pubic symphysis. Acta Orthop Scand 55:203, 1984

Weismantel A: Evaluation and treatment of sacroiliac joint problems. Bull Orthop Sect Am Phys Ther Assoc 3(1):5, Spring 1978

Wilder DG, Pope MH, Frymoyer JW: The functional topography of the sacroiliac joint. Spine 5(6):575, 1980

19

Surgical Treatment of the Hip

DAVID ROUBEN

The differential diagnosis of pain in and around the pelvis and the low back is a confusing and persistently perplexing problem. Pain to the thigh and anterior groin region can be referred from the knee. Pathology in and around the patellofemoral joint, degenerative changes, or synovitic inflammation of the right knee can refer pain to the quadriceps musculature and up through the thigh in general. Patients can complain of persistent discomfort while ambulating, subjectively describing the pain in and around the thigh and upper femoral region. A complete physical examination and assessment is imperative to determine the difference. Pain perceived in the "hip" (i.e., the buttocks) can also be referred pain from the back. Pain along the lateral aspect of the upper femur is usually a soft tissue bursitic or mechanical inflammatory pain from the abductor musculature or the fascia lata rubbing against the prominent trochanteric aspect of the proximal femur. As a general rule, pain perceived in the anterior aspect of the thigh is referred pain from the lumbar facet joints, the hip joints, or neural pain from an irritated anterior lateral femoral cutaneous nerve.

A careful history identifying where the pain comes from and when the pain is produced can often untangle these confusing issues. A careful examination of what manipulations of what joints and muscle groups in and around the area reproduce the pain can also help to determine just where the pain seems to arise. Focal palpatory pain to the buttocks or the lower sacral or lumbar region usually emanates from the area in and around the bony or soft tissue aspects of the lumbosacral articulation. Firm palpation over the trochanteric prominence of the

lateral aspect of the proximal femur usually reproduces pain emanating from soft tissue irritation in that region. Gentle, passive, internal and external rotation under no gravitational stress usually reproduces the pain if it emanates from the hip joint itself.

Nevertheless, sometimes more extreme examinations must be performed to confirm whether the pain is coming from the hip joint. If the patient is supine, the pain is often not elicited except in abduction or adduction positions with associated internal and external rotation. Sometimes flexion must be added to elicit pain emanating from the hip joint region. Nevertheless, in most cases, reproducible pain is pain perceived in the anterior aspect of the proximal pelvis-thigh articulation (the groin).

Appropriate to any discussion of the evaluation and treatment of pain in and around the hip joint is a consideration of the numerous causes of those conditions that may necessitate operative intervention to afford the patient a return to normal ambulation; therefore, the following section discusses each cause briefly.

HIP JOINT PATHOLOGY AND DYSFUNCTION

Trauma

Traumatic injuries to the hip joint occur in every age group. Children involved in motor vehicle accidents, in spite of early operative reduction and intervention, may still sustain partial or total avascular necrosis and subsequent collapse of the femoral head. This would certainly be the case in older age groups as well. Dislocations and fracture dislocations of the hip joint can traumatically affect the vascular supply of the femoral head as well as cause either the femoral head or the acetabulum irreparable injury, necessitating further reconstructive intervention.

Vascular Compromise

In addition to trauma, vascular compromise of the femoral head can be caused by Legg-Perthes' disease in the young, congenital metabolic disorders such as Gaucher's disease, chronic alcoholism, sickle cell disease, nitrogen gas occlusion syndrome (diver's disease),[1,2] or idiopathic disorders.

Metaplastic Lesions

Any number of tumorous metaplastic lesions can afflict the femoral head or the acetabulum. Among these, chondroblastoma and osteogenic sarcoma are seen in the young, Giant Cell tumor in early adulthood and middle age, and metastatic cancer and Paget's disease in mature individuals.[3]

Collagen Vascular Disease

Collagen vascular diseases such as ankylosingspondylitis and rheumatoid arthritis have been shown to cause degenerative changes if not ankylosis, necessitating operative reconstruction. Rheumatoid arthritis in the young as well as in the old can necessitate progressive reconstructive arthroplastic procedures around the hip joint.

Congenital Hip Disorders

Congenital afflictions of the hip joint such as congenital dislocation or acetabulum dysplasia may make reconstructive procedures in and around the hip necessary as the patient matures.

Infections

Patients who have sustained significant destruction of the hip joint as a result of cured or quiescent infections often require reconstructive surgery to repair damage.

SURGICAL INTERVENTION

Each patient who, for whatever reason, may require reconstructive surgery in and around the hip joint must be evaluated and treated individually. The best treatment option for one patient is not necessarily the best treatment option for another, even though the same pathology may be present in both. As orthopaedic research progresses, our armamentarium of treatment options grows as well. Each patient must be evaluated and provided with treatment option that offers the greatest chance of lone-term, painfree, ambulatory success. This is never a straightforward or easy decision. A careful assessment taking into account the age and the medical, emotional, physiologic, physical, and intellectual stability of the patient must be made, and the long-term goals and desires of each patient must be respected.

Before modern metals made implantations and reconstruction of the hip joint anatomically feasible, a number of seemingly aggressive and definitive treatments were used on a rather commonplace basis. Two of these procedures, resection arthroplasty and joint fusion, are still used today for various reasons.

Arthroplasty

Resection arthroplasty, commonly known as the "girdlestone procedure," involves the surgical excision of the femoral neck with no purposeful soft tissue interposition.[1,2] Indications for resection arthroplasty include, in addition to incurable infection, postradiation necrosis of the involved bone of the proximal femur, and absence of any bone to reconstruct. The procedure is also indicated for patients whose medical status is so compromised that any more definitive procedure to alleviate pain due to developmental structural deformities would likely result in death.[1,2,4,5]

The patient is placed postoperatively in skeletal traction for approximately 2 weeks and then is progressively taught ambulatory skills. This is done initially with the patient in a nonweightbearing status, progressing to weightbearing as tolerated over a 6-month period. The procedure results in up to 5 inches of shortening of the limb, but once soft tissue healing is accomplished, the patient is able to ambulate with the use of an assistive device with a noticeable limp but minimal disability and no pain.

Arthrodesis

Arthrodesis of the hip accomplished by any number of techniques (Fig. 19-1) is most often indicated in young adults and teenagers, more often in males than in females, where total hip replacement is not indicated because of premature age. These patients, if adequately taught, postoperatively, can attain the ambulatory skills to participate in aggressive athletics during their youth, and can ambulate with a minimal limp. As one might expect, they compensate for the loss of hip motion through increased motion at the lumbosacral region of the spine. These patients show evidence of early radiographic degenerative changes, if not outright symptomatology to the lumbosacral spine after 20 to 30 years, however. These hip fusions are amenable to reconstruction at a later age, but present the surgeon, therapist, and patient with unique rehabilitative hurdles to overcome postoperatively.

Prosthesis

As our technical knowledge and skill with metals progressed, the first successful proximal femoral replacements were devised; they have been used successfully now for 30 to 40 years. Complete transec-

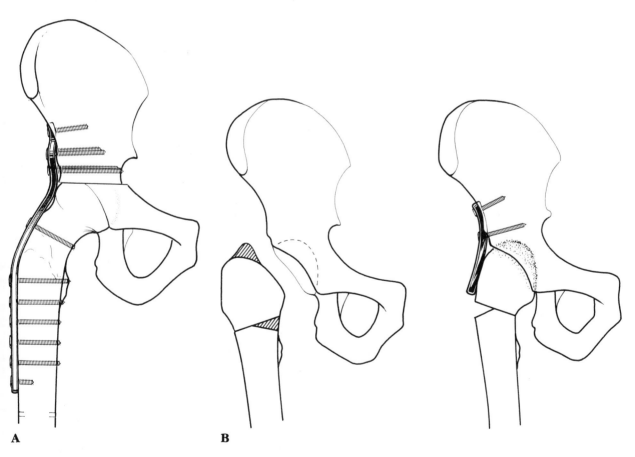

A   **B**

Fig. 19-1. (A) Hip arthrodesis with rigid internal compression fixation (Schneider's cobra head plate, 1966); **(B)** arthrodesis of a girdle stone hip. (From Liechti,[11] with permission.)

tion and excision of the femoral head at the femoral neck, with insertion of a metal stem into the cancellous aspect of the shaft of the proximal femur, seems to offer patients one more chance at reattaining ambulatory skills when afflicted with those conditions that destroy at least the femoral head. Today, these prostheses are most often used in elderly patients, whose fractures in and about the femoral neck preclude closed or open reduction and internal fixation of their femoral neck fractures. The prostheses most often used are the Thompson and Austin Moore types.[1,2,4-6] Insertion of these prostheses is accomplished from either an anterior or a posterior approach.[4,5,7]

Postoperative patients are protected from adduction, internal rotation, and flexion maneuvers. They are allowed to ambulate using a walker, crutch, or cane. Either partial, toe-touch, or non-weightbearing status is prescribed for a period of time at the discretion of the operative surgeon. (Refer to the section on "Hip Arthroplasty" for a discussion of postoperative ambulatory problems that might persist after these types of hip procedures.)

Osteotomy

Most often advocated and popularized recently in Europe is the utilization of a varus or valgus osteotomy to buy the patient some time before more aggressive joint reconstructive arthroplasties are undertaken. Prerequisites for osteotomy include subluxation, reasonable congruity, at least one-half of the normal cartilage thickness, and at least 60 percent of the normal range of motion, particularly flexion and abduction. Good to excellent results are seen, affording the patient as well as the operative clinician additional time to assess, evaluate, and suggest the best and longest lasting treatment[1,2] (Fig. 19-2).

Varus intertrochanteric osteotomy is rarely indicated in patients with advanced arthritic changes, although there is a place for patients with coxa

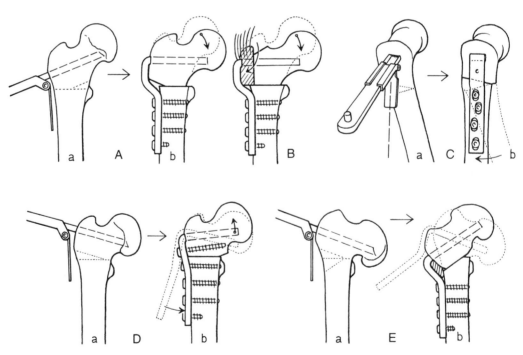

Fig. 19-2. The five main types of intertrochanteric osteotomies. **(A)** Adduction osteotomy; **(B)** adduction osteotomy with distal displacement of the greater trochanter; **(C)** extension osteotomy before and after fixation; **(D)** abduction osteotomy of 50 degrees, fixed with a double-curved 120 degree blade plate, with bone graft between the plate and the proximal fragment. (From Muller,[12] with permission.)

magna to undergo a valgus osteotomy of the proximal femur. Osteotomies in young people with structural hip abnormalities play an important part in prophylactically precluding early degenerative changes as a result of that structural deformity. On the other hand, it is very difficult to talk parents of young patients into having their child undergo significant operative procedures when the patients are largely asymptomatic.

Hip Arthroplasty

John Charnley in the early 1960s successfully popularized what is now known as the total hip arthroplasty. Continued advancements in biologically compatible metals, surgical implantation technique, and modifications to attain the most biologically efficient structural shapes have made total hip arthroplasty the state of the art for patients with painful incongruent hip joint disease.

In the recognition that standard hip arthroplasty requires resection of the femoral head and neck and structural resurfacing of the acetabulum, early attempts were made at surface replacement procedures (Fig. 19-3). Young children with disruption of hip articular congruity and associated pain were treated with cup arthroplasties (Fig. 19-4). These were simply interposition metal cups placed over the top of the femoral head. In many cases these

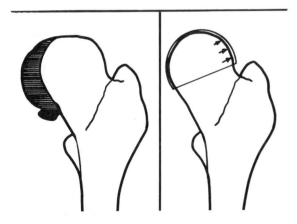

Fig. 19-3. Correct preparation of the femoral head component. Excess bone is excised with a chisel, and the femoral head is rounded with a reamer. (From Wagner,[13] with permission.)

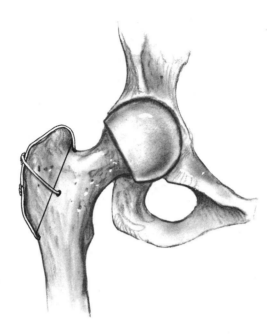

Fig. 19-4. Cup arthroplasty. (From Goldstein and Dickerson,[14] with permission.)

time-buying procedures afforded the adolescent patient a chance at attaining adulthood before more radical reconstructive procedures were indicated.[1,2,4,5]

In a further attempt to avoid massive bony resection, modifications of this basic approach were tested during the 1970s. These procedures have nevertheless fallen by the wayside because of "statistical evidence to support femoral loosening, with or without osteonecrosis of the underlying femoral head, femoral neck fracture and acetabular loosening."[1]

As our understanding grows of what structural configurations of femoral and acetabular implants are best tolerated, and as our technical skill in implantation has progressed, complications of previous total hip arthroplasties showing significant femoral and acetabular loosening, or failure within a 10-year period after the implantation, have certainly lessened significantly. The theoretical and biomechanical benefits of the differing structural designs that a surgeon may choose are many, and are beyond the scope of this chapter. Research and re-evaluation of many of the metals and designs are continuing. No one design is universally accepted. The state of the art and the most accepted practice for total joint arthroplasty remains methylmethacrylate cement fixation for both the femoral and acetabular components.

A routine anterior or posterior approach is utilized. The choice of approach is determined by the technical experience and expertise of the surgeon. Some research supports the notion that posterior approaches are more inclined to result in dislocation posteriorly; however, this is a controversial issue. The anterior approach and the anterior lateral approach are considered to be more technically demanding, however.[4,5,7]

The basic procedure for total hip arthroplasty is as follows. Once the soft tissue exposure to the proximal femur and acetabulum has been accomplished, formal resection of the head and neck is performed. Trochanteric osteotomies were utilized routinely in early total hip arthroplasty procedures. They are now relegated primarily to very complex reconstructive arthroplasty procedures necessitating a wide and extensive exposure, and to revision arthroplasties. Preparation of the proximal femoral medullary canal is performed, and the acetabular articular bony surface is prepared with the appropriate rasping and articular cartilage débridement tools. The methylmethacrylate cement is prepared and placed into the acetabulum, and the acetabulum component is placed in the appropriate angular alignment, closely approximating the true angulation of the anatomic acetabulum.

Once the cement has hardened, the same procedure is performed with respect to the insertion of the femoral component.[4,5,8,9]

Reduction and testing of the structural stability of the hip are performed prior to soft tissue closure. The capsule may or may not be resected or retained. If it is retained, it may or may not be left open or repaired. The soft tissues are approximated in an anatomic fashion.

Postoperative care is as important as the decision of which prosthesis to use. The regimen is determined by the prior training of the operative surgeon and by the surgeon's appreciation of the existing literature. Some surgeons allow upright ambulation without weightbearing or with toe-touch as soon as the patient can tolerate it. Some surgeons suggest a longer period of bed rest. There is a wide area of divergence among surgeons as to when the patient can be weaned off of ambulatory aids. A close relationship with the physical therapist is certainly necessary in these and all cases of ambulatory rehabilitation following surgery. It is imperative that the therapist understand the anatomic approach utilized in the procedure so as best to appreciate what muscles will be temporarily structurally impaired. The physical therapist must also recognize what range of motion will most likely compromise the structural stability of the hip joint. The posterior approach presents the greatest chance of posterior dislocation in an adducted, flexed, and internally rotated position. An anterior approach is most likely to result in anterior dislocation when the hip is adducted, extended, and externally rotated.

It is imperative that the therapist have a thorough understanding of the operative surgeon's goals so as not to confuse the patient during the ambulatory rehabilitative period. During the early 1980s, interest was directed toward modifying the basic total hip design. This interest was based on early evaluations of the initial 10 years' experience of total hip arthroplasty. A review of some of the unhappy findings of our initial experience spurred attempts to avoid the utilization of methylmethacrylate.

Bipolar Reconstructive Prosthesis

The bipolar reconstructive prosthesis allows the physician to implant a proximal femoral replacement of the same type utilized in standard total joint arthroplasty, but to insert a metallic interposition cup into the bony acetabulum with a high-density polypropylene plastic inner bearing to articulate with the metal proximal femoral ball. This type of arthroplasty component system is used by many surgeons. It allows the operative surgeon to use cemented or cementless proximal femoral techniques. It also lets the surgeon avoid destruction of the bony acetabulum and makes possible further reconstructive acetabulum procedures if clinically indicated without compromise of the bony architecture of the acetabulum.[1,2]

Cementless Fixation

During the 1970s, primarily in Europe, research was undertaken to develop a cementless acetabular component that accomplished fixation by the use of large peripheral threads that simply screwed into the bony acetabular architecture. Early follow-up of these components has demonstrated reasonably good results; however, should revision be necessary, the significant loss of acetabular bony architecture necessary to insert one of these components presents formidable problems.

In the early 1980s, interest in the United States centered on development of a porous surface for both acetabular and femoral implant components. A pore diameter of somewhere between 50 and 400 microns was desired. Research into the type of coating and the metal most efficaciously accepted by the human body is still under way. Theoretical excitement about porous implants centered around the body's ability to grow bone from the normal medullary canal through the interstices of the beaded surface, affording a biologically firm interlock.[1,2]

Surgical Revisions

In spite of our attempts to develop better surgical techniques, and to invent enhanced metals and structural designs to afford greater long-term acceptance, total hip arthroplasties intermittently continued to fail for any number of reasons. Failure necessitates re-exploration of the hip joint through a more dramatic approach, virtually always utilizing a trochanteric osteotomy. The failed component is removed, and all of its biologic and nonbiologic fixation tissue is completely excised.

The size of the replacement prosthesis as well as the type of fixation is in a state of continued development. Most revisions use cement and long-stemmed proximal femoral replacements. Yet these continue to show a certain incidence of failure. Investigations are now being directed toward biologic means of fixation. Experience is accumulating in the use of autograft and allograft bone in the form of fresh, fresh-frozen, or freeze-dried bone. The results of this experience are not yet conclusive.[10]

Postoperative care after revision must be critically planned and designed for the unique demands of the patient and the revision devices. A close working relationship and understanding of what has been done must be developed through direct communication between the treating therapist and the operative surgeon.

SUMMARY

More innovative progress has been accomplished in the treatment and care of hip joint disorders over the last 20 years than in any other period of time. The field continues to develop on a year-to-year basis. What seems to be most efficacious one year is not necessarily proven to be so the next. Conclusions with respect to cementless fixation, in both virgin and revision joint arthroplasty, are still premature. However, three points must be understood by the therapist treating a patient after surgery of the hip: First, the therapist must understand why the hip failed to begin with. Second, the therapist must understand what was done surgically and how it was done. Finally, the therapist must have a comfortable professional relationship with the patient and the treating physician. Only then can the therapist offer the patient the greatest chance of achieving a pain-free, quality, ambulatory life.

REFERENCES

1. American College of Orthopaedic Surgeons. Orthopaedic Knowledge Update I. p. 287. American College of Orthopaedic Surgeons, Chicago, 1984
2. American College of Orthopaedic Surgeons. Orthopaedic Knowledge Update II. pp. 357, 383. American College of Orthopaedic Surgeons, Chicago, 1987
3. Enneking WF: Clinical Musculoskeletal Pathology. Storter Printing, Gainesville, Florida, 1986
4. Crenshaw AH: Campbell's Operative Orthopaedics. Vol. II. pp. 1091, 1213. CV Mosby, St. Louis, 1987
5. Crenshaw AH: Campbell's Operative Orthopaedics. Vol. III. p. 1719. CV Mosby, St. Louis, 1987
6. Rockwood CA, Green DP (eds): Fractures in Adults. Vol. II. p. 1211. JP Lippincott, Philadelphia, 1984
7. Hoppenfield S, de Boer P: Surgical Exposures in Orthopaedics. p. 302. JB Lippincott, Philadelphia, 1984
8. Evarts CM: The hip. In Evarts CM (ed): Surgery of the

Musculoskeletal System. Churchill Livingstone, New York, 1983

9. Figgie H: Current Concepts and Total Hip Arthroplasty. Orthopaedic Surgery Update Series. p. 154. Case Western Reserve University, Cleveland, 1986

10. Turner RH, Scheller AO: (eds): Revision Total Hip Arthroplasty. Grune & Stratton, New York, 1982

11. Liechti R: Hip arthrodesis. p. 6:99. In Evarts CM (ed): Surgery of the Musculoskeletal System. Churchill Livingstone, New York, 1983

12. Muller ME: Intertrochanteric osteotomies. p. 6:57. In Evarts CM (ed): Surgery of the Musculoskeletal System. Churchill Livingstone, New York, 1983

13. Wagner H: Surface replacement arthroplasty of the hip. p. 6:401. In Evarts CM (ed): Surgery of the Musculoskeletal System. Churchill Livingstone, New York, 1983

14. Goldstein LA, Dickerson RC: Atlas of Orthopaedic Surgery. 2nd Ed. CV Mosby, St. Louis, 1981

20

Dysfunction, Evaluation, and Treatment of the Knee

ROBERT M. POOLE
TURNER A. BLACKBURN, JR.

ANATOMY OF THE KNEE

The foundation for understanding the knee joint is comprehension of its anatomy. Although individual variations may occur, the functional components of knee anatomy remain unchanged.

Structural Foundation

The knee joint lies between the femur and the tibia, two of the largest and strongest levers in the human body. It is exposed to severe angular and torsion stresses, especially in athletes. The knee is basically a ligament-controlled joint, reinforced by the quadriceps, hamstring, and gastrocnemius muscle groups. These structures provide the main stabilizing influences for the knee joint.[1-3]

The distal end of the femur has an expanded medial and lateral condyle. The proximal end of the tibia is flared to create a plateau with medial and lateral sections to accommodate the medial and lateral femoral condyles (Fig. 20-1). These sections are divided by the tibial spine. Located in the medial and lateral sections are the menisci, which deepen the contour sections to ensure proper contact with the corresponding femoral condyle. The expanded femoral and tibial condyles are designed for weightbearing and to increase contact between the bones. The shape of the femoral condyles is also important in the movement of the tibia on the femur.

In addition to the tibiofemoral joint, there is the patellofemoral joint, which consists of the patella and its articulating surface on the femur. The patella, the largest sesamoid bone in the body, is embedded in the quadriceps tendon. Its location allows greater mechanical advantage for the extension of the knee. The patellar groove on the distal end of the femur covers the anterior surfaces of both condyles and takes the shape of an inverted U (Fig. 20-2). The articular surface of the patella can be divided into a larger lateral part and a smaller medial part, which fit into the corresponding groove on the femur.[4]

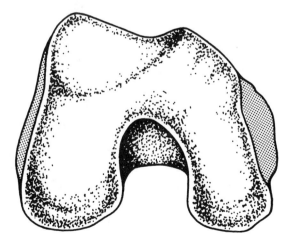

Fig. 20-1. Distal end of femur with expanded medial and lateral condyles.

493

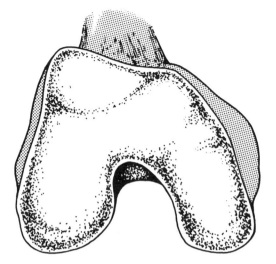

Fig. 20-2. Distal end of femur showing patellar groove and anterior condylar surface.

Extensor Mechanism

The extensor mechanism of the knee consists of the quadriceps femoris muscle, which has four parts: the rectus femoris, the vastus intermedius, the vastus lateralis, and the vastus medialis. The vastus medialis muscle is further divided into the vastus medialis longus and the vastus medialis obliquus (Fig. 20-3A). These muscles come together to form a common tendon that continues from the quadriceps group to the tuberosity of the tibia and is called the ligamentum patellae or patellar tendon. The patella itself is used by the muscles to provide a greater mechanical advantage for the extension of the knee. The articularis genu muscle is also included in the extensor mechanism (Fig. 20-3B). This small muscle is attached to the suprapatellar bursa and synovial membrane of the knee and provides support for these structures during movements of the knee.

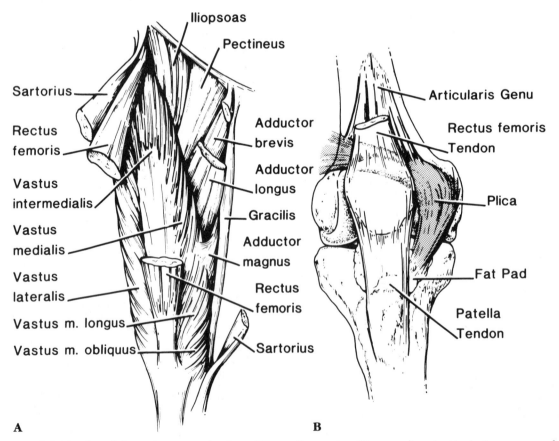

Fig. 20-3. (A) Muscles of the extensor mechanism; **(B)** patellar tendon (ligament) and articularis genu muscle.

Other structures are included in the extensor mechanism. The patellar fat pad lies beneath the patellar tendon running from the inferior pole of the patella to the tibial tubercle. The patellofemoral and patellotibial ligaments, which are thickenings of the extensor retinaculum, also help to cover the anterior portion of the knee and stabilize the patella. The entire knee joint is surrounded by a synovial membrane that is one of the most extensive and complex in the human body (Fig. 20-3).

Medial Compartment

The medial compartment of the knee is supported by the extensor retinaculum and the muscles of the thigh. The pes anserinus group, composed of the sartorius, gracilis, and semitendinosus muscles (Fig. 20-4), crosses the posteromedial aspect of the joint and attaches to the anteromedial part of the tibia at the level of the tibial tubercle. The adductor magnus muscle attaches to the medial femoral condyle at the adductor tubercle. The most important of these stabilizers is the semimembranosus muscle, which has five components; the principal component is attached to the tubercle on the posterior aspect of the medial tibial condyle. The semimembranosus is an important medial stabilizer of the knee; fibers from the other four slips of this muscle

support the posterior capsule and posterior medial capsule, and also attach to the medial meniscus to pull it posteriorly from the joint as the knee flexes[5] (Fig. 20-5).

The C-shaped medial meniscus has an intimate attachment to the capsular ligament along its periphery. The capsular ligaments are divided into meniscofemoral and meniscotibial components.[6] The medial capsular ligaments can be further divided into anterior, middle, and posterior thirds (Fig. 20-6). The posterior third is often referred to as the posterior oblique ligament and is important in controlling anteromedial rotatory instability.[7] Lying superficial to these ligaments is the tibial collateral ligament. It originates at the medial condyle of the femur, medially below the adductor tubercle, and attaches distally to the medial condyle on the medial surface of the shaft of the tibia below the pes anserinus group.

The posterior cruciate ligament is also included in the medial compartment. It has often been referred to as the key to the stability of the knee.[8] It is attached to the posterior intercondylar area of the tibia and to the posterior extremity of the lateral meniscus, passing upward, forward, and medially as a broad band to attach to the lateral surface of the medial condyle of the femur. The ligament is composed of the main posterolateral band and a smaller

Fig. 20-4. Muscles of the pes anserinus group, medial aspect of the knee.

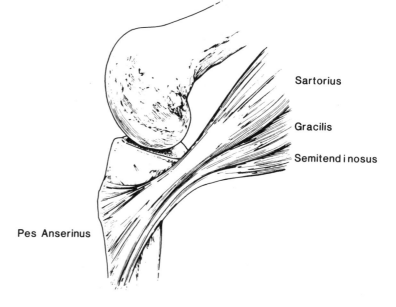

Sartorius

Gracilis

Semitendinosus

Pes Anserinus

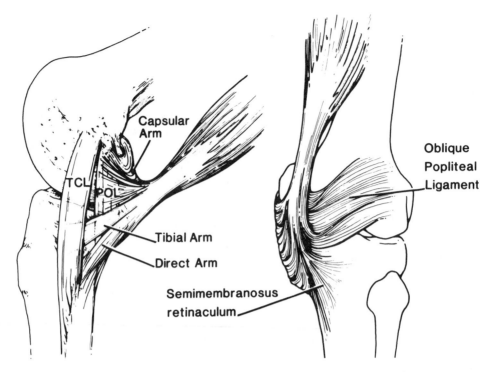

Fig. 20-5. The five components of the semimembranosus muscle.

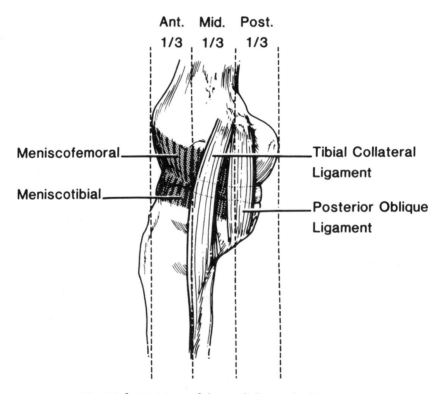

Fig. 20-6. Divisions of the medial capsular ligaments.

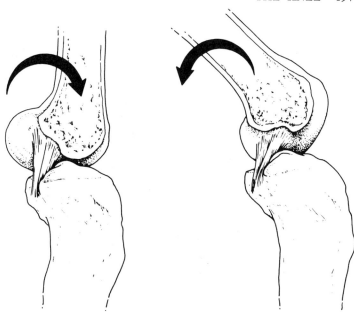

Fig. 20-7. Attachment of the posterior cruciate ligament. The different bundles change in tension as the knee moves from extension to flexion.

anteromedial band. Tension within each band varies as the knee moves from flexion to extension (Fig. 20-7).

Lateral Compartment

The structures of the lateral compartment of the knee are somewhat similar to those of the medial compartment. Muscular support for lateral struc-tures is provided by the tensor fasciae latae, which can be separated into two functional components: the iliopatellar band and the iliotibial tract.[9] These structures attach anterolaterally to Gerdy's tubercle on the lateral aspect of the tibia (Fig. 20-8). Also providing support for the lateral side are the two heads of the biceps femoris. The long head and the short head form a common tendon (lateral ham-string), which splits around the fibular collateral

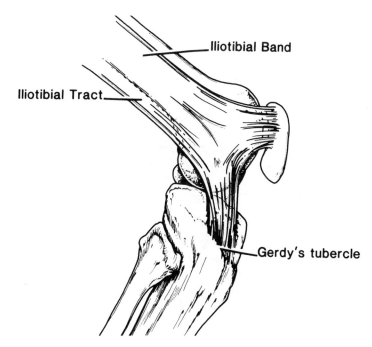

Fig. 20-8. Iliotibial band and iliotibial tract and their attachment to Gerdy's tu-bercle.

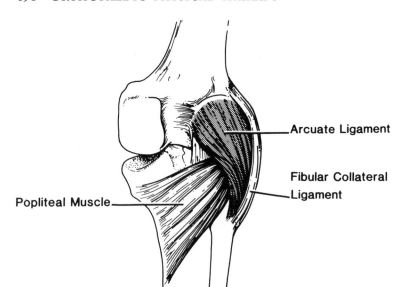

Fig. 20-9. The popliteus muscle forms the deep floor of the popliteal fossa.

ligament and attaches to the head of the fibula.

The triangular and flat popliteus muscle forms the deep floor of the lower part of the popliteal fossa (Fig. 20-9). The larger part of the fossa arises on the lateral condyle of the femur and helps support the fibrous lateral capsule adjacent to the lateral meniscus. The popliteus muscle inserts in the posteromedial edge of the tibia and serves to reinforce the posterior third of the lateral capsular ligament. The fibular collateral ligament appears on the lateral aspect of the knee as a large rounded cord, which is attached to the lateral epicondyle of the femur and below to the head of the fibula; it has no attachment to the lateral meniscus (Fig. 20-10).

The lateral capsular ligaments attach to the lateral meniscus in much the same way that the medial capsular ligaments attach to the medial meniscus. The lateral capsular ligaments can also be divided into meniscofemoral and meniscotibial sections. These can be further subdivided into anterior, medial, and posterior thirds. The middle third of the lateral capsular ligament provides support against

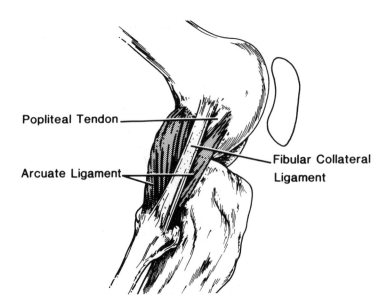

Fig. 20-10. The fibular collateral ligament and the arcuate ligament. Components of the arcuate complex.

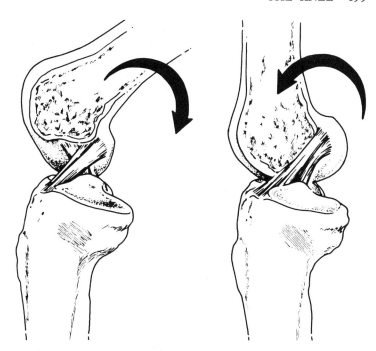

Fig. 20-11. The attachments of the anterior cruciate ligament. The bundles change in tension as the knee moves from flexion to extension.

anterior lateral rotatory instability. The posterolateral third of the lateral compartment is also supported by the arcuate ligament. The arcuate ligament consists of a Y-shaped system of capsular fibers, the stem of which is attached to the head of the fibula. The two branches of the upper portion extend medially to the posterior border of the intercondylar area of the tibia and anteriorly to the lateral epicondyle of the femur (Figs. 20-9, 20-10). Collectively, the posterior third of the lateral capsular ligament, the fibular collateral ligament, the arcuate ligament, and the aponeurosis of the popliteus muscle

are known as the arcuate complex. The arcuate complex provides lateral support for the knee joint.

The anterior cruciate ligament is also included in the lateral compartment. It consists of an anteromedial bundle, an intermediate bundle, and a posterolateral bundle. The anteromedial bundle originates on the posterior superior medial surface of the lateral femoral condyle and inserts on the medial aspect of the intercondylar eminence of the tibia. The posterolateral bundle lies more anterior and distal to the anteromedial bundle on the medial surface of the lateral femoral condyle and inserts later-

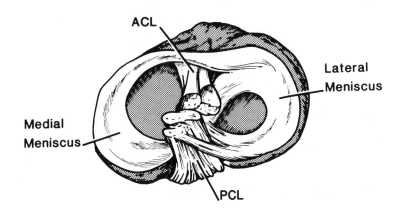

Fig. 20-12. Cross-sectional view of the knee joint showing the medial and lateral menisci and bundles of the anterior and posterior cruciate ligaments.

ally to the midline of the intercondylar eminence. The intermediate bundle lies between these two bundles. Tension on these bundles is altered as the knee moves from flexion to extension (Figs. 20-11, 20-12).

EVALUATION OF THE ACUTELY INJURED KNEE

Evaluation of an acutely injured knee should be completed as soon as possible after injury.[8,10,11] A detailed history and description of the mechanism of injury are vital components of the initial evaluation. It is also very important to complete the evaluation before muscle spasm begins, in order to determine accurately the extent of damage to the knee.

Pain parameters—the existence of pain, the onset of pain, and whether the patient can walk without pain—are good indicators of the extent of injury. Another important indicator is the extent of fluid accumulation in the joint. Fluid accumulation within 2 hours of injury indicates the possibility of a hemarthrosis, which could result from an anterior cruciate ligament tear, an osteochondral fracture, a peripheral meniscus tear, or an incomplete ligament sprain. Fluid accumulation that occurs 24 hours after injury is usually a synovial fluid buildup, which is indicative of meniscal tear, a tear of the capsular lining of the knee joint, or a subluxated fat pad. With a major tear of knee tissues, there is no fluid accumulation; rather the fluid extravasates into the soft tissues. This is usually associated with extensive capsular tears or tears of the posterior cruciate ligament. Palpation of the knee for areas of tenderness or local edema may help to isolate the site of injury. It is always important to establish pulses and the status of sensation around the joint since surrounding neurovascular structures may be damaged in any knee injury.

Diagnostic Tests

Once the history and mechanism of injury have been determined, along with the neurovascular status, there are a number of special tests that should be performed to complete the examination (Table 20-1). All tests should be performed on the normal

Table 20-1. Diagnostic Tests for Knee Instabilities

Instability	Tear	Test
Straight medial	Medial compartment, and posterior cruciate ligament	Abduction stress in full extension
Straight lateral	Lateral compartment and posterior cruciate ligament	Adduction stress in full extension
Straight posterior	Posterior cruciate ligament, posterior oblique, and arcuate complex	Posterior drawer
Straight anterior	Posterior cruciate ligament	Anterior drawer
AMRI	Medial compartment, posterior oblique, anterior cruciate ligament	Abduction stress test at 30 degrees, anterior drawer with external rotation
ALRI	Middle third lateral capsular, anterior cruciate ligament	Anterior drawer in neutral, Adduction stress test at 30 degrees (may be normal or only mildly positive)
PLRI	Arcuate complex	Adduction stress test at 30 degrees, external rotation recurvatum test
Combined ALRI/PLRI	All lateral compartments (with or without iliotibial band)	Anterior and posterior drawer tests in neutral
Combined ALRI/AMRI	Medial and lateral capsular ligaments	Anterior drawer in neutral, abduction/adduction stress tests at 0 degrees, jerk test
Combined ALRI/AMRI/PLRI	Both medial and lateral capsular ligaments	Anterior drawer in neutral, posterior drawer, abduction/adduction stress test at 30 degrees

AMRI, anteromedial rotatory instability; ALRI, anterolateral rotatory instability; PLRI, posterolateral rotatory instability.

knee first. This helps to establish a baseline of stability in a normal joint and helps to gain the patient's confidence and allow him to be more relaxed. The patient should be positioned comfortably supine on the examining table, head down on a pillow and hands relaxed.

Abduction Stress Test

The extremity is slightly abducted at the hip and extended so that the thigh is resting on the surface of the examination table. The knee should be flexed to 30 degrees over the side of the table, with one of the examiner's hands placed on the lateral aspect of the knee while the other hand grasps the foot. A gentle abduction stress is applied to the knee while the examiner's hand on the foot provides a gentle external rotation. By repeating this test in a consistent manner, the examiner can gradually increase the stress up to the point of pain and maximum laxity without producing a muscle spasm. A comparison between the injured and uninjured knee is made. The abduction stress test is always performed with each knee in full extension and in 30 degrees of flexion (Fig. 20-13).

A positive abduction stress test at full extension indicates injury to the posterior cruciate ligament and medial compartment; therefore, a rotatory instability cannot be classified. A negative test at full extension but a positive test at 30 degrees of flexion indicates a tear of the ligaments of the medial compartment, and a diagnosis of anteromedial rotatory instability can be made.

Adduction Stress Test

By simply changing hands, moving the hand to the medial aspect of the knee, and applying an adduction force at both 30 degrees and full extension, the examiner can perform the adduction stress test. A positive adduction stress test at 30 degrees indicates anterolateral rotatory instability (Fig. 20-14).

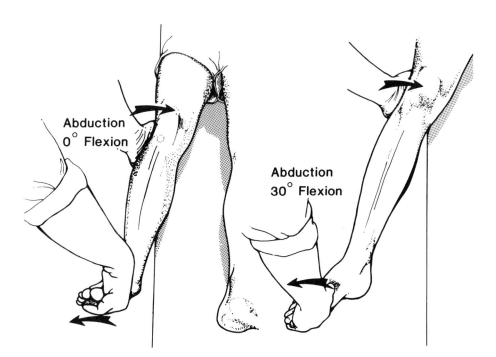

Fig. 20-13. Abduction stress test.

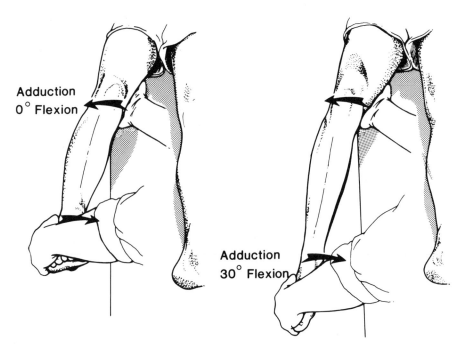

Fig. 20-14. Adduction stress test.

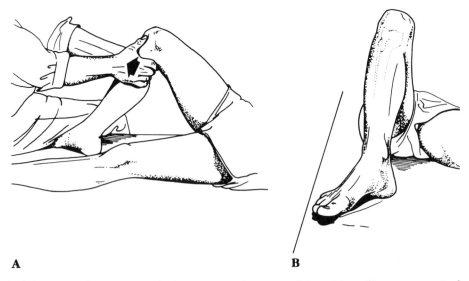

A

B

Fig. 20-15. **(A)** Anterior drawer test with tibia in external rotation; **(B)** position of lower extremity for anterior drawer test with tibia in external rotation.

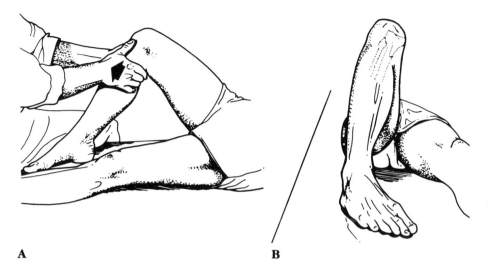

Fig. 20-16. **(A)** Anterior drawer test with tibia in internal rotation; **(B)** position of lower extremity for anterior drawer test with tibia in internal rotation.

Anterior Drawer Test

In the anterior drawer tests, the patient's actively raising his head produces hamstring tightening, which can alter the results of the test. The lower extremity should be flexed at the hip to 45 degrees and the knee flexed to 80 or 90 degrees with the foot flat on the table. The examiner sits on the table, positioning his or her buttocks on the dorsum of the foot to fix it firmly. The examiner's hands are placed about the upper part of the tibia, with the forefingers positioned to palpate the hamstrings to ensure that they are relaxed. The thumbs are positioned at the anterior joint line both medially and laterally. The examiner provides a gentle pull repeatedly in an anterior direction. This test should be performed first with foot and leg externally rotated beyond the neutral position (Fig. 20-15), then internally rotated as much as possible (Fig. 20-16), and finally in the neutral position (Fig. 20-17). Each lower extremity is tested and results are compared.

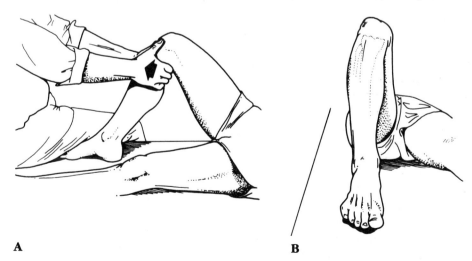

Fig. 20-17. **(A)** Anterior drawer test with tibia in neutral position; **(B)** position of lower extremity for anterior drawer test with tibia in neutral position.

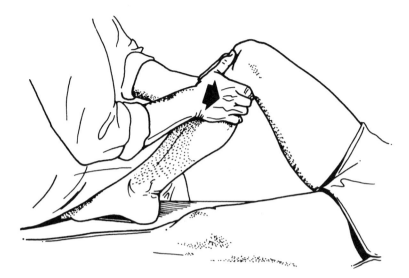

Fig. 20-18. Posterior drawer test for posterolateral instability.

A positive anterior drawer test with the foot in external rotation indicates anteromedial rotatory instability; with the foot in the neutral position a positive test indicates anterolateral rotatory instability, and with the foot in internal rotation a posterior cruciate tear.

Posterior Drawer Test

In the posterior drawer test the hip is flexed to 45 degrees, the knee is flexed to 90 degrees, and the foot is placed flat on the table. Again the examiner sits on the dorsum of the foot to fix it firmly. The hands are positioned so that the middle fingers can palpate the hamstrings; the thumbs are placed along the tibia at the joint line. The examiner pushes straight back gently. Movement of the tibia on the femur is noted with a positive posterior drawer test (Fig. 20-18). A positive posterior drawer sign can often be misinterpreted as a positive anterior drawer sign. For additional clarification of the posterior instability test, a gravity test may be helpful. With the patient supine and the knees together and flexed to approximately 80 degrees, and the feet planted together on the table, posterior displacement of the tibial tuberosity can be seen when viewed from the side (Fig. 20-19A). Another gravity test that may be helpful is the external rotation recurvatum test.[12] The patient's extended legs are lifted together by the toes, and an increase in recurvatum is noted in a positive test (Fig. 20-19B).

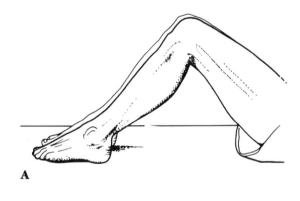

A

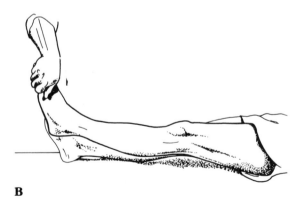

B

Fig. 20-19. **(A)** Gravity test for posterolateral instability; **(B)** external rotation recurvatum test.

Jerk Test

The examiner supports the lower extremity and flexes the hip to about 45 degrees and the knee to 90 degrees while at the same time internally rotating the tibia. If the right knee is being examined, the foot should be in the examiner's right hand internally rotating the tibia while the left hand is placed over the proximal end of the tibia and fibula. The left hand is used to exert a valgus stress. The knee is gradually extended, maintaining the internal rotation and valgus stress. With a positive jerk test, a subluxation of the lateral femoral condyle on the tibia occurs at about 20 degrees of flexion. With further extension, a spontaneous relocation occurs. This relocation is described in engineering terms as a "jerk," which is a sudden change in the rate of acceleration between surfaces. In this case, it would be the change in the velocity of the tibia in relation to the femur (Fig. 20-20). A positive jerk test indicates anterolateral rotatory instability.

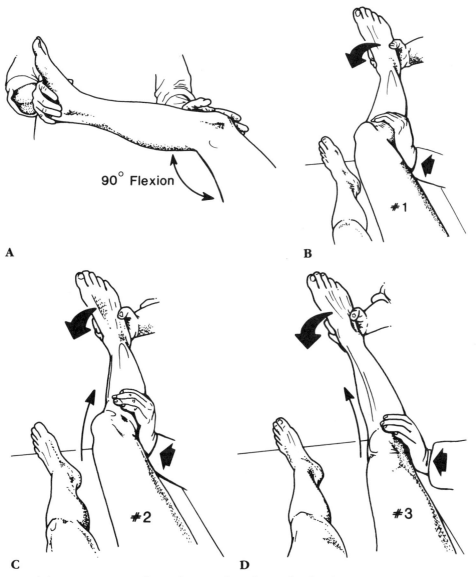

Fig. 20-20. **(A)** Starting position for performing the jerk test; **(B,C)** jerk test sequence; **(D)** ending position of jerk test.

Anterior Drawer-in-Extension Test (Lachman-Ritchey)

The anterior drawer-in-extension test is performed with the patient's knee in approximately 20 degrees of flexion. The examiner uses one hand to stabilize the femur by grasping the distal thigh just proximal to the patella. With the other hand the examiner grasps the tibia distal to the tibial tubercle. A firm pressure is applied to the posterior aspect of the tibia, in an effort to produce an anterior subluxation (Fig. 20-21). This test is one of the most sensitive methods of diagnosing anterior cruciate ligament injury.

CLASSIFICATION OF INSTABILITY

Given the clinical findings of the tests just described, and using the system of classification of knee ligament instabilities of Hughston et al.,[8,13] knee ligament instabilities can be classified as either straight (nonrotatory) or rotatory. Rotatory instabilities may be further subclassified as simple or combined.

Straight Instability

There are four types of instabilities that involve no rotation of the tibia on the femur. They are as follows:

1. Medial instability: a tear in the medial compartment ligaments with an associated tear of the posterior cruciate ligament. It is demonstrated by a positive abduction stress test with the knee in full extension.
2. Lateral instability: a tear in the lateral compartment ligaments and the posterior cruciate ligament. This is demonstrated by a positive adduction stress test with the knee in full extension.
3. Posterior instability: a tear in the posterior cruciate ligament and laxity in both the posterior oblique ligament and the arcuate complex. This is demonstrated by a positive posterior drawer test in which both tibial condyles subluxate posteriorly by an equal amount with no rotation.
4. Anterior instability: a torn anterior cruciate ligament, medial and lateral capsular ligaments, and a torn posterior cruciate ligament. This is demonstrated by a positive anterior drawer sign in which both tibial condyles subluxate anteriorly by an equal amount with no rotation.

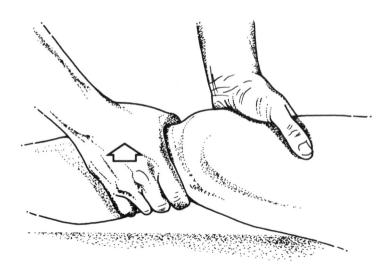

Fig. 20-21. Anterior drawer in extension test.

Simple Rotatory Instability

There are three types of simple rotatory instability. Each demonstrates a rotatory component of the tibia on the femur involving either the medial or the lateral tibial condyle.

1. Anteromedial rotatory instability: a tear of the medial compartment ligaments including the posterior oblique and/or the middle third of the medial capsular ligament. The anterior cruciate ligament may or may not be torn. The abduction stress test at 30 degrees of flexion is positive, as is the anterior drawer test with the tibia externally rotated.
2. Anterolateral rotatory instability: a tear of the middle third of the lateral capsular ligament and possibly the anterior cruciate ligament. It is demonstrated by a positive jerk test and positive anterior drawer test with the tibia in the neutral position. The adduction stress test with the knee at 30 degrees of flexion may be normal or only mildly positive. Lachman test is positive.
3. Posterolateral rotatory instability: a tear of the arcuate complex. The adduction stress test at 30 degrees of knee flexion is positive.

Combined Rotatory Instabilities

Three types of combined rotatory instability have been described.

1. Combined anterolateral and posterolateral instability: a tear of the lateral compartment capsular ligaments, which may or may not include a tear of the iliotibial band. The posterior cruciate ligament remains intact. The posterior drawer test, with the tibia in neutral position, shows that the lateral tibial plateau rotates forward and backward as stress is applied. An adduction stress test with the knee in full extension is positive. What seems to be a straight lateral opening is actually external rotation and posterolateral subluxation with a varus displacement of the knee. An adduction stress test with the knee at 30 degrees of flexion is only mildly positive because of migration of the iliotibial band posteriorly during flexion.
2. Combined anterolateral and anteromedial rotatory instabilities: tears of the medial and lateral capsular ligaments in the middle third. The posterior cruciate ligament again remains intact. The anterior drawer test with the tibia in the neutral position is positive, with both tibial condyles subluxating anteriorly. The anterior drawer test is also positive when performed with the tibia externally rotated. Both abduction and adduction stress tests are positive although they may be only mildly so. The jerk test is also positive.
3. Combined posterolateral, anterolateral, and anteromedial rotatory instability: tears of the lateral capsular ligament, anterior cruciate ligament, arcuate complex, and medial capsular ligaments. In a knee with these lesions, anterior drawer tests with the tibia in the neutral position and in external rotation are positive. A posterolateral drawer test is positive and causes the tibia to rotate externally and backward. Adduction and abduction stress tests are positive with the knee at 30 degrees of flexion, but negative with it at full extension. The jerk test is also positive.

SURGICAL INTERVENTION FOR ROTATORY INSTABILITIES

Surgical treatment of rotatory instability should always be directed toward restoring the normal anatomy by correcting the pathologic anatomy. There are far too many surgical procedures to attempt to review them in this work. Understanding surgical procedures and surgical philosophy provides a starting point for restoring normal function through an effective rehabilitation program in the knee-injured patient.[14]

Basic surgical philosophy mandates the repair of acutely torn structures.[15,16] This may include a direct repair of the anterior cruciate ligament itself or a repair with augmentation. Acute repair of capsular ligaments may also be performed. In chronic situations, extra-articular reconstruction using capsular reefings, tendon transfers, and tenodesis as well as anterior cruciate intra-articular grafts is necessary. These materials may be composed of autografts (the body's own tissue, e.g., the patellar or semitendinosus tendon), allografts (tissue from cadaver sources), or prosthetic tissues (manmade materials, e.g., Gor-tex or LAD).

REHABILITATION FOR KNEES WITH ROTATORY INSTABILITY

With the refinement of diagnostic skills and the addition of complex new surgical techniques, the rehabilitation of knee injuries has become proportionately more complex. Rehabilitation programs should always be based on sound biomechanical principles and directed toward restoring a functionally stable knee that will meet the demands of the patient's sport or activity. Proper strength, flexibility, endurance, proprioception, agility, skill, and speed should be combined in an exercise program to meet this goal.[17,18] Maintenance of strength in the uninjured leg and upper extremity should also be included in any rehabilitation program.[19]

Paulos et al.[20,21] stated two principles of rehabilitation: First, the effects of immobility must be minimized, and second, healing tissues must never be overloaded. Immobility of a joint can lead to contracture, histochemical changes, and a decrease in ligamentous strength. Joint contracture is manifested mechanically in the amount of torque required to move the knee joint. The torque may have to be increased ten times over the force normally required to move the joint. The ligament-bone complex also reacts to immobility. Not only is the ligament itself weakened, but its body attachment has been found to be weakened by as much as 40 percent after only 8 weeks of immobility. Noyes and colleagues[22] found that after 8 weeks of immobization the joint required reconditioning for at least 1 year before 90 percent of strength could be expected to return. Histochemically, a selective atrophy of type I fibers, which are slow-twitch or red muscle fibers, has been shown to decrease total muscle mass by as much as 30 to 47 percent with immobilization.

The second principle concerns protecting the healing tissues from excessive overload. In the early phases of rehabilitation, healing tissues should be protected from abnormal joint displacement, such as twisting or falling on the knee. The second form of common mechanical failure is caused by subjecting the healing tissues to cyclic forces. This causes a fatigue-like failure, which may be avoided by protecting the healing tissues from repetitive complete range of motion. A third form of overload is induced by stretching the healing tissues past their elastic limit. Proper surgical technique is probably the most important means of prevention of this type of ligamentous failure. However, high forces over an extended period of time can produce this type of failure; for example, when extending the knee rapidly from 30 degrees to full extension, an anterior drawer effect creates a strain on the anterior cruciate ligament and weakens the repair if sufficient healing has not occurred. For this reason, it is vitally important to consider the surgical procedure employed along with the other variables when formulating the rehabilitation program.

The patient who has just undergone an intra-articular anterior cruciate ligament reconstruction is placed in a cast brace with extension locked at 30 degrees. As the patient becomes more comfortable, he is allowed more flexion in the brace. Gait is nonweightbearing to touchdown weightbearing for 3 weeks, followed by partial weightbearing to full weightbearing as tolerated. As noted earlier, the patient should be protected from overload of the healing structures. A slow progression is essential to produce a good end result with an intra-articular procedure. Motion can be started as early as possible, and a continuous passive motion (CPM) machine may also be used within the first week. Quadriceps work is limited to 45 degrees of extension in the brace. Straight leg raises, with the patient still in the brace, as well as hip flexion exercises and hamstring curls, may be started during the first week as well. There is a gradual increase in repetition and weight as tolerated.[23] After 3 weeks, the patient is allowed to begin partial weightbearing with the cast brace locked at 10 degrees. The patient may gradually increase weightbearing and wean himself off the crutches over a period of several weeks. Stationary bicycling may begin as soon as tolerated. Straight leg raises, terminal knee extensions, and full arc exercises are started at 3 weeks. Weight is gradually progressed to 10 pounds and maintained until 6 months after surgery.

Three months after surgery the cast brace is discarded, and the patient is placed in a Lenox Hill or a carbon-titanium brace for activity. His activities are progressed with the addition of side step-ups, sitting leg press, and full extensions with low weight as tolerated, depending on the healing restraints of the knee. The patient may also begin swimming in order to increase the endurance of the muscles, and the patient is encouraged to walk to help strengthen and recondition the legs. Walking up and down stairs has been noted to be effective. Running and other advanced activities are allowed as tolerated after 7 months. Isokinetic and functional testing may be used to determine when the operated leg is ready for more functional activity and return to play.

The patient who has undergone an extra-articular reconstruction with iliotibial tract tenodesis may be in a cast for approximately 6 weeks. He is encouraged to do quadriceps setting and active-assisted straight leg raises. Hamstring contraction, co-contraction sets, and ankle pumps are begun as tolerated. Gait is nonweightbearing.

Some patients are placed in a cast brace following extra-articular repair. Motion in the cast brace is limited to from 40 to 70 degrees for the first 3 weeks. After 3 weeks the flexion stop is eliminated, and the patient is allowed to gain as much flexion as possible. At 6 weeks, with the patient still nonweightbearing, active-assisted flexion range-of-motion exercises are begun in an attempt to reach an active flexion of 120 degrees. The patient is encouraged to continue to work on quadriceps setting. Flexion-to-extension exercises at 90 to 45 degrees, with a progressive increase to 5 pounds and the addition of hamstring curls and hip flexion strengthening exercises, are performed in the period from 6 weeks to 12 weeks after surgery.

Twelve weeks after surgery, the patient is encouraged to begin to work on active full extension. Terminal knee extensions, straight leg raises, and other active extension exercises are used to achieve this goal. No passive extension is used. The other exercises continue as well. The patient gradually progresses from partial weightbearing to full weightbearing as tolerated. At full weightbearing, he is allowed to progress to advanced activities such as side step-ups and leg presses. The patient should use a toe-heel gait to encourage extension of the knee. Bicycling and swimming may also start at this

point. At 6 months postsurgery, the patient may begin agility and competitive preparation exercises. These are expected to help the patient progress back to his sport activities and should be designed to be the same type of activities he will use in his sport.

When prosthetic ligaments are used, the biomechanics and healing restraints that normally are a big factor in the postsurgical rehabilitation process are less important. The patient is again placed in a cast brace or a long leg brace, which is locked at 45 degrees for the first 3 days. The patient's gait is nonweightbearing. He is allowed to work on exercises out of the brace and work on active extension with straight leg raises, terminal knee extensions, and flexion-to-extension exercises as well as active-assisted flexion. Hamstring strengthening and hip strengthening begin during the first 3 weeks. After 1 week, the cast brace is reset to minus 15 degrees extension, and partial weightbearing is allowed. At the end of 6 weeks, the brace is returned to full extension. At 12 weeks, the patient is allowed to progress off his crutches but must continue to wear his cast brace until 4 months after surgery. No running is allowed until after muscle strength has returned to 80 percent of normal. Isokinetic testing is again helpful in making this assessment.

For the patient who will return to athletic endeavors, the advanced rehabilitation program should contain functional and specific exercises that will imitate the motions demanded of the patient by his sport. Bicycling is a good means for building endurance and aerobic capacities for the patient who will be returning to an active sport. Straight leg raises should be continued until the patient can lift 10 pounds. Range-of-motion activities should continue until the range of motion in the operated leg is close to that of the normal extremity.

Once 10 pounds of weight can be lifted with a high number of repetitions, various weight machines can be used to supplement the high repetition-low weight program. Hamstring curl and leg press machines are recommended for increasing the bulk of the leg. When an athlete can walk up and down stairs for 30 minutes, ride a bicycle for an hour, and has 80 percent of his quadriceps strength as measured with isokinetic testing, and proper healing has taken place, a running program can be initiated. When the patient can run 2 miles with no swelling, pain, or limp, he can begin to sprint. Once the athlete can sprint at nearly full speed, various cutting activities can be performed. These cutting activities promote agility and should be similar to the situations that the athlete would encounter in his sport.

Proprioception and balance are usually lost following major knee injury and/or surgery. Balancing activities such as standing on one foot with the eyes open and with the eyes closed, and standing on the toes with the eyes opened and eyes closed, should be included in the advanced rehabilitation process.

One other factor is important in the advanced rehabilitation of the athlete. The athlete has to be psychologically ready to return to play. After any major knee injury and subsequent surgery, the rehabilitation process is never complete until the athlete is confident that he can again participate in his sport without being reinjured. A well-planned program of exercise with reasonably set goals will help the athlete to return to his sport with the confidence that he needs to participate without the lingering doubts caused by his previous injury.

The illustrations that follow demonstrate the techniques discussed. As with any exercise program, a great deal depends on communication among the therapist, the surgeon, and the patient. Each must be aware of the biomechanical and healing restraints following an injury, and all must be willing to do their part in order to produce a good result following an injury.

Quadriceps Setting Exercise

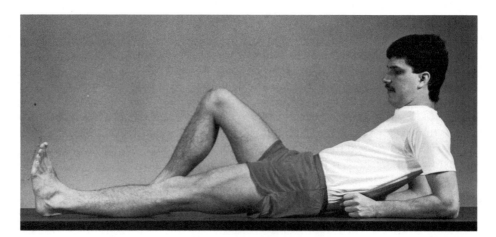

Fig. 20-22. Quadriceps setting exercise. An isometric contraction of the quadriceps muscle. The leg should be straightened as much as possible, and the patella should track proximally. Hold the contraction for at least 5 counts and perform about 50 times per hour.

Straight Leg Raise

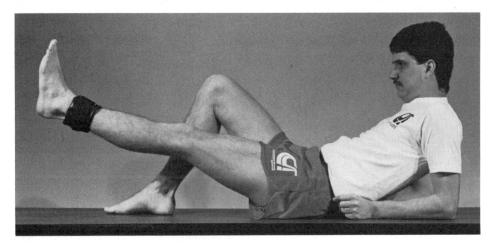

Fig. 20-23. Straight leg raise. The patient is positioned supine with the oposite leg flexed to 90 degrees and the foot planted flat next to the involved knee. The quadriceps muscle is contracted and the leg lifted to approximately 45 degrees and no higher than the thigh of the opposite leg. The leg is held there for at least 5 counts and is then slowly lowered to the floor; relax for at least 2 counts and repeat this exercise. Ten sets of 10 lifts are completed with a 1-minute rest in between each set of 10. Straight leg raises are done 3 times a day. Once the patient can complete 10 sets of 10, 3 times a day, ankle weights are added for resistance. Begin with a 1-pound weight and progress slowly to 5 pounds, still maintaining 10 sets of 10 lifts. Weights are increased according to the patient's tolerance.

Terminal Knee Extension

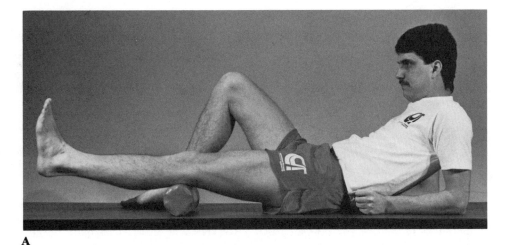

A

Fig. 20-24. Terminal knee extension. A support is placed beneath the knee to be exercised. The quadriceps muscle is again contracted, and the heel is lifted from the floor in a short arc range of motion. Five sets of 10 of this exercise are completed 3 times a day. *(Figure continues.)*

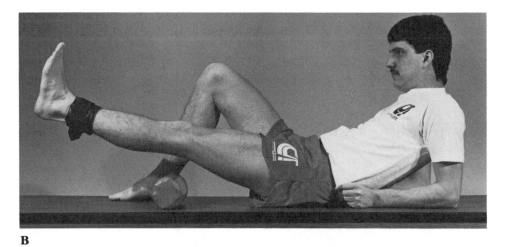

B

Fig. 20-24 *(continued)*. Resistance can be added as tolerated. The terminal knee extension can be incorporated with the straight leg raise to assist in bringing the knee out to full extension.

Hamstring Stretching

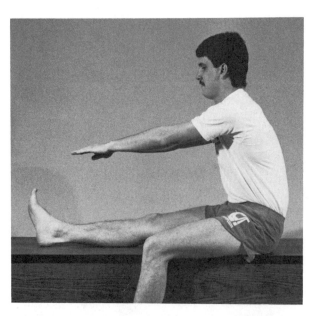

Fig. 20-25. Hamstring stretching. The patient is in a sitting position with one leg off the exercise table. The back is straight, and the leg to be stretched is straight. The patient reaches forward slowly and holds for count of 10. At least 5 minutes of stretching is performed 3 times a day. The patient should be cautioned not to bounce when stretching.

Hamstring Curls

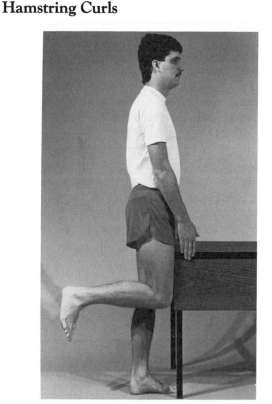

Fig. 20-26. Hamstring curls. The patient stands with the thigh pressed against a wall or table to block hip flexion. The knee is flexed to its maximum position and held for a count of 5. The foot is then lowered to the floor. Five sets of 10 of this exercise are done 3 times a day. Resistance can be added progressively according to the patient's tolerance from 1 to 5 pounds.

Active Range of Motion for Flexion

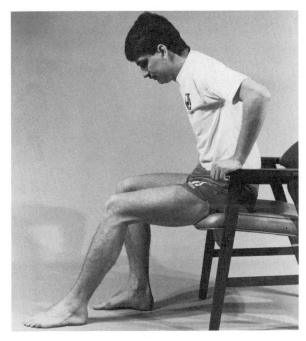

Fig. 20-27. Active range of motion for flexion. The patient is seated with feet flat on the floor. The injured leg is allowed to actively slide back along the floor, keeping the foot flat on the floor. The foot is planted, and the hips are allowed to slide forward over the affected leg, providing some extra stretch. This exercise may be repeated 30 times, 3 times a day. The stretch is held for at least a count of 10.

Flexion-to-Extension Exercise

Fig. 20-29. Flexion-to-extension exercise. The starting position is with the patient sitting with feet resting on the floor. The knee is then extended and held in as full extension as possible for a count of 5 and then gently lowered to the floor. This exercise can be repeated up to 10 sets of 10, 3 times a day. Resistance can be added as tolerated, from 1 to 5 pounds.

Hip Flexion Exercise

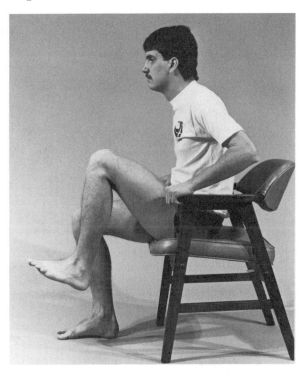

Fig. 20-28. Hip flexion exercise. The patient is sitting with feet resting on the floor. The knee is lifted toward the chest at a 45 degree angle and held there for a count of 5. The knee is lowered gently, and the foot is placed on the floor. Five sets of 10 repetitions of this exercise are done 3 times a day, and resistance can be added at the knee as the patient tolerates it, from 1 to 5 pounds.

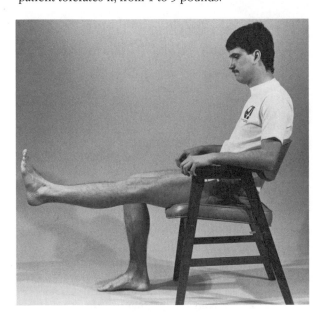

Hip Abduction Exercises

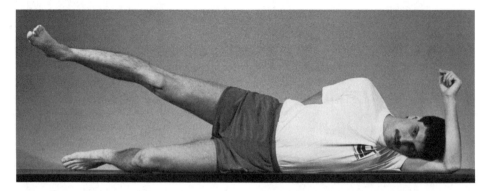

Fig. 20-30. Hip abduction exercises. The patient is positioned side-lying with the unaffected knee flexed to 90 degrees and the hip flexed at 45 degrees. The affected leg is straight, and the body weight is shifted forward. The leg is lifted and held for a count of 5 and gently lowered back to the starting position. Resistance can be added at the ankle, from 1 to 5 pounds. This exercise should be done in 5 sets of 10, 3 times a day.

Adductor Stretching

Heel Cord Stretching

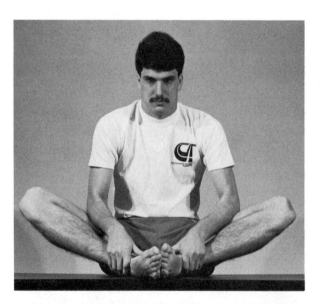

Fig. 20-31. Adductor stretching. The patient should sit with the soles of the feet together and slide them back toward the buttocks as far as possible. With the elbows positioned on the leg, the patient pushes down toward the floor and holds for a count of 10. This should be repeated for approximately 5 minutes, 3 times a day.

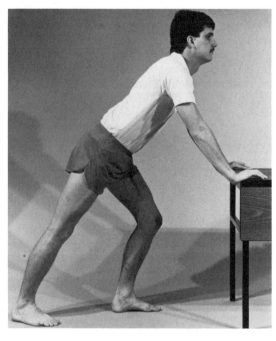

Fig. 20-32. Heel cord stretching. The patient stands with the toes slightly pointed in and the heels on the floor. The knees are kept straight. The patient leans forward, stretching the muscles. The stretch should be held for a count of 10 and repeated for 5 minutes, 3 times a day. The soleus muscle can also be stretched in this position.

Adduction Leg Raise

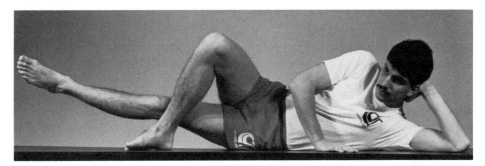

Fig. 20-33. Adduction leg raise. The patient is again side-lying with the affected leg against the table. The leg is lifted into adduction and held for a count of 5. This exercise can be repeated in 5 sets of 10 and resistance added as tolerated, from 1 to 5 pounds.

Quadriceps Femoris Stretching

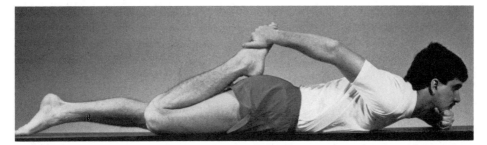

Fig. 20-34. Quadriceps femoris stretching. The patient is positioned prone, and the heel is pulled toward the buttocks. The position is held for a count of 10 and then released. The patient should stretch for 5 minutes, 3 times a day.

Hip Flexor Stretching

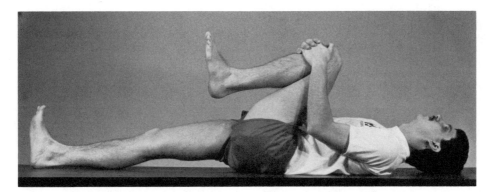

Fig. 20-35. Hip flexor stretching. With the patient lying supine, one knee is pulled toward the chest while the opposite leg is held as straight as possible. The patient should hold this stretch for a count of 10 and then release; 5 minutes, 3 times a day is preferred.

Exercise Bicycling

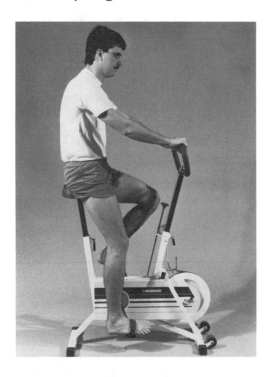

Fig. 20-36. Use of the exercise bicycle is a good method to increase endurance, strength, and range of motion for knee-injured patients. The patient should be positioned on the bicycle with a high seat, with about a 15 degree bend in the knee when the foot is at the bottom of the pedal stroke. Toe clips can be used to help exercise both the quadriceps and the hamstring muscles. The patient should progress from 10 minutes at minimum resistance to 1 hour twice a day.

Side Step-up

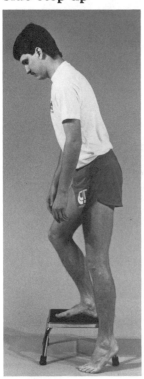
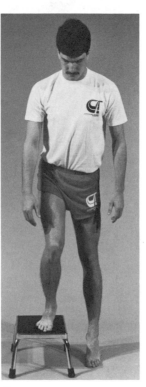

A   B

Fig. 20-37. Side step-up. The patient should stand sideways with the involved foot flat on a step. The body weight is lifted with the involved leg. The patient is allowed to push off with his uninvolved foot. Once the patient is able to complete this exercise 100 times once a day, the patient is progressed from a 4-inch step to a 7-inch step.

Side Step-up

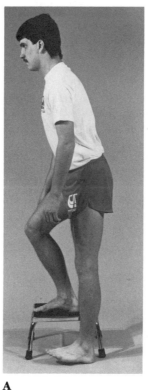
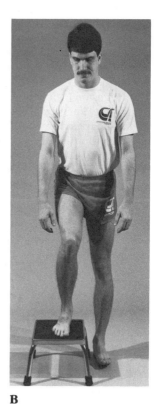

Fig. 20-38. Side step-up. The progression of the side step-up exercise shows the patient again standing with his involved leg on the step; however, in this exercise, he is now allowed to push off with his uninvolved foot. He must push off with the uninvolved heel touching the floor only. Again, 100 of these exercises, or 10 sets of 10, should be done once a day.

A   **B**

ACKNOWLEDGMENTS

The authors would like to thank Carol Capers for her illustrations and Kathy Scrantom for her photography, which add so much to this work; also Margaret Anderson, Betty Clements, and Carol Binns for their technical expertise in research; and Dr. Carol Walker for the motivation to write.

REFERENCES

1. Blackburn T, Craig E: Knee anatomy: a brief review. Phys Ther 60:1556, 1980
2. Harty M, Joyce J: Surgical anatomy and exposure of the knee joint. p. 206. In AAOS Instructional Course Lectures. Vol. 20. CV Mosby, St. Louis, 1971
3. Kaplan E: Some aspects of functional anatomy of the human knee joint. Clin Orthop 23:18, 1962
4. Williams P, Warwick R, (eds): Gray's Anatomy. 36th Ed. Churchill Livingstone Company, Edinburgh, 1980
5. Brantigan O, Voshell A: The mechanics of the ligaments and menisci of the knee joint. J Bone Joint Surg 23:1, 1941
6. Heller L, Langman J: The meniscofemoral ligaments of the human knee. J Bone Joint Surg 46:2, 1964
7. Hughston J, Eilers A: The role of the posterior oblique ligament in repairs of acute medial collateral ligament tears of the knee. J Bone Joint Surg 55:5, 1973
8. Hughston J, Andrews J, Cross M, Moschi A: Classification of knee ligament instabilities. Part I. The medial compartment and cruciate ligaments. J Bone Joint Surg 58:2, 1976
9. Terry G, Hughston J, Norwood L: The anatomy of the iliopatellar band and iliotibial tract. Am J Sports Med 14:1, 1986
10. Bonnarens F, Drez D: Clinical examination of the knee for anterior cruciate ligament laxity. In Jackson D, Drez D (eds): The Anterior Cruciate Deficient Knee. CV Mosby, St. Louis, 1987

11. Hughston J: Acute knee injuries in atheletes. Clin Orthop 23:114, 1962

12. Hughston J, Norwood L: The posterolateral drawer test and external rotational recurvation test for posterolateral rotatory instability of the knee. Clin Orthop 147:82, 1980

13. Hughston J, Andrews J, Cross M, Moschi A: Classifications of knee ligament instabilities. Part II. The lateral compartment. J Bone Joint Surg 58:173, 1976

14. Hughston J: Knee surgery. A philosophy. Phys Ther 60:63, 1980

15. Hughston J, Barrett G: Acute anteromedial rotatory instability: Long term results for surgical repair. J Bone Joint Surg 65:2, 1983

16. Hughston J, Bowden J, Andrews J, et al: Acute tears of the posterior cruciate ligament. Results of operative treatment. J Bone Joint Surg 62:438, 1980

17. Blackburn T: Rehabilitation of anterior cruciate ligament injuries. Orthop Clin North Am 16:241, 1985

18. Montgomery J, Steadman J: Rehabilitation of the injured knee. Clin Sports Med 4:333, 1985

19. Malone T, Blackburn T, Wallace L: Knee rehabilitation. Phys Ther 66:54, 1980

20. Paulos L, Noyes F, Grood E, et al: Knee rehabilitation after anterior cruciate ligament reconstruction and repair. Am J Sports Med 9:140, 1981

21. Paulos L, Payne F, Rosenburg T: Rehabilitation after anterior cruciate ligament surgery. p. 291. In Jackson D, Drez D (eds): The Anterior Cruciate Deficient Knee. CV Mosby, St. Louis, 1987

22. Noyes F, Torvik P, Hyde W, et al: Biomechanics of ligament failure. II. An analysis of immobilization, exercise, and reconditioning effects in primates. J Bone Joint Surg 56:1406, 1974

23. Delorme T: Restoration of muscle power by heavy resistance exercise. J Bone Joint Surg 27:645, 1945

21
Surgery of the Knee

RICK HAMMESFAHR

The methods for successfully treating knee injuries have undergone rapid change in the last several years. With advances in research have come new surgical procedures, a better understanding of the function of the knee, and new approaches to the rehabilitation of knee injuries. Fifteen years ago, who would have suspected that the philosophy of orthopaedic medicine would shift to emphasize the simultaneous healing and rehabilitation of an injury? Because of this change in philosophy, it is now essential that orthopaedic surgeons have an understanding of biomechanics and an understanding of physical therapy. It is equally important that the therapist have a better understanding of matters that have traditionally been the domain of the orthopaedic surgeon. Since aggressive therapy protocols are now routinely being prescribed in the early postoperative period, it is incumbent upon the therapist to have a basic understanding of the healing process, of biomechanics, and of the many factors that affect the outcome of any injury. In the past, when physical therapy was instituted only after satisfactory healing had occurred, the likelihood of therapy-induced injuries was very low. This is no longer true. This chapter describes the biomechanics of the knee and enumerates some of the concerns that orthopaedists have during the period of combined healing and therapy.

The orthopaedic literature is replete with confusing and contradictory statements concerning the effect of meniscectomy on the knee. At one extreme is the dire prediction that degenerative joint disease is the inevitable result if total meniscectomy is not performed for a meniscal tear. Other reports indicate that meniscectomy is a benign procedure because the meniscus is a vestigial remnant of muscle serving no function. Sutton in 1897 described the meniscus as the functionless remains of the leg muscle.[1] As late as the mid-1970s, when the five-in-one reconstruction for knee instability was described, the meniscus was sacrificed to provide exposure, as no long-term complication was anticipated from its loss.[2]

The longevity of meniscectomy has often been questioned. Smilley stated that total excision of a meniscus is invariably followed by replacement with a structure consisting of fibrous tissue that is almost a replica of the original.[3] Sir Robert Jones noted that "in cases that have come to me with a history of removal of a cartilage, I have found no trace of any new structure even ten years after the operation."[4]

Into this confusing picture of meniscal excision, regrowth, and function are introduced the relatively new concepts of partial meniscectomy and repair. This chapter reviews the mechanical function of the meniscus, the biomechanical alterations of total and subtotal meniscectomy, and the vascular basis for repair.

FUNCTIONS OF THE MENISCUS

The meniscus is a biconcave (C-shaped) fibrocartilaginous piece of tissue interposed between the tibia and the femur (Fig. 21-1).[5] It is now realized that the menisci are integral components of the complex biomechanics of the knee.

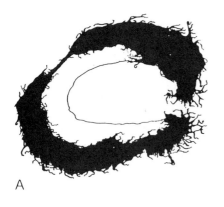

A

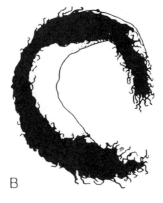

B

Fig. 21-1. Superior view of the medial **(A)** and lateral **(B)** meniscus. The general shape of the medial aspect is oval; the lateral aspect is rounder. The vascular supply of the peripheral margins extends into the horns. (From Mangine and Price,[57] with permission.)

Stability

Because of their triangular cross-sectional geometry, the menisci are deep in the tibia and render the knee joint more congruous to the bulbous femoral condyles.[6] Therefore, stability of the knee increases in both the anteroposterior and the rotatory plane.[7] Cadavers with an intact anterior cruciate ligament had a 14 percent increase in rotatory laxity after medial and lateral meniscectomy.[8]

Instability depends on many factors: muscular coordination, joint laxity, and joint geometry. All are altered after meniscectomy. Although coordination may be restored with rehabilitation, the altered joint geometry is permanent, as are the changes of joint laxity. Studies indicate that the effect of meniscectomy on joint laxity depends on the presence of concomitant knee ligament injuries.[9–13] The study by Levy et al.[12] nicely demonstrated the effects of meniscectomy on anteroposterior stability of the knee. Briefly, anterior drawer tests were performed on knees that had undergone meniscectomies and anterior cruciate ligament sectioning, in different combinations. Whereas loss of anterior cruciate ligament integrity increased laxity in the anteroposterior plane, meniscectomy failed to do so in the presence on an intact anterior cruciate ligament. This demonstrates that the primary function of the anterior cruciate ligament is to resist anterior laxity. However, when the anterior cruciate ligament was sectioned and meniscectomies were performed, laxity greatly increased. This finding indicates a poor prognosis for the patient with an anterior cruciate ligament-deficient knee who undergoes meniscectomy, and implies a secondary role of the meniscus in stability of the knee.[12]

Lubrication and Nutrition

The meniscus also is involved in the lubrication[14] and nutrition[15] of the knee. The meniscus has been demonstrated to act as a spacer between the tibia and the femur, so that actual tibiofemoral contact is decreased. This is reflected by a 20 percent rise in the coefficient of friction between the tibia and the femur after meniscectomy.[16] MacConaill has stated that the menisci aid in joint lubrication.[14] Radin and Bryan stated that the menisci may help spread synovial fluid, but joint motion alone would probably suffice.[17] It has been postulated that prolonged contact between the articular surfaces would interfere with the diffusion of nutrients from the synovial fluid.[18] The work of Lutfi pointed out the increased proximity of the femoral and tibial articular surfaces after meniscectomy. He felt that it was reasonable to assume that there was increased friction between the opposing articular surfaces.[19]

Protection of Synovial Tissue

It has been postulated that the spacer effect of the meniscus also serves to prevent synovial tissue impingement.[20]

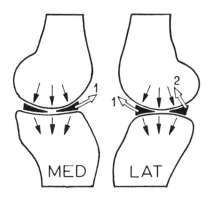

Fig. 21-2. Extension buffer action of the meniscus. (From Kapandji,[58] with permission.)

Extension Buffer

With extension, the anterior horns go forward, acting as buffers to hyperextension and dampening the pendulum effect of the leg during the swing-through phase of gait (Fig. 21-2).[20]

Shock Absorption

Undoubtedly the most controversial role of the meniscus is that of shock absorption; its importance has only been proven lately.[21-23] As early as 1948, Fairbank noted radiographic changes after meniscectomy including (1) narrowing of the joint space, (2) flattening of the femoral condyles, and (3) osteophyte formation. He attributed these changes to the loss of the weightbearing function of the menisci (Fig. 21-3).[24]

BIOMECHANICAL ALTERATIONS IN MENISCUS REPAIR

Shrive demonstrated loss of weightbearing function by placing a cadaveric knee in a compressive machine and measuring the joint space narrowing before and after meniscectomy. His work demonstrated the intact knee to have a joint space of 1 mm at a pressure of two body weights. With a medial and lateral meniscectomy, the narrowing doubled.[25]

This narrowing is due to two different mechanical functions: (1) loss of spacer action allowing tibiofemoral contact, and (2) reduction in the contact area with the absence of the meniscus.[26] When the cartilage is removed, the contact area drops to 40 percent of normal. The larger contact area with the intact meniscus results in decreased contact stress (contact force/contact area) on the articular cartilage. By decreasing the contact stress and increasing the contact area, the menisci lower stress in the articular cartilage, preventing mechanical damage to chondrocytes and the matrix; thus, after meniscectomy, there is increased stress due to decreased contact area.[21,22,27]

Fukabayashi used pressure-sensitive films to measure the contact stresses of the knee. With increasing load, the contact area of the knee increases. However, after meniscectomy, the overall contact area decreased relative to the normal knee.[21,27] This study supports Seedhom's hypothesis that the increased stress after meniscectomy is due to an applied force acting only in the decreased contact area.[23]

To understand the effects of partial meniscec-

Fig. 21-3. Load distribution function of the meniscus. **(A)** The contact area and stress with an intact meniscus. **(B)** The reduced areas of contact and stress after meniscectomy, which lead to increased deformation of the articular cartilage and eventual flattening of the bony condyles. (From Mangine and Price,[57] with permission.)

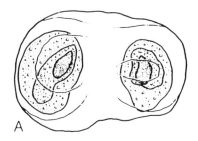
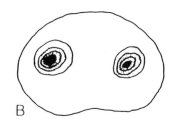

tomy as it affects load transmission across the remaining meniscus and hence the joint, it is necessary to understand the structural anatomy of the meniscus.[28,29] The majority of collagen fibers are oriented circumferentially. Bullough's studies of meniscal strength show the largest strength in samples elongated parallel to fiber direction. When a force is applied perpendicular to the fiber direction, the strength of the meniscus decreases to less than 10 percent because collagen fibers function primarily to resist tensile forces along the direction of the fibers (i.e., circumferentially).[30]

The compression of the menisci by the tibia and the femur generates forces that act outward to push the menisci out from between the bones.[25] This outward force is counteracted by the circumferential or hoop tension that develops in the meniscus. These hoop forces are transmitted to the tibia through the strong anterior and posterior attachments of the menisci. In addition, the extra-articular tissues (capsule, collateral ligaments, etc.) aid in keeping the meniscus in place (Fig. 21-4). These tissues offer a force opposite in direction to that of the outward component of the compressive force. The constraining action of the tissues prevents the menisci from popping out of place when the joint is compressed. Thus, the hoop tension appears to be only one factor in securing the menisci so that they

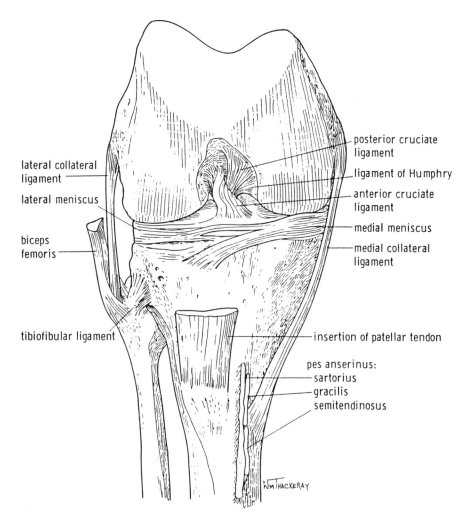

Fig. 21-4. Partially dissected knee joint, showing the location of the ligaments and meniscus. **(A)** Anterior view. **(B)** Posterior view. (From Insall,[59] with permission.)

lateral collateral ligament

lateral meniscus

biceps femoris

tibiofibular ligament

posterior cruciate ligament

ligament of Humphry

anterior cruciate ligament

medial meniscus

medial collateral ligament

insertion of patellar tendon

pes anserinus:
sartorius
gracilis
semitendinosus

WmThackeray

A

may transmit the compression forces applied to each other, and in fact these two systems function in conjunction with one another.[25,26,30]

Shrive has reported that the hoop tension is lost when a single radial cut is made out to the capsular margin,[25] and that a single radial cut through the meniscus is equivalent to a meniscectomy in load-bearing terms. With the menisci intact, the joint load is transmitted through the meniscus and through direct contact between the cartilage surfaces. When a radial cut is made, the meniscus expands because of the loss of the hoop tension force, allowing the compression force to be transmitted through direct cartilage contact. Thus, in performing a subtotal me-

niscectomy, it is obvious that preservation of the meniscal rim becomes very important in preventing articular cartilage pressure. Confirming this is the further work of Ahmed and Burke,[28] who studied the contact stresses for a bucket handle tear where the peripheral rim is left intact. Contour maps, which reflect the tibiofemoral contact stresses, indicate that an undisplaced bucket handle tear functions similarly to an intact meniscus as long as the bucket handle fragment remains in a normal anatomic position (Fig. 21-5). However, the contour map of the meniscus following removal of the bucket handle portion indicates that there is an increase in contact stress. This stress is not as great as the increase noted

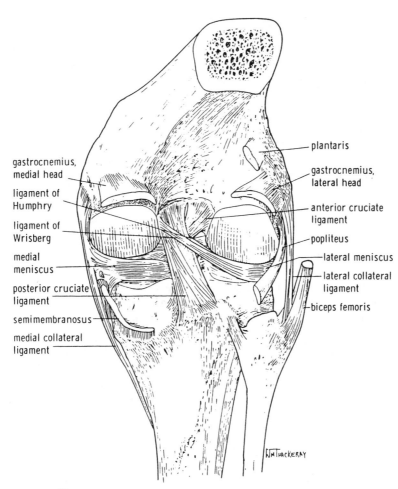

gastrocnemius, medial head

ligament of Humphry

ligament of Wrisberg

medial meniscus

posterior cruciate ligament

semimembranosus

medial collateral ligament

plantaris

gastrocnemius, lateral head

anterior cruciate ligament

popliteus

lateral meniscus

lateral collateral ligament

biceps femoris

B

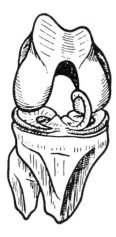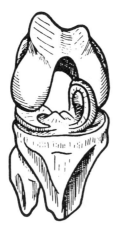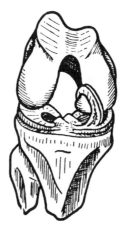

Fig. 21-5. Bucket handle tear. (From Kapandji,[58] with permission.)

after a total meniscectomy. They concluded that the remaining portion of the meniscus continues to transmit contact forces.[28]

In summary, then, the menisci do in fact serve an important function in the knee, and by increasing the contact area, the menisci reduce contact stresses, thus protecting the joint articular cartilage.[31] Meniscal function depends upon the circumferential hoop tension and the extra-articular tissues that anchor the menisci.[25] Partial segmental meniscectomy, which disrupts the rim, also destroys the hoop tension, thus reducing the ability of the menisci to perform their weightbearing function.[25] If this loss of function is combined with an injury to the capsule and collateral ligaments, then function may be totally lost as the meniscus is partially displaced toward the peripheral aspect of the knee.

A partial meniscectomy, in contrast, leaves a rim of tissue in place and maintains significant stress protection for the articular cartilage.[21,25,27,31] A total meniscectomy, in the absence of regeneration, is associated with increased cartilage degeneration, alterations in bone geometry, joint narrowing, and osteophyte formation.[19,24] Thus, we have set the stage for exploring the possibility of doing something to preserve the meniscus rather than just doing a partial meniscectomy. Obviously, what we are about to explore is the possibility of meniscal repair.

VASCULAR BASIS FOR MENISCUS REPAIR

The vascular supply to the medial and lateral portions of the knee originates predominantly from the medial and lateral genicular arteries. Branches from these vessels give rise to a perimeniscal capillary plexus with the synovial and capsular tissues of the knee joint.[32,33] This plexus is a network of vessels that supplies the peripheral border of the meniscus throughout its attachment to the joint capsule (Fig. 21-1). These perimeniscal vessels are oriented in a predominantly circumferential pattern paralleling the collagen fibers, with radial branches directed toward the center of the joint.[32] Anatomic studies have shown that the degree of peripheral vascular penetration is 10 to 30 percent of the width of the medial meniscus and 10 to 25 percent of the width of the lateral meniscus, except for the posterolateral corner of the lateral meniscus, which has an absence of vessels at the popliteus hiatus.[32]

The vascular supply of the meniscus is an essential element in determining its potential for repair. Of equal importance is the ability of this blood supply to support the inflammatory response that is characteristic of wound repair. Recent papers have demonstrated that the peripheral meniscal vascular supply is capable of producing a reparative response similar to that seen in other connective tissues.[34]

Following injury within the peripheral vascular zone, the normal healing response occurs with a fibrin clot forming. The clot, rich in inflammatory cells, allows blood vessels from the capillary plexus to proliferate through this fibrinous scaffold. Eventually, the lesion is filled with a cellular fibrovascular scar tissue, which holds the wound edges together and appears continuous with the adjacent normal meniscal fibrocartilage. The vessels from the capillary plexus as well as a proliferative vascular pannus from the synovial fringe penetrate the fibrous scar to provide a marked inflammatory response with subsequent healing. Experimental studies in animals have shown that complete radial lesions of the meniscus are completely healed with fibrovascular scar tissue by 10 weeks.[34,35] However, the conversion of the scar tissue into normal-appearing fibrocartilage requires several months.

The ability of these lesions to heal has provided the rationale for repair of peripheral meniscal injuries. Early reports indicate excellent results following primary or delayed repair of these very peripheral lesions. Postoperative arthroscopic examination reveals a process of repair similar to that noted in the animal models.[35-37]

Mulholland has advocated recognizing the zonal system of vascularity when evaluating a torn meniscus for possible repair. Zone I tears have a vascular supply to both sides of the tear; hence their classification of "red-on-red." Zone II lesions have a vascular supply on only one side and are therefore termed "red-on-white." A "white-on-white" tear is one that is completely avascular, and constitutes a zone III injury.[38] Initial enthusiasm for repair was limited to those zone I lesions that had a definite vascular supply. Later, it became apparent that lesions in zone II could also be repaired. However, exciting experimental evidence indicates that lesions in zone III, the avascular area, can also be repaired, assuming some means of vascular access to the area is provided.[34] Experimental and clinical observations show that if the longitudinal lesions and the avascular portion of the meniscus are connected to the peripheral vasculature by a vascular access channel, then these lesions are capable of healing through a

process of fibrovascular scar proliferation similar to that described earlier in this chapter. Using Arnoczky's technique, a full-thickness vascular access channel was made at the midportion of the longitudinal lesion, connecting it with the vessels of the perimeniscal capillary plexus. These vessels are then able to proliferate through the vascular access channels into the lesion, filling it with a fibrovascular scar tissue.[34]

A number of studies have investigated the feasibility of a peripheral meniscal repair. One of the more recent by Gillquist indicates that there is a 20 percent retear rate following meniscal repair.[37] In his series, 8 percent of the patients retore the meniscus at the site of the original repair. Three of these four patients had an untreated deficiency of the anterior cruciate ligament. An additional 4 percent (two patients) sustained a second tear at a site removed from the original repair. An additional 8 percent (four patients) sustained a new tear at the site of the healed tear. When Gillquist further analyzed the tears by the time from the tear to surgery, he discovered that among the tears greater then 2 weeks old there was an overall retear rate of 20 percent, with 11 percent being reruptures and 9 percent new tears. When the acute tears (less than 2 weeks old) were analyzed, only 1 of 15 cases sustained a new tear, and this was at a site distant from the original repair.[37] Thus, it is reasonable to expect that there is a role for partial meniscectomy and also for peripheral repair.

IMPLICATIONS FOR REHABILITATION IN MENISCECTOMY AND MENISCAL REPAIR

It becomes important to understand the potential for meniscal repair, the differences between meniscal repair and meniscectomy, and how a patient's rehabilitation is affected by the type of procedure performed. Unfortunately, the exercises used during a standard postmeniscectomy knee rehabilitation program are often detrimental to a meniscal repair. Because the mechanical clearances within the knee are very small, no abnormal motion can be tolerated in the healing meniscus, as this motion may be disruptive to the success of the repair. The site of the meniscal repair must heal without any abnormal laxity. Since the menisci have a normal anteroposterior excursion with knee motion, a full range of motion may place undue stress upon the sutures and the repair site. Thus the "scar" may elongate, allowing for failure of the repair.[39,40] Weightbearing, because of the transmission loads at the menisci, likewise may allow for enough microscopic motion to interfere with adequate healing. Postoperative serous effusions may be the result of several different factors, acting individually or in unison. Among the factors responsible for this phenomenon are an overly aggressive rehabilitation program, postoperative inflammatory synovitis, or an overuse synovitis. The result is an increase in the enzymes that are responsible for clot lysis. The normal healing response requires blood clot formation at the repair site for subsequent differentiation to fibrous scar tissue. Therefore any event that promotes the dissolution of a blood clot would be disruptive to the meniscal repair.

Similarly, if range-of-motion exercises are initiated too early, or if an aggressive knee manipulation program is instituted, the stresses placed upon the sutures or the suture line may disrupt healing.

Specific rehabilitation programs are covered in Chapter 20. It is imperative that the therapist approach each patient with the goal of individualizing that patient's rehabilitation program. For the therapist to do this successfully, an understanding of the biomechanics of the joint, of the healing process, and of the biomechanics of the rehabilitation program is absolutely essential. Not only must these factors be understood and taken into consideration for the specific site of injury, but they must also be recognized for other areas around the knee. It does no good to have a successful surgical procedure, such as a meniscal repair, if the patient develops another problem. One of the more common disorders that becomes symptomatic after any type of knee injury is a patellofemoral pain syndrome. But why does this happen?

Perhaps the patient had pre-existing subclinical asymptomatic chondromalacia, which became symptomatic because of the injury-induced quadri-

ceps atrophy. It is important that any rehabilitation program also be directed at preventing the development of patellofemoral pain syndromes, lateral facet syndromes, symptomatic medial plicas, chondromalacia, or other problems.

There is no reason why a patient should not be placed on a rehabilitation program that incorporates the appropriate therapy for the treatment, or for the prevention, of patellofemoral disease. It has been shown that a significant majority of the patellofemoral pain syndromes stem from a biomechanical abnormality.[41] The quadriceps atrophy leads to increased patellofemoral contact stresses, the minimal lateral subluxation of the patella secondary to vastus medialis obliquus (VMO) atrophy, the resultant alteration in the facet contact forces and the facet articular cartilage nutrition. The persistent lateral subluxation, even though minimal, allows for lateral retinacular contracture. Eventually all of these changes allow for the development of symptomatic patellofemoral disease.[41] In the protocols that are used by the author, all patients are routinely started on a prophylactic patellofemoral rehabilitation program, which is then modified to incorporate a therapeutic program specific for the injury. Obviously, this requires close supervision by the therapists and, most importantly, observation for the development of any factors that may be detrimental to the patient's recovery. Only if these factors are identified can the rehabilitation program be modified early to allow for the continued successful treatment of the patient.

ANTERIOR CRUCIATE LIGAMENT REPAIR

Anterior cruciate ligament injuries also require an individualized rehabilitation program. Again, the therapist must institute a procedure-specific protocol and then modify it to suit the specific patient's needs. Because of the duration of the therapy necessary to recover from anterior cruciate ligament surgery, the process of modification is a constant one, requiring frequent updates, frequent activity changes, and close observation.

The outcome of anterior cruciate ligament surgery is highly dependent upon the therapist. At the time of surgery, the reconstructed knee is stable and has a full range of motion. During the postoperative course, patient-physician contact occurs at best weekly and usually only every few weeks. However, during this course of time, patient-therapist contact is often several times a week. Thus it is the therapist who plays the major role in identifying those clinical changes that develop during the postoperative course that may interfere with the patient's rehabilitation and expected course of recovery.

Although no physician expects the therapist to specifically diagnose and initiate treatment, it is reasonable to expect the therapist to be aware of the expected course of recovery, to identify any deviation from that course, and to make the necessary rehabilitation modifications, after consultation with the physician. The lines of communication must be kept open between the doctor and the therapist because, although the therapist may correctly diagnose a development during the course of rehabilitation, the significance of that development must be put into proper perspective. For example, the development of patellar pain in a patient who has undergone a central third bone-tendon-bone graft for an anterior cruciate ligament reconstruction may represent an early patellofemoral pain syndrome that only requires modification of the rehabilitation program, or it may represent a patellar stress fracture at the donor site of the graft. Only the close interaction of the physician-therapist team will allow the correct diagnosis to be made and the proper course of action taken.

The anterior cruciate ligament is composed of two major structural bands: the anteromedial and the posterolateral.[8,33,42,43] The anteromedial band is taut both in flexion and in extension, and the posterolateral is taut in extension only.[8,42,43] The ligament originates at the posteromedial wall of the lateral femoral condyle, passes obliquely through the joint, and inserts at the anteromedial aspect of the tibial spine. The exact points of attachment and anatomy have been well described by others.[8,33,42,43] The vascular supply of the ligament arises from the middle genicular artery and passes from the proximal aspect of the ligament to the distal aspect, coursing through the synovial membrane of the anterior cruciate ligament.[43,44] The anterior cruciate ligament seems to be the most lax from 30 degrees to 60 degrees of flexion.[43]

Biomechanically, the anterior cruciate ligament is the primary anterior stabilizer of the knee and a major secondary stabilizer of rotary instability. In general, the anterior cruciate ligament will stretch approximately 57 percent, relative to its normal resting length, before its ultimate failure.[45]

Since there are two functionally separate bands, it is possible to have a partial tear of the ligament. This explains why a patient may have a history consistent with the diagnosis of a torn anterior cruciate ligament, the pertinent physical finding of an acute hemarthrosis,[47,48] and an equivocal physical examination. If the anteromedial band is torn, and the posterolateral band is intact, the patient may have a negative Lachman test and a positive anterior drawer. Conversely, if the posterolateral band is disrupted, the patient may have a negative anterior drawer test and a positive Lachman test. The presence of a hemarthrosis is associated with a torn anterior cruciate ligament approximately 72 percent of the time.[47,48]

Noyes et al. did a biomechanical analysis of human ligament grafts and discovered that the central third bone-patellar tendon-bone graft had a strength that was approximately 168 percent of the normal anterior cruciate ligament. Among the other tissues tested were the semitendinosus (70 percent), the gracilis (49 percent), and the quadriceps-patellar retinaculum-patellar tendon graft (21 percent).[48] Although many procedures[23] have been developed for the reconstruction of the anterior cruciate ligament, and since the reconstructions are being performed both with an arthrotomy and with arthroscopy, rather than attempt to address the multitude of reconstructions, the author will briefly discuss the bone-tendon-bone central third reconstruction[49] and the iliotibial band tenodesis.[50]

The popularity of the central third bone-patellar tendon-bone intra-articular reconstruction is in large part due to the strength of the graft.[48] This procedure was initially reported in 1963,[51] and later modified by Clancy.[49] The surgical procedure may be done with a medial arthrotomy, a lateral arthrotomy, or with an arthroscope. It consists of harvesting the central third of the patellar tendon, with a bony block at each end of the graft (Fig. 21-6). Thus the donor site includes a portion of the tibial tubercle and a part of the nonarticular portion of the patella.

After sizing the graft to determine the appropriate diameter of the drill holes, a tunnel is drilled from the anteromedial border of the tibia, exiting intra-articularly at a point anterior and medial to the axis of the insertion of the anterior cruciate ligament on the tibial plateau. A second drill hole is placed through the lateral femoral condyle. This hole exits the medial wall of the intra-articular portion of the lateral femoral condyle, deep in the femoral notch, at a point posterior and superior to the anatomic center of origin of the anterior cruciate ligament from the lateral femoral condyle. A femoral notch-plasty is performed to remove any potential impingement of the notch on the anterior cruciate ligament as the knee comes to a position of full extension. The graft is then passed through the two drill holes and securely fixed to the tibia and to the femur. The knee examination is then performed to ensure that stability has been restored and that full motion of the knee is possible. The incisions are closed, the dressings applied, and the rehabilitation is then initiated.

Rather than do an intra-articular reconstruction or augmentation, the surgeon may elect to perform an extra-articular reconstruction. Again, a large number of these procedures have been devised. The iliotibial tenodesis, devised and popularized by Andrews,[50] is aimed at stabilizing the knee by using the iliotibial band to replace the function of the injured anterior cruciate ligament. Briefly, the iliotibial band is split at the posterolateral aspect of the knee, and suture material is used to create two bundles of tissue. An isometric point of attachment on the lateral femoral condyle, between the linea aspera and the lateral femoral epicondyle, is then chosen. This area of the bone is then shingled, using osteotomes, and the suture material is then passed through the distal aspect of the femur. The sutures are then pulled taut and tied medially. The knee examination is performed to ensure that full range of motion is possible and that stability has been achieved. During the range-of-motion testing, attention is directed to the two bundles of tissue that have been tenodesed. The posterior bundle is seen to become tight as the knee comes to full extension, much as the posterolateral bundle of the normal anterior cruciate ligament does. The surgically created anterior bundle becomes tight as the knee goes into a position of flexion, duplicating the function of the

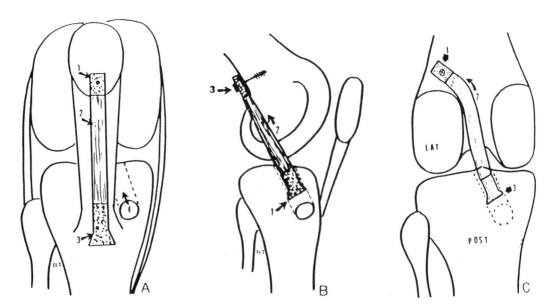

Fig. 21-6. Bone-tendon-bone central third reconstruction. (From James,[60] with permission.)

anteromedial bundle of the normal anterior cruciate ligament. Following completion of the procedure, the appropriate physical therapy protocols are instituted.

All of the rehabilitation protocols must address the need for immobilization versus the benefit of motion.[14,15,18,52-54] In general, prolonged immobilization has been advocated in the past to allow for sufficient healing of the tissue and to allow for protection of the tissue while in the healing phase. Unfortunately, this type of treatment has been shown to result in decreased cartilage nutrition,[15,18] increased accumulation of the lysozomal enzymes which are detrimental to soft tissue healing, and increased soft tissue stiffness.[13] In addition, the well-documented reduction of muscle strength occurs.[13,55]

Fortunately, with the development of newer cast braces, and with the results of research, it is now apparent that early motion is beneficial provided that the motion is applied in such a fashion that physiologically tolerable stresses are applied to the joint and to the repair site.[55] In effect, the benefits of protected rehabilitation are now recognized. It is now possible to design a program that will allow for healing while participating in a rehabilitation process, rather than the traditional method of allowing healing to occur and then initiating the period of therapy.[55,56]

However, it is crucial that the therapist be cognizant of the specific surgical pathology and of the technical details of the procedure prior to instituting therapy. Obviously the program for an isolated intra-articular anterior cruciate ligament reconstruction would differ from that needed for an intra-articular anterior cruciate ligament reconstruction and meniscal repair. Among the technical details that should be considered are location of the arthrotomy, security of fixation of the graft, quality of the graft, range of motion possible without placing undue tension on the graft, isometricity of graft placement, associated conditions such as articular surface chondral fractures, presence or absence of patellofemoral disease, presence of any predisposing factors for the later development of patellofemoral disease (tight lateral retinaculum, lateral subluxation, abnormally increased Q angle[41]), any additional surgical procedures performed, and the need for immobilization versus the benefits of mo-

bilization. Ideally, only after this type of information has been obtained can the rehabilitation program be modified successfully to allow for the most rapid progress without jeopardizing the outcome.

REFERENCES

1. Sutton JB: Ligaments, Their Nature and Morphology. 2nd Ed. HK Lewis, London, 1897
2. Nicholas JA: The five-one reconstruction for anteromedial instability of the knee. J Bone Joint Surg 55:899, 1973
3. Smillie IS: Injuries of the Knee Joint. E & S Livingston, Edinburgh, 1946
4. Jones R: Notes on derangements of the knee. Ann Surg 50:969, 1909
5. Welsh RP: Knee joint structure and function. Clin Orthop 147:7, 1980
6. Torg JS, Conrad W, Kalen V: Clinical diagnosis of anterior cruciate ligament instability in the athlete. Am J Sports Med 4:84, 1976
7. Wang CJ, Walker PS: Rotary laxity of the human knee joint. J Bone Joint Surg 56A:161, 1974
8. Tapper EM, Hoover NW: Late results after meniscectomy. J Bone Joint Surg 51A:517, 1969
9. Butler DL, Noyes FR, Grood ES: Ligamentous restraints to anterior-posterior drawer in the human knee. J Bone Joint Surg 62A:259, 1980
10. Hsieh H, Walker PS: Stabilizing mechanisms of the loaded and unloaded knee joint. J Bone Joint Surg 58A:87, 1976
11. Hughston JC: A simple meniscectomy. Am J Sports Med 3:179, 1975
12. Levy IM, Torzilli PA, Warren RF: The effect of medial meniscectomy on anterior-posterior motion of the knee. J Bone Joint Surg 64A:883, 1982
13. Wills CA, Caiozzo VJ, Rasukawa DI, et al: Effects of immobilization on human skeletal muscle. Orthop Rev 11:57, 1982
14. MacConaill MA: The movements of the bones and joints. 3. The synovial fluid and its assistants. J Bone Joint Surg 32B:244, 1950
15. Salter RB, Field P: The effects of continuous compression on living articular cartilage. J Bone Joint Surg 42A:31, 1960
16. MacConaill MA: The function of intra-articular cartilages, with special reference to the knee and inferior radio-ulnar joints. J Anat 66:210, 1932
17. Radin EL, Bryan RS: The effect of weight-bearing on

regrowth of the medial meniscus after meniscectomy. J Trauma 12:169, 1970

18. Salter RB, Bell RS, Keeley FW: The protective effect of continuous passive motion on living articular cartilage in acute septic arthritis: an experimental investigation in the rabbit. Clin Orthop 159:223, 1981

19. Lutfi AM: Morphological changes in the articular cartilage after meniscectomy. J Bone Joint Surg 57B:525, 1975

20. Distefano VJ: Function, post-traumatic sequelae and current concepts of knee meniscus injuries: a review. Clin Orthop 151:143, 1980

21. Fukubayashi T, Kurosawa H: The contact area and pressure distribution pattern of the knee. A study of normal and osteoarthritic knee joints. Acta Orthop Scand 51:871, 1980

22. Fukubayashi T, Torzilli PA, Sherman MF, Warren RF: An in vitro biomechanical evaluation of anterior-posterior motion of the knee. Tibial displacement, rotation, and torque. J Bone Joint Surg 64A:258, 1982

23. Seedhom BB, Dowson D, Wright V: Functions of the menisci—a preliminary study. In Proceedings of the British Orthopaedic Research Society. J Bone Joint Surg 56B:381, 1974

24. Fairbank TJ: Knee joint changes after meniscectomy. J Bone Joint Surg 30B:664, 1948

25. Shrive NG, O'Conner JJ, Goodfellow JW: Loadbearing in the knee joint. Clin Orthop 131:279, 1978

26. Grood ES: Meniscal function. Adv Orthop Surg 7:193, 1984

27. Kurosawa H, Fukubayashi T, Nakajima H: Load bearing mode of the knee joint. Clin Orthop 149:283, 1980

28. Ahmed AM, Burke DL: In vivo measurement of static pressure distribution in synovial joints. Part I: tibial surface of the knee. J Biomech Eng 105:201, 1983

29. Bullough PG, Munuera L, Murphy J, Weinstein AM: The strength of the menisci of the knee as it relates to their fine structure. J Bone Joint Surg 52B:564, 1970

30. Sisk D: Campbell's Operative Orthopaedics. p. 2299. CV Mosby, St. Louis, 1987

31. Hargreaves DJ, Seedhom BB: On the bucket handle tear: partial or total meniscectomy? A quantitative study. In Proceedings of the British Orthopaedic Research Society. J Bone Joint Surg 61B:381, 1979

32. Arnoczky SP, Warren RF: Microvasculature of the human meniscus. Am J Sports Med 10:90, 1982

33. Arnoczky SP: The anatomy of the anterior cruciate ligament. Clin Orthop 172:19, 1983

34. Arnoczky SP, Warren RF: The microvasculature of the meniscus and its response to injury: an experimental study in the dog. Am J Sports Med 11:131, 1983

35. Cabaud HE, Rodkey WG, Fitzwater JE: Medial meniscus repairs: an experimental and morphologic study. Am J Sports Med 9:129, 1981

36. Cassidy RE, Shaffer AJ: Repair of peripheral meniscus tears. Am J Sports Med 9:209, 1981

37. Hamberg P, Gillquist J, Lysholm J: Suture of new and old peripheral meniscus tears. J Bone Joint Surg 65A:193, 1983

38. Mulholland J: Presented at Techniques in Arthroscopic Surgery, Emory University, Atlanta, 1983

39. LaBan MM: Collagen tissue: implications of its response to stress in vitro. Arch Phys Med Rehab 43:461, 1962

40. Stromberg D, Wiederhielm CA: Viscoelastic description of a collagenous tissue in simple elongation. J Appl Physiol 26:857, 1969

41. Ficat R, Hungerford D: Disorders of the Patello-femoral Joint. Williams & Wilkins, Baltimore, 1977

42. Girgis FG, Marshall JL, Al Monajem ARS: The cruciate ligaments of the knee joint. Anatomical, functional and experimental analysis. Clin Orthop 106:216, 1975

43. Kennedy JC, Weinberg HW, Wilson AS: The anatomy and function of the anterior cruciate ligament. J Bone Joint Surg 56A:223, 1974

44. Resines C, Munuera L, Calvo M, et al: The blood supply of the cruciate ligaments and the effect of trauma (abstract). J Bone Joint Surg 61B:120, 1979

45. Noyes FR, DeLucas JL, Torvik PJ: Biomechanics of anterior cruciate failure: an analysis of strain-rate sensitivity and mechanism of failure in primates. J Bone Joint Surg 56A:236, 1974

46. DeHaven KE: Diagnosis of acute knee injuries with hemarthrosis. Am J Sports Med 8:9, 1980

47. Noyes FR, Bassett RW, Grood ES, Butler DL: Arthroscopy in acute traumatic hemarthrosis of the knee. Incidence of anterior cruciate tears and other injuries. J Bone Joint Surg 62A:687, 1980

48. Noyes FR, Butler DL, Grood ES, et al: Biomechanical analysis of human ligament grafts used in knee-ligament repairs and reconstructions. J Bone Joint Surg 66A:344, 1984

49. Clancy WG, Nelson DA, Reider B, Narechania RG: Anterior cruciate ligament reconstruction using one-third of the patellar ligament, augmented by extra-articular transfers. J Bone Joint Surg 64A:352, 1982

50. Andrews JR, Sanders R: A "mini-reconstruction" technique in treating anterolateral rotatory instability (ALRI). Clin Orthop 172:93, 1983

51. Jones KG: Reconstruction of the anterior cruciate ligament. J Bone Joint Surg 45A:925, 1963

52. Cabaud HE, Feagin JA, Rodkey WG: Acute anterior

cruciate ligament injury and augmented repair. Am J Sports Med 8:395, 1980

53. Haggmark T, Eriksson E: Cylinder or mobile cast brace after knee ligament surgery. Am J Sports Med 7:48, 1979

54. Noyes FR: Functional properties of knee ligaments and alterations induced by immobilization — a correlative biomechanical and histological study in primates. Clin Orthop 123:210, 1977

55. Dickson A, Bennett M: Therapeutic exercise. Clin Sports Med 4(4):417, 1985

56. Markey K: Rehabilitation of the ACL deficient knee. Clin Sports Med 4:513, 1985

57. Mangine RE, Price S: Innovative approaches to surgery and rehabilitation. p. 191. In Mangine RE (ed): Physical Therapy of the Knee. Churchill Livingstone, New York, 1988

58. Kapandji IA: The Physiology of the Joints. Vol. 2. The Lower Limb. p. 115. Churchill Livingstone, Edinburgh, 1974

59. Insall JE: The anatomy of the knee. p. 1. In Insall JE (ed): Surgery of the Knee. Churchill Livingstone, New York, 1984

60. James SL: Knee ligament reconstruction. p. 7:31. In Evarts CM (ed): Surgery of the Musculoskeletal System. Vol. 3. Churchill Livingstone, New York, 1983

22

Dysfunction, Evaluation, and Treatment of the Foot and Ankle

JOHN C. GARBALOSA
ROBERT DONATELLI
MICHAEL J. WOODEN

This chapter briefly reviews the anatomy and normal and abnormal biomechanics of the foot and ankle. Various foot and ankle pathologies are also discussed with respect to pathomechanics, evaluation, and treatment. The pathologies include entrapment syndromes, traumatic injuries to the foot and ankle, and foot deformities. The biomechanical evaluation of the foot and ankle is also described.

NORMAL BIOMECHANICS

Anatomy

Some 33 bones comprise the skeletal structure of the foot and ankle.[1-5] This osseous structure can be broken down into a forefoot and a rearfoot section. In the rearfoot, the osseous structures of clinical importance are the distal ends of the fibula and tibia, the talus, and the calcaneus. These four bones interact to serve as supportive structures and pulley systems for the various tendons that pass over the bones.[6]

The tibia, the fibula, and the talus together form a hinge joint: the talocrural joint. Two types of motion occur at this joint: osteokinematic and arthrokinematic.[2-7] Osteokinematic movement is the overall movement of two bones without reference to the motion occurring at the joint between the bones (i.e., flexion and extension). Arthrokine-

matic movement is the motion actually occurring at the joint between the two bones (i.e., roll and spin).[5]

Plantar flexion and dorsiflexion are the osteokinematic motions occurring at the talocrural joint. Osteokinematic movement at the talocrural joint is governed and restricted primarily by the bony configuration of the joint surfaces. The arthrokinematic joint motions of the talocrural joint are roll and slide. Several ligaments help restrict the arthrokinematic joint movements found at the talocrural joint. These ligaments are the anterior tibiofibular, the anterior and posterior talofibular, the deltoid, and the calcaneofibular.[2-7]

A second joint found in the rearfoot, the subtalar joint, is composed of the calcaneus inferiorly and the talus superiorly.[2-8] Since the axis of the subtalar joint is located in three planes, a complex series of supination and pronation motions occurs there.[6] Supination is defined as inversion, plantar flexion, and adduction of the calcaneus on the talus in the open kinetic chain. Pronation, on the other hand, is defined as eversion, dorsiflexion, and abduction of the calcaneus on the talus.[4,6-8] These joint motions are governed by ligamentous tension and bony restraint mechanisms. The deltoid, anterior and posterior talofibular, and calcaneofibular ligaments prevent excessive motion from occurring at the subtalar joint.[3-5,7,9]

533

The rearfoot is separated from the forefoot by the midtarsal joint, which is composed of the cuboid and navicular bones, the calcaneus and the talus.[1-5] As in the subtalar joint, the triplane motions of supination and pronation occur in the midtarsal joint. Triplanar motions at the midtarsal joint occur about two joint axes: the longitudinal and the oblique. The motions of eversion, during pronation, and inversion, during supination, in an open kinetic chain occur about the longitudinal axis. About the oblique midtarsal joint axis, the open kinetic chain motions of plantar flexion and adduction occur during supination and dorsiflexion, and abduction occurs during pronation.[6,7,10] Ligamentous structures restraining the motions of supination and pronation are the bifurcate ligament, the spring ligament, the short and long plantar ligaments, and the plantar aponeurosis.[3-6]

The remaining osseous structures of the forefoot are the three cuneiforms, the five metatarsals, the two plantar sesamoids of the first metatarsal, and the 14 phalanges. These bones form several joints, of which only the metatarsophalangeal (MTP) and interphalangeal (IP) joints will be briefly discussed. The MTP joint is an ellipsoidal joint, which allows the osteokinematic motions of abduction, adduction, flexion, and extension to occur. The IP joints are pure hinge joints and allow the osteokinematic motions of flexion and extension to occur. Both joints have proper joint capsules with accompanying supportive ligamentous structures.[1-5,7]

There are several muscles of clinical importance in the foot. The role many of these muscles play in the production of pathology in the foot is covered in the discussion of foot pathologies. Some of these muscles are the gastrocsoleus-tendoachilles complex, the peroneus brevis and longus, and the tibialis posterior and anterior.[2-5] These muscles are crucial in the rehabilitation of the foot and ankle.

Important neurovascular structures passing through and terminating in the foot are the posterior (which divides into the medial and lateral plantar nerves) and anterior tibial nerves, the musculocutaneous nerve, the sural nerve, the dorsalis pedis artery, and the posterior tibial artery (which divides into the medial and lateral plantar arteries).[2-5] The effect these structures have on foot pathology is further discussed in the section on entrapments.

For a more detailed discussion of the anatomy of the foot, refer to various textbooks on the subject.[3-5]

Open Kinetic Chain

According to Lemkuhl and Smith, in an open kinetic chain the distal segment of the chain is free (e.g., when a person is not bearing weight on an extremity).[11] During open kinetic chain motion at the subtalar joint, movement occurs about a fixed talus. The calcaneus will evert, dorsiflex, and abduct, and invert, plantar flex, and adduct about the talus during pronation and supination, respectively.[6,12-17] The lack of talar motion in the open kinetic chain is due to the absence of direct muscular attachments on the talus.[4,6,12]

During pronation, open kinetic chain motion at the midtarsal joint consists of eversion about the longitudinal axis and abduction and dorsiflexion about the oblique axis. During supination, inversion occurs about the longitudinal axis, and adduction and plantar flexion occur about the oblique axis.[6,7,10,14,15,18] The extent of permissible movement at the midtarsal joint depends upon the position of the subtalar joint. Supination of the subtalar joint causes a decrease in the available motion of the midtarsal joint; pronation at the subtalar joint causes an increase.[6,15,18-21]

MTP joint motion, in an open kinetic chain, can affect the amount of available joint motion seen in the forefoot and rearfoot joints. MTP joint extension will cause the forefoot and rearfoot joints to be placed in a closed-packed position. Therefore, a cinching up of the joints of the foot occurs. This cinching up is described as the "windlass effect."[4,13,22-24] It is produced by the attachments of the plantar aponeurosis onto the bases of the MTP joints and the calcaneus.[4,22] A minimum of 60 degrees of MTP extension is needed for normal MTP function during gait.[4,6,13,25]

Closed Kinetic Chain

A closed kinetic chain exists when the distal segment of an extremity is fixed (e.g., when the foot is in contact with the ground).[11] There are some differences between closed and open kinetic chain motion in the foot and ankle. These differences are a result of the gravitational and ground reaction forces imparted upon the foot and ankle.[6,13,16,24]

One such difference between the two kinetic chains is in the motion occurring at the subtalar joint. In the closed kinetic chain, during supination, the calcaneus inverts while the talus dorsiflexes and abducts.[6,14,16,17,24] During pronation the calcaneus everts while the talus plantar flexes and adducts.[6,14,16,17,24] The chief difference between the two kinetic chains is the presence of talar motion in the closed kinetic chain and its absence in the open kinetic chain.

During the gait cycle the events of closed kinetic chain motion in the lower extremity can be observed. At heel-strike the subtalar joint is in a neutral to slightly supinated position, while the talocrural joint is in dorsiflexion. As the talocrural joint begins to plantar flex, the subtalar joint begins to pronate. Both of these motions occur as a result of body weight forcing the subtalar joint to pronate. Muscular eccentric contraction of the evertors and dorsiflexors of the talocrural and subtalar joints control this motion of pronation. When the gait cycle reaches the foot-flat phase, the subtalar joint is fully pronated and the talocrural joint has reached the joint's extent of plantar flexion.[4,6,8,16,24]

As the gait cycle continues, the subtalar joint begins to resupinate at midstance, reaching maximum supination at toe-off. The talocrural joint goes through a cycle of dorsiflexion-plantar flexion-dorsiflexion from the midstance to the swing phase of gait. Resupination activity at the subtalar joint results from concentric muscle activity of the plantar flexors and invertors of the subtalar joint, and external rotation of the lower limb. The dorsiplantar-dorsiflexion activity of the talocrural joint is due to eccentric and concentric activity of the plantar flexors of the talocrural joint.[4,6,8,16,24]

Midtarsal joint motion, as in the open kinetic chain, is dependent upon the position of the subtalar joint. Supination at the subtalar joint decreases the amount of available motion at the midtarsal joint. The midtarsal joint locks with subtalar joint supination. Pronation of the subtalar joint unlocks the midtarsal joint, causing the forefoot to become an unstable "loose bag of bones."[4,6,8,16,18–21]

Midtarsal joint pronation is seen from foot-flat to midstance of the gait cycle. The pronating motion consists of eversion along the longitudinal axis and dorsiflexion and abduction along the oblique axis of the midtarsal joint. Supination of the midtarsal joint is seen from just after midstance to toe-off in the gait cycle. Inversion about the longitudinal axis and plantar flexion and adduction along the oblique axis are seen during midtarsal joint supination.[4,6,16,24]

Midtarsal joint pronation is caused by eccentric muscle action of the invertors of the foot and concentric activity of the evertors. Supination is caused by concentric muscle activity of the invertors of the foot and ankle.[4,6] The extent of supination and pronation movements also depends on the subtalar joint position.

Both supination and pronation are necessary for normal function of the lower extremity. Concurrent pronation of the midtarsal and subtalar joints allows the foot to adapt to uneven surfaces and to dissipate and transmit ground reaction forces.[4,6,13,16,24] Supination transduces the foot and ankle into a rigid lever to transfer the vertical forces of propulsion to the ground from the lower extremity, thus reducing the shear forces transmitted directly to the forefoot during propulsion.[4,6,13,16,24] Supination and pronation of the subtalar joint also serve to convert the transverse plane rotations of the trunk and lower limb into sagittal plane rotations.[8,13] During normal gait activity the trunk and lower limb rotate internally at heel-strike, and externally at heel-off. The subtalar joint, in response to these transverse plane rotations, pronates during internal rotation and supinates during external rotation, thus acting as a torque convertor for the lower kinetic chain.[6,13]

The chief activity at the MTP joints during closed kinetic chain activity is the dorsiflexion-plantar flexion motion of the toes. As heel-off occurs, the toes passively dorsiflex, then actively plantar flex as toe-off occurs. Passive dorsiflexion during heel-off tightens the plantar aponeurosis and cinches up the tarsal and metatarsal bones. This cinching up assists in the transduction of the foot into a rigid lever for propulsive activities. Plantar flexion of the phalanges, mainly the hallux, during toe-off acts as the chief propeller of the lower extremity.[4,6,22,24] Several sources in the literature provide in-depth discussions of the normal mechanics of the foot.[6,13,16,24]

ABNORMAL BIOMECHANICS

Abnormal biomechanics will be discussed in reference to a closed kinetic chain. The adverse effects of abnormal biomechanics are usually seen during the weightbearing phase of gait. In the foot and ankle these adverse effects are usually the result of either excessive pronation or excessive supination.[6]

Excessive Pronation

Excessive pronation is defined as pronation that either occurs for too long a time or is of too great an amount.[6] This excessive pronation takes place at the subtalar joint. When pronation occurs for too long a time, the subtalar joint remains pronated after the foot-flat phase of gait. If the subtalar joint exhibits more than 30 degrees of calcaneal eversion from foot-flat to the midstance phase of gait, too great an amount of pronation is present.[6]

Excessive pronation can be attributed to congenital, neuromuscular, and/or acquired factors. Only the acquired factors are discussed in this chapter. For further readings regarding neuromuscular or congenital factors see Jahss' textbook on disorders of the foot.[26]

Acquired factors causing excessive pronation can be divided into extrinsic and intrinsic causes. Extrinsic causes are those due to events occurring outside of the foot and ankle region, in the lower leg or knee.[6] Two examples of extrinsic causes are gastrocsoleus tightness and rotational deformities of the lower extremity (e.g., femoral anteversion and tibial varus).

Intrinsic causes of excessive pronation are those that occur within the foot and ankle region.[6] These causes are usually fixed deformities of the subtalar and midtarsal joints.[6] Examples of intrinsic causes are forefoot varus, and ankle joint equinus.

Both intrinsic and extrinsic causes can produce excessive compensatory subtalar joint pronation. The response to the extrinsic or intrinsic cause of excessive pronation varies from person to person depending on the number of intrinsic and extrinsic factors present and the mobility of the subtalar, midtarsal, and other foot joints.

An alteration in the normal mechanics of the lower kinetic chain occurs with excessive pronation at the subtalar joint.[6] Pronation during the push-off portion of gait causes the foot to be unstable at a time when the foot needs to be a rigid lever.[4,6,16,17,24] If unstable, the foot will be unable to transmit the forces encountered during push-off.[4,6,24] This inability to transmit forces may lead to tissue breakdown within the foot (e.g., Morton's neuroma).[6] An added effect of an excessively long pronatory phase is a disruption of the normal transverse rotatory cycle of the lower extremity, possibly causing pathology at the knee and hip.[4,6,19,24]

Excessive Supination

Excessive supination is much the same as excessive pronation; supination can occur for too long a time period or be of too great a quantity.[6] As in excessive pronation, a myriad of causes ranging from congenital to acquired deformities may result in excessive supination.

An excessively supinated foot prevents the foot and ankle mechanism from absorbing shock.[4,6,24] The foot and ankle therefore transmit this stress up the kinetic chain to the hip, knee, or back, possibly causing pathology.[6,13,17] Also, the foot remains a rigid structure at a time when it needs to become a mobile, adaptable structure (i.e., from heel-strike to foot-flat). Therefore, the foot is unable to adapt to uneven terrain, and the result is a loss of equilibrium (a possible perpetuating factor in repeated ankle sprains in the athlete).[6]

Excessive supination can also alter the normal transverse rotational events of the lower kinetic chain.[6,19] This hindrance of normal rotational events may cause damage in the foot and ankle, as well as be detrimental to the remainder of the kinetic chain.

DYSFUNCTIONS AND PATHOLOGIES

Entrapments

Tarsal Tunnel

Tarsal tunnel syndrome is an entrapment of the posterior tibial nerve and artery as they pass through a fibrous osseous tunnel located posteromedial to the medial malleolus.[27-31] The roof of the tunnel is composed of the flexor retinaculum (the laciniate ligament), and the floor is comprised of the underlying bony structures. A decrease in the available space of the tunnel may cause compression of the posterior tibial nerve and artery, resulting in symptoms.[29,30] The decrease in space may be due to external or internal pathology.

Excessive pronation of the subtalar joint is an external pathology that tends to compress the tunnel. The laciniate ligament is stretched during excessive pronation, thereby decreasing the diameter of the tunnel.[28-30] Tendinitis of the posterior tibial, the flexor digitorum longus, and/or the flexor hallucis longus tendon is an example of internal pathology causing a decrease in the diameter of the tarsal tunnel.[27,29,30] Misalignment of the bony structures of the talocrural joint secondary to fracture can be considered a combination of internal and external pathologies causing a diminished tarsal tunnel diameter. All of these pathologies may compromise the tunnel either by occupying or decreasing the space of the tunnel.[27,30]

Another purported cause of tarsal tunnel symptoms is entrapment of the posterior tibial nerve by the abductor hallucis muscle as the nerve gains entrance to the plantar aspect of the foot. The entrapment is caused by a tethering of the nerve, as the nerve gains entrance to the foot, by the abductor hallucis and the underlying bone.[31] This tethering stretches the posterior tibial nerve during gait activities.

Neuromas

Neuromas are fibrotic proliferations of the tissue surrounding the neurovascular bundles located between the metatarsals. The fibrotic proliferation is usually due to abnormal shearing forces between the metatarsal heads and the underlying tissues. An ischemic response of the neurovascular bundles is the end result of the tissue proliferation, ultimately leading to the symptoms felt by the patient.[6,27,31]

The pathomechanics involved in the formation of a neuroma are usually the result of abnormal pronation during the propulsive phase of gait.[6] Normally the neurovascular bundles lie plantar to and between the metatarsals. During abnormal pronation,

the metatarsal heads of the first, second, and third metatarsals move in a lateroplantar direction while the fifth metatarsal head moves in a dorsomedial direction.[6,32] At the same time, the soft tissues on the plantar surface of the foot are fixed by ground reaction forces and the patient's shoe. A shear and a compressive force are established by the metatarsal head motion. The compressive force is due to the metatarsal heads lying over the neurovascular bundles.[6] The result of these compressive and shear forces is fibrotic proliferation of the surrounding tissue in an effort to protect the neurovascular bundles.[6,27,31]

Trauma

Fractures

Talocrural fractures are the result of four basic types of abnormal forces: compression, inversion, eversion, and/or torsion.[33-35] Inversion and eversion fractures are usually accompanied by a torsional component.[34,35] An inversion or eversion fracture, with or without a torsional component, results in damage to the soft tissues and osseous structures about the talocrural and subtalar joints.[28,33-35] Depending on the severity of the injury and on whether the forefoot is in supination or pronation, a fracture of the medial and/or the lateral malleolus can be seen.[34-36] A possible concomitant injury is osteochondral fracture of the talar dome.[33-36] Disruption of the inferior tibiofibular syndesmosis may also be a consequence of an eversion or inversion fracture.[33-36]

Compression fractures of the talocrural joint are usually the result of a jumping incident.[28,33,36] In this type of fracture there is direct damage to the talus as a result of the applied force. A secondary event may be disruption of the inferior tibiofibular syndesmosis as in an eversion or inversion injury.[33,36]

Metatarsal fractures generally involve either the first or the fifth metatarsal and can be a result of either trauma or excessive stress.[37] Traumatic fractures of the first metatarsal usually involve an abduction and hyperflexion or hyperextension mechanism of injury.[28,33] The mechanism of injury in a traumatic fracture of the fifth metatarsal is normally an avulsion fracture of the insertion of the peroneus brevis muscle during an inversion injury.[28,33] During an inversion injury the peroneus brevis attempts to prevent the excessive inversion, thus avulsing the styloid process of the fifth metatarsal.[28,33]

Stress fractures are usually the result of hyperpronation of the midtarsal and subtalar joints.[6,28,38] The hyperpronation prevents the foot from locking. Instead of the forces of propulsion being transmitted up the kinetic chain, the forces are dissipated within the foot, which is incapable of handling the extra stress of the propulsive forces.[6,38] Stress fractures can also be a result of a lack of pronation in the subtalar joint (the supinated foot). The subtalar joint is unable to pronate, and therefore does not allow the forces of compression to be absorbed properly.[6]

Sprains

The mechanism of a talocrural sprain is either lateral or medial, with or without a torsional force component. In a lateral injury the mechanism of injury involves an inversion force. The injury may involve ligamentous damage occurring in the following order: the anterior talofibular, calcaneofibular, posterior talofibular, and tibiofibular ligaments. As more ligaments are involved, the severity of the injury increases.[27,28,39]

Medial mechanisms of injury are the result of eversion forces. The deltoid and tibiofibular ligaments are usually torn in this type of injury.[27,28,39] An associated fracture of the fibula is a usual complication of an eversion injury.[27,28,33,36,39] Medial injuries are rare compared to lateral ligamentous injuries.

Metatarsophalangeal sprains normally involve a hyperflexion injury to the joint. Capsular tearing, articular cartilage damage, and possible fracturing of the tibial sesamoid are seen in MTP joint sprains.[27,28] This type of injury is thought to be a causative factor in hallux limitus deformities.[6]

Tibiofibular sprains are frequently a secondary involvement of talocrural injuries or a result of a compression injury.[27] Fracture of the dome of the talus or of the distal end of the fibula is a possible complication.[27,36] The mechanism of injury often involves a rotational or a compressive force with a concomitant dorsiflexion force.[27,28,36]

Pathomechanics

Hallux Abductovalgus

By definition, hallux abductovalgus is adduction of the first metatarsal with a valgus deformity of the proximal and distal phalanges of the hallux.[6,40] Hallux abductovalgus may be a result of hypermobility of the first metatarsal in a forefoot adductus, rheumatoid inflammatory disease, neuromuscular disease, or a result of postsurgical malfunction.[6,41,42] In all of these, a subluxation of the first MTP joint occurs initially followed by dislocation.[6,41,42]

Classically, there are four stages of progression of this hallux deformity. The predisposing factor is a hypermobility of the first metatarsal.[6,41,42] This hypermobility allows the hallux to abduct and the first metatarsal to adduct and invert upon the tarsus and the hallux. Abnormal pronation is usually the cause of the hypermobility of the first metatarsal.[6,40-42] Any structural or neuromuscular problem causing abnormal pronation or a laterally directed muscular force may lead to a hallux abductovalgus deformity.[6,41,42]

In stage one a lateral subluxation of the base of the proximal phalanx is seen on the roentgenogram. Abduction of the hallux, with indentation of the soft tissues laterally, is seen once stage two is reached. Metatarsus adductus primus, an increase of the adduction angle between the first and the second metatarsal, is the hallmark of stage three of the deformity. Stage four is noted by a subluxation or dislocation of the first MTP joint with the hallux riding over or under the second toe.[6]

Hallux Rigidus and Hallux Limitus

Hallux rigidus is a hypomobility of the first MTP joint. Hallux limitus is an ankylosing of the first MTP joint. A rigidus deformity may be a precursor to a limitus deformity.[6,28,40]

There are several etiologies of hallux limitus deformity. Hypermobility of the first ray associated with abnormal pronation and calcaneal eversion, immobilization of the first MTP joint, degenerative joint disease of the first MTP joint, trauma causing an inflammatory response of the joint, metatarsus primus elevatus, and an excessively long first metatarsal may all be precursors.[6,27,28] All of these precursors cause an immobilization of the first MTP joint. As a result of this immobilization of a synovial joint, a limitus deformity occurs.[43-46]

The pathomechanics of a hallux limitus deformity are due to two problems: an inability of the first metatarsal to plantar flex or of the first MTP joint to dorsiflex. Abnormal pronation of the subtalar joint prevents the first metatarsal from plantar flexing because of the effect of ground reaction forces on the metatarsal. Ground reaction forces dorsiflex the first metatarsal during abnormal pronation. An excessively long first metatarsal can also prevent the metatarsal from plantar flexing.

Any trauma or inflammatory disease that causes bony deformation of the first MTP joint can prevent normal MTP joint motion. If this type of immobilization continues untreated, the end result will be a rigidus (or ankylosed) deformity of the first MTP joint.[6,27,47]

Tailor's Bunion

Tailor's bunion is the mirror image of an abductovalgus deformity of the first ray occurring at the fifth MTP joint.[6] An adduction of the fifth toe and abduction of the fifth metatarsal is seen in this deformity.[6,31] Four causes of tailor's bunion are abnormal pronation, uncompensated forefoot varus, congenitally dorsiflexed fifth metatarsal, and congenitally plantar flexed fifth metatarsal.

Abnormal pronation is reported to be a factor in the etiology of tailor's bunion.[6] For abnormal pronation to cause a tailor's bunion, one of the other etiologic factors noted above must also be present.[6] Abnormal pronation causes a hypermobility of the fifth metatarsal. This hypermobility produces internal shearing between the metatarsal and the overlying soft tissue. As the deformity progresses, the events described in the hallux abductovalgus deformity occur.[6]

Uncompensated forefoot varus, exceeding the range of motion of pronation of the subtalar joint, causes the fifth metatarsal to bear excessive weight. This excessive weightbearing forces the fifth metatarsal to dorsiflex and evert. The dorsiflexion and eversion cause the fifth metatarsal to abduct and the proximal phalanx of the fifth toe to adduct, resulting in a tailor's bunion.[6]

Congenital plantar flexion of the fifth metatarsal prevents the fifth metatarsal from dorsiflexing beyond the transverse plane of the other metatarsal heads. This plantar flexed attitude and abnormally pronating foot cause the fifth metatarsal to become unstable. Ground reaction forces force the fifth metatarsal to evert, abduct, and dorsiflex. Eventually the fifth metatarsal subluxates and is no longer functional.[6]

The last cause of a tailor's bunion is a congenitally dorsiflexed fifth metatarsal. The only visual abnormality present is a dorsally located bunion. The dorsal attitude of the fifth toe causes abnormal shearing between the bone and the overlying dorsal soft tissues. This abnormal shearing is due to the firm fixation of the soft tissues by the shoe.[6]

Hammer Toes

In a hammer toe deformity, the MTP and distal interphalangeal (DIP) joints are in extension while the proximal interphalangeal joint (PIP) is in flexion.[6,31,48,49] Plantar flexed metatarsals, loss of lumbrical function, imbalance of interossei function, paralysis of the extensors of the toes, shortness of a metatarsal, forefoot valgus, hallux abductovalgus, trauma to the MTP joint causing instability, and subluxation of the fifth toe into pronation are all possible causes of a hammer toe deformity.[6,31] The common denominator among all of these pathologies is the production of a force imbalance across the MTP joint. This force imbalance may lead to a joint instability of the MTP or an imbalance of the muscles crossing the MTP joint.[4,6,31]

Claw Toes

A claw toe deformity occurs when the MTP joint is in extension and the DIP and PIP joints are in flexion.[6,31,48,49] The possible etiologic factors are forefoot adductus, congenitally plantar flexed first metatarsal, arthritis, spasm of the long and short toe flexors, weak gastrocnemius, forefoot supinatus, and pes cavus.[6,31]

Forefoot adductus, congenitally plantar flexed first ray, forefoot supinatus, and pes cavus all have the same pathomechanical effect on the toes.[6] The adduction angle of the metatarsals and the abduction angle of the phalanges increase. Instability of the MTP joints ensues as a result of this malalignment. The function of the lumbricales and flexors of the toes is altered as a result of the combined effect of instability and poor joint position. The alteration of these muscle groups instigates extension of the MTP and flexion of the DIP and PIP joints of all the digits of the foot.[6]

Arthritis of the MTPs leads to an overstretching of the restraining mechanisms of the extensor tendons of the toes, much the same as in arthritic conditions of the hand. This overstretching allows the tendons to drift laterally and alter their line of pull. Again the alteration of the line of pull causes the toes to be abducted, and the claw toe deformity ensues.[6,31]

During heel-lift and toe-off an increase in the activity of the long toe flexors occurs to compensate for a weak gastrocnemius. The increased toe flexor activity overpowers the extensors of the toes, resulting in a claw toe deformity. Spasm of the long and short toe flexors can cause a claw toe deformity in a similar fashion.[6]

Mallet Toes

The DIP joints of one or more toes are in a flexed attitude in a mallet toe deformity. The flexed attitude may be fixed or malleable. The etiology of mallet toe deformity is unknown as yet. Some authors speculate the condition to be congenital or due to improper shoe wear (the shoe not being long enough).[6,31]

Plantar Fasciitis

Plantar fasciitis involves an overstressing of the plantar fascia causing an inflammatory reaction, usually near the fascia's calcaneal attachment. The plantar fascia is overstretched, with pronation and extension of the MTP joint occurring simultaneously. Any individual who abnormally pronates during the push-off phase of gait is at risk to develop plantar fasciitis. The presence of a pes cavus foot also predisposes the individual to this condition, because in pes cavus the plantar fascia is already on stretch even when the foot is at rest.[50-53]

General Evaluation

Musculoskeletal

A foot and ankle evaluation begins with a visual inspection of the lower extremity as a whole. Any muscular imbalances affecting structural alignment and possibly altering normal mechanics are noted. The examiner then focuses on the foot and ankle. Areas of redness, ecchymosis, effusion, edema, bony angulation, and callus formation are noted.[9,48,49] The visual inspection is followed by a palpatory examination. Any areas of tenderness and increased tissue tension are discerned.[9,48,49]

Next a range-of-motion evaluation noting the amount of dorsiflexion and plantar flexion of the talocrural and MTP joints is performed.[9,48,49,54] For normal function of the lower extremity there should be at least 10 degrees of dorsiflexion and 30 degrees of plantar flexion of the talocrural joint.[6,9,55] There should be at least 60 degrees of dorsiflexion for normal function of the first MTP joint.[13,25,56]

A gross manual muscle test is performed next.[9,48,49] The musculature about the ankle is tested. For a more quantitative test of ankle muscle strength, an isokinetic evaluation can be performed. The examiner should expect to see normal absolute peak torque values at 30 degrees per second and at 120 degrees per second for all muscle groups tested. Peak torque values for ankle evertors and invertors should be around 21 foot-pounds for men and 15 foot-pounds for women at 30 degrees per second. At 120 degrees per second the torque values should be around 15 foot-pounds for men and 10 foot-pounds for women.[57,58]

A general overview of the neurovascular structures ends the general screening evaluation. Areas of decreased sensation as well as areas of hyperesthesia are noted. A general circulatory examination is performed to establish circulatory integrity of the arterial supply to the foot and ankle. The dorsalis pedis and posterior tibial pulses are established.[9,48,49]

Specific Evaluative Procedures

Tarsal tunnel entrapment may be discerned by two specific manual tests: hyperpronation and Tinel's sign.[28,30,48] Hyperpronation of the subtalar joint decreases the diameter of the tarsal tunnel. During the hyperpronation test, the subtalar joint is maintained in excessive pronation for 30 to 60 seconds. A positive test results in the reproduction of the patient's symptoms on a consistent basis.[30] In Tinel's sign the examiner taps the posterior tibial nerve proximal to its entrance to the tarsal tunnel. A positive test again results in the reproduction of the patient's symptoms.[28]

Along with these two manual tests, manual muscle and sensory testing are performed to determine the extent of nerve trunk compression. Weakness, as determined by a manual muscle test, of the muscles innervated by the medial and lateral plantar nerves may be indicative of a peripheral nerve entrapment at the tarsal tunnel.[28,30] Sensory tests are performed to determine the presence and extent of areas of hypoesthesia. These areas should correspond to the particular area of innervation of the involved nerves.[27,28,30]

Electromyographic studies can be performed to further document the presence of tarsal tunnel entrapment. Latencies greater than 6.2 and 7.0 seconds to the abductor hallucis and the abductor digiti quinti, respectively, are indicative of entrapment of the posterior tibial nerve at the tarsal tunnel.[27]

The history taken by the clinician will usually elicit complaints of burning, tingling, or pain in the medial arch or the plantar aspect of the foot. These symptoms usually are aggravated by increased activity. The patient may complain of nocturnal pain with proximal or distal radiation of symptoms.[27,28,30]

During the general evaluation, the clinician may notice a valgus attitude of the calcaneus during static standing. This attitude of the calcaneus may be a predisposing, perpetuating, or precipitating factor in tarsal tunnel entrapment. One other evaluative procedure, a biomechanical foot evaluation, is also performed. In this evaluation other predisposing, perpetuating, or precipitating factors of tarsal tunnel may be discovered (e.g., excessive subtalar joint motion).[6,27,28,30] This portion of the evaluation is discussed in detail later in this chapter.

Patients with neuroma typically render a history of acute episodes of radiating pains and/or paresthesias into the toes. The onset of the pain is sudden and cramp-like in nature. Initially, the symptoms occur only when the patient is wearing shoes that compress the toes; with time the pain may become intractable. The patient reports that the symptoms are or were alleviated by the removal of shoes and massaging of the toes.[6,27-31]

The chief physical therapy evaluative procedures in a patient with neuroma are a biomechanical gait analysis and a general lower kinetic chain evaluation to determine the perpetuating, predisposing, and precipitating factors for the development of a neuroma.

Fractures and sprains of the talocrural and MTP joints are evaluated in much the same manner. The major difference is that the clinician must wait until a fracture has healed sufficiently before proceeding with any evaluative tests, whereas in a patient who has sustained a sprain, the clinician may apply the evaluative tests immediately. The evaluation generally consists of obtaining a history, performing range-of-motion measurements and strength testing, noting the presence of edema or effusion, and noting the presence of any residual deformity in the foot and ankle.[28,33,36]

The osteokinematic motion of the involved joint is first assessed by range-of-motion testing. The joint itself as well as the joints proximal and distal to it are assessed. For example, in a talocrural fracture the range of motion of the MTP joints and the knee as well as of the ankle is evaluated. Once the osteokinematic motion has been assessed, the arthrokinematic movements of any joints previously noted to be restricted are assessed.[28,33,36,59,60] In addition, intermetatarsal joint play motion should also be assessed to determine any lack of mobility secondary to immobilization.

Strength is evaluated using manual muscle testing techniques and/or isokinetic procedures. As in the range-of-motion testing, the joints proximal, distal, and at the site of injury are all tested.[28] If isokinetic tests are performed, the involved joint is tested at both slow and fast speeds.[58]

Circumferential measurements of the foot and ankle are taken to document the presence of effusion or edema. The flexibility of the heel cord is assessed to rule out heel cord tightness. A biomechanical foot evaluation may also be beneficial in assessing the impact any foot deformities may have on the patient's lower kinetic chain.[28,33,36]

There are two added components in the evalua-

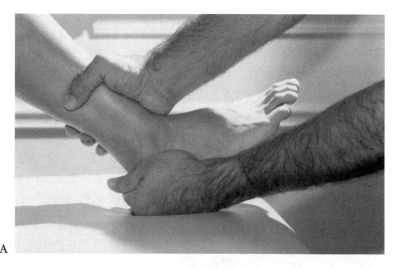

A

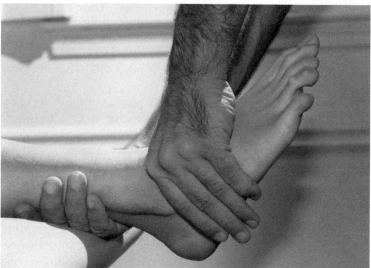

B

Fig. 22-1. (A) Anterior drawer test. **(B)** Posterior drawer test.

tion of talocrural and tibiofibular sprains: ligamentous laxity and talar mobility tests. There are three ligamentous laxity tests used to evaluate the integrity of the talocrural ligaments. The first is the anterior and posterior drawer test (Fig. 22-1) to determine the integrity of the anterior and posterior talofibular ligaments.[9,28] The others are the inversion and eversion stress tests (Fig. 22-2). These tests evaluate the integrity of the calcaneofibular and the deltoid ligaments.[28] Talar mobility tests consist of medial and lateral stress tests (Fig. 22-3). These tests evaluate the integrity of the inferior talofibular syndesmosis. Palpation may also be helpful in isolating the ligamentous tissues at fault.[9,28]

In pathomechanical conditions, the major portion of the assessment consists of a biomechanical foot and ankle evaluation and a proper medical work-up. The medical work-up is necessary to rule out systemic or neurologic causes for the presenting deformity.[6] Obtaining a good history from the patient may also be helpful initially as well as later in assessing the effects of any treatments.

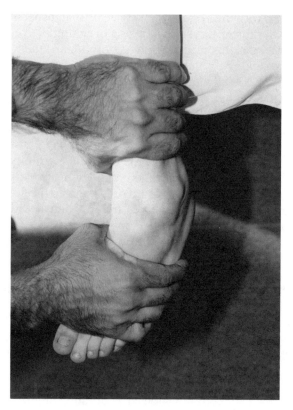

Fig. 22-2. Inversion stress test.

Biomechanical Evaluation

The biomechanical assessment of the foot involves several steps. The evaluation begins with the visual inspection of the patient in a static standing posture, followed by static supine-lying, static prone-lying, static standing, and dynamic gait analyses.

Visual Inspection

The biomechanical evaluation begins with a visual inspection of the lower extremities while the patient is standing, feet shoulder-width apart. The clinician needs to have visual access to the patient's entire lower quarter. From a frontal view, the clinician will note the presence of tibial or genu varus or valgus disorders, toe deformities or attitudes, and the position of the forefoot. A posterior view of the

One pathomechanical entity requiring a slightly different evaluative procedure is plantar fasciitis. Along with a history, medical work-up, and biomechanical evaluation, the clinician needs to perform a palpatory evaluation of the calcaneal area. In the history, the patient will complain of pain and tenderness localized to the plantar aspect of the foot. The pain may radiate forward along the plantar aspect of the foot. Usually the pain is noted upon awakening in the morning and worsens as the client increases the distance he walks or runs.

Upon visual inspection of a patient with plantar fasciitis, the clinician may note the presence of a cavus foot. Edema of the medial plantar aspect of the heel may also be seen on visual inspection. Palpation may reveal point tenderness localized to the medial aspect of the calcaneus.[28,50-52] Passive toe extension may also reproduce the patient's pain.[53]

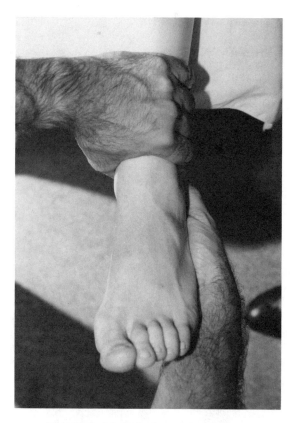

Fig. 22-3. Medial talocrural stress test.

client may reveal the presence of heel, tibia, or genu varus or valgus and the position of the talus (or subtalar joint).

Static Supine-Lying

During the supine-lying portion of the evaluation, the first step is to observe the foot for the presence of any callosities or deformities. Next, the range of motion of the first MTP joint is noted (Fig. 22-4). The angle of pull of the quadriceps muscle (Q angle) is discerned at this time. This angle is determined by aligning one arm of the goniometer with an imaginary line drawn from the anterior superior iliac crest to the center of the knee joint, and the other arm with the anterior border of the tibia. The axis of the goniometer will lie at the center of the knee joint. Finally, the amount of intermetatarsal mobility is evaluated by applying inferosuperior force and assessing the degree of resistance that is met by the clinician's hands. The above measurements are compared to those of the other limb for any dissimilarities.[6,28,48,60,61]

Static Prone-Lying

The patient is positioned in a prone-lying attitude with both lower extremities over the edge of a supporting surface so that the malleoli of the ankles are even with the edge of the surface. Visual inspection of the lower extremity consists of noting the presence of callosities and bony deformities of the foot and ankle.[6,28,48] Next, the range of motion of talocrural dorsiflexion and plantar flexion is evaluated with the knee in extension (Fig. 22-5).

One of the client's lower extremities is placed by the clinician in slight knee flexion and abduction, flexion and external rotation of the hip (Fig. 22-6). This posture ensures that the opposite extremity is in a plane parallel with the ground and supporting surface, keeping the foot at a right angle to the floor. Longitudinal bisection lines are now drawn with a fine tip marker along the posterior aspect of the lower third of the calf and the heel of the lower extremity.[61,62] It is extremely important to draw these bisection lines accurately. The clinician should make every effort to consistently choose the same anatomic landmarks to ensure the reliability of present and future measurements. One study in the literature has determined this procedure to be reliable if the clinician makes the effort to ensure the consistency of the anatomic landmarks.[62]

Using the bisection lines, the clinician then measures the amount of subtalar joint range of motion. The clinician grasps the heel and the calf as indicated in Figure 22-7. The heel is moved in one direction (into inversion or eversion) until maximal re-

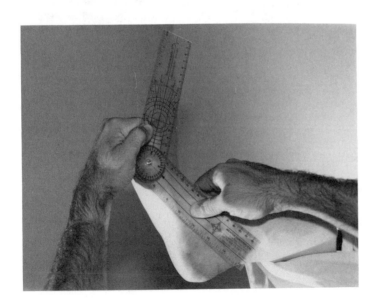

Fig. 22-4. Goniometric measurement of MTP joint flexion.

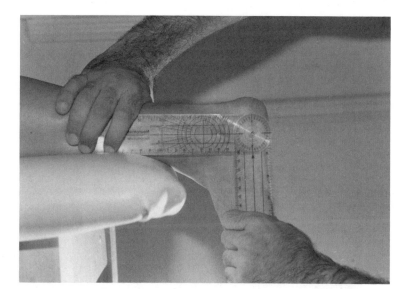

Fig. 22-5. Goniometric measurement of talocrural joint dorsiflexion.

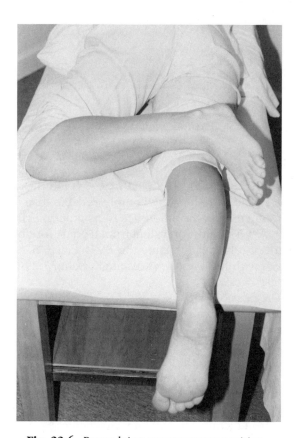

Fig. 22-6. Prone-lying measurement position.

sistance is felt, and the angular displacement of the heel is recorded. The same method is repeated in the opposite direction.[61,62]

The eversion and inversion angles are summed to give the total subtalar joint range of motion. The total range of motion is divided by three, and the quotient is subtracted from the average calcaneal eversion angle to arrive at the calculated subtalar joint neutral position (Fig. 22-8). From the subtalar neutral position, a minimum of 4 degrees of eversion and 8 degrees of inversion of the calcaneus in the frontal plane (or total subtalar joint motion) is needed for normal function of the foot.[23,61,62]

The subtalar joint is now placed in the calculated subtalar joint neutral position by grasping the distal third of the shaft of the fifth metatarsal and everting or inverting the foot. Great care must be taken to ensure that the foot is not dorsiflexed during this maneuver, as this may alter the forefoot-rearfoot frontal plane angular relationship. Once the subtalar joint is in the neutral position, the frontal plane forefoot-to-rearfoot posture is determined by aligning one of the arms of a goniometer along the plane of the metatarsal heads and the other arm perpendicular to the bisection line of the heel (Fig. 22-9).[61,62] One study, using a goniometer and a forefoot measuring device, noted that the most prevalent forefoot-to-rearfoot attitude in the normal pop-

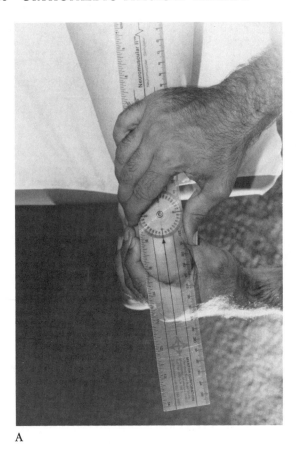 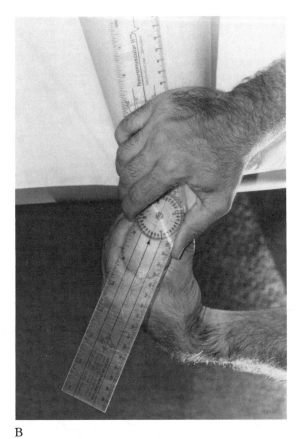

A   B

Fig. 22-7. Calcaneal measurements. **(A)** Eversion. **(B)** Inversion.

ulation is one of varus. The next most prevalent attitude is one of valgus. The least common attitude is the neutral condition. A normal forefoot varus attitude, as measured by a goniometer, is 7.82 degrees, and a normal valgus attitude is 4.69 degrees.[62]

One other instrument, cited in the literature, that can be used to measure the forefoot-rearfoot frontal plane angular relationship is the forefoot measuring device (FMD).[61-63] The preliminary measurement steps (e.g., subtalar joint positioning) are the same for the FMD as for the goniometer. The frontal plane relationship is measured with the FMD by aligning the slit on the posterior part of the FMD with the bisection line on the posterior surface of the cal-caneus. The plateau on the front part of the FMD is placed on the plantar surface of the foot, even with

the fifth metatarsal (Fig. 22-10).[61,62] Two studies report the FMD to be slightly more reliable than the goniometer, but the difference is insignificant clinically.[62,63] The most prevalent frontal plane forefoot-rearfoot relationship using the FMD is also one of varus, with the average varus angle being 7.24 degrees.[62]

The possible influence of the gastrocsoleus complex on the subtalar joint can also be determined in the prone-lying position. Dorsiflexion at the talocrural joint with the knee in extension is compared to dorsiflexion with the knee in flexion. A dramatic increase in the range of motion of the talocrural joint with the knee in flexion as compared to extension is an indication that the gastrocsoleus complex may be affecting subtalar joint mechanics.[6]

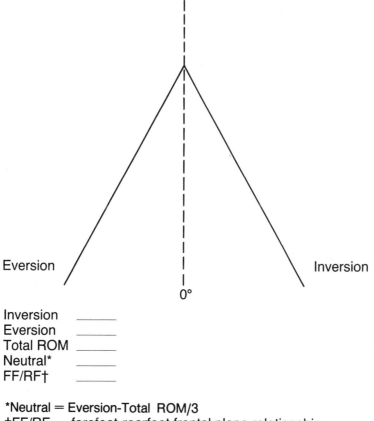

Eversion   Inversion

0°

Inversion   _____
Eversion   _____
Total ROM _____
Neutral*   _____
FF/RF†   _____

*Neutral = Eversion-Total ROM/3
†FF/RF = forefoot-rearfoot frontal plane relationship.

Fig. 22-8. Static biomechanical foot evaluation form.

Static Standing

The amount of tibial and heel valgus or varus is measured with the patient in the static standing position, the feet shoulder-width apart. The clinician uses a goniometer to measure the angle of heel varus or valgus. The arms of the goniometer are aligned with the longitudinal bisection line of the heel and parallel to the ground to measure the amount of heel varus or valgus. To measure the amount of tibial varus or valgus, the arms of the goniometer are aligned with the longitudinal bisection line on the posterior aspect of the tibia and parallel to the ground.[6,28,48,61,64]

Gait Analysis

All of the above information is correlated with a dynamic gait analysis. The patient is instructed to ambulate on a treadmill or floor, with and without shoes. The speed of gait should be slow at first and progressively increased. The markings on the heel allow the clinician to observe the patient for variances from the normal sequence of gait. Recall that from heel-strike to foot-flat the subtalar joint pronates (the calcaneus everts). From foot-flat to heel-off, the subtalar joint resupinates (the calcaneus inverts). The relationship of the lower extremity to the body should also be noted. As the speed of gait

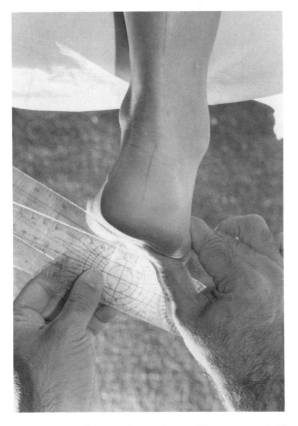

Fig. 22-9. Forefoot-rearfoot relationship as measured by a goniometer.

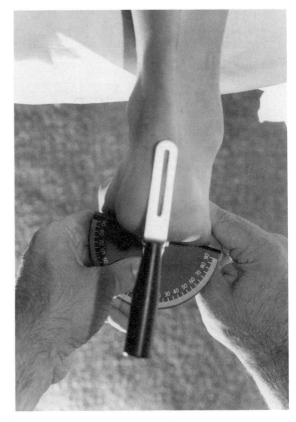

Fig. 22-10. Forefoot-rearfoot relationship as measured by an FMD.

increases, the lower extremity of the client should adduct slightly. Gait analysis is discussed further in Chapter 13.

Summary of Evaluative Procedures

The presence of a particular pathology is not based solely upon the findings from any one of the above evaluative procedures. Instead, the findings from all of the procedures should be correlated, and a decision on the particular type of or approach to treatment should then be made. For instance, the presence of a forefoot deformity (e.g., forefoot valgus or varus) by itself is not indicative of a pathology. The subtalar joint may be capable of compensating for the forefoot deformity. When the forefoot deformity is present with some other factor (e.g., tight gastroc-

soleus complex), the subtalar joint may now be unable to compensate for the deformity. At this time the decision to treat the forefoot deformity by the use of biomechanical orthotics is made.[59,62,65]

TREATMENT

Entrapments

Treatment for tarsal tunnel entrapments should address the predisposing and perpetuating causes of the entrapment. Permanent biomechanical orthotics to control the perpetuating and predisposing factors of excessive pronation is an excellent method of treatment.[6,28] In cases where the tarsal tunnel symptoms are due to internal causes (e.g., tendinitis of the posterior tibialis tendon), the use of an anti-inflammatory medicine may be prescribed by a physician. The physician may opt to inject the area with medication or prescribe the use of iontophoresis or phonophoresis with an anti-inflammatory cream (such as 1 percent hydrocortisone cream).[66,67]

Conservative treatment of patients with neuromas of the foot consists of proper shoe wear. The patient is advised to wear wider shoes. Accommodative orthotics may be prescribed to relieve metatarsal head pressure on the neuroma as well as correct the precipitating factor of abnormal pronation. Nonconservative treatment measures consist of surgical removal of the neuroma. For optimal results, nonconservative measures should be combined with treatments addressing the precipitating or perpetuating factors (e.g., biomechanical orthotics).[6,27,28,31]

Trauma

Treatment of traumatic injuries consists of three phases: acute, subacute, and postacute rehabilitation.

The acute phase of treatment follows the basic principles of protection from further injury, rest, ice, and compression and elevation of the injured site.[28,58,68] For the most part, the acute phase of treatment is a passive stage for the patient. This phase of treatment begins immediately after injury. Its duration is roughly the same for both fractures and sprains of the foot and ankle: 24 to 48 hours. Control and reduction of the inflammatory process are of the utmost importance during the acute stage.

The subacute phase of treatment is slightly different for fractures and sprains of the foot and ankle. Stability of the fracture site is still of paramount importance. Control and reduction of edema and effusion, prevention of muscle atrophy, and maintenance of cardiovascular fitness are key goals for the rehabilitation program during this phase of treatment of foot and ankle fractures. Elevation of the involved extremity, isometric exercises of the immobilized muscles, and the use of upper extremity ergometers are all recommended. The strengthening of uninvolved extremities, to prevent disuse atrophy, is also recommended.[28,58,69]

Treatment of sprains differs from that of fractures in that mobility is encouraged during the subacute phase of the rehabilitation program.[28,58] The patient is encouraged to begin sagittal plane exercises and movement. These exercises promote increased circulation as well as prevent excessive joint stiffness. Compressive supports (i.e., air splints) are used to provide stability and prevent an increase in edema when the involved lower extremity is in a dependent position. Partial weightbearing using axillary crutches is also encouraged. Isometric exercises with the peroneal muscles may also be of some benefit. As in the subacute phase of traumatic fractures, the control of effusion and edema and the maintenance of cardiovascular fitness are emphasized during the subacute phase of sprains.[28,58,68]

The postacute phase of traumatic injuries to the foot and ankle emphasizes the improvement of mobility and strength of the adjacent and involved joints and muscles. Once again, the treatment of fractures and the treatment of sprains parallel each other. The only difference between the two types of injuries is in the areas of emphasis in the initial periods of treatment. The initial emphasis with fractures is on the improvement of range of motion, both osteokinematic and arthrokinematic, of the involved joint, whereas the initial emphasis with sprains during the postacute phase is on improving the strength of the surrounding musculature and the proprioceptive ability of the injured joint. The strength of the invertors, evertors, dorsiflexors, and plantar flexors of the ankle are increased by the use of isokinetic exercises at high and low speeds. As previously mentioned, other involved muscle groups of the lower kinetic chain may also need strengthening. The end rehabilitation stage of both types of injury is a progression into functional activities. For the athlete the end stage is a progression into skill and agility exercises (e.g., figure-eights).[28,58,70–72]

Specific treatments of talocrural fractures include mobilization of the talocrural, inferior tibiofibular, midtarsal, intermetatarsal, and MTP joints. Initially, the arthrokinematic motions of roll and glide are restored through various mobilization techniques.[28,58,73] Two mobilization techniques used in treating the talocrural joint are posterior glide of the tibia and fibula on the talus and long axis distraction of the talocrural joint (see Chapter 24).[59,60,73] The glide technique is used to assist in restoring the osteokinematic motion of dorsiflexion and plantar flexion. A general capsular stretch is provided by the distractive technique. Osteokinematic motions are also performed along with the arthrokinematic motions. Usually the osteokinematic motions can be performed while the patient is in a whirlpool. The warmth of the water in the whirlpool can assist in pain control and promotion of tissue plasticity. Heel cord stretching is also emphasized during treatment.[28,58,73]

Along with the improvement of movement and strength, the joint proprioceptors must also be retrained. This retraining consists of tilt board and unilateral weightbearing exercises with the eyes shut and opened.[70-72] Finally, in some cases the prescription of a biomechanical orthotic may be of assistance in controlling any abnormal pronatory or supinatory forces that may be present. The use of orthotics may be of most use in those patients who have experienced a stress fracture of the metatarsals.

Specific treatment of MTP sprains consists of icing to reduce the inflammatory process, protective wrapping, and a nonweightbearing gait initially. Exercises that do not increase discomfort in conjunction with a graduated return to painfree activity program will follow. Mobilization of the MTP joint is performed when stiffness indicates this procedure to be of value.

Pathomechanical Conditions

As with entrapments, the treatment of pathomechanical conditions addresses the predisposing and perpetuating factors of the condition. These two factors are usually handled by the use of biomechanical orthotics, which control the abnormal pronation or supination occurring at the subtalar joint. Also, the orthotics will support varus or valgus deformities of the forefoot, if present.[6]

Other forms of treatment that accommodate or attempt to control the predisposing or perpetuating factors are heel lifts and accommodative shoes. For instance, decreasing the heel height has been recommended for individuals who abnormally pronate because of intrinsic foot factors. Increasing the heel height of the shoe has been recommended for individuals who abnormally pronate to compensate for extrinsic muscle problems (e.g., gastrocnemius tightness). Both of these heel height corrections have been recommended in the treatment of hallux abductovalgus conditions.[6,42,51]

Some pathomechanical conditions may require other forms of treatment in addition to the use of biomechanical orthotics or shoe inserts. Mobilization of any joints exhibiting limitation of movement, thereby causing abnormal pronation or supination, may be needed. Such techniques may be useful in the treatment of a plantar flexed fifth metatarsal in a tailor's bunion, a limitus deformity of the first MTP joint, and mallet toe deformity. In conjunction with the mobilization techniques, the use of appropriate heating modalities has been shown to be effective in the treatment of joint hypomobility.[6,47]

Adjunct treatments for inflammatory conditions of the foot and ankle include the use of cryotherapy to control any edema present. Iontophoresis or phonophoresis with 10 percent hydrocortisone cream can also be used to control the inflammatory reaction that is present with plantar fasciitis and alleviate the presenting symptoms.[28,66]

Of course, surgical correction of any deformities that are present is a promising alternative.[6,27] Surgery may also be the most effective treatment in cases where the predisposing factor is an excessively long metatarsal or elevatus condition.[6,43] Tenotomies of the flexor tendon with relocation of the tendon onto the dorsal surface of the foot are also alternative forms of treatment in such cases as mallet toes.[6]

Isokinetic strengthening of weak musculature, if present, is also advocated in pathomechanical conditions. Isokinetic exercises may also be needed in patients who have required surgery to prevent disuse atrophy from occurring during the recuperative period.

SUMMARY

A review of the anatomy and biomechanics, both abnormal and normal, has been presented. Various pathologic entities and their pathophysiology, evaluation, and treatment have been described. A common bond among all the entities presented has been in the areas of treatment and evaluation. When treating these conditions, the clinician must be aware of adjacent areas that may require treatment. These adjacent areas are discovered through a comprehensive evaluation of the lower kinetic chain.

Much research, both demographic and cause-and-effect, needs to be done in the area of the foot and ankle. Future research should address the effectiveness of various treatments on the pathologic entities treated. An attempt should also be made to establish normative data regarding the various lower extremity relationships and strength values. The foundation of a sound treatment program is sound research.

REFERENCES

1. Bojsen-Moller F: Anatomy of the forefoot, normal and pathological. Clin Orthop 142:10, 1979
2. Jaffe WL, Laitman JT: The evolution and anatomy of the human foot. p. 1. In Jahss M (ed): Disorders of the Foot. Vol. 1. WB Saunders, Philadelphia, 1982
3. Moore KL: The lower limb. p. 491. In Clinically Oriented Anatomy. Williams & Wilkins, Baltimore, 1980
4. Sarafian SK: Anatomy of the Foot and Ankle: Descriptive, Topographic, Functional. JB Lippincott, Philadelphia, 1983
5. Warwick R, Williams PL: Gray's Anatomy. WB Saunders, Philadelphia, 1973
6. Root ML, Orien WP, Weed JH: Normal and Abnormal Function of the Foot: Clinical Biomechanics. Vol. 2. Clinical Biomechanics Corp, Los Angeles, 1977
7. Steindler A: The mechanics of the foot and ankle. p. 373. In Steindler A: Kinesiology of the Human Body Under Normal and Pathological Conditions. Charles C Thomas, Springfield IL, 1955
8. Perry J: Anatomy and biomechanics of the hindfoot. Clin Orthop 177:9, 1983
9. Fetto JF: Anatomy and examination of the foot and ankle. p. 371. In Nicholas JA, Hershman EB (eds): The Lower Extremity and Spine in Sports Medicine. Vol. 1. CV Mosby, St. Louis, 1986
10. Elftman H: The transverse tarsal joint and its control. Clin Orthop 16:41, 1960
11. Lemkuhl LD, Smith LK: Mechanical principles: kinematics. p. 7. In Lemkuhl LD, Smith LK: Brunnstrom's Clinical Kinesiology. 2nd Ed. FA Davis, Philadelphia, 1983
12. Digiovani JE, Smith SD: Normal biomechanics of the adult rearfoot: a radiographic analysis. J Am Podiatr Assoc 66(11):812, 1976
13. Donatelli R: Normal biomechanics of the foot and ankle. J Orthop Sports Phys Ther 7(3):91, 1985
14. Green DR, Whitney AK, Walters P: Subtalar joint motion: a simplified view. J Am Podiatr Assoc 69(1):83, 1979
15. Manter JT: Movements of the subtalar and transverse tarsal joints. Anat Rec 80(4):397, 1941
16. McPoil TG, Knecht HG: Biomechanics of the foot in walking: a functional approach. J Orthop Sports Phys Ther 7(2):69, 1985
17. Subotnick SI: Biomechanics of the subtalar and midtarsal joints. J Am Podiatr Assoc 65(8):756, 1975
18. Hicks JH: The mechanics of the foot. I: The joints. J Anat 87:345, 1953
19. Morris JM: Biomechanics of the foot and ankle. Clin Orthop 122:10, 1977
20. Inman VT: UC-BL dual axis ankle control system and UC-BL shoe insert: biomechanical considerations. Bull Prosthet Res 10–11:130, 1969
21. Phillips RD, Phillips RL: Quantitative analysis of the locking position of the midtarsal joint. J Am Podiatr Assoc 73(10):518, 1983
22. Hicks JH: The mechanics of the foot. II: The plantar aponeurosis and the arch. J Anat 88:25, 1954
23. Wright DG, Desai SM, Henderson WH: Action of the subtalar ankle joint complex during the stance phase of walking. J Bone Joint Surg 48A(2):361, 1964
24. Mann RA: Biomechanics of the foot and ankle. p. 1. In Mann RA (ed): Surgery of the Foot. 5th Ed. CV Mosby, St. Louis, 1986
25. Bojsen-Moller F, Lamoreux L: Significance of free dorsiflexion of the toes in walking. Acta Orthop Scand 50:471, 1979
26. Jahss M (ed): Disorders of the Foot. Vols. 1 and 2. WB Saunders, Philadelphia, 1982
27. Singer KM, Jones DC: Soft tissue conditions of the ankle and foot. p. 498. In Nicholas JA, Hershman EB (eds): The Lower Extremity and Spine in Sports Medicine. Vol. 1. CV Mosby, Philadelphia, 1986
28. Roy S, Irwin R: Sports Medicine: Prevention, Evaluation, Management, and Rehabilitation. Prentice-Hall, Englewood Cliffs NJ, 1983
29. Koppell HP, Thompson WAL: Peripheral Entrapment Neuropathies. 2nd Ed. Robert E Krieger, Malabar FL, 1976
30. Kushner S, Reid DC: Medial tarsal tunnel syndrome: a review. J Orthop Sports Phys Ther 6(1):39, 1984
31. Viladot A: The metatarsals. p. 659. In Jahss M (ed): Disorders of the Foot. Vol. 1. WB Saunders, Philadelphia, 1982
32. Oldenbrook LL, Smith CE: Metatarsal head motion secondary to rearfoot pronation and supination: an

anatomical investigation. J Am Podiatr Assoc 69(1):24, 1979

33. Glick J, Sampson TG: Ankle and foot fractures in athletics. p. 526. In Nicholas JA, Hershman EB (eds): The Lower Extremity and Spine in Sports Medicine. Vol. 1. CV Mosby, Philadelphia, 1986

34. Segal D, Yablon IG: Bimalleolar fractures. p. 31. In Yablon IG, Segal D, Leach RE (eds): Ankle Injuries. Churchill Livingstone, New York, 1983

35. Lauge-Hansen N: Fractures of the ankle. II. Combined exploration-surgical and exploration-roentgenographic investigation. Arch Surg 60:957, 1950

36. Turco VJ, Spinella AJ: Occult trauma and unusual injuries in the foot and ankle. p. 541. In Nicholas JA, Hershman EB (eds): The Lower Extremity and Spine in Sports Medicine. Vol. 1. CV Mosby, Philadelphia, 1986

37. O'Donoghue DH: Injuries of the foot. p. 747. In O'Donoghue DH: Treatment of Injuries to Athletes. 3rd Ed. WB Saunders, Philadelphia, 1976

38. Hughes LY: Biomechanical analysis of the foot and ankle for predisposition to developing stress fractures. J Orthop Sports Phys Ther 7(3):96, 1985

39. Leach RE, Schepsis A: Ligamentous injuries. p. 193. In Yablon IG, Segal D, Leach RE (eds): Ankle Injuries. Churchill Livingstone, New York, 1983

40. Mann RA, Coughlin MJ: Hallux valgus and complications of hallux valgus. p. 65. In Mann RA (ed): Surgery of the Foot. 5th Ed. CV Mosby, St. Louis, 1986

41. Greensburg GS: Relationship of hallux abductus angle and first metatarsal angle to severity of pronation. J Am Podiatr Assoc 69(1):29, 1976

42. Subotnick SI: Equinus deformity as it affects the forefoot. J Am Podiatr Assoc 61(11):423, 1971

43. Akeson WH, Amiel D, Woo S: Immobility effects of synovial joints: the pathomechanics of joint contracture. Biorheology 17:95, 1980

44. Enneking W, Horowitz M: The intra-articular effects of immobilization on the human knee. J Bone Joint Surg 54A:973, 1972

45. Woo S, Matthews JV, Akeson WH, et al: Connective tissue response to immobility: correlative study of biomechanical and biochemical measurements of normal and immobilized rabbit knees. Arthritis Rheum 18:257, 1975

46. Donatelli R, Owens-Burkart H: Effects of immobilization on the extensibility of periarticular connective tissue. J Orthop Sports Phys Ther 3(2):67, 1981

47. Kelikan H: The hallux. p. 539. In Mann RA (ed): Surgery of the Foot. 5th Ed. CV Mosby, St. Louis, 1986

48. Hoppenfeld S: Physical examination of the foot and ankle. p. 197. In Hoppenfeld S (ed): Physical Examination of the Spine and Extremities. Appleton-Century-Crofts, New York, 1976

49. Mann RA: Principles of examination of the foot and ankle. p. 31. In Mann RA (ed): Surgery of the Foot. 5th Ed. CV Mosby, St. Louis, 1986

50. Marshall RN: Foot mechanics and joggers' injuries. NZ Med J 88:288, 1978

51. Aronson NG, Winston L, Cohen RI, Tarr RP: Some aspects of problems in runners: treatment and prevention. J Am Podiatr Assoc 67(8):595, 1977

52. Leach RE, DiIorio E, Harney RA: Pathologic hindfoot conditions in the athlete. Clin Orthop 177:116, 1983

53. Turek SL: The foot and ankle. p. 1407. In Turek SL: Orthopaedics: Principles and Their Applications. 4th Ed. Vol 2. JB Lippincott, Philadelphia, 1984

54. Stolov WC, Cole TM, Tobis JS: Evaluation of the patient: goniometry; muscle testing. p. 17. In Krusen FH, Kottke FJ, Ellwood PM (eds): Physical Medicine and Rehabilitation. WB Saunders, Philadelphia, 1971

55. Adelaar RS: The practical biomechanics of running. Am J Sports Med 14(6):497, 1986

56. Boissonault W, Donatelli R: The influence of hallux extension on the foot during ambulation. J Orthop Sports Phys Ther 5(5):240, 1984

57. Wong DLK, Glasheen-Wray M, Andrew LF: Isokinetic evaluation of the ankle invertors and evertors. J Orthop Sports Phys Ther 5(5):246, 1984

58. Davies GJ: Subtalar joint, ankle joint, and shin pain testing and rehabilitation. p. 123. In Davies GJ (ed): A Compendium of Isokinetics in Clinical Usage and Clinical Notes. S&S Publishers, LaCrosse WI, 1984

59. Maitland GD: Peripheral Manipulation. 2nd Ed. Butterworths, Boston, 1977

60. Mennell JM: Joint Pain; Diagnosis and Treatment Using Manipulative Techniques. Little, Brown, Boston, 1964

61. Root ML, Orien WP, Weed JH: Biomechanical Examination of the Foot. Vol. 1. Clinical Biomechanics Corp, Los Angeles, 1971

62. Garbalosa JC, McClure M, Catlin PA, Wooden MJ: Normal angular relationship of the forefoot to the rearfoot in the frontal plane. Submitted for publication, 1987

63. Cantu R, Catlin PA, Wooden MJ: A comparison of two measurement tools and two techniques for measuring the forefoot/rearfoot relationship. Unpublished data. 1987

64. Lohmann KN, Rayhel HE, Schneirwind WP, Danoff JV: Static measurement of tibia vara: Reliability and effect of lower extremity position. Phys Ther 67(2):196, 1987

65. Murphy P: Orthoses: not the sole solution for running ailments. Phys Sportsmed 14(2):164, 1986

66. Harris PR: Iontophoresis: clinical research in musculoskeletal inflammatory conditions. J Orthop Sports Phys Ther 4(2):109, 1982

67. Boone DC: Applications of iontophoresis. p. 99. In Wolf S (ed): Clinics in Physical Therapy. Vol 2: Electrotherapy. Churchill Livingstone, New York, 1981

68. Sims D: Effects of positioning on ankle edema. J Orthop Sports Phys Ther 8(1):30, 1986

69. Nicholas JA, Hershman EB (eds): The Lower Extremity and Spine in Sports Medicine. Vols. 1 and 2. CV Mosby, Philadelphia, 1986

70. DeCarlo MS, Talbot RW: Evaluation of ankle joint proprioception following injection of the anterior talofibular ligament. J Orthop Sports Phys Ther 8(2):70, 1986

71. Rebman LW: Ankle injuries: clinical observations. J Orthop Sports Phys Ther 8(3):153, 1986

72. Smith RW, Reischl SF: Treatment of ankle sprains in young athletes. Am J Sports Med 14(6):465, 1986

73. Kessler RM, Hertling D: The ankle and hindfoot. p. 448. In Kessler RM, Hertling D (eds): Management of Common Musculoskeletal Disorders: Physical Therapy Principles and Methods. Harper & Row, Philadelphia, 1983

23

Reconstructive Surgery of the Foot and Ankle

STANLEY KALISH
GEORGE VITO

Podiatric medicine has progressed well beyond attending to nails and bunions, to include surgery of the foot and leg. The study of deformities of the ankle and leg, in addition to those of the foot, forms a major part of the education of podiatrists today. This chapter presents four common deformities of the foot that podiatrists treat regularly by surgical intervention.

THE KALISH BUNIONECTOMY

Hallux abductovalgus is one of the most common structural deformities seen in the lower extremity.[1] The primary predisposing factor in the formation of hallux abductovalgus is excessive pronation of the foot during the stance phase of gait.[1]

Hallux abductovalgus presents with a medial eminence or bunion deformity on the medial surface of the first metatarsal. Lateral deviation of the great toe can be noted in more severe cases, with the possibility of dislocation of the metatarsalphalageal (MPJ) joint with an associated overlapping or underlapping of the second toe. This is considered the hallux abductus angle (Fig. 23-1). The first metatarsal may be displaced medially with respect to the second (metatarsal primus adductus); the angle formed between them is referred to as the intermetatarsal angle (Fig. 23-2). The normal measurements of these angles are 0 to 8 degrees and 15 degrees, respectively.

Approaches to hallux abductovalgus surgery have ranged from proximal or distal metaphyseal correction to joint destructive procedures. The indications for hallux abductovalgus surgery include pain of the first MPJ joint, and deformity of the first MPJ joint along with a high intermetatarsal angle or a high hallux abductus angle. In 1962 Dale Austin first performed a distal osteotomy of the first metatarsal.[2] The operation was a horizontally directed 60 degree V displacement osteotomy. This has become a very successful operation with few complications. The complications that have occurred include displacement of the osteotomy, delayed union or nonunion, K-wire tract infections, and limitation of first MPJ joint range of motion.

The Kalish modification of this procedure addresses the complications of the original Austin procedure by using a 55 degree V, which reduces the possibility of displacement along with the possibility of delayed union or nonunion. Pin tract infections are eliminated by the use of two 2.7-mm cortical screws. Range-of-motion exercises along with immediate ambulation decrease limitation of the MPJ joint's range-of-motion.

Indications for the Kalish bunionectomy are as follows:

1. Hallux abductus angle greater than 15 degrees
2. Metatarsus primus abductus angle less than or equal to 15 degrees

555

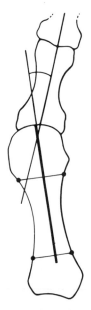

Fig. 23-1. The relationship shown between the first metatarsal and the proximal phalanx is termed the Hallux abductus angle.

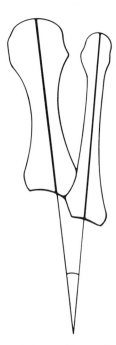

Fig. 23-2. The angle formed by the first and second metatarsals is termed the intermetatarsal angle.

3. Pain of the first MPJ through the range of motion
4. Absence of degenerative joint disease.

Description of the Procedure

An incision is made over the first MPJ joint. The incision is deepened to the level of the joint capsule and carried down to the level of the transverse metatarsal ligament of the first interspace. The adductor hallucis tendon is released. Dissection of the medial side of the joint is performed to the plantarmost aspect of the joint.

An inverted-L capsular incision is then performed. This is done to maximize exposure of the joint and for easier closure of the joint capsule after the procedure. Resection of the medial eminence of the first metatarsal head is then performed. At this point a 0.045 K-wire is directed medially to laterally through the cortices of the first metatarsal head to serve as an apical axis guide. This is done so that a proper bone cut can be performed. With proper placement of this apical axis guide, the surgeon is able to plantar flex, dorsiflex, or maintain the current level of the first metatarsal head. Elongation or shortening can also be achieved by proper placement of the apical axis guide (Fig. 23-3).

A 55 degree V-osteotomy with an elongated dorsal wing is then performed so as to accommodate two 2.7-mm cortical screws. Distal traction is then placed on the first metatarsal head, and the capital fragment is displaced laterally one-fourth to one-half the width of the first metatarsal shaft.

Once the metatarsal head is displaced, a 0.045 K-wire is placed distally across the osteotomy in a dorsolateral to plantar-medial direction to temporally fixate the osteotomy.

After prefixation has been performed using the K-wire, primary fixation is attempted. Two 2.7-mm cortical screws are placed through the osteotomy. After screw fixation has been performed, the first wire is removed (Fig. 23-4).

Complications

Complications of this procedure are the same as in any procedure involving an osteotomy: nonunion, delayed union, and bone infection. Hallux varus is a

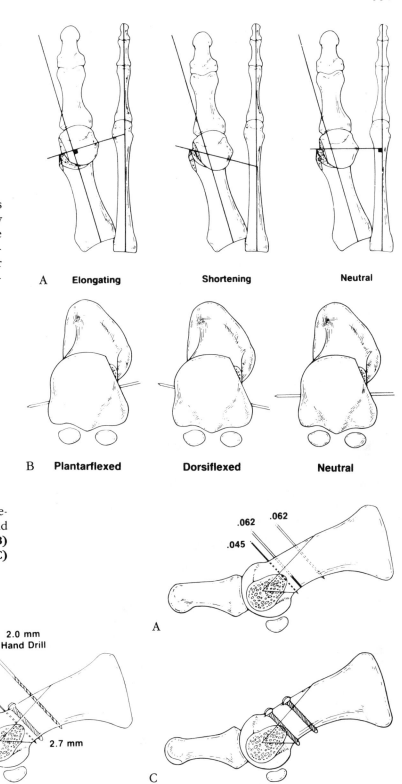

Fig. 23-3. Placement of the apical axis guide can determine **(A)** if the osteotomy will elongate, shorten, or maintain the length of the first metatarsal; **(B)** if the osteotomy will plantar flex, dorsiflex, or maintain the position of the first metatarsal.

A   Elongating   Shortening   Neutral

B   Plantarflexed   Dorsiflexed   Neutral

Fig. 23-4. Kalish bunionectomy. **(A)** Placement of K-wires for stabilization of and screw direction at the osteotomy site; **(B)** 2.0-mm drill in place for proximal hole; **(C)** the osteotomy with fixation completed.

definite possibility because of the large amount of metatarsus primus adductus correction. This deformity occurs when the hallux faces in a medial direction rather than the normal slightly lateral position (Fig. 23-5). It is very important that the first metatarsal and the tibial sesamoidal positions be evaluated intraoperatively to avoid hallux varus. Intraoperative fracture of the elongated dorsal wing of the metatarsal head is one of the more common complications. This fracture occurs at the most proximal portion of the dorsal wing secondary to improper placement of the proximal screw.

Physical Therapy

Physical therapy can be initiated postoperatively with passive range of motion of the hallux. The patient is to refrain from weightbearing for 1 week in a post-op shoe. Hydrotherapy, active range-of-motion exercises, and weightbearing in regular shoes can be initiated 1 to 2 weeks postoperatively, keeping the incision site covered and dry for the first week.

The goal of physical therapy is to achieve 50 to 60

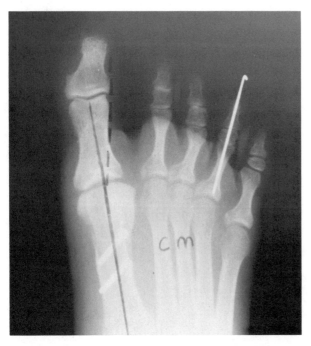

Fig. 23-5. Radiograph showing the proximal phalanx of the hallux facing in the medial direction (hallux varus).

degrees of passive dorsiflexion of the MTP so that proper propulsion may be achieved in the final phase of stance.

HEEL SPUR SURGERY

Obese individuals are most at risk for calcaneal tuberosities or heel spurs. However, obesity is not the only major factor.[3] Mechanical heel pain is usually present in individuals who place increased tension on the plantar structures inserting into the inferior aspect of the heel bone. Abnormal biomechanical forces such as those caused by pronated foot, cavus foot, and compensation for equinus can lead to heel pain. Overuse secondary to jogging or aerobics is very common. People who work extended periods of time standing on hard surfaces also suffer from chronic heel pain.

Most patients present with a chief complaint of pain in the heels after getting up in the morning or upon standing after sitting for an extended period of time. Clinical examination reveals pain on the inferior aspect of the heel. The symptoms are reproduced by dorsiflexing the foot on the leg and extending the digits on the forefoot. This places tension on the plantar fascia and intrisic muscles. Pain is most noticeable at the anterior inferior medial aspect of the medial calcaneal tubercle, the point of attachment of the long plantar ligament.

With chronic abnormal pull of the plantar fascia on the calcaneus, symptoms are produced. Initially an inflammatory response occurs at the attachment of the plantar fascia to the heel. Calcification occurs inferiorly and anteriorly along the pull of the plantar fascia.[3] Hypertrophy of the connective tissue develops and differentiates into fibrocartilage and later osseous tissue. The pain that is produced is due not to the development of osseous tissue, but to the fasciitis, periostitis, or adventitious bursitis that develops.[4] Any foot exposed to chronic microtrauma from pull of the plantar fascia at the heel may become symptomatic.

Radiographic evaluation will usually show an enlarged portion of the anterior-inferior shelf of the calcaneus. The size of the shelf generally depends on the chronicity of the disorder. However, size is not related to the degree of pain.

Description of the Procedure

Surgical treatment is reserved for the 5 percent of patients who have recurrent heel pain that is not relieved by conservative treatments such as orthotics, padding, steroid injections, and strappings. The procedure is performed with the patient in a supine position under local anesthesia or using a thigh tourniquet with general anesthesia. A 4- to 6-cm medial incision is placed at the level of the medial calcaneal tubercle and directed distally in a line inferior to the abductor hallucis muscle belly and superior to the medial band of the plantar fascia. Subcutaneous dissection will reveal multiple fibrous septa that run between this layer and the deep fascia. These septa form part of the highly organized, complex chambers of the inferior heel fat pad.

A retractor is used to retract subcutaneous tissues from the plantar fascia. Sharp dissection is used to free the medial plantar aponeurosis from the abductor muscle fascia. The aponeurosis is separated from the inferior calcaneus, and sharp dissection is used to dissect the plantar fascia cleanly from the inferior aspect of the calcaneus. The spur should be evident at this level (Fig. 23-6). It is resected with a bone rongeur, bone forceps, or osteotome. The remaining bone is rasped smooth. Removal of 1 to 2 cm of the plantar fascia at its attachment to the bone is performed to reduce any chances of recurrence of spur and soft tissue inflammation (Fig. 23-7).

Postoperative Care

Postoperatively, ice is applied to the surgical site for 2 to 3 days, and the leg is elevated above the hip when sitting and above the heart while reclining. Guarded weightbearing with a surgical shoe and crutches is allowed 3 days after the surgery. Drains are removed 48 hours after the procedure, and the sutures 21 days postoperatively. Two weeks after the procedure, increased weightbearing is allowed and the patient decreases the use of the crutches. By the third or fourth week tennis shoes or oxfords with foot orthotics are allowed.

Complications

Heel pain affects 5 percent of our population.[4] Pain can and does occur in any foot type. Most complications are avoidable with accurate preoperative assessment, atraumatic operative technique, and proper postoperative care. Patients should be made aware that surgery is not a cureall for their heel pain and is only attempted after all metabolic or arthritic causes have been ruled out and aggressive conservative treatment methods have been exhausted.

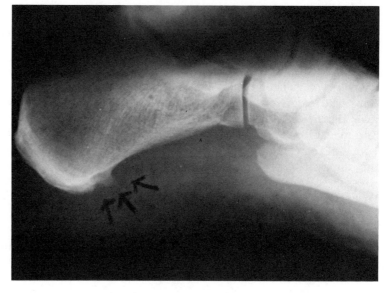

Fig. 23-6. Radiograph showing a heel spur on the plantar surface of the calcaneus.

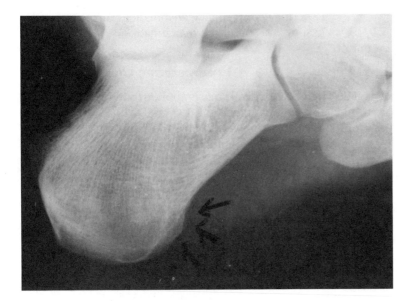

Fig. 23-7. Radiograph showing removal of the heel spur.

ANKLE STABILIZATION

The split peroneus brevis lateral ankle stabilization (SPBLAS) procedure was developed to restore stability to the lateral complex of the ankle. This procedure was developed for the patient with chronic inversion ankle instability and weakness; it is also used when it is determined intraoperatively that the ligamentous structures are insufficient for a primary repair.

Chronic instability can be demonstrated by stress radiographs. These views should be done only when the initial scout radiographs (normal standard views consisting of an anteroposterior view, a mortise view, and a lateral view) fail to reveal any fractures. The stress views reveal the integrity of the two main ligaments of the lateral complex of the ankle. The two stress views presently used at the Atlanta Foot and Leg Clinic are the talar tilt (Fig. 23-8) and the anterior drawer test (Fig. 23-9). These views stress the calcaneal fibular and the anterior talofibular ligament, respectively.

Functional instability and a history of multiple sprains with negative stress views along with chronic pain are also indications for the SPBLAS procedure.[5] The advantage of this procedure is that it does not sacrifice the entire peroneus brevis muscle and tendon as do other procedures, leaving the peroneus longus to overpower the foot. The procedure is a double ligament repair with no osseous involvement and can be performed within an hour. This procedure is mainly indicated for the young patient with chronic ankle instability. The peroneus brevis tendon is split from above the ankle mortise proximally to the base of the fifth metatarsal distally. The tendon is rerouted through the fibula from anterior to posterior and inserted into the calcaneus (Fig. 23-10).

Description of Procedure

The patient is placed in the lateral position with both knees bent. A thigh tourniquet is used to maintain hemostasis and decrease the exposure time of the patient.

The insertion of the peroneus brevis tendon is identified at the base of the fifth metatarsal. The lateral wall of the calcaneus posterior to the posterior facet of the subtalar joint is marked where the trephine plug (round bone peg) will be removed for implantation of the split tendon.

With the foot held perpendicular to the leg, a

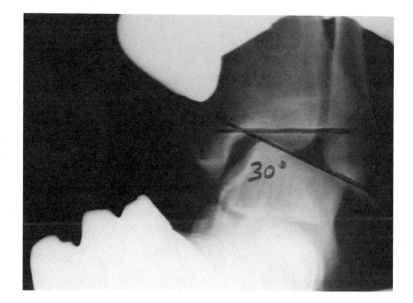

Fig. 23-8. The relationship shown between the superior surface of the talus and the inferior surface of the tibia with varus stress of the calcaneus on an anteroposterior view is termed a talar tilt.

piece of umbilical tape is used to measure the length of split tendon needed. One end of the tape is held at the fifth metatarsal base. This end represents the insertion of the peroneus brevis tendon, and this insertion is maintained throughout the procedure. The tape is aligned from the posterior margin of the fibula to the point marked on the skin representing the trephine location in the lateral wall of the calcaneus. This will be the length of tendon taken for the transfer.

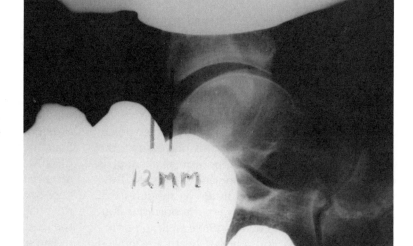

Fig. 23-9. Drawer test reveals anterior displacement of the talus with respect to the ankle mortise on a lateral radiograph.

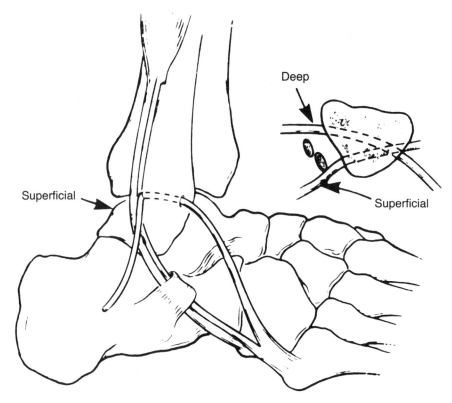

Fig. 23-10. Route of the peroneus brevis through the fibula from anterior to posterior and its insertion into the calcaneus.

Care is taken to preserve the sural nerve throughout the procedure and especially at closure. A small trephine hole is made from the anterior margin of the fibula just proximal to the origin of the anterior talofibular ligament. The trephine is approximately perpendicular to the fibula and exits posteriorly at the peroneal groove.

The skin and superficial fascia are retracted posteriorly, and a periosteal incision is placed over the lateral calcaneal wall. A subperiosteal channel is created between the fifth metatarsal base and the anterior fibular trephine hole. A subperiosteal channel is also created between the posterior fibular trephine hole and the calcaneal trephine hole.

The deep fascia and tendon sheath are incised proximally over the peroneus longus and brevis. At this level the peroneus longus lies superficially, and

it is retracted to expose the peroneus brevis. The tendons are isolated and functionally tested to ensure identification.

At this level the peroneus brevis tendon is quite thin and broad. As one moves distally, the tendon thickens and the muscle mass diminishes as it contributes tendinous fibers.[5] The tendon is encircled proximally with 2-0 suture, and the integrity of the fibers is maintained as the peroneus brevis is split distally. The tagged end of the tendon is pulled distally through its tendon sheath with uterine forceps or a curved hemostat. Care is taken to preserve the attachments of both the harvested tendon and the intact brevis tendon at the fifth metatarsal base.

The split peroneus brevis tendon is then rerouted subperiosteally to the anterior margin of the fibula, through the fibular trephine hole, and subperiosteally to the calcaneal trephine hole. It is very important to hold the foot perpendicular to the leg and the subtalar joint in a neutral position throughout the remainder of the procedure until a compression dressing can be applied. A closed suction drain can be used after the deep fascial incision is closed and before the superficial fascia is closed.

Postoperative Care and Rehabilitation

The ankle is kept from bearing weight for 4 weeks and is then placed in a weightbearing cast for an additional 2 weeks.[5] At this time the ankle is placed in an air cast. This facilitates the rehabilitation process for the therapist and the patient. It allows the patient to proceed with hydrotherapy, range-of-motion exercises, progressive resistance exercises, and isokinetic testing and training.

GASTROCNEMIUS TENDON RECESSION

The distal recession of the gastrocnemius aponeurosis is a common procedure for the correction of gastrocnemius equinus.[6] The etiology of gastrocnemius equinus can be attributed to muscular spasm, congenital shortness, or acquired shortness.[7]

Spastic equinus is found in the majority of cases in association with neuromuscular diseases such as cerebral palsy.[7] The posterior crural musculature can be partially or wholly spastic and can overpower the weaker anterior musculature entirely.

Congenital shortness of the posterior crural musculature presents with toe walking, especially in the child. The child may exhibit toe-to-toe gait but is able to lower his heels to the ground.

Acquired shortness of the posterior crural musculature, creating an ankle equinus, can result from many sources. Situations that create prolonged or repeated plantar flexed or equinus positions of the ankle can result in ankle equinus due to musculature contracture.[8] Examples range from prolonged casting with the ankle joint plantar flexed to repeated use of higher heeled shoes. Acquired shortness can also result from post-traumatic tendoachilles rupture or iatrogenic causes.[9]

Description of the Procedure

The surgical approach is through a 6- to 7-cm linear incision placed medial to the midline of the lower third of the leg. Once the superficial fascia is exposed, the surgeon must avoid the sural nerve and the small saphenous vein. Dissection is carried to the level of the deep fascia. The deep fascia and the paratenon are incised in a linear fashion, exposing the underlying gastrocnemius aponeurosis. With the foot in a plantar flexed position, the medial and lateral thirds of the gastrocnemius aponeurosis are severed proximally (Fig. 23-11). One must be careful to protect the underlying soleus muscle when attempting the proximal cuts. The foot is then maximally dorsiflexed, and the middle third of the gastrocnemius is incised in a fashion to allow sliding of the aponeurosis to a lengthened position when the foot is dorsiflexed on the leg with the knee joint fully extended.[9]

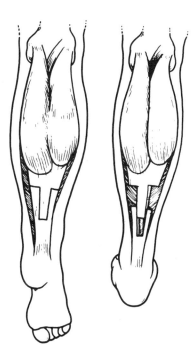

Fig. 23-11. Gastrocnemius tendon recession. *(A)* The gastrocnemius is severed proximally; *(B)* The gastrocnemius is shown in a lengthened position after dorsiflexion of the ankle.

When adequate lengthening has been achieved, the margins of the cut gastrocnemius tendon may be loosely sutured with an absorbable suture to provide approximation of the ends of the gastrocnemius aponeurosis in a lengthened position. The deep fascia and paratenon are closed together with an absorbable suture, as are the subcutaneous and superficial fascial layers. The skin is closed in a subcuticular fashion (the suture being passed through the dermal layer of the skin) to prevent a hypertrophic scar. Steri-strips and a dry compressive dressing are applied, followed by a below-the-knee cast with the subtalar joint held in a neutral position and the foot at a right angle to the leg.

Postoperative Care and Rehabilitation

Postoperative care includes a below-the-knee cast for 4 to 6 weeks followed by the use of compressive elastic bandaging, which helps decrease the normal swelling following cast removal. Hydrotherapy, ultrasound, and isokinetic training can be started at this time. Stringent physical activity such as running, walking, or standing for a prolonged period of time is avoided until muscle strength has returned, which is usually within 10 to 12 weeks.

REFERENCES

1. Ruch JA, Merrill TJ, Banks AS: First ray hallux abducto valgus and related deformities. p. 133. In McGlamry ED (ed): Comprehensive Textbook of Foot Surgery. Vol. 1. Doctors Hospital Podiatry Institute, Tucker GA, 1987
2. Kalish SR, Bernbach MR: Modification of the Austin bunionectomy. p. 86. In McGlamry ED (ed): Reconstructive Surgery of the Foot and Leg. Doctors Hospital Podiatry Institute, Tucker GA, 1987
3. Baxter DE, Thigpen CM: Heel pain—operative results. Foot Ankle. 5:16, 1984
4. Jimenez LA, Malay SD: Heel spur surgery. p. 118. In McGlamry ED (ed): Surgery of the Foot and Leg. Doctors Hospital Podiatry Institute, Tucker GA, 1986
5. Kalish SR, Merrill T: Ankle stabilization procedure. p. 156. In McGlamry ED (ed): Doctors Hospital Surgical Seminar Syllabus. Doctors Hospital Podiatry Institute, Tucker GA, 1987
6. Whitney AK, Green DR: Pseudoequinus. J Am Podiatr Assoc 72:365, 1982
7. Banks HH: The management of spastic deformities of the foot and ankle. Clin Orthop 122:70, 1977
8. McGlamry ED, Kitting RW: Equinus foot: an analysis of the etiology, pathology and treatment techniques. J Am Podiatr Assoc 63:165, 1973
9. Downey M: Tricep surae contractures and equinus deformities of the ankle. In McGlamry ED (ed): Doctors Hospital Podiatry Institute, Tucker GA, 1985

SELECTED READINGS

Austin DW, Leventen EO: A new osteotomy for hallux valgus. Clin Orthop 157:25, 1981

Brand RL, Collins MF: Operative management of ligamentous injuries to the ankle. Clin Sports Med 1:117, 1982

Brantigan JW, Pedegana LR, Lippert FG: Instability of the subtalar joint. J Bone Joint Surg 59A:322, 1977

Craig JJ, Van Vuren J: The importance of gastrocnemius recession in the correction of equinus deformity in cerebral palsy. J Bone Joint Surg 58B:84, 1976

Evans GA, Frenyo SD: The stress-tenogram in the diagnosis of ruptures of the lateral ligament of the ankle. J Bone Joint Surg 61B:347, 1979

Fulp MJ, McGlamry ED: Gastrocnemius tendon recession: tongue in groove procedure to lengthen gastrocnemius tendon. J Am Podiatr Asso 64:163, 1974

Kelikian H: Osteotomy, Hallux Valgus, Allied Deformities of the Forefoot and Metatarsalgia. p. 163. WB Saunders, Philadelphia, 1965

Leach RE, Namiki O, Paul R, Stockel J: Secondary reconstruction of the lateral ligaments of the ankle. Clin Orthop Rel Res No. 160, 1981

Mann RA, DuVries HL: Major surgical procedures for disorders of the forefoot. p. 590. In Mann RA (ed): DeVries' Surgery of the Foot. 4th Ed. CV Mosby, St Louis, 1978

Mechetti ML, Jacobs SA: Calcaneal heel spurs: etiology and treatment, and a new surgical approach. J Foot Leg Surg 22:234, 1983

Ruch JA: Comprehensive evaluation and treatment of the lateral ankle sprain. p. 179. In Schlefman B (ed): Doctors Hospital Surgical Seminar Syllabus. Doctors Hospital Podiatry Institute, Tucker GA, 1982

Vahvanen V, Westerlund M, Nikku R: Lateral ligament injury of the ankle in children. Acta Orthop Scand 55:21, 1984

24
Mobilization of the Lower Extremity

MICHAEL J. WOODEN

The lower extremity mobilization techniques described in this chapter are by no means all of those that exist. Rather, these are the techniques that the author has found to be safe, easy to apply, and effective.

The reader is referred to Chapter 12 for a discussion of the definitions, indications, and contraindications of mobilization. Also, Chapter 14 and Chapters 18 through 23 contain descriptions of anatomy, mechanics, pathology, and evaluation of the lower limb joints.

TECHNIQUES

For each technique illustrated, patient position, the therapist's hand contacts, and the direction of movement are described. Table 24-1 lists each technique along with the physiologic movement it theoretically enhances.

Table 24-1. Summary of Lower Extremity Techniques

Joint	Mobilization Technique	Movement Promoted	Figure No.
Hip	Long axis distraction	General	24-1
	Distraction in flexion	Flexion	24-2
	Lateral distraction	General	24-3
	Lateral distraction in flexion	Flexion	24-4
	Posterior capsule stretch	Flexion	24-5
	Anterior capsule stretch	Extension	24-6, 24-7
	Medial capsule stretch	Abduction	
Patellofemoral	Superior glide	Extension	24-8A
	Interior glide	Flexion	24-8B
	Lateromedial glide	General	24-9
Tibiofemoral	Anterior glide	Extension	24-10, 24-12, 24-13, 24-14
	Posterior glide	Flexion	24-11, 24-13, 24-14
	Medial rotation	Medial rotation, flexion	24-15A, 24-16
	Lateral rotation	Lateral rotation, extension	24-15B, 24-16
	Long axis distraction	General	24-17
	Distraction in flexion	Flexion	24-18, 24-19
Superior tibiofibular	Anteroposterior glides	General	24-20, 24-21
	Downward glide	Downward glide of fibula	24-22
	Upward glide	Upward glide of fibula	24-23
Inferior tibiofibular	Tib-fib glide	Fibular movement, ankle plantar flexion and dorsiflexion	24-24

(Table continues.)

Table 24-1. *(continued)*

Joint	Mobilization Technique	Movement Promoted	Figure No.
Ankle mortice	Distraction	General	24-25, 24-26, 24-27
	Anterior glide	Plantar flexion	24-28, 24-29, 24-31
	Posterior glide	Dorsiflexion	24-28, 24-30
Subtalar	Distraction	General	24-32, 24-33, 24-34
	Distraction with calcaneal rocking	Inversion, eversion	24-35
Midtarsal	Talonavicular glide	Pronation, supination	24-36
	Calcaneocuboid glide	Pronation, supination	24-37
Intermetatarsal (anterior arch)	Glides	General	24-38
Metatarsophalangeal	Distraction	General	24-39
	Dorsal glide	Dorsiflexion	24-40A, 24-42
	Plantar glide	Plantar flexion	24-40B, 24-42
	Mediolateral glide and tilt	General	24-41
Interphalangeal	Distraction	General	24-43
	Dorsoplantar glides	Dorsiflexion, plantar flexion	24-43

THE HIP

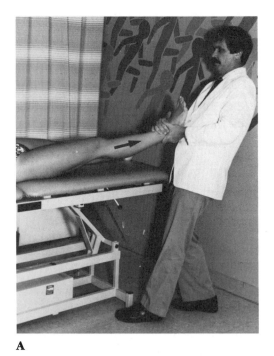
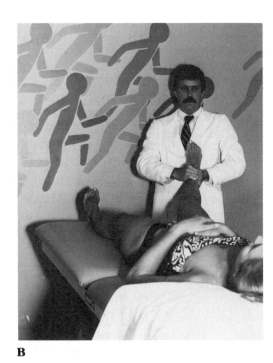

A   **B**

Fig. 24-1. Long axis distraction.
Patient position: supine, leg extended.
Contacts: grasp the leg with both hands around the malleoli, elbows flexed; the leg is held in slight flexion **(A)** and abduction **(B)**.
Direction of movement: the therapist leans backward and pulls along the long axis of the leg.

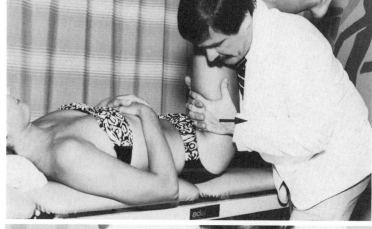

Fig. 24-2. Distraction in flexion.
Patient position: supine, hip and knee flexed to 90 degrees.
Contacts: the back of the knee rests on the therapist's shoulder; hands grasp the anterior aspect of the proximal thigh with fingers interlocked.
Direction of movement: the femoral head is pulled inferiorly.

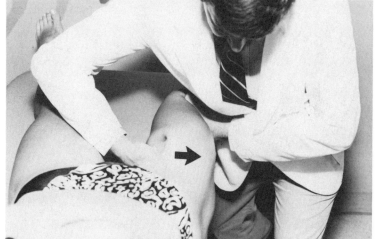
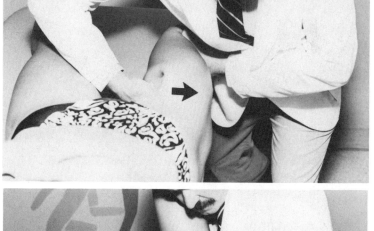

Fig. 24-3. Lateral distraction.
Patient position: supine, leg extended.
Contacts: one hand stabilizes the lateral aspect of the femur above the knee; the other hand contacts the first web space against the medial aspect of the proximal femur.
Direction of movement: the femoral head is distracted laterally.

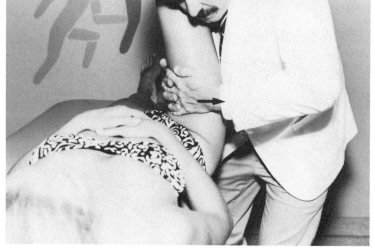

Fig. 24-4. Lateral distraction in flexion.
Patient position: supine, hip and knee flexed to 90 degrees.
Contacts: the back of the knee rests on the therapist's shoulder; hands grasp the medial aspect of the proximal thigh with fingers interlocked.
Direction of movement: the femoral head is distracted laterally.

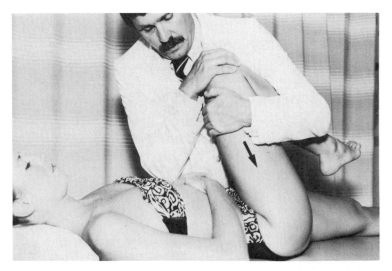

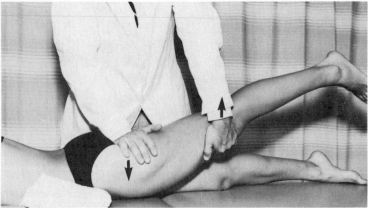

A

Fig. 24-5. Posterior capsule stretch.

Patient position: supine, hip flexed to at least 100 degrees.

Contacts: the medial aspect of the knee rests against the therapist's chest; hands grasp the distal femur and over the patella.

Direction of movement: push downward along the long axis of the femur posteriorly, inferiorly, and slightly laterally.

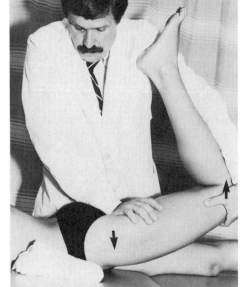

B

Fig. 24-6. Anterior capsule stretch.

Patient position: prone, leg extended, small towel roll under the anterior superior iliac spine.

Contacts: one hand cradles the anterior aspect of the distal femur; the heel of the other hand is against the posterior aspect of the hip joint.

Direction of movement: simultaneously lift the knee while pushing the femoral head anteriorly **(A)**; with the knee flexed, the same maneuver also stretches the rectus femoris **(B)**.

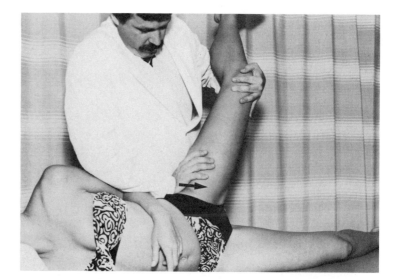

Fig. 24-7. Medial capsule stretch.
Patient position: side-lying, hip at end-range abduction.
Contacts: one hand cradles the medial aspect of the knee to stabilize; the heel of the other hand contacts the lateral aspect of the hip at the greater trochanter.
Direction of movement: push the femoral head inferiorly.

THE KNEE
The Patellofemoral Joint

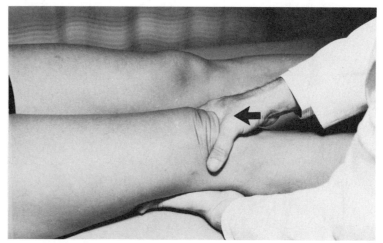

A

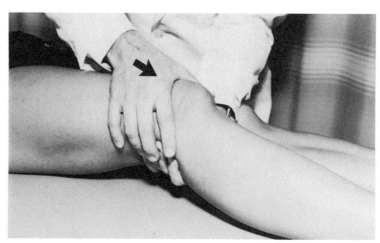

Fig. 24-8. Superoinferior glide.
Patient position: supine.
Contacts: support the knee in slight flexion; contact the patella with the first web space, at the base (superior) or the apex (inferior).
Direction of movement: glide superiorly **(A)** or inferiorly **(B)**.

B

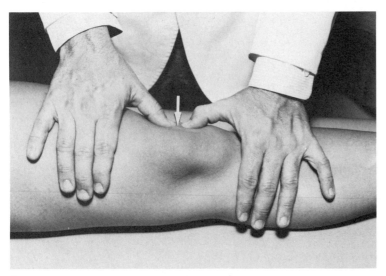

A

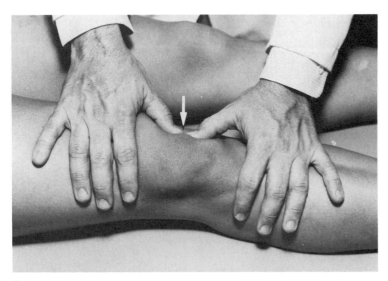

B

Fig. 24-9. Lateromedial glide.
Patient position: supine.
Contacts: use thumbtips against the medial or lateral patellar borders.
Direction of movement: glide medially **(A)** or laterally **(B)**.

The Tibiofemoral Joint

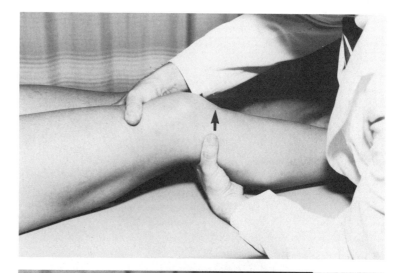

Fig. 24-10. Anterior glide.
Patient position: supine, knee in slight flexion.
Contacts: stabilize the anterior aspect of the distal femur; grasp the posterior aspect of the proximal tibia.
Direction of movement: glide the tibia anteriorly on the femur.

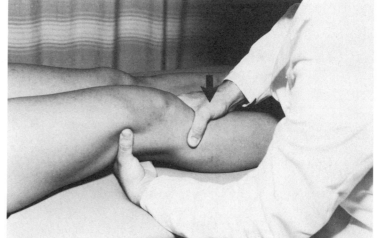

Fig. 24-11. Posterior glide.
Patient position: supine, knee in slight flexion.
Contacts: stabilize the posterior aspect of the distal femur; grasp over the tibial tubercle.
Direction of movement: glide the tibia posteriorly.

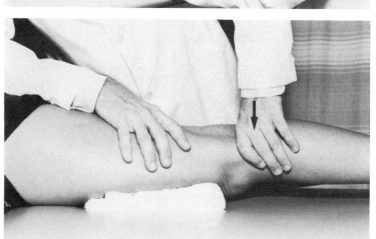

Fig. 24-12. Anterior glide.
Patient position: prone, knee extended.
Contacts: the anterior aspect of the femur is stabilized with a small towel roll; the first web space contacts the posterior aspect of the proximal femur.
Direction of movement: glide the tibia anteriorly.

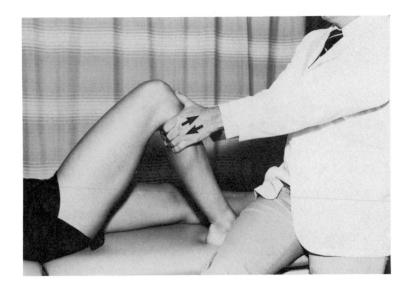

Fig. 24-13. Anteroposterior glide.
Patient position: supine, knee flexed to 90 degrees.
Contacts: grasp the proximal aspect of the tibia, thumbs anterior.
Direction of movement: glide the tibia anteriorly and posteriorly.

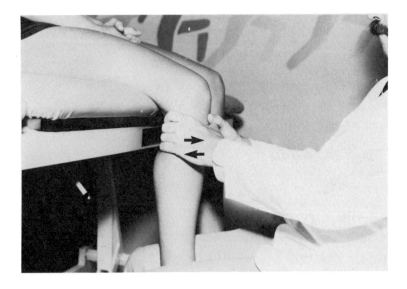

Fig. 24-14. Anteroposterior glide.
Patient position: sitting, knee flexed to 90 degrees.
Contacts: grasp the proximal aspect of the tibia, thumbs anterior.
Direction of movement: glide the tibia anteriorly and posteriorly.

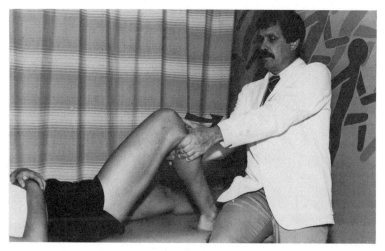

A

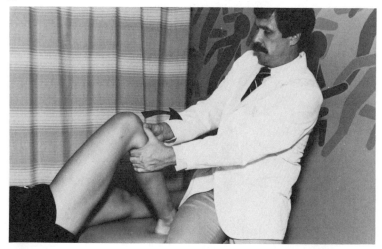

Fig. 24-15. Mediolateral rotation.
Patient position: supine, knee flexed to 90 degrees.
Contacts: grasp the proximal aspect of the tibia, thumbs anterior.
Direction of movement: combine anterior glide with medial (A) and lateral rotation (B).

B

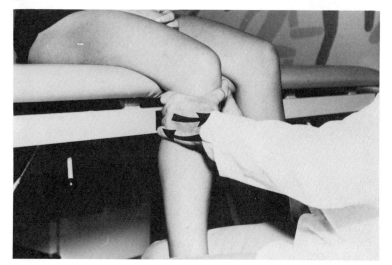

Fig. 24-16. Mediolateral rotation.
Patient position: sitting, knee flexed to 90 degrees.
Contacts: grasp the proximal aspect of the tibia, thumbs anterior.
Direction of movement: combine anterior and posterior glide with medial and lateral rotation.

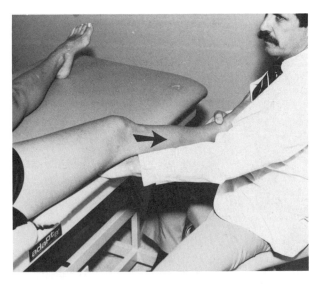

Fig. 24-17. Long axis distraction.
Patient position: supine, slight flexion.
Contacts: stabilize with hand behind the knee; the other hand grasps the lower leg around the malleoli
Direction of movement: pull along the long axis of the lower leg.

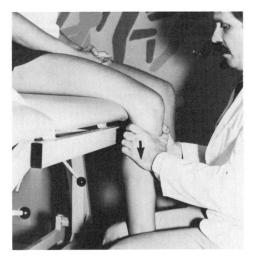

Fig. 24-18. Distraction in flexion.
Patient position: sitting, knee flexed to 90 degrees.
Contacts: grasp the proximal aspect of the tibia, thumbs anterior.
Direction of movement: distract the lower leg downward; distraction can be assisted by the therapist holding the malleoli between the knees. Note: In this position, anteroposterior glides and rotations can also be applied while distracting.

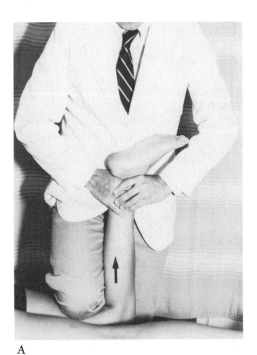

A

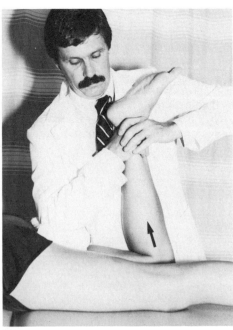

B

Fig. 24-19. Distraction in flexion.
Patient position: prone, knee flexed to 90 degrees or more.
Contacts: grasp the distal femur with hands around the malleoli; stabilize the posterior aspect of the femur with the knee **(A)** or elbow and a towel roll **(B)**.
Direction of movement: **(A)** distract by pulling the leg upward; **(B)** distract by flexing the leg toward the stabilizing arm and simultaneously lifting the leg upward.

The Superior Tibiofibular Joint

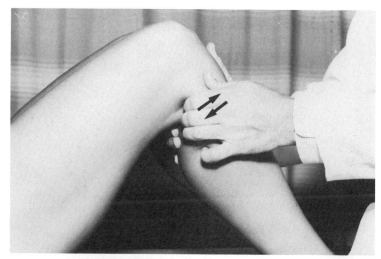

Fig. 24-20. Anteroposterior glide.
Patient position: supine, knee flexed to 90
  degrees.
Contacts: stabilize the medial aspect of the
  tibia; grasp the fibular head with thumb
  and forefinger.
Direction of movement: glide the fibular
  head anteriorly and posteriorly.

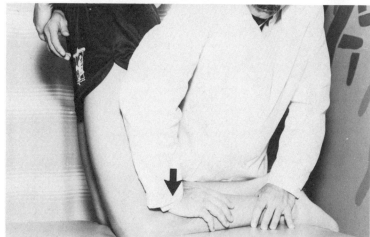

Fig. 24-21. Anterior glide.
Patient position: kneeling.
Contacts: stabilize lower leg on the table;
  the carpal tunnel contacts the posterior
  aspect of the fibular head.
Direction of movement: glide the fibular
  head downward (anteriorly).

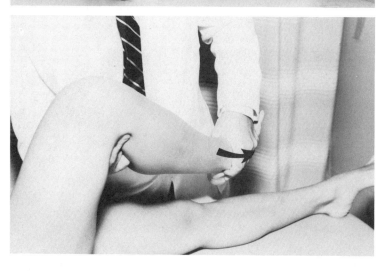

Fig. 24-22. Downward glide.
Patient position: supine, hip and knee
  flexed to about 90 degrees.
Contacts: support the knee posteriorly
  while palpating the head of the fibula;
  the other hand grasps the leg above the
  ankle with the index finger hooked
  around the lateral malleolus.
Direction of movement: simultaneously
  invert the ankle and pull the lateral malleolus downward.

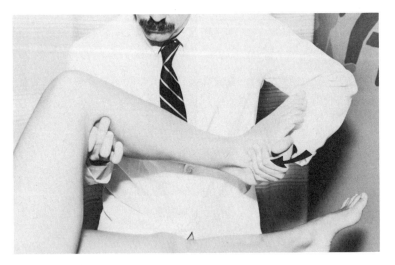

Fig. 24-23. Upward glide.
Patient position: supine, hip and knee flexed to about 90 degrees.
Contacts: support the knee posteriorly while palpating the head of the fibula; the heel of other the hand contacts the lateral aspect of the plantar surface of the foot.
Direction of movement: evert the foot sharply to push the fibula upward.

THE FOOT AND ANKLE
Distal Tibiofibular Joint

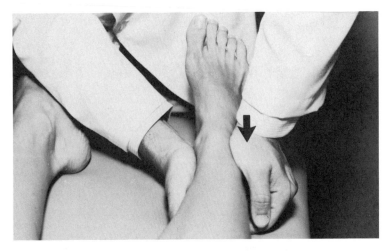

A

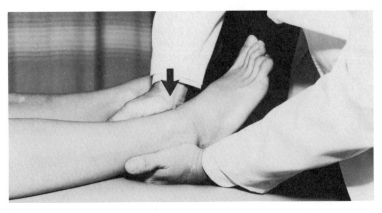

B

Fig. 24-24. Fibular glides.
Patient position: supine.
Contacts: stabilize the medial malleolus against the carpal tunnel of the hand resting on the table; the carpal tunnel of the other hand contacts the anterior aspect of the lateral malleolus.
Direction: glide the fibula posteriorly on the tibia **(A)**; reverse hand positions to glide the tibia posteriorly **(B)**.

The Talocrural (Mortice) Joint

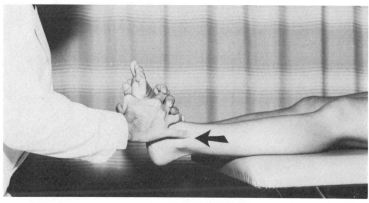

A

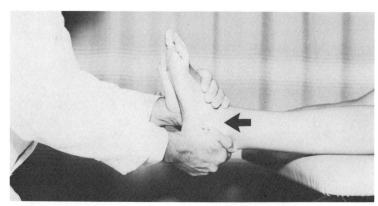

Fig. 24-25. Distraction.
Patient position: supine.
Contacts: grasp the foot with the second, third, and fourth fingers of both hands interlocked over the dorsum, thumbs plantar **(A)**, or grasp with one hand dorsomedially while the other hand holds the calcaneus laterally **(B)**.
Direction of movement: distract the talus from the mortise.

B

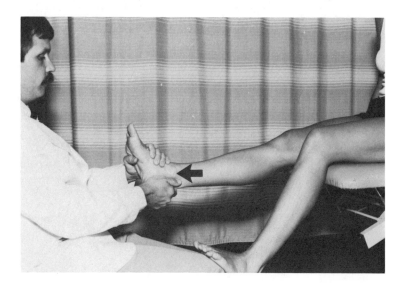

Fig. 24-26. Distraction.
Patient position: sitting at the end of the table; the therapist is also sitting.
Contacts: same as in Fig. 24-25; the patient adds stability by resting the opposite foot on the therapist's knee.
Direction of movement: distract the talus from the mortise.

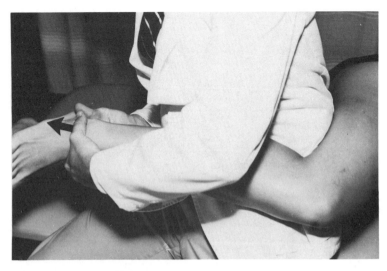

Fig. 24-27. Distraction.
Patient position: side-lying.
Contacts: the posterior aspect of the femur is stabilized against the therapist's hip and iliac crest; the first web spaces grasp anterior and posterior to the talus.
Direction of movement: distract the talus from the mortise.

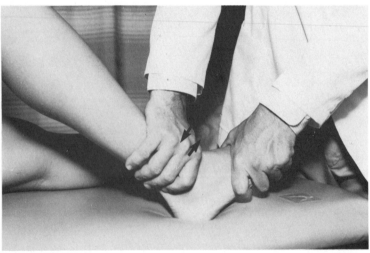

Fig. 24-28. Anteroposterior glide.
Patient position: supine, knee flexed with heel resting on the table.
Contacts: stabilize the foot by grasping dorsolaterally; the other hand grasps the anterior aspect of the lower leg above the malleoli.
Direction of movement: glide the tibia and fibula anteriorly and posteriorly on the talus.

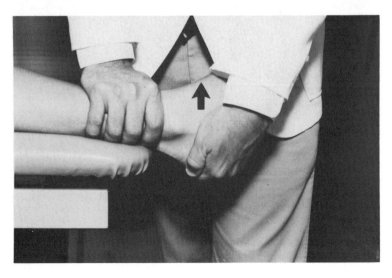

Fig. 24-29. Anterior glide.
Patient position: supine, leg extended with the foot off the end of the table.
Contacts: stabilize the tibia and fibula by holding them against the table; the other hand cradles the calcaneus laterally.
Direction of movement: glide the calcaneus and talus upward (anteriorly).

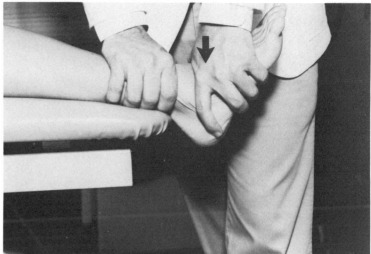

Fig. 24-30. Posterior glide.

Patient position: supine, leg extended with the foot off the edge of the table.

Contacts: stabilize the tibia and fibula by holding them against the table; the other hand grasps the foot dorsolaterally with the first web space against the anterior aspect of the talus.

Direction of movement: glide the talus posteriorly.

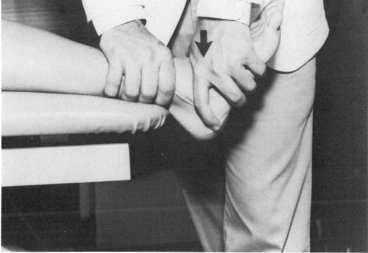

Fig. 24-31. Anterior glide.

Patient position: prone, foot off the end of the table.

Contacts: stabilize the tibia and fibula by holding them against the table; the first web space of the other hand contacts the posterior aspect of the ankle.

Direction of movement: glide the calcaneus and talus downward (anteriorly) on the mortise.

The Subtalar Joint

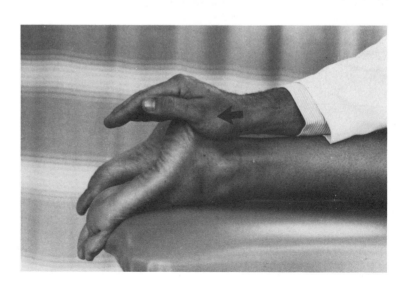

Fig. 24-32. Distraction.

Patient position: prone, ankle plantar flexed, toes off the end of the table.

Contacts: the therapist's carpal tunnel contacts the posterior aspect of the calcaneus near the insertion of the tendo Achillis.

Direction of movement: distract the calcaneus from the talus by pushing caudally.

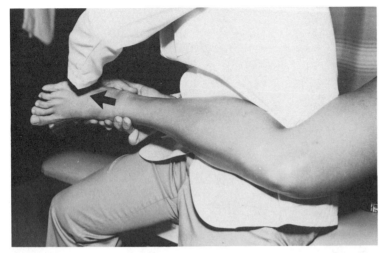

A

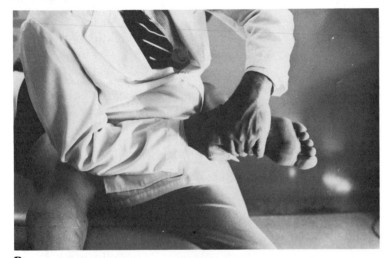

B

Fig. 24-33. Distraction.
Patient position: side-lying.
Contacts: the posterior aspect of the femur is stabilized against the therapist's hip and iliac crest **(A)**; first web spaces grasp the posterior and plantar aspects of the calcaneus **(B)**.
Direction of movement: distract the calcaneus from the talus.

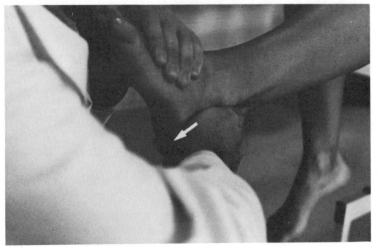

Fig. 24-34. Distraction.
Patient: supine or sitting, foot off the end of the table.
Contacts: stabilize the foot by grasping it dorsomedially; the other hand grasps the calcaneus laterally.
Direction of movement: distract the calcaneus from the talus.

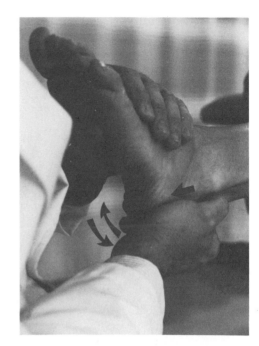

Fig. 24-35. Distraction with calcaneal rocking.
Patient position: supine or sitting, foot off the edge of the table.
Contacts: same as in Fig. 24-34.
Direction of movement: while distracting the calcaneus, invert and evert it on the talus.

The Talonavicular Joint (Medial Aspect of the Midtarsal Joint)

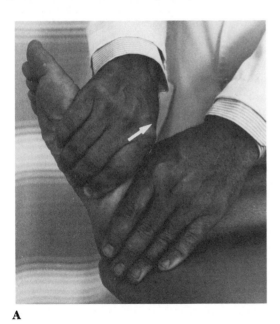

A

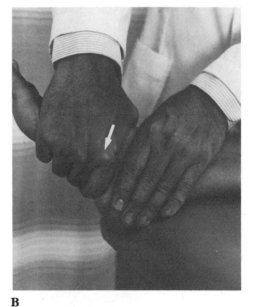

B

Fig. 24-36. Talonavicular glide.
Patient position: supine.
Contacts: with hands on the medial aspect of the foot, stabilize the talus and grasp the navicular with the first web space.
Direction of movement: glide the navicular in dorsal **(A)** and plantar **(B)** directions.

The Calcaneocuboid Joint (Lateral Aspect of the Midtarsal Joint)

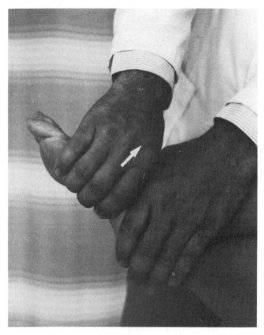

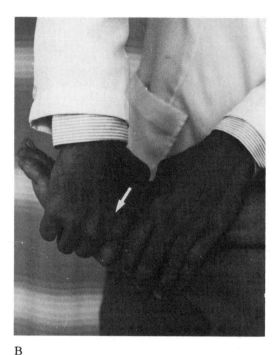

A

B

Fig. 24-37. Calcaneocuboid glide.
Patient position: supine.
Contacts: with hands on the lateral aspect of the foot, stabilize the calcaneus and grasp the cuboid with the first web space.
Direction of movement: glide the cuboid in dorsal **(A)** and plantar **(B)** directions.

The Intermetatarsal Joints

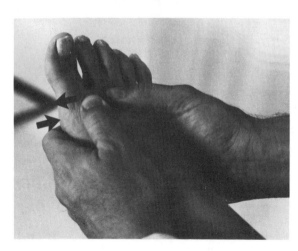

Fig. 24-38. Intermetatarsal glides.
Patient position: supine.
Contacts: with thumbs and forefingers, grasp the first and second metatarsal heads; stabilize the second metatarsal head.
Direction of movement: glide the first metatarsal head in dorsal and plantar directions; repeat at the second, third, and fourth interspaces.

The First Metatarsophalangeal (MTP) Joint

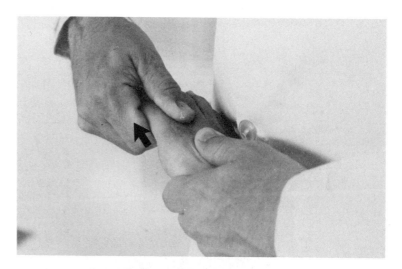

Fig. 24-39. Distraction.

Patient position: supine.

Contacts: stabilize the first metatarsal head; the other hand grasps the proximal phalanx on its dorsal and plantar aspects.

Direction of movement: distract the phalanx from the metatarsal.

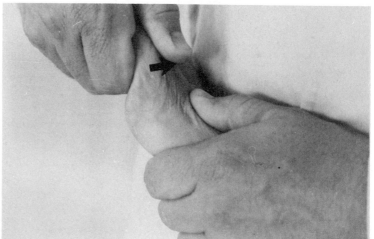

A

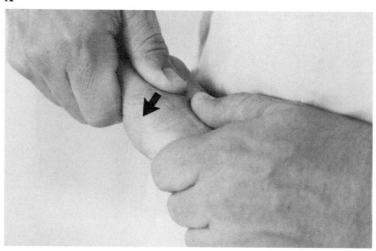

Fig. 24-40. Dorsoplantar glides.

Patient position: supine.

Contacts: stabilize the first metatarsal head; the other hand grasps the dorsal and plantar aspects of the proximal phalanx.

Direction of movement: glide the phalanx in dorsal **(A)** and plantar **(B)** directions.

B

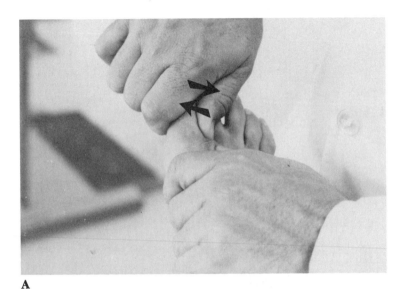

A

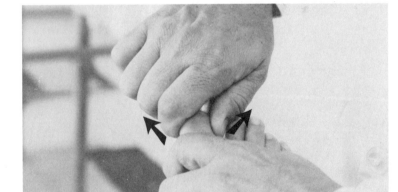

B

Fig. 24-41. Mediolateral glide and tilt.
Patient position: supine.
Contacts: stabilize the first metatarsal head; the other hand grasps the medial and lateral aspects of the proximal phalanx.
Direction of movement: glide the phalanx medially and laterally **(A)**; tilt the phalanx medially and laterally **(B)**.

The Second to Fifth MTP Joints

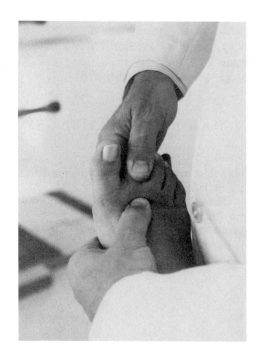

Fig. 24-42. Distraction and dorsoplantar glides.
Patient position: supine.
Contacts: stabilize the second metatarsal head; the other
hand grasps the dorsal and plantar aspects of the proximal phalanx.
Direction of movement: distract or glide the phalanx (as
in Figs. 24-39 and 24-40); repeat at the third, fourth, and
fifth MTP joints.

The Interphalangeal Joints

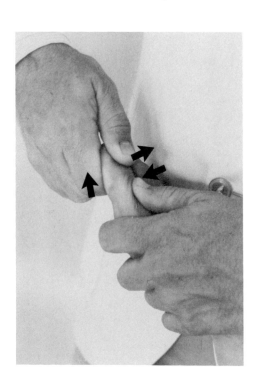

Fig. 24-43. Distraction and dorsoplantar glides.
Patient position: supine.
Contacts: stabilize the proximal phalanx; grasp the dorsal
and plantar aspects of the distal phalanx.
Direction of movement: distract and glide in the dorsal
and plantar directions; repeat for all interphalangeal
joints.

ACKNOWLEDGMENTS

The author thanks Janie Wise, MMSc, PT (the photographer), Amelia Haselden, PT (the model), and the Physical Therapy Department at Emory University Hospital for their valuable assistance.

SUGGESTED READINGS

Basmajian JV, MacConail C: Arthrology. In Warwick R, Williams P (eds): Gray's Anatomy. 35th British Ed. WB Saunders, Philadelphia, 1973

Corrigan B, Maitland GD: Practical Orthopaedic Medicine. Butterworths, London, 1985

Cyriax J: Textbook of Orthopaedic Medicine. Vol. I: Diagnosis of Soft Tissue Lesions. Balliere Tindall, London, 1978

Cyriax J, Russell G: Textbook of Orthopaedic Medicine. Vol. II: Treatment by Manipulation, Massage and Injection. 9th Ed. Balliere Tindall, London, 1977

Cyriax J, Cyriax P: Illustrated Manual of Orthopaedic Medicine. Butterworths, London, 1983

Hoppenfeld S: Physical Examination of the Spine and Extremities. Appleton-Century-Crofts, New York, 1976

Kapandji IA: The Physiology of the Joints. Vol. II: The Lower Limb. Churchill Livingstone, Edinburgh, 1982

Maitland G: Peripheral Manipulation. 2nd Ed. Butterworths, London, 1978

Mennell JM: Joint Pain: Diagnosis and Treatment Using Manipulative Techniques. Little, Brown, Boston, 1964

Paris SV: Extremity Dysfunction and Mobilization. Institute Press, Atlanta, 1980

Index

Page numbers followed by *f* indicate figures; those followed by *t* indicate tables

587